AF530529

Phytobiotics and Animal Production

Phytobiotics and Animal Production

Dr. Pankaj Kumar Singh
Department of Animal Nutrition
Bihar Veterinary College
Bihar Animal Sciences University
Patna-800014, (Bihar), India

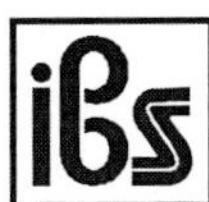

International Books & Periodical Supply Service
(Publisher of Scientific Books)
38, NISHANT KUNJ, PITAM PURA MAIN ROAD
DELHI-110034 (India)
Phone : 011-27352078, Mobile : 09810146811, E-mail : hkjain1975@yahoo.com

Published by :

International Books & Periodical Supply Service

(Publisher of Scientific Books)
38, NISHANT KUNJ, PITAM PURA MAIN ROAD
DELHI-110034 (India)
Phone : 011-27352078, Mobile : 09810146811, E-mail : hkjain1975@yahoo.com

ISBN 978-81-93906-57-6

Composed, Designed & Printed in India

Dedicated

to

My Teachers

&

Parents

Foreword

The world's population is expected to increase to 9.5 billion people by 2050. The demand for animal food products is likely to double. Modern intensive livestock and poultry production has achieved phenomenal gains but maximum economic gain from livestock production with minimum stress to the animals is major concern of the present society. Extensive research work has been conducted for reducing the feed cost encompassing judicious use of available feed resources, precise nutrient supply and augmenting nutrient utilization through feed processing and supplementation with suitable feed additives. The concept of using chemical feed additives is being practised to augment production of livestock in economic manner. Use of antibiotics in animal feed is either banned or under severe scrutiny in many countries due to burgeoning problem of antimicrobial resistance and chemical residue in animal products. The development of microbial resistance to various drugs has necessitated research interests towards the use of phytochemicals as feed additives replacing synthetic drugs.

Phytobiotic feed additives are plant-derived natural bioactive compounds that can be incorporated into diets to improve the productivity of livestock through modulation of feed properties, promotion of the animal's performance, and improving the quality of food derived from these animals. Due to their holistic and broad-spectrum efficacy, phytogenic feed additives are moving further into spotlight among nutritionists, feed manufactures and farmers. There is immense scope of use of phytobiotics in livestock and poultry feed to improve health, production and reproduction. However, Phytobiotics are a relatively new class of feed additives and scientific knowledge is still limited regarding the mode of action of specific additives and aspects of their application.

In this book *'Phytobiotics and Animal Production'*, the editor has included most of the herbal feed additives that are being used or researched for use in livestock and poultry. Each chapter of the book imparts latest information on individual phytobiotic supported with good amount of experimental evidence and references. In my opinion, the book covers theoretical and practical aspects of phytobiotics in a systematic and comprehensive manner to enlighten the significance of major phytobiotics in sustainable livestock and poultry production.

I complement the editor and authors for their sincere effort in bringing out this publication for the benefit of animal nutrition. This book will serve as an important reference volume for the students, teachers and researchers.

(Rameshwar Singh)
Vice-Chancellor
Bihar Animal Sciences University,
Patna, (Bihar), India

Preface

Phytogenic feed additives are plant-derived bioactive compounds that can be incorporated into diets to improve the productivity of livestock through amelioration of feed properties, promotion of the animal's production performance, and improving the quality of food derived from those animals. Phytochemicals present in plants exhibit antioxidant, antibacterial, antiviral and antifungal activities against a wide range of pathogenic and non-pathogenic microorganisms. The growing concerns over bacterial resistance to antibiotics and chemical residues in animal derived foods have led to a resurgence of interests to use phytochemicals as alternatives to growth promoting antibiotic feed additives. Phytogenic additives present a plausible alternative of antibiotic growth promoter as they enhance a number of important processes in the animal body. A rapid development in the potential use of phybiotics feed additives has occurred mainly due to the 2006 European Union ban on the use of antimicrobial substances as growth stimulators. Despite mounting and convincing evidence that phytobiotics are very useful for economic and eco-friendly livestock and poultry production, most of the phytobiotics are not very popular to use. A part of the reason for this relative paucity may be the lack of complete and easily available information on phytobitoics. The growing interest in phytogenic feed additives provoked an enormous attempt to understand systematic effects and underlying mechanisms of action of particular phytocompounds and plant extracts on animal performance.

It has been experienced that information about the recent concept on different herbal feed additive have not been presented in a single book so that readers can understand their intricacy and practical applications in livestock and poultry. However, reviews on different feed additives are distributed in diverse journals that are sometimes physically and financially out of reach of most of the students. Therefore, the need for the hour is to compile all the necessary information pertaining to phytobiotics in a single publication and update the students, researchers, pharmaceutical companies and feed manufacturing agencies with current knowledge on this topic.

This book on *Phytobiotics and Animal Production* deals with updated information on the use of different herbs as feed additive in livestock and poultry. This is the first book of its kind to deal with the significance of different phytobiotics in livestock and poultry. In preparing this reference book, authors from major teaching and research establishments, who have an enviable tract record in their respective specialism, have been selected. The book contains 30 chapters to cover almost all researched herbs like garlic, turmeric, ginger, thyme, neem, black cumin, holy basil, Indian goose berry, cumin, ajwain, coriander, artimisia, pepper mint, wheat grass, giloy, fenugreek, wormwood, shatavari, yucca, etc. herbal feed additives.

Each chapter contains taxonomy, geographical distribution, nutritional composition, quality and quantity of active principles, and effects of herbs or phytobiotics on livestock production, health, immunity and reproduction. Content of each chapter of the book is supported with good amount of the experimental evidence and references which will enable the research workers to obtain information quickly, when necessary. The information included in this book would be extremely valuable to students of animal sciences at undergraduate and post-graduate levels of animal science, professors, animal nutritionists, veterinarians and personnel of pharmaceutical and feed industry.

The book is dedicated to all the authors who contributed their expertise and valuable time to write their comprehensive and authoritative chapters. I acknowledge and express my thanks to my teachers, parents and family members, friends and well-wishers, who have been incredibly supportive to bring this book. I also acknowledges the staff of the publisher for their support and supervision in completion of this book.

Pankaj Kumar Singh
Patna, (Bihar), India

List of Contributors

Amitava Bhattacharya Department of Poultry Science, UP Pt. Deen Dayal Pashu ChikitsaVigyanVishwavidyalya, Mathura-281001, Uttar Pradesh, India

Amlan Kumar Patra Department of Animal Nutrition, West Bengal University of Animal and Fishery Sciences, Kolkata-700037, West Bengal, India

Amrish Kumar Tyagi Animal Nutrition Division, ICAR-National Dairy Research Institute, Karnal-132001, Haryana, India

Anamika Department of Animal Nutrition, Khalsa College of Veterinary & Animal Sciences, Amritsar-143001, Punjab, India

Anshu Rahal Department of Animal Nutrition, G B Pant University of Agriculture & Technology, Pantnagar-263145, Uttarakhand, India

Ashok Kumar Patil Department of Animal Nutrition, Nanaji Deshmukh Pashu Veterinary Science University, Jabalpur-482001, Madhya Pradesh, India

Avinash Kumar Department of Animal Nutrition, UP Pt. Deen Dayal Pashu ChikitsaVigyanVishwavidyalya, Mathura-281001, Uttar Pradesh, India

Bikas Chandra Debnath Department of Animal Nutrition, West Bengal University of Animal and Fishery Sciences, Kolkata-700037, West Bengal, India

Brishketu Kumar Department of Animal Science, College of Agriculture, Nevsari Agricultural University, Bharuch-392011, Gujarat, India

Debashis Roy Department of Animal Nutrition, UP Pt. Deen Dayal Pashu ChikitsaVigyanVishwavidyalya, Mathura-281001, Uttar Pradesh, India

Deben Sapcota Debarment of Poultry Science, Assam Agricultural University, Khanapara Campus, Guwahati-781022, Assam, India

Deepak Upadhyay Plant Animal Relationship Division, ICAR-Indian Grassland and Fodder Research Institute, Jhansi-284003, Uttar Pradesh, India

Dinesh Jain Department of Animal Nutrition, Rajasthan University of Veterinary and Animal Sciences, Bikaner-334001, Rajasthan, India

Dinesh Kumar Department of Veterinary Science & Animal Husbandry, Jawahar Lal Nehru Krishi Vishwavidyalaya, Tikamgarh-472001, Madhya Pradesh, India

Garima Shukla Department of Poultry Science, U P Pt. Deen Dayal Pashu Chikitsa VigyanVishwavidyalya, Mathura-281001, Uttar Pradesh, India

Guru Prasad Mandal Department of Animal Nutrition, West Bengal University of Animal and Fishery Sciences, Kolkata-700037, West Bengal, India

Hujaz Tariq Animal Nutrition Division, ICAR-National Dairy Research Institute, Karnal-132001, Haryana, India

Jaya Bharati Department of Veterinary Physiology and Biochemistry, Banaras Hindu University, Varanasi-221005, Uttar Pradesh, India

Jyoti Palod Department of Livestock Production Management, GB Pant University of Agricultural University, Pantnagar-263145, Uttarakhand, India

K. Merina Devi Research Scholar, Department of Poultry Science, Assam Agricultural University, Guwahati-781022, Assam, India

Kaushal Kumar Department of Veterinary Pathology, Bihar Animal Sciences University, Patna-800014, Bihar, India

Kaushalendra Kumar Department of Animal Nutrition, Bihar Animal Sciences University, Patna-800014, Bihar, India

Kaushik Pal Krishi Vigyan Kendra, West Bengal University of Animal and Fishery Sciences, Ashok Nagar-743223, West Bengal, India

Lipismita Samal Post-Graduate Department of Poultry Science, Orissa University of Agriculture & Technology, Bhubaneswar-751003, Odisha, India

Madhu Mishra Research Scholar, Division of Veterinary Bacteriology, ICAR-Indian Veterinary Research Institute, Izatnagar-243122, Uttar Pradesh, India

Melody Lalhriatpuii Department of Animal Nutrition, College of Veterinary Sciences and Animal Husbandry, Agartala-799008, Tripura, India

Mohd. Nayeem Ali Senior Research Fellow, ICAR-National Dairy Research Institute, Karnal-132001, Haryana, India

Muzaffar Ahmed Naik Research Scholar, Animal Reproduction Division, ICAR-National Dairy Research Institute, Karnal-132001, Haryana, India

N.C. Behura Post-Graduate Department of Poultry Science, Orissa University of Agriculture & Technology, Bhubaneswar-751003, Odisha, India

Neha Sharma Research Scholar, Department of Animal Nutrition, Rajasthan University of Veterinary and Animal Sciences, Bikaner-334001, Rajstahan, India

Nishant Kumar Animal Reproduction Division, ICAR-National Dairy Research Institute, Karnal-132001, Haryana, India

Pankaj Kumar Singh Department of Animal Nutrition, Bihar Animal Sciences University, Patna-800014, Bihar, India

Pramod Prabhakar Department of Animal Husbandry, Mandan Bharti Agriculture College, Bihar Agricultural University, Saharsa-852201, Bihar, India

Prasanta Kumar Choudhury Animal Nutrition Division, ICAR-National Dairy Research Institute, Karnal-132001, Haryana, India

Punita Kumari Research Scholar, Division of Animal Nutrition, ICAR-Indian Veterinary Research Institute, Izatnagar-243122, Uttar Pradesh, India

R.P.S. Baghel Department of Animal Nutrition, Nanaji Deshmukh Pashu Veterinary Science University, Jabalpur-482001, Madhya Pradesh, India

Ravindra Kumar Division of Animal Nutrition and Product Technology, ICAR-Central Institute for Research on Goats, Makhdoom-281122, Uttar Pradesh, India

S.S. Lathwal Livestock Production and Management Division, ICAR-National Dairy Research Institute, Karnal-132001, Haryana, India

Sachin Kumar Animal Nutrition Division, ICAR-National Dairy Research Institute, Karnal-132001, Haryana, India

Satish Kumar Research Scholar, Division of Animal Genetics and Breeding, ICAR-Indian Veterinary Research Institute, Izatnagar-243122, Uttar Pradesh, India

Shabir Ahmed Lone Research Scholar, Division of Animal Reproduction, Indian Veterinary Research Institute, Izatnagar-243122, Uttar Pradesh, India

Shalu Kumari Pathak Research Scholar, Divission of Animal Genetics and Breeding, Indian Veterinary Research Institute, Izatnagar-243122, Uttar Pradesh, India

Sheikh Adil Hamid Division of Livestock Production and Management, Sher-e-Kashmir University of Agricultural Sciences and Technology, Srinagar-190006, Jammu & Kashmir, India

Srobana Sarkar Animal Nutrition Division, ICAR-National Dairy Research Institute, Karnal-132001, Haryana, India

Sunil Nayak Department of Animal Nutrition, Nanaji Deshmukh Pashu Veterinary Science University, Jabalpur-482001, India

Tara Bothra Department of Livestock Production and Management, Rajasthan University of Veterinary and Animal Sciences, Bikaner-334001, Rajasthan, India

Umesh Kumar Prajapat Department of Animal Nutrition, Rajasthan University of Veterinary and Animal Sciences, Bikaner-334001, Rajasthan, India

Yasir Afzal Beigh Division of Animal Nutrition, Faculty of Veterinary Sciences & Animal Husbandry, Sher-e-Kashmir University of Agricultural Sciences and Technology, Srinagar-190006, Jammu & Kashmir, India.

About the Author

Dr. Pankaj Kumar Singh is working as Assistant Professor in Animal Nutrition Department of Bihar Animal Sciences University, Patna, India, and has a teaching and research experience of 16 years. Earlier, he served as Assistant Professor in Faculty of Veterinary and Animal Sciences of Sher-e-Kashmir University of Agricultural Sciences & Technology, Srinagar, Jammu and Kashmir, India, and contributed significantly in the field of Animal Nutrition and Feed Technology.

He has authored 5 books, 6 laboratory manuals and 30 book chapters on animal nutrition, which are very well accepted by the students, teachers and researchers. He has published more than 55 research articles and 45 technical articles in journals of high repute. He is editorial board member and referee of several reputed journals worldwide.

He has been involved in 15 externally funded and institutional projects as principal investigator and associated scientist and guided a number of postgraduate students for the master's degree programme. His research interests are feed additives, feed supplements, nutraceuticals, phytobiotics, unconventional feeds and feed technology for livestock and poultry.

Dr. Singh is recipient of prestigious 'Dr. S. K. Ranjhan Best Ph.D thesis Award' from Animal Nutrition Society of India, 'Young Scientist Award' from Uttarakhand State Council of Science & Technology, 'Excellence in Research Award' from Society of Agriculture & Development, India. He has also been awarded the Junior and Senior Research Fellowship Award of Indian Council of Agricultural Research, India. He is an executive member of Animal Nutrition Association of India and Animal Nutrition Society of India. He is life member of Indian Association for the Advancement of Veterinary Research and Blue Cross Society of India.

Contents

Part I:
Overview of Phytobiotics

Chapter 1

Phytobiotics and Animal Production: An Overview

Pankaj Kumar Singh

Department of Animal Nutrition, Bihar Animal Sciences University, Patna-800014, India, E-mail: vetpank@gmail.com

ABSTRACT

Recently, the growing occurrences of multi-drug resistant strains of bacteria and the appearance of strains with decreased susceptibility to antibiotics have led to a resurgence of research interests in the discovery of novel antimicrobial agents from natural sources for therapeutic and preventive purposes against microbial diseases and feed additives in the animal industry. Phytobiotics or phytogenic feed additives are plant–derived natural bioactive compounds that can be incorporated into diets to improve the productivity of livestock through amelioration of feed properties, promotion of the animal's production performance, and improving the quality of food derived from those animals. The active compounds of phytobiotics are secondary plant constituents, which have variety of functions, including antimicrobial, anthelmentic, anticoccidial, antiviral, antioxidative, immune-modulatory, anti-inflammatory, hypocholesteremic effects and improvement in the palatability of feed and gut health. Phytobiotics are used in livestock and poultry feed as natural growth promoters due to their beneficial effect on gut health and immunity and growth performance. Besides the inconsistent results and inconclusive mechanisms of using phytogenic feed additives in animal feed, the challenges of using phytogenic compounds in animal feed may also include side effects, regulatory obstacles and cost-effectiveness.

Keywords : Phytobiotics, Growth promoter, Antioxidant, Antimicrobial, Livestock.

1.1 Introduction

Global economic pressures have driven a tendency of the livestock production to produce more products per unit cost. Undoubtedly, modern intensive livestock and poultry production has achieved phenomenal gains in the efficient and economical production of high quality and safe animal products and by-products. At the same time as making gains in production and efficiency, the industry has had to maximize the health and well-being of the livestock and minimize the impact of the industry on the environment. The use of feed additives has been an important part of achieving this success. In the modern feeding practices, feed additives are assuming a position of prime importance in livestock production. Antibiotics have long been used at sub-therapeutic levels in swine, poultry, aquaculture and ruminant diets to maximize the efficiency of production, product quality and to control diseases. However, the use of antibiotics as growth promoters in animal feed is now restricted due to public concerns regarding antibiotic residue in animal tissue and development of antibiotic–resistant bacteria in humans. The practice without using antibiotic growth promoters in food animal production has been implemented in the European Union countries since 2006 and more countries are expected to follow. There are a number of challenges after the withdrawal of antibiotics from feed. The cost- effectiveness in substituting antibiotics with alternatives is the most challenging one, which remains critical for ensuring the long-term sustainable animal production. There have been a significantly increased number of studies focused on searching alternatives to antibiotics with similar antimicrobial and growth-promoting effects without inducing bacterial resistance and potential side effects to animals. Organic acids (Eckel *et al.*, 1992), enzymes (Bedford and Cowieson, 2012), probiotics (Musa *et al.*, 2009), prebiotics (Gibson *et al.*, 2004), antimicrobial peptide (Choi *et al.*, 2013) and phytogenic compounds (Windisch et al. 2008; Gong *et al.*, 2014) have been widely recognized as potential alternatives to antibiotics in feed. Due to their holistic and broad-spectrum efficacy, phytogenic feed additives are moving further into the spotlight among scientists, nutritionists, feed manufactures, producers and farmers. Therefore, there are immense scope of use of phytobiotics in livestock and poultry feed to improve health, production and reproduction.

Phytobiotics or phytogenic feed additives are plant–derived natural bioactive compounds that can be incorporated into diets to improve the productivity of livestock through amelioration of feed properties, promotion of the animal's production performance, and improving the quality of food derived from those animals. Phytobiotics comprises very wide range of substances with respect to biological origin, formulation, chemical description and purity. Windisch *et al.*, (2008) have recommended some other commonly used terms to classify different phytogenic compounds based on their origin and processing, including herbs (flowering, non-woody and non-persistent plants), botanicals (entire or processed parts of a plant, e.g. root, leaves, bark), spices (herbs with an intensive smell or taste commonly added to human food), essential oils (hydro distilled extracts of volatile plant compounds) and oleoresins (extracts derived by non-aqueous solvents). Examples of herbal feed additives are garlic, turmeric, cumin, black cumin, clove, aloe vera, thyme, cumin, neem, etc.

1.2 Phytochemicals and Phytobiotics

Phytochemicals (from the Greek word phyto, meaning plant) are biologically active, naturally occurring chemical compounds found in plants, which provide health benefits for humans further than those attributed to macronutrients and micronutrients (Hasler and Blumberg, 1999). They protect plants from disease and damage and contribute to the plant's colour, aroma and flavour. In general, the plant chemicals that protect plant cells from environmental hazards such as pollution, stress, drought, UV exposure and pathogenic attack are called as Phytochemicals. There are more than thousand known and many unknown Phytochemicals like alkaloids, sterols, terpenes, volatile oils, tannins, saponins, flavonoids, anthraquinones, terpenoids, steroids, carbohydrates, glycosides etc. (Edeoga *et al.*, 2005). Phytochemicals accumulate in different parts of the plants, such as in the roots, stems, leaves, flowers, fruits or seeds . Many phytochemicals, particularly the pigment molecules, are often concentrated in the outer layers of the various plant tissues. Levels vary from plant to plant depending upon the variety, processing, cooking and growing conditions. They may be available in solid, dried, and ground forms, or as extracts (essential oils). A common feature of phytobiotics is that they are a very complex mixture of bioactive components. Phytochemicals can be divided into many major classes depending upon the chemical structures, botanical origins, biosynthesis pathways or biological properties. The most phytochemical classification scheme is based on chemical structures such as phenolics, alkaloids, saponins, terpenoids and so on. Theses Phytochemicals have have biological properties such as antioxidant activity, antimicrobial effect, modulation of detoxification enzymes, stimulation of the immune system, decrease of platelet aggregation and modulation of hormone metabolism and anticancer property, etc. While phytochemicals are classified by function, an individual compound may have more than one biological function.

1.3 Mechanism of Action of Phytobiotics

Plant products have been used for centuries by humans as food and to treat ailments. Natural medicinal products originating from herbs and spices have also been used as feed additives for farm animals in ancient cultures for the same length of time. Mechanism of the action of these additives is not completely clear, however, there are various positive effects of phytobiotics on health, production and reproduction of livestock and poultry. Some plant extracts influence digestion and secretion of digestive enzymes and besides, they exhibit antibacterial, antiviral and antioxidant (Cross *et al.*, 2007). Wenk (2003) reported that herbs, spices and their extracts can stimulate appetite and endogenous secretions such as enzymes or have antimicrobial, coccidiostatic or anthelmintic activities in monogastric animals. Phytobiotics, especially those from the group of essential oils are often claimed to improve flavour and palatability of feed and hence, to raise performance of monogastrics livestock through stimulation of feed intake. Increased feed intake and digestive secretions are also observed in animals offered phytobiotic-supplemented feed (Windisch and Kroismayr, 2006). A wide range of phytobiotics are known to exert pharmacological actions within the digestive tract, such as laxative and spasmolytic effects. Some phytobiotics act also as antioxidant and may, thus indirectly stabilize the nutritional and sensorial feed quality.

The active compounds of phytobiotics are secondary plant constituents, which have variety of functions, including antimicrobial, anthelmentic, anticoccidial, antiviral, antioxidative, immune-modulatory, anti-inflammatory, hypocholesteremic effects and improvement in the palatability of feed and gut health. A common feature of phytobiotics is that they are a very complex mixture of bioactive components. The herbs and plant extracts used as feed additives include many different bio-active ingredients such as essential oils, alkaloids, flavonoids, glycosides, mucilage, saponins and tannins, etc. (Wang *et al.*, 1998; Wenk, 2003). Therefore, the effects of herbs and plant extracts also vary. They may exert multiple functions in the animal body. Research trials have demonstrated that herbal feed additives have significant positive effect on growth performance and milk production, milk quality, health and reproduction without any side effects neither for animal performance nor consumers.

The mode of action of most phytogenic feed additives is still not fully understood. However, the following are some of the potential mechanisms by which they may improve performance.

1.3.1 Antimicrobial Action

There are a large number of herbs which have antibacterial activities (Cowan, 1999). In recent years, the use of phytogenic compounds has gained momentum for their potential role as natural alternatives to antibiotic growth promoters in animal nutrition (Lee *et al.*, 2014). Numerous secondary metabolites formed by plants serve as defence agents against physiological and environmental stressors, predators and pathogenic micro-organisms. Essential oils are commonly used as an alternative of antiobiotic growth promoter due to their anti-microbial properties. The actions of essential oils on microbial cells vary by the location of their functional hydroxyl or alkyl groups. The hydroxyl group of the phenolic terpenoids and the presence of delocalized electrons are important elements for their antimicrobial action. The locations of the functional groups such as hydroxyl groups in these molecules usually determine the level of their activity on different bacteria. Helander *et al.* (1998) reported that thymol and carvacrol had prominent outer membrane-disintegrating properties, mainly due to their enhanced ability to release lipo-polysaccharides, which acted more like detergents for sensitization. Because of the lipopolysaccharide release properties, both thymol and carvacrol have shown superior antimicrobial properties against some G″ bacteria than other phytogenic compounds. Several *in vitro* studies showed strong antimicrobial activity of certain plant extracts against Gram negative and Gram positive bacteria. Pasqa *et al.* (2006) found a change in long chain fatty acid profile in the membranes of *E. coli* grown in the presence of limonene or cinnamaldehyde. Similar observations were made with *Salomonella enterice* grown in the presence of carvacrol or eugenol and with *Bronchotrix thermosphacta* grown in the presence of limonene, cinnamaldehyde, carvacrol or eugenol. In the case of *Pseudomonas fluorescens* in *Staphylococcus* aureus none of the tested phytochemicals changed the fatty acid profile. The changes in fatty acid composition can affect surviving ability of micro-organisms.

It was reported that herbs and spices act as antimicrobial agents by changing the characteristics of cell membranes, and causing ion leakage, thus making microbes less virulent (Windisch *et al.*, 2008). The exact antimicrobial action of herbs and spices in *in vivo* situations is hard to evaluate, because of the very complex and balanced microbial populations in gastrointestinal tract and the interaction of active components from herbs and spices with other nutrients. Castillo *et al.* (2006) reported that the mixture of cinnamaldehyde, capsicum oleoresin and carvacrol enhances the growth of lactobacilli, and so increases the ratio of lactobacilli to enterobacteria. So, herbs and spices do not possess only the antimicrobial activity, but also modulate the composition of microbial population. Phytobiotics can selectively influence micro-organisms through antimicrobial activity, or by a favourable stimulation of the eubiosis of the microflora. This leads to better utilization and absorption of nutrients resulting in higher performance.

1.3.2 Anti -Inflammatory Action

Inflammation is a complex pathophysiological process mediated by a variety of signaling molecules produced by leukocytes, macrophages and mast cells as well as by the activation of complement factors. Plant's secondary metabolites have provided an important source of drugs since ancient times and now around half of the practical drugs used are derived from natural sources (Wang *et al.*, 2008). Many of these herbal constituents are being prescribed widely for the treatment of inflammatory conditions (Bagul *et al.*, 2005). Extracts of turmeric, red pepper, black pepper, cumin, cloves, nutmeg, cinnamon, mint and ginger showed anti-inflammatory effect in the studies on rats (Srinivasan, 2005). The major active molecules with anti-inflammatory action are terpenoids and flavonoids. These molecules suppress the metabolism of inflammatory prostaglandins. Flavonoids were investigated in models of inflammation in rats and were found to possess significant activity in both proliferative and exudative phases of inflammation. Flavonoids showed anti-inflammatory activity and inhibited the development of the induced granuloma, mostly when a catechol or guaiacol-like B ring is contained in the compound structure (Park *et al.*, 2007). Some flavonoids, such as quercetin, blocked both the cyclooxygenase and lipooxygenase pathways at relatively high concentrations, while at lower concentrations; the lipooxygenase pathway was the primary target of inhibitory anti-inflammatory activity (Rodrigo *et al.*, 2010).

1.3.3 Antioxidative Action

Many active components of herbs and spices can prevent lipid peroxidation through quenching free radicals or through activation of antioxidant enzymes like superoxide dismutase, catalase, glutathione peroxidise and glutathione reductase. Main molecules responsible for the antioxidative properties of herbs and spices are phenolic substances (flavonoids, hydrolysable tannins, proanthocianidins, phenolic acids, phenolic terpenes) and some vitamins (A, C and E). Phenolics exhibit several properties beneficial to humans and its antioxidant properties are important in determining their role as protecting agents against free radical-mediated disease processes. Often used herbs rich in phenolics are: rosemary, thyme, garlic, oregano, sage, green tea and marigold. The health promoting effect of antioxidants from plant is thought to arise from their protective effects by counteracting reactive oxygen species. Antioxidants are compounds that help delay and inhibit lipid oxidation and when added to foods tend to minimize rancidity, retard the formation of toxic oxidation products, and help maintain the nutritional quality (Aghsaghali, 2012). Herbs and spices can protect the feed against oxidative deterioration during storage. This is a widely used practice in pet food and human food industry. The herb commonly used for feed/food preservation is rosemary (*Rosmarinus officinalis*). It can be used alone or in combination with tocopherols or synthetic antioxidants (Jacob, 2008).

1.3.4 Immunostimulant Function

The immune system generally benefits from the herbs and spices rich in flavonoids, vitamin C and carotenoids. Polysaccharides derived from many plants play an important role in stimulating the growth of immune organs, such as the spleen, thymus and bursa, increasing the number and activities of many interdependent cell types such as T, B lympocytes, macrophages and natural killer (NK) cells, and enhancing cellular and humoral immune response. It is also known that certain plant polysaccharides act as immunostimulatory (adjuvant effect) substances (Paulsen, 2002; Chen *et al.*, 2003). The plants containing molecules which possess immunostimulatory properties are echinacea, liquorice, garlic and cat's claw. These plants can improve the activity of lymphocytes, macrophages and NK cells, they increase phagocytosis or stimulate the interpheron synthesis (Craig, 1999).

1.4 Phytobiotics as Feed Additives

Phytobiotics are natural growth promoters that have been growing in popularity as feed additives, due to their beneficial effect on gut health and immunity and growth performance. The beneficial effects of phytobiotics in livestock and poultry may arise from the activation of feed intake and the secretion of digestive enzymes, immune stimulation, antibacterial, coccidiostatic, anthelmintic, antiviral or anti-inflammatory activity, or from antioxidant properties. As a result of these beneficial effects, they lead to an increase in performance.

Feed additives with growth promoting activity increase stability of feed and beneficially influence the gastrointestinal ecosystem mostly through growth inhibition of pathogenic micro-organism's growth. Due to improved health status of digestive system, animals are less exposed to the toxins of microbiological origin. Consequently herbs and spices help to increase the resistance of the animals exposed to different stress situations and increase the absorption of essential nutrients, thus improving the growth of the animals (Windisch *et al.*, 2008).

Antimicrobial activity and immune enhancement probably are the two major mechanisms by which phytobiotics exert positive effects on the growth performance and health of animals. Phytochemicals in phytobiotics are well known to have antimicrobial ability (Cowan, 1999). Polysaccharide components are considered to be the most important immune active components (Xue and Meng, 1996). Oligosaccharides and polysaccharides such as inulin (fructan), fructo-oligosaccharides and arabinogalactans, which are extracted from plants, and sulfated fructans, which are extracted from seaweeds, are potential substitutes for currently used antibiotic growth promoting compounds (Tringali, 1997; Iji and Tivey, 1998). Growth enhancement through the use of phytobiotics is probably the result of the synergistic effects among complex active molecules existing in phytobiotics (Gauthier, 2002). Another field of phytobiotic actions comprises astringent and denaturizing properties in ruminants.

Herbs develop their initial activity in the feed as flavour and, therefore, influence eating patterns, the secretion of digestive fluids and total feed intake. Stimulation of digestive secretions, including saliva, digestive enzymes, bile and mucus is often considered to be one of the important actions of phytobiotics. Turmeric, garlic, black cumin, Aloe vera, wheat grass have been shown to improve feed intake in poultry. When considering supplementing the feed with herbs and spices or their extracts to stimulate the appetite, we have to know the taste preferences of different animal species. Janz *et al.* (2007) found that pigs preferred the feed supplemented with garlic or rosemary over the feed supplemented with oregano or ginger. Due to the wide variety of active components, different herbs and spices affect digestion processes differently. Most of them stimulate the secretion of saliva. Curcuma, pepper, ginger, anis, mint, onions, fenugreek, and cumin enhance the synthesis of bile acids in the liver and their excretion in bile, what beneficially effects the digestion and absorption of lipids.

Some bioactive substances from plants act as antimicrobial agents and exert their effects by modulating the cellular membrane of microbes (Kamel, 2000). Various essential oil mixtures, which contain natural polyphenolic compounds or flavonoids as major active ingredients, have been identified as potential antimicrobial and antioxidant agents (Cruickshank, 2001; Friedman *et al.*, 2004). Thus, supplementation of broiler diets with essential oil mixtures can create a healthier gut microflora, aiding optimum digestion and improving bird performance (Cruickshank, 2001).

Various plant extracts, especially essential oils, have been studied for their antimicrobial properties. Phytogenic substances derived from thyme, oregano, especially the major active substances thymol and carvacrol, are known to exert antimicrobial and bacterial actions *in vitro*, while eugenol, a component of the essential oil from cloves, has been shown to inhibit *Salmonella typhimurium*. Blends of oil containing thymol, eugenol, curcumin and piperin could be used to control *Clostridium perfringens*, the bacterium that causes necrotic enteritis in broiler chickens.

Phytobiotics are natural antioxidants. Turmeric, Black cumin, garlic, Aloevera, Indian gooseberry, ginger, etc., and its extract, is well known as a powerful antioxidant. One of the major roles of phyto-antioxidants in poultry production is on lipid oxidation in meat and meat products. Plant oils containing natural antioxidants contribute to the improved oxidative stability of meat and meat products containing higher levels of polyunsaturated fatty acid. The results of the investigation by Fallah *et al.* (2013) showed that adding phytobiotic compounds as artichoke leaves meal and menthe extract in broiler diets caused a decrease in HDL and LDL concentration. Essential oils function mainly as antimicrobials and antioxidants; their antimicrobial ability may modulate the gut ecosystem to affect fat digestibility (Lee *et al.*, 2004), starch or/and protein digestibility of feeds (Hernandez *et al.*, 2004).

The stimulatory effect of phytogenics on feed intake is due to the improvement in palatability of the diet resulting from the enhanced flavour and odour, especially with the use of essential oils. A product from rhizomes of *Sanguinaria canadensis* is frequently used in Europe for pigs and poultry. With other herb mixtures or botanicals effects on feed intake as well as growth performance in piglets and growing finishing pigs as well as poultry could be achieved. In has been concluded that in both species (piglet and broiler) a slight increase in feed intake could be observed at least partly at low levels and then a dramatic decrease at higher levels of a particular herb. Similar observations were made in laying hens with turmeric, a powder of the rhizome of *Curcuma longa,* a spice that is frequently used in the south Asian kitchen (Wenk, 2003) 0.25% Turmeric improved feed intake. At higher levels upto 1% feed intake returned to the control treatment without supplementation.

Herbs develop their initial activity in the feed of farm animals as flavour and can, therefore, influence the eating pattern, secretion of digestive fluids and total feed intake. Herbs or the phytochemicals can influence selectively the micro-organisms by an anti-microbial activity or by a favourable stimulation of the eubiosis of the microflora. The consequence can be a better nutrient utilization and absorption or the stimulation of the immune system. Finally herbs can contribute to the nutrient requirements of the animals and stimulate the endocrine system and intermediate nutrient metabolism. Most of the prelisted spices stimulate the function of pancreatic enzymes (lipases, amylases and proteases), some also increase the activity of digestive enzymes of gastric mucosa (Srinivasan, 2005). Besides the effect on bile synthesis and enzyme activity, extracts from herbs and spices accelerate the digestion and shorten the time of feed/food passage through the digestive tract (Platel and Srinivasan, 2001).

1.5 Challenges of Using Phytogenic Compounds in Animal Feed

Phytogenic compounds have multiple functions as whole, including antimicrobial and antioxidant activities as well as digestion and immune-enhancing properties. To define the specific effect and target site (either animal host or its microbiota) of individual phytogenic compounds is difficult and this limits widespread application of phytogenic compounds in animal feed. Fully understanding the mechanism of action of active principles of phytobiotics is very critical. A better understanding of the effects and mechanisms of action of various phytobiotics will guide the designs for more effective phytogenic additives to improve feed efficiency and promote animal growth. Use of phytobiotic compounds have been investigated extensively. Research into their mechanisms of action, compatibility with diet needs to be done before they can be applied more extensively in animal feed. In addition, challenges in using phytogenic compounds as animal feed additives may include potential side effects (toxic, unpleasant odour/taste), regulatory affair concerns and possible interactions with other feed ingredients (Friedman *et al.*, 2002; Cheng *et al.*, 2014).

Phytobiotics contain many pharmacologically active components which play a major role in the defense system of the plant. Phytobiotics are generally assumed as GRAS (Generally Recognized as Safe); however safety concerns cannot be excluded (Mathe, 2009). Toxicity and safety assessment (based on the fact that some phytobiotic might have harmful substances) needs to be done before they can be applied more extensively in poultry feed. Phytobiotics may contain ingredients which may be harmful to both animals and humans. Furthermore, undesired residues may not be excluded in a natural product. In several experiments, it was observed that bioactive ingredients or their metabolites may be transferred to tissues (Windisch *et al.*, 2009). Some, concerns are reported for capsaicin (cancer causing), cyanide containing ingredients, carvacrol (in oregano) and glycosides. Also, it is difficult to conduct systematic and comprehensive evaluations toward the efficacy and safety of phytogenic compounds due to their complex composition. There have hardly been developed analytical methods to identify and quantify the traceability of phytogenic compounds in feeds and animal tissues.

The results related to use of phytobiotics in animal feed from previous studies are highly variable. Ingredients of phytobiotics may vary distinctly due to climatic conditions, soil, species, time of harvest, degree of maturation, included parts, etc. This holds mainly for products of dried whole plants or parts. Extracts of essential oils or oleoresins show less variation. In animal feeding, phytobiotics are used as single preparations or as mixtures of plant extracts, herb mixes, spice mixes, oil blends). There appear to be four reasons associated with the inconsistency: (i) variations in the composition of phytogenic compounds due to plant growing locations, manufacturing methods and the storage conditions (Yang *et al.*, 2009) (ii) variations in the dosages that may not be efficacious (Cross *et al.*, 2007) (iii) the lack of efficacy of phytogenic compounds; (iv) varied conditions during the trials such as environment, animal age, genetics, feeds and health status (Giannenas *et al.*, 2003). In addition, the minimum inhibition concentration (MIC) values of most phytogenic compounds are significantly higher than the levels to be acceptable in animal production from the viewpoint of cost-effectiveness, since the acceptance by the industry to use feed additives to optimize the animal performance and health is largely dependent on feed input costs.

Some phytogenic compounds are very volatile and can evaporate rapidly, leading to largely varied final concentrations in the products (Lambert *et al.*, 2001). The stability of phytogenic compounds during feed processing is often questionable. In addition, some phytobiotics may be absorbed to feed components, leading to a reduced activity (Si *et al.*, 2006). Therefore, without proper protection, most essential oils will be lost during feed processing and delivery to the animal gut and thus may not be able to reach the lower gut of animals, where most pathogens reside and propagate. It will reduce the profitability of feed eventually and become one of major barriers for essential oils application in feed.

Effective method of delivery of phytobiotics is also an issue of concern. To improve efficacy, effective and practically feasible delivery method for the use of the phytobiotics is essential. Microencapsulation has become one of the most popular methods to solve the issue (Piva *et al.*, 1997). A commonly used method is the microencapsulation of essential oils in a lipid matrix that could dissolve as it passes along the small intestine (Piva *et al.*, 1997). However, other methods are to be explored. A study indicated that alginate-whey protein microparticles could be used as a target delivery carrier in feed to enhance the gut delivery of carvacrol in broiler chickens, the effect of encapsulated carvacrol on reducing necrotic enteritis in *Clostridium perfringens*-challenged broilers was comparable to that of antibiotics in feed (Zhang *et al.*, 2014). Thus, it is clear that proper microencapsulation technologies can lower the required effective dosage of a phytogenic compound in feed and reduce the feed cost.

Besides the inconsistent results and inconclusive mechanisms, the challenges of using phytogenic compounds in animal feed may also include side effects, regulatory obstacles and cost-effectiveness. Nevertheless, application of novel technologies integrating research to simultaneously examine genomes, metagenomes, transriptomes and proteomes should help to better understand the modes of action of phytogenic compounds and subsequently lead to the development of feasible and cost-effective ways to use phytogenic compounds in animal feed.

References

Bagul MS, Srinivasa H, Kanaki NS, Rajani M (2005) Antiinflammatory activity of two Ayurvedic formulations containing guggul. Indian J Pharma 37: 399-400

Bedford MR, Cowieson AJ (2012) Exogenous enzymes and their effects on intestinal microbiology. Anim Feed Sci Technol 173: 76–85

Castillo M, Martin-Orue SM, Roca M, Manzanilla EG, Badiola I, Perez JF, Gasa J (2006) The response of gastrointestinal microbiota to avilamycin, butyrate, and plant extracts in early-weaned pigs. J Anim Sci 84: 2725–2734

Chen YJ, Kim IJ, Choi JH, Yoo JS, Wang Q, Wang Y, Huang Y (2008) Evaluation of dietary L-carnitine or garlic powder on growth performance, dry matter and nitrogen digestibilities, blood profiles and meat quality in finishing pigs. *Anim Feed Sci Technol* 141(1): 141-152

Cheng G, Hao H, Xie S, Wang X, Dai M, Huang L, Yuan Z (2014) Antibiotics alternatives: The substitution of antibiotics in animal husbandry? Front Microbiol 5: 217-222

Choi SC, Ingale SL, Kim JS, Park YK, Kwon IK, Chae BJ (2013) An antimicrobial peptide-A3: Effects on growth performance, nutrient retention, intestinal and faecal microflora and intestinal morphology of broilers. Br Poult Sci 54: 738–746

Cowan MM (1999) Plant products as antimicrobial agents. Clin Microbiol Rev 12: 564-582

Craig WJ (1999) Health-promoting properties of common herbs. Am J Clin Nutr 70: 491S-499S

Cross DE , McDevitt RM, Hillman K, Acamovic T (2007) The effect of herbs and their associated essential oils on performance, dietary digestibility and gut microflora in chickens from 7 to 28 days of age. Br Poult Sci 48: 496-506

Cruickshank G (2001) Botanical growth enhancers offer natural option for broiler growers. Poult World 10: 19–22

Eckel B, Kirchgessner M, Roth, FX (1992) Influence of formic acid on daily weight gain, feed intake, feed conversion rate and digestibility. J Anim Physiol Anim Nutr 67: 93–100

Edeoga HO, Okwu DE, Mbaebie BO (2005) Phytochemical constituents of some Nigerian medicinal plants. Afr J Biotechnol 4(7): 685-688

Fallah R, Kiani A, Azarfar A (2013) Effect of Artichoke leaves meal and menthe extract (*Mentha piperita*) on immune cells and blood biochemical parameters of broilers. Global Veterinarian 10(1): 99-102

Friedman M., Henika, PR, Mandrell, RE (2002) Bactericidal activities of plant essential oils and some of their isolated constituents against *Campylobacter jejuni, Escherichia coli, Listeria monocytogenes* and *Salmonell enterica*. J Food Protection 65: 1545–156

Gauthier R (2002) Poultry Therapeutics: New alternatives. Accessed on 5 April, 2017. http://www.jefo.ca/pdf/ALA2003_en.pdf

Giannenas A I, Florou-Paneri P, Papazahariadou M, Christaki E, Botsoglou N A, Spais A B (2003) Dietary oregano essential oil supplementatio non-performance of challenged with *Eimeria tenella*. Arch Anim Nutr 57: 99–106

Gibson GR, Probert HM, Loo JV, Rastall RA, Roberfroid MB (2004) Dietary modulation of the human colonic microbiota: Updating the concept of prebiotics. Nutr Res Rev 17: 259–275

Gong J, Yin F, Hou Y, Yin Y (2014) Chinese herbs as alternatives to antibiotics in feed for swine and poultry production: Potential and challenges in application. Can J Anim Sci 94: 223–241

Hasler CM, Blumberg JB (1999) Symposium on Phytochemicals: Biochemistry and Physiology. J Nutr 129: 756S-757S

Helander I M and Mattila-Sandholm T, (2000) Permeability barrier of the Gram-negative bacterial outer membrane with special reference to nisin. International J Food Microbiol 60: 153–161

Hernandez F, Madrid J, Garcia V, Orengo J, Megias MD (2004) Influence of two plant extracts on broiler performance, digestibility and digestive organ size. Poult Sci 83: 169-174.

Iji P A and Tivey D R (1998) Natural and synthetic oligosaccharides in broiler chicken diets. World's Poult Sci, 29–143

Jacobsen C, Undeland I, Storrø I, Rustad T, Hedges N, Medina I (2008) Preventing lipid oxidation in seafood, in Improving Seafood Products for the Consumer: Improving seafood products for the consumer, T. Borresen (Ed),. Cambridge, Woodhead Publishing. pp. 426-460.

Janz JAM, Morel PCH, Wilkinson BHP and Purchas R W (2007) Preliminary investigation of the effects of low-level dietary inclusion of fragrant esential oils and oleoresins on pig performance and pork quality. Meat Sci 75: 350–355

Kamel C (2000) Natural plant extracts: Classical remedies bring modern animal production solutions. In: Proceedings of the III Conference of Feed Manufacturers of the Mediterranean: Feed manufacturing in the Mediterranean region improving safety: From feed to food, pp. 31–38 (ed. J. Brufau). Institut Agronomique Mediterraneen de Zaragoza, Reus, Spain.

Lambert RJW, Skandamis PN, Coote PJ, Nychas GJE (2001) A study of the minimum inhibitory concentration and mode of action of oregano essential oil, thymol and carvacrol. Appl Microbiol 91: 453–462

Lee KW, Ecerts H, Beynen AC (2004) Essential oils in broiler nutrition. Int J Poult Sci 3: 738-752

Musa HH, Wu S L, Zhu C H, Seri H I, Zhu G Q (2009) The potential benefits of probiotics inanimal production and health. J Anim Vet Adv 8: 313–321

Park EK, Rhee H I, Jung HS, Ju SM, Lee YA, Lee SH, Hong SJ, Yang HI, Yoo MC, Kim KS (2007) Anti-inflammatory effects of a combined herbal preparation (RAH13) of Phellodendron amurense and Coptis chinensis in animal models of inflammation. Phytotherapy Res 21(8): 746-50

Pasqua RD, Hoskins NB, Mauriello G (2006) Changes in membrane fatty acids composition of microbial cells induced addition of thymol, carvacrol, limonene, cinnamaldehyde, and eugenol in the growing media. J Agric Food Chem 54(7): 2745–2749

Paulsen BS (2002) Biologically active polysaccherides as possible lead compounds. Phytochem Rev 1: 379-387.

Piva A, Anfossi P, Meola E, Pietri A, Panciroli A, Bertuzzi T, Formigoni A, (1997) Effect of micro-encapsulation on absorption processes in the pig. Livest Prod Sci 51: 53–61

Platel K, Srinivasan K (2001). Influence of dietary spices and their active principles on pancreatic digestive enzymes in albino rats. Food Nahrung 44: 42-46

Rodrigo G, Ana LC, Adriano LS, Helton CS, Claire L, Jacqueline AL, Virginia SL, Mauro M (2010) The flavonoid dioclein reduces the production of proinflammatory mediators *in vitro* by inhibiting PDE4 activity and scavenging reactive oxygen species. European J Pharm 63: 85–92

Si W Gong J, Chanas C, Cui S, Yu H, Caballero C (2006) *In vitro* assessment of antimicrobial activity of carvacrol, thymol and cinnamaldehyde towards *Salmonella serotype Typhimurium* DT104: Effects of pig diets and emulsification in hydrocolloids. J Appl Microbiol 101: 1282–1291.

Tringali C (1997) Bioactive metabolites from marine algae: recent results. Current Organic Chem 1: 375–394

Wang S, Xiang-Yu-Lan, Xiao J, Yang J, Kao J, Chang S (2008) Anti inflammatory activity of Lindera erythrocarpa fruits. Phyto Res 22: 213-216.

Wang R, Li D, Bourne S (1998) Can 2000 years of herbal medicine history help us solve problems in the year 2000? In: Biotechnology in the Feed Industry. Proceedings of Alltech's 14th Annual Symposium, ed. Lyons TP and Jacques KA. pp. 273-291

Wenk C, (2003) Herbs and Botanicals as feed additives in Monogastric animals. Asian Aust J Anim Sci 6(2): 282-289

Windisch W, Kroismayr A (2006) The effects of phytobiotics on performance and gut function in monogastrics.. www.feedinfo.com. Accessed in April 07, 2017

Xue M, Meng XS (1996). Review on research progress and prosperous of immune activities of bioactive polysaccharides. J TradVet Med 3: 15-18

Yang Y, Iji PA, Choct M (2009) Dietary modulation of gut microflora in broiler chickens: A review of the role of six kinds of alternatives to feed antibiotics. Worlds Poult Sci 65: 97–114

Zhang Y, Gong J, Yu H, Guo Q, Defelice C, Hernandez M, Yin Y, Wang Q (2014) Alginate-whey protein dry powder optimized for target delivery of essential oils to the intestine of chickens. Poult Sci 93: 2514–2525.

❑❑❑

Chapter 2

Phytochemicals: Mode of Action

Kaushalendra Kumar and Pankaj Kumar Singh

Department of Animal Nutrition, Bihar Animal Sciences University, Patna-800014, India, E-mail: kaushalivri@gmail.com

ABSTRACT

The non-nutrient chemical compounds of plant origin or bioactive components are often referred as phytochemicals. These phyto-constituentsare responsible for protecting the plant against microbial infections or infestations by pests and its over exploitation. Phytochemicals can be divided into different classes depending upon the chemical structures, botanical origins, biosynthesis pathways and its biological properties. The most phytochemical classification is based on chemical structures such as phenolics, alkaloids, saponins, terpenoids, essential oil, etc.Mechanism of action of these bioactive plant constituentsmay be multiple in nature. These phytochemicals reduce oxidation, reduce inflammationand stimulateimmune systemagainst viruses, bacteria and other disease causing agents. Plants also contain a wide variety of free radicals scavenging molecules including phenols, flavonoids, vitamins, terpenoids, etc. having very good antioxidant activity.

Keywords : Phytochemical, Phenolics, Alkaloids, Saponins, Terpenoids, Essential oils.

2.1 Introduction

Phytochemicals literally mean plant chemicals. The non-nutrient plant chemical compounds or bioactive components are often referred to as phytochemicals (phyto- from Greek - *phyto* meaning 'plant') or phytoconstituents and are responsible for protecting the plant against microbial infections or infestations by pests (Doughari *et al.*, 2009). The study of natural products on the other hand is called phytochemistry. Phytochemicals have been isolated and characterized from fruits such as grapes and apples, vegetables such as broccoli and onion, spices such as turmeric, beverages such as green tea and red wine, as well as many other sources (Doughari and Obidah, 2008; Doughari *et al.*, 2009). Researchers have identified thousands of different phytochemicals, found in vegetables, fruits, beans, whole grains, nuts and seeds. Eating lots of plant foods rich in phytochemicals may help to prevent several life threatening serious ailments such as heart disease, cancer, etc.

The ethnopharmacologists, botanists, microbiologists and natural-product chemists are constantly in search of medicinal efficacy of plants and their phytochemicals, since the reported data so far available on plants are comparatively meager compared to the vast number of plant population. The structures of close to 40,000 compounds have already been elucidated and there are perhaps hundreds of thousands of such compounds in plants (Pichersky and Gang, 2000). Only a few of these are part of 'primary' metabolic pathways (those common to all organisms). The rest are secondary metabolites or phytochemicals whose biosynthesis is restricted to selected plant groups. Phytochemicals can be divided into many major classes depending upon the chemical structures, botanical origins, biosynthesis pathways or biological properties. The most phyto-chemical classification scheme is based on chemical structures such as phenolics, alkaloids, saponins, terpenoids and so on.

2.2 Mechanism of Action of Different Classes of Phytochemicals

2.2.1 Alkaloids

Alkaloids have been defined as N-heterocyclic basic metabolites, although the definition does not clearly separate from other N-containing compounds. Alkaloids have been classified in many ways depending upon biogenic precursors or carbon skeleton characteristics. They have a great structural diversity compared with other classes of phytochemicals. Alkaloids are generally known according to their carbon skeleton structures. Pyridine (e.g. piperine), piperidine, quinoline, indole, pyrrolidine, quinazoline, isoquinoline, glyoxaline, lupinane, tropan, phenanthridine, imidazoline, alkaloidal amines and terpenoid types of alkaloids are commonly found in plants (Hegnauer, 1988). The alkaloids are usually with potent activity and bitter taste. They are of limited distribution in the plant kingdom. The various groups have diverse clinical properties.Tropane alkaloids are present in Solanaceae (nightshade family), Atropa belladonna (deadly nightshade), Datura spp (thorn apples) and Hyoscyamus niger (henbane). The compounds have anticholinergic activity (muscarine receptor antagonists) and are used medically to reduce smooth muscle spasms, hypersecretion and pain. Pyrrolizidine alkaloids are produced in Asteraceae (daisy family), particularly in Senecio spp. (Ragworts) and in Boraginaceae (borage family). Their adverse effect in man and animals are hepatotoxicity after bioactivation. Papaveraceae (poppy family) and Berberidaceae (barberry family) produce isoquinoline alkaloids which have a range of biochemical effects relevant for medical use, as inhibition of various conditions as pain, cancer cells and bacteria, and stimulation of bone marrow leucocytes as well as myocardial contractility. The main producers of methylxanthine alkaloids are *Coffea arabica* (coffee) and Theobroma cacao (cacao). Methylxanthines to a various extent bind to adenosine receptor and elicit neurological effects in man and animals which may be regarded stimulating at low to moderate intake. Compounds called pseudoalkaloids have chemical properties close to alkaloids and are produced by species in Apiaceae (carrot family) for instance, *Cicuta virosa* (cowbane) and *Conium maculatum* (hemlock), and in Taxaceae (yew family) for instance Taxus baccata (yew). The pseudo-alkaloids in *Cicuta virosa* and Conium maculatum have effects on the central nervous system.

In nature, the alkaloids exist in large proportions in the seeds and roots of plants and often in combination with vegetable acids. Alkaloids have pharmacological applications as anaesthetics and CNS stimulants (Madziga *et al.*, 2010). More than 12,000-alkaloids are known to exist in about 20% of plant species and only few have been exploited for medicinal purposes. The name alkaloid ends with the suffix *-ine* and plant-derived alkaloids in clinical use include the analgesics morphine and codeine, the muscle relaxant tubocurarine, the antibiotics sanguinafine and berberine, the anticancer agent vinblastine, the antiarrythmic ajmaline, the pupil dilator atropine, and the sedative scopolamine. Other important alkaloids of plant origin include the addictive stimulants caffeine, nicotine, codeine, atropine, morphine, ergotamine, cocaine, nicotine and ephedrine. Amino acids act as precursors for biosynthesis of alkaloids with ornithine and lysine commonly used as starting materials.

2.2.2 Glycosides

The glycosides consist of various categories of secondary metabolites bound to a mono- or oligosaccharide or to uronic acid. The saccharide or uronic acid part is called glycone, and the other part the aglycone. The main groups of glycosides are cardiac glycosides, cyanogenic glycosides, glucosinolates, saponins and anthraquinone glycosides. Furthermore, flavonoids frequently occur as glycosides. Glycosides in general, are defined as the condensation products of sugars (including polysaccharides) with a host of different varieties of organic hydroxy (occasionally thiol) compounds (invariably monohydrate in character), in such a manner that the hemiacetal entity of the carbohydrate must essentially take part in the condensation. Glycosides are colourless, crystalline carbon, hydrogen and oxygen-containing (some contain nitrogen and sulfur) water-soluble phytoconstituents, found in the cell sap. Chemically, glycosides contain a carbohydrate (glucose) and a non-carbohydrate part (aglycone or genin) (Kar, 2007; Firn, 2010). Glycosides are neutral in reaction and can be readily hydrolyzed into its components with ferments or mineral acids. Glycosides are classified on the basis of type of sugar component, chemical nature of aglycone or pharmacological action. The rather older or trivial names of glycosides usually has a suffix 'in' and the names essentially included the source of the glycoside, for instance: strophanthidin from *Strophanthus*, digitoxin from *Digitalis*, barbaloin from *Aloes*, salicin from *Salix*, cantharidin from *Cantharides*, and prunasin from *Prunus.*

However, the systematic names are invariably coined by replacing the "ose" suffix of the parent sugar with "oside". This group of drugs are usually administered in order to promote appetite and aid digestion. Glycosides are purely bitter principles that are commonly found in plants of the Genitiaceae family and though they are chemically unrelated but possess the common property of an intensely bitter taste. The bitters act on gustatory nerves, which results in increased flow of saliva and gastric juices. Chemically, the bitter principles contain the lactone group that may be diterpene lactones (e.g. *andrographolide*) or triterpenoids (e.g.*amarogentin*). Some of the bitter principles are either used as astringents due to the presence of tannic acid, as antiprotozoan, or to reduce thyroxine and metabolism. Cardiac glycosides (acts on the heart), anthracene glycosides (purgative, and for treatment of skin diseases), chalcone glycoside (anticancer), amarogentin, gentiopicrin, andrographolide, ailanthone and polygalin. Sarker and Nahar (2007) reported that extracts of plants that contain cyanogenic glycosides are used as flavouring agents in many pharmaceutical preparations. Amygdalin has been used in the treatment of cancer (HCN liberated in stomach kills malignant cells), and also as a cough suppressant in various preparations. Excessive ingestion of cyanogenic glycosides can be fatal. Some foodstuffs containing cyanogenic glycosides can cause poisoning (severe gastric irritations and damage), if not properly handled (Sarker and Nahar, 2007).

The aglycones of cardiac glycosides have a steroidal structure. Their effect is inhibition of Na+/K+-ATPase-pumps in the cell membranes. These pumps are concentrated in and critical for the functioning of the cardiac cells and the effects from these compounds are very pronounced in the heart, resulting in increased contractility and reduced rate. The cardiac glycosides are present in plants of *Scrophulariaceae* (figwort family) particularly *Digitalis purpura* (foxglove) and in *Convallariaceae* (convall family) with *Convallaria majalis* (lily of the valley) as a typical example.The cyanogenic glycosides have aglycones derived from amino acids. Several of these compounds can interfere with the iodine utilisation and result in hypothyroidism. The other important effect is via their release of hydrogen cyanide, which is very toxic being lethal at high dosages. Cyanogenic glycosides are present in species of Rosaceae (rose family) in particular in Prunus spp.The glucosinolates contain sulphur-containing, pungent amino acid-derived aglycones. The compounds show a complex set of effects on cytochrome P450 isoforms in various cells and tend to decrease hepatic bio activation of environmental procarcinogens. The glucosinolates can be skin irritating and also induce hypothyroidism and goitre. The Brassicaceae (brassica family) is the family mainly associated with glucosinolate production. Anthraquinone glycosides show a relatively limited distribution within the plant kingdom. In Polygonaceae (dock family), they are present for instance, in *Rumex crispus* (curly dock) and Rheum spp (rhubarbs). Their primary effect is induction of water and electrolyte secretion as well as peristalisis in colon. It may induce detoxification of carcinogens, limit production of cancer elated hormones, block carcinogens and prevent tumour growth and work as antioxidants.

2.2.3 Flavonoids

Flavonoids are important group of polyphenols widely distributed among the plant flora. They have significant antioxidant properties, which are beneficial for health. The compounds are derived from parent compounds known as flavans. These polyphenolic compounds are constructed basically with an A and C ring of benzo-1-pyran-4-quinone and a B ring. The main classes of flavonoids are: (1) flavones (basic structures), e.g. luteolin, apigenin, diosmetin, chrysoeriol, tangeretin, sinensetin, gardenin, vitexin and baicalein; (2) flavonols (having a hydroxyl group at the 3-position), e.g. kaempferol, quercetin, galangin, datiscetin, morin, robinetin, isorhamnetin, tamarixetin, quercetagetin and myricetin; (3) flavanones (2-3 bond saturated), e.g. hesperetin, taxifolin, eriodictyol and naringenin; (4) flavan-3-ol, e.g. catechin and epicatechin; (5) isoflavone, e.g. genistein, daidzein and coumestrol; (6) anthocyanidins: cyanidin, delphinidin, pelargonidin and peonidin (Crozier *et al.*, 2006). The majority of flavonoids commonly remain conjugated with sugars as glycosides.It may inhibit inflammation and tumour growth; may aid immunity and boost production of detoxifying enzymes in the body.

All compounds contain phenol-groups involved in an effect as general antioxidant. Other actions are diverse several structures reduce inflammation or carcinogenicity. The group isoflavones are primarily known as phytoestrogens. Flavonoids and proanthocyanidins are all pigments occurring in a long range of plant families. Isoflavones are produced by species of Fabaeceae (bean family). A recent study by Berger *et al.* (2012) showed that rumen microbes enhanced the bioavailability of flavonoid rutin (quercetin-3-O-rutinoside) by degradation of glycosidic linkage. This degradation resulted in libration of quercetin. Further, the quercetin and its methylated (isorhamnetin, tamarixetin) and dehydroxylated (kaempferol) derivatives were detected in plasma of nonlactating cows. Similarly, a recent study compared the bioavailability of quercetin in the aglycone and glucorhamnoside forms through duodenal administration in German Holstein cows. Their results showed higher intestinal bioavailability of quercetin in the aglycone form as compared to the glucorhamnoside form.Epigallocatechin gallate exerted strong antibacterial growth against Gram-positive bacteria than against Gram-negative bacteria (Yoda *et al.*, 2004; Engels *et al.*, 2009). It has been stated that Gram-positive bacteria absorb more epigallocatechin gallate into their peptidoglycan cell wall and aggregate its presence, while Gram-negative bacteria do not aggregate and absorb less epigallocatechin gallate (Ikigai *et al.*, 1993; Engels *et al.*, 2009) because of the repulsive negative charge of lipopolysaccharides on the surfaces of Gram-negative bacteria. The binding of epigallocatechin gallate to peptidoglycan disrupts its function in osmotic protection, cell division, and cell wall biosynthesis (Yoda *et al.*, 2004).

2.2.4 Phenolics

Phenolic compounds are a group of phytochemicals, which have a phenol structure, i.e. an aromatic benzene ring bearing at least one hydroxyl substituent (Robbins, 2003; Vermerris and Nicholson, 2006). Phenolic compounds are commonly found throughout the plant kingdom, where they protect the plants from microbial infections, ultraviolet radiation and chemical stressors. This large and diverse group of phytochemicals is classified into many subclasses depending upon chemical structures and occurrence in plants. The commonly categorized subclasses of phenolic compounds are simple phenolics (resorcinol and phloroglucinol), phenolic acids and aldehydes, coumarins, flavonoids, chalcones, aurones, benzophenones, xanthones, stilbenes, benzoquinones, naphthaquinones, anthraquinones, betacyanins, lignans and polyphenols (proanthocyanidin, galloyl, hexahydroxydiphenylester, hydroxy cinnamic acid, and phloroglucinol derivatives) (Vermerris and Nicholson, 2006; Handique and Baruah, 2002). The detailed structures and chemistry of these phenolic compounds are presented elsewhere (Vermerris and Nicholson, 2006). Foods containing phenolics are becoming an important part of diets due to their potential anti-oxidative properties. Besides, these compounds have also potent anti-microbial properties. A number of simple phenols and phenolic acids possess antibacterial, antiviral and antifungal activities against a wide range of microbes, but at different concentrations.

Phenolic compounds are usually poorly absorbed in the small intestine, and thus, most of the dietary phenolics accumulate in the colon (Clifford, 2004; van Duynhoven *et al.*, 2011). Therefore, higher concentrations of phenolic acids may reach in the intestine than the concentrations in diets. Phenolics may selectively suppress or stimulate the growth of certain members of intestinal microbiota, which may influence microbial population dynamics in the gastrointestinal tract (Tzounis *et al.*, 2008). In general, antibacterial activity of phenolic acids is stronger against gram-positive bacteria than Gram-negative bacteria

(Merkl *et al.*, 2010; Cueva *et al.*, 2010). The outer membrane of gram-negative bacteria provides them with a hydrophobic surface structure that is able to exclude certain hydrophilic molecules, making them inherently resistant to many antimicrobial agents including phenolic acids (Alakomi *et al.*, 2007; Cueva *et al.*, 2010).

Phenolics in plants are mostly synthesized from phenylalanine via the action of phenylalanine ammonia lyase. They are very important to plants and have multiple functions. The most important role may be in plant defence against pathogens and herbivore predators, and thus, are applied in the control of human pathogenic infections (Puupponen- Pimia *et al.*, 2008). They are classified into: (i) phenolic acids and (ii) flavonoid polyphenolics (flavonones, flavones, xanthones and catechins) and (iii) non-flavonoid polyphenolies. Caffeic acid is regarded as the most common of phenolic compounds distributed in the plant flora followed by chlorogenic acid known to cause allergic dermatitis among humans (Kar, 2007). Phenolics essentially represent a host of natural antioxidants, used as nutraceuticals, and found in apples, green-tea, and red-wine for their enormous ability to combat cancer and are also thought to prevent heart ailments to an appreciable degree and sometimes are anti-inflammatory agents. Sources are green tea, grapes, wine, berries, citrus fruits, apples, whole grains and peanuts. It may prevent cancer formation, prevent inflammation and work as antioxidants.

2.2.5 Saponins

The term 'saponin' is derived from *Saponaria vaccaria* (*Quillaja saponaria*), a plant, which abounds in saponins and was once used as soap. Saponins, therefore, possess 'soaplike' behaviour in water, i.e. they produce foam. On hydrolysis, an aglycone is produced, which is called sapogenin. There are two types of sapogenin: steroidal and triterpenoidal. Usually, the sugar is attached at C-3 in saponins, because in most sapogenins, there is a hydroxyl sugar molecule is combined with triterpene or steroid aglycone. There are two major groups of saponins and these include: steroid saponins and triterpene saponins. Saponins are soluble in water and insoluble in ether, and like glycosides on hydrolysis, they give aglycones. Saponins are extremely poisonous, as they cause heamolysis of blood and are known to cause cattle poisoning (Kar, 2007). They possess a bitter and acrid taste, besides causing irritation to mucous membranes. They are mostly amorphous in nature, soluble in alcohol and water, but insoluble in non-polar organic solvents like benzene and n-hexane. Saponins are also important therapeutically as they are shown to have hypolipidemic and anticancer activity. Saponins are also necessary for activity of cardiac glycosides. The two major types of steroidal sapogenin are diosgenin and hecogenin. Steroidal saponins are used in the commercial production of sex hormones for clinical use. For example, progesterone is derived from diosgenin. The most abundant starting material for the synthesis of progesterone is diosgenin isolated from *Dioscorea* species, formerly supplied from Mexico, and now from China (Sarker & Nahar, 2007). Other steroidal hormones, e.g. cortisone and hydrocortisone, can be prepared from the starting material hecogenin, which can be isolated from Sisal leaves found extensively in East Africa (Sarker & Nahar, 2007).

In tropical countries, crop residues and poor quality hays and pastures form a major part of the animal diets. Urea ammoniation has been used extensively for enhancing the digestibility and in turn intake and nutrient utilisation from these low quality roughages. However, a major disadvantage of the ammoniation process is the loss of nitrogen in the form of ammonia that occurs during fermentation. Saponins are considered to bind ammonia. In one of our studies (Makkar *et al.*, 1999), *Quillaja saponaria* bark saponins and Yucca schidigera plant extract rich in saponins were added during urea-ammoniation to reduce ammonia loss to the air. As some methanogens (10% to 20% of total) live in association with protozoa (Newbold *et al.*, 1997), it was expected that reducing protozoa would also reduce methanogens, thus reducing methane production. Saponins may kill or inactivate protozoa (Makkar *et al.*, 1998b), resulting in a lower predation of bacteria by protozoa and a larger bacterial population, slowing protein turnover in the rumen. The slower protein turnover should lead to an increase in bacterial nitrogen flow to the duodenum and increase in productivity (Wallace *et al.*, 2002; Hess *et al.*, 2004).

2.2.6. Tannins

Tannins are widely distributed in plant flora. They are phenolic compounds of high molecular weight. Tannins are soluble in water and alcohol and are found in the root, bark, stem and outer layers of plant tissue. Tannins have a characteristic feature to tan, i.e. to convert things into leather. They are acidic in reaction and the acidic reaction is attributed to the presence of phenolics or carboxylic group

(Kar, 2007). They form complexes with proteins, carbohydrates, gelatine and alkaloids. Tannins are divided into hydrolysable tannins and condensed tannins. Hydrolysable tannins, upon hydrolysis, produce gallic acid and ellagic acid and depending on the type of acid produced, the hydrolysable tannins are called gallotannins or egallitannins. On heating, they form pyrogallic acid. Tannins are used as antiseptic and this activity is due to presence of the phenolic group. Common examples of hydrolysable tannins include theaflavins (from tea), daidezein, genistein and glycitein. Tannin rich medicinal plants are used as healing agents in a number of diseases. In Ayurveda, formulations based on tannin-rich plants have been used for the treatment of diseases like leucorrhoea, rhinnorhoea and diarrhoea.

These are considered to have both adverse and beneficial effects depending on their concentration and nature as well as other factors such as animal species, physiological state of the animal and composition of the diet. Some of the beneficial effects of tannins are enhancement of rumen undegradable protein and making feed protein available post-ruminally for production purposes, enhancement of efficiency of microbial protein production, and protection of ruminants from bloat. Some tannin is also known to have strong anticarcinogenic and antioxidant activities (Riedl *et al.*, 2002).

Skatole and indole are flavour compounds formed in the rumen, which exert negative effects on meat flavour and quality. These compounds originate from deamination and decarboxylation of the amino acid tryptophan by rumen microbes and are present in meat fat. Rumen bacteria that produce a range of indolic compounds have recently been described (Attwood *et al.*, 2006). In *in vitro* studies, condensed tannins from *Lotus corniculatus* have been demonstrated to reduce the production of skatole, and this was attributed to decreased rumen protein degradation by lotus tannins (Schreurs *et al.*, 2004). Condensed tannins from Dorycnium rectum also inhibited skatole and indole formation in the in vitro rumen system (Tavendale *et al.*, 2005). Further studies are needed to verify, if tannins could play a role in decreasing fat skatole and indole in meat from animals. In addition, these effects lead to protein-sparing effects in ruminants and decreased methane emissions and nitrogen excretion to the environment, thereby reducing emission of environmental pollutants despite producing more meat, milk and wool.

Tannins isolated from leaves of various multipurpose trees and browses have anticarcinogenic activity (Perchellet *et al.*, 1996). Proanthocyanidins (condensed tannins), both in free form and bound to proteins, have been shown to have free radical scavenging abilities (Hagerman *et al.*, 1999) and decrease the susceptibility of healthy cells to toxic agents. Most polyphenols have strong antioxidant properties and inhibit lipid peroxidation and peroxygenases. Pistafolia A, a gallotannin, has strong free radical scavenging properties (Wei *et al.*, 2002). A number of hydrolysable tannins including ellagitannins and 1-o-galloyl castalagin and casuarinin (present in *Eugenia jambos*) have been shown to have activity against cell carcinomas and tumour cell lines (Yang *et al.*, 2000). Catechins, polyhydroxylated flavonoids, are present in a wide distribution of browses and tree leaves. These undergo considerable microbial and tissue biotransformations, which are present in blood. Oligomeric CT fractions did not have any influence on both strains, as determined by methane production measurements. The polymeric fraction completely inhibited methane production.Besides, direct inhibitory to methanogens, tannins have been shown to lower protozoal numbers (Patra and Saxena, 2011), which may also decrease protozoal associated methanogenesis (Finlay *et al.*, 1994).

Tannins also protect ruminants from bloat and have anthelmintic effects (Kahn and Diaz-Hernandez, 2000). Tannins have also been found to affect meat colour and quality. Feeding tannin-containing acacia or sulla leaves or carob pulp has been found to produce meat of lighter colour. The addition of PEG, a tannin-inactivating agent, reversed this effect, suggesting that the lighter colour produced is due to tannins (Priolo *et al.*, 2005). Decrease in blood haemoglobin and myoglobin and iron utilisation by tannins (Bhatta *et al.*, 2002) could contribute to the lightness of the meat (Priolo *et al.*, 2000). The lighter meat produced as a result of feeding tannin could favour consumer preference in some regions. Fatty acid composition is associated with the risk or the prevention of several human illnesses. Herbages containing low amount of tannins increased n-3 fatty acid and conjugated linoleic acid (9-cis 11-trans C18:2; CLA) in lamb meat, compared with lambs fed concentrate (Priolo *et al.*, 2005), enhancing meat nutritional properties for human consumption.Rumen microbes are capable of degrading hydrolysable tannins. The toxicity, therefore, appears to be due to absorption of degraded products of hydrolysable tannins and higher loads of phenols in the blood stream, which is beyond the capability of liver to detoxify them.

Parasitism by gastrointestinal nematodes is one of the major constraints on livestock production, especially when the nutritional status of the animals is poor. In subtropical and tropical areas of the world where the animals are on low quality feeds and have poor nutritional status, mortality and morbidity due to nematode infection are widespread (Singh *et al.*, 2003). There is a growing realisation that chemical anthelmintic treatment, on its own, may not provide a long-term strategy for managing parasites in grazing animals. The widespread development and prevalence of resistant strains of nematode parasites and public concern over drug residues excreted in animal products have stimulated efforts to identify and use plant-based anthelmintic compounds.

The customary mode of control of GIN has been based on the use of chemical anthelmintics. However, *H. contortus* drug resistance has become an important issue in small ruminant husbandry, especially when anthelmintics are applied at high levels and increasing frequency and inappropriate doses (Pandey *et al.*, 2001). Thus, environment friendly sustainable novel strategies are required, which could reduce the exclusive reliance on chemical anthelmintic treatments. Use of phytochemicals like CT may offer more efficacious control than chemical anthelmintics to treat *H. contortus* (Chaichisemsari *et al.*, 2011; Hassanpour *et al.*, 2011). The CT could complex with nutrients and inhibit nutrient availability for larval growth or decrease GIN metabolism directly through inhibition of oxidative phosphorylation (Scalbert, 1991), causing larval death (Athanasiadou *et al.*, 2001). This raises the possibility that feeding locally available plant species containing CT may prove to be a successful and economical alternative method for controlling *H. contortus* infections.

2.2.7 Essential Oils

Essential oils are the odourous and volatile products of various plant and animal species. Essential oils have a tendency evaporate on exposure to air even at ambient conditions and are, therefore, also referred to as volatile oils or ethereal oils. They mostly contribute to the odouriferous constituents or *'essences'* of the aromatic plants that are used abundantly in enhancing the aroma of some spices (Martinez *et al.*, 2008). Essential oils are either secreted either directly by the plant protoplasm or by the hydrolysis of some glycosides and structures such as directly plant structures associated with the secretion of essential oils include: Glandular hairs (Lamiaceae e.g. *Lavandula angustifolia*), Oil tubes (or vittae) (Apiaceae e.g. *Foeniculum vulgare*, and *Pimpinella anisum* (Aniseed), modified parenchymal cells (Piperaceae e.g. *Piper nigrum* - Black pepper), Schizogenous or lysigenum passages (Rutaceae e.g. *Pinus palustris* - Pine oil. Essential oils have been associated with different plant parts including leaves, stems, flowers, roots or rhizomes. Chemically, a single volatile oil comprises of more than 200 different chemical components, and mostly the trace constituents are solely responsible for attributing its characteristic flavour and odour (Firn, 2010). Essential oils can be prepared from various plant sources either by direct steam distillation, expression, extraction or by enzymatic hydrolysis. Examples of volatile oils include amygdaline (volatile oil of bitter almond), sinigrin (volatile oil of black mustard), and eugenol occurring as gein (volatile oil of *Geum urbanum*).

The actions of essential oils on microbial cells vary by the location of their functional hydroxyl or alkyl groups. For example, thymol and carvacrol, the two common terpenoids, have similar antimicrobial effects but act differently against G^+ or $G^{''}$ bacteria based on the locations of one or more functional groups in these two molecules. The hydroxyl group of the phenolic terpenoids and the presence of delocalized electrons are important elements for their antimicrobial action. The locations of the functional groups such as hydroxyl groups in these molecules usually determine the level of their activity on different bacteria. Helander *et al.* (1998) reported that thymol and carvacrol had prominent outer membrane-disintegrating properties, due mainly to their enhanced ability to release lipo-polysaccharides, which acted more like detergents for sensitization. Because of the lipo-polysaccharide release properties, both thymol and carvacrol have shown superior antimicrobial properties against some $G^{''}$ bacteria than other phytogenic compounds.

Essential oils might inhibit the Hyper-Ammonia Producing (HAP) bacteria in the rumen, which results in decreased amino acids deamination (Wallace, 2004; Patra and Saxena, 2011). The main effects of essential oils in the rumen have been suggested to be due to reduction of protein and starch degradation and an inhibition of amino acid degradation due to selective action on certain rumen micro-organisms, specifically some bacteria (Hart *et al.*, 2008). One mode of action suggested for essential oils is an effect on the pattern of bacterial colonisation of particular starch rich substrates as they enter the rumen. A second possible mode of action is the inhibition of HAP bacteria involved in amino acid deamination. As essential oils inhibit HAP bacteria in the rumen, the concentrations of ammonia and deaminase activities sometimes decreases. The HAP bacteria comprise only around 1% of the rumen bacterial populations, but they possess a very high deamination activity (Wallace, 2004). This could decrease the rate of ammonia production in the rumen, which may be beneficial nutritionally by increasing the efficiency of protein utilization in the rumen (Wallace *et al.*, 2002).

However, it is known that phenols in essential oils target bacterial cell membrane by changing its structure and function, resulting in swelling and thus, increasing the membrane permeability. The damage to the cell membrane might explain the observed additive effects, since the phenolic compounds could cause sublethal injury to cell membranes, increasing the susceptibility of the bacteria to acidic environment. Moreover, at low pH the hydrophobicity of an essential oils increases, enabling it to more easily dissolve in the lipids of the cell membrane of target bacteria.

2.2.8 Terpenes

Terpenes are among the most widespread and chemically diverse groups of natural products. They are flammable unsaturated hydrocarbons, existing in liquid form commonly found in essential oils, resins or oleoresins (Firn, 2010). Terpenoids includes hydrocarbons of plant origin of general formula (C5H8)n and are classified as mono- , di-, tri- and sesquiterpenoids depending on the number of carbon atoms. Examples of commonly important monoterpenes include terpinen-4-ol, thujone, camphor, eugenol and menthol. *Diterpenes (C20)* are classically considered to be resins and taxol, the anticancer agent, is the common example. The t*riterpenes (C30)* include steroids, sterols, and cardiac glycosides with anti-inflammatory, sedative, insecticidal or cytotoxic activity. Common triterpenes: amyrins, ursolic acid and oleanic acid *sesquiterpene (C15)* like monoterpenes, are major components of many essential oils (Martinez *et al.*, 2008). The sesquiterpene acts as irritants when applied externally and when consumed internally, their action resembles that of gastrointestinal tractirritant. A number of sesquiterpene lactones have been isolated and broadly they have antimicrobial (particularly antiprotozoal) and neurotoxic action. The sesquiterpene lactone, palasonin, isolated from *Butea monosperma* has anthelmintic activity, inhibits glucose uptake and depletes the glycogen content in *Ascaridia galli*. Terpenoids are classified according to the number of isoprene units involved in the formation of these compounds. Their actions vary greatly, a range of which have been utilised in herbal remedies. Of particular importance are antineoplastic, antibacterial, antiviral effects as well as gastrointestinal stimulation. However, they are not associated with toxicity unless they are concentrated as volatile oils. The plant family best known for these compounds is Lamiaceae (thyme family) but are also present in a range of other families.Terpenes such as perillyl alcohol, limonene and carnosol. Sources are cherries, citrus fruit peel, rosemary may protect cells from becoming cancerous, slow cancer cell growth, strengthen immune function, limit production of cancer related hormones, fight viruses, work as antioxidant.

2.2.9 Lignans

Lignans are composed of two phenylpropanoid units to form an 18-carbon skeleton, with various functional groups connected. They are generally lipophilic and have structural functions within the plant cell membranes. Lignans are present at highest concentrations in oil seeds, but are also found in other parts of a long range of plants of different families. Several lignans show clinical activity as phytoestrogenic, cathartic or antineoplastic effects.

2.2.10 Carotenoids

Carotenoids such as beta carotene, lycopene, lutein and zeaxanthin. Sources are red, orange and green fruits and vegetables including broccoli, carrots, cooked tomatoes, leafy greens, sweet potatoes, winter squash, apricots, cantaloupe, oranges and watermelon. It may inhibit cancer cell growth, work as antioxidants and improve immune response.

2.2.11 Resins

The resins are complex lipid-soluble mixtures-usually both non-volatile and volatile compounds. The non-volatile fraction may consist of diterpenoid and triterpenoid compounds, and mono- and sequiterpenoids predominate in the volatile fraction. Most typical are resins secreted by wood structures, but resins are also present in herbaceous plants. They are all sticky and the fluidity depends on their contents of volatile compounds. When exposed to air, they harden. Most resins are antimicrobial and wound healing, but their actions depend on the composition of the chemical mixture. Resins are generally safe, but contact allergy may occur.

2.2.12 Steroids

Plant steroids (or steroid glycosides) also referred to as 'cardiac glycosides' are one of the most naturally occurring plant phyto-constituents that have found therapeutic applications as arrow poisons or cardiac drugs (Firn, 2010). The cardiac glycosides are basically steroids with an inherent ability to afford a very specific and powerful action mainly on the cardiac muscle, when administered through injection into man or animal. Steroids (anabolic steroids) have been observed to promote nitrogen retention in osteoporosis and in animals with wasting illness (Maurya *et al.*, 2008; Madziga *et al.*, 2010). Caution should be taken when using steroidal glycosides as small amounts would exhibit the much needed stimulation on a diseased heart, whereas excessive dose may cause even death. Diosgenin and cevadine (from *Veratrum veride*) are examples of plant steroids.

2.2.13 Proteins and Peptides

Proteins from plants are an important source in food and feed. Amino acids thereof are absorbed from the intestine of man and animals and are built up into adapted proteins. Nevertheless, there are also plant proteins and peptides with bioactivity. They are often not hydrolysed in the digestive tract, but may to a certain extent be absorbed and exert their specific action in the body. Euphorbiaceae (spurge family) include plants producing such proteins, for instance, ricin in seeds of *Ricinus communis* (castor bean). The very potent little protein (lectin) ricin inhibits protein synthesis and induce systemic effects in animals and humans, with gastrointestinal symptoms dominating. Far less potent lectins are also present in seeds of several species of Fabaceae (bean family). Colic and other gastrointestinal symptoms may occur, if seeds are eaten without sufficient heat treatment, which inactivates many lectins.

2.3 Multiple Effects of Phytochemicals

Multiple molecular targets of dietary phytochemicals have been identified, from pro- and anti-apoptotic proteins, cell cycle proteins, cell adhesion molecules, protein kinases, transcription factors to metastasis and cell growth pathways (Aggarwal and Sisodia, 2006). Phytochemicals such as epigallocatechin- 3-gallate (EGCG) from green tea, curcumin from turmeric, and resveratrol from red winetend to aim at a multitude of molecular targets. It is because of these characteristics that definitive mechanisms of action are not available despite decades of research (Francis *et al.*, 2002). The multi-target nature of phytochemicals may be beneficial in overcoming cancer drug resistance. This multi-faceted mode of action probably hinders the cancer cell's ability to develop resistance to the phytochemicals. It has also been demonstrated that EGCG has inhibitory effects on the extracellular release of verotoxin (VT) from *E. coli* 0157: H7 (Voravuthikunchai and Kitpipit, 2003). Ethanol pericarp extracts from *Punica granatum* was also reported to inhibited VT production in periplasmic space and cell supernatant. Mechanisms responsible for this are yet to be understood, however, the active compounds from the plant are thought to interfere with the transcriptional and translational processes of the bacterial cell (Voravuthikunchai and Kitpipit, 2003). More work is needed to be done in order to establish this assumption. Phytochemicals may also modulate transcription factors (Andreadi *et al.*, 2006), redox-sensitive transcription factors (Surh *et al.*, 2005), redox signalling, and inflammation. As an example, nitric oxide (NO), a signalling molecule of importance in inflammation, is modulated by plant polyphenols and other botanical extracts. Many phytochemicals have been classified as phytoestrogens, with health-promoting effects resulting in the phytochemicals to be marketed as nutraceuticals (Moutsatsou, 2007).

The quantity and quality of protein flowing to the intestine is one of the major factors determining the productivity of ruminant livestock. The flow of protein from the rumen to abomasum depends on proteolysis by rumen micro-organisms and the efficiency of microbial protein synthesis in the rumen. Tannins may improve the protein metabolism in the rumen by reducing protein degradation via formation of insoluble tannin-protein complexes and decreasing the solubility of protein (Min *et al.*, 2000). An increase in dietary protein flow to the abomasum may also be due to the inhibitory effects of tannins on proteolytic bacteria and proteolytic enzyme activity. Besides, tannins might sometime also affect the efficiency of microbial protein synthesis. The changes in the activities of proteolytic bacteria and the protease enzyme by tannins could mediate nitrogen metabolism in the rumen. A reduction in proteolysis might be attributed to the direct effects of CT on microbial proteolytic enzyme activity or to the indirect effects on rumen metabolite concentration that can regulate proteolytic activity in some bacteria (Waghorn *et al.*, 1994). Rate of proteolysis by bacteria varies among bacterial species in the presence of CT.

2.4 Role of Phytochemicals in Diseases Prevention

- Stimulate the immune system, the body's defence against viruses, bacteria and other disease causing agents.
- Block the potential for carcinogens (cancer causing substances) to be formed in the body from substances we eat, drink and absorb from the environment.
- Reduce oxidation, the damage to cells that occurs with aging and exposure to pollution. Oxidation, caused by molecules called free radicals, can cause abnormalities in cells that may eventually lead to cancer.
- Slow the growth rate of cancer cells.
- Reduce inflammation that provides a setting favourable for cancer growth.
- Trigger death (a process known as apoptosis) of damaged cells that may be precursors to cancer.
- Prevent DNA damage and help with DNA repair mechanisms.
- Help to regulate hormones, such as oestrogen and insulin. Excess levels of these hormones are linked with increased risk for breast and colon cancer.

2.5 Future Prospects and Conclusions

It is matter of facts that there are some disadvantages associated with natural products. These include difficulties in access and supply, complexities in chemistry and inherent slowness of working as well as intellectual property rights concerns. Despite these limitations, various feeding trials, clinical trials and projects are going on throughout the world. However, more extensive collections of plants could provide many novel chemicals for use in drug discovery essays on different aspects. The chemical diversity of natural products is a better match to that of successful drugs or additive supplements than the diversity of collections of synthetic compounds due to global emergence of multidrug resistant pathogens. There will be further developments in the use of novel natural products and chemical libraries based on natural products in drug discovery campaigns. Therefore, there is a need to explore the unknown chemistry and exact mode of action of various plants photochemical and there are better opportunities to explore the biological activity of previously inaccessible sources of natural products.

References

Aggarwal BB, Sisodia S (2006) Molecular targets of dietary agents for prevention and therapy of cancer. Biochem Pharm 71: 1397-1421

Alakomi HL, Puupponen-Pimia R, Aura AM, Helander IM, Nohynek L, Oksman-Caldentey, KMS,Aarela M (2007) Weakening of salmonella with selected microbial metabolites of berry derived phenolic compounds and organic acids. J Agric Food Chem55: 3905-3912

Andreadi CK, Howells LM, Atherfold PA, Manson MM (2006) Involvement of Nrf2, p38, B-Raf, and nuclear factor-kappaB, but not phosphatidylinositol 3-kinase, in induction of haemeoxygenase-1 by dietary polyphenols. Mol Pharm 69: 1033-1040

Athanasiadou S, L Kyriazakis, FJackson and RL Coop (2001) Direct anthelmintic effects of condensed tannins towards different gastrointestinal nematodes of sheep: *in vitro* and *in vivo* studies. Vet Parasitol 99: 205-209

Attwood GLD, Pacheco D, Tavendale M (2006) Production of indolic compounds by rumen bacteria isolated from grazing ruminants. J Appl Micro 100: 1261-1271

Berger RG, Lunkenbein S, Strohle A, Hahn A (2012) Antioxidants in food: mere myth or magic medicine. Crit.Rev Food Sci Nutr 52: 162–171

Bhatta R, Shinde AK, Vaithiyanathan S, Sankhyan SK, Verma DL (2002) Effect of polyethylene glycol-6000 on nutrient intake, digestion and growth of kids browsing Prosopis cineraria. Anim. Feed Sci Tech 101: 45-54

Chaichisemsari M, Eshratkhah B, Maherisis N, Sadaghian M, Hassanpour S (2011) Evaluation of total protein, albumin, globulin and blood urea nitrogen concentrations in gastrointestinal nematodes infected sheep. Global Vet 6: 433-437

Clifford MN (2004) Diet-derived phenols in plasma and tissues and their implication for health. Planta Med 70: 1103-1114

Crozier LG, Zabel RW (2006) Climate impacts at multiple scales: evidence for differential population responses in juvenile Chinook salmon. J Ani Eco 75: 1100–1109

Cueva C Moreno Arribas MV, Martín Alvarez PJ, Bills G, Vicente MF, Basilio A, Rivas CL, Requena T, Rodríguez JM and Bartolome B (2010) Antimicrobial activity of phenolic acids against commensal, probiotic and pathogenic bacteria. Res Microbiol 161: 372-382

Doughari JH, Obidah JS (2008) Antibacterial potentials of stem bark extracts of Leptadenia lancifolia against some pathogenic bacteria. Pharmacol online 3: 172-180

Doughari JH, Human IS, Bennade S and Ndakidemi PA (2009) Phytochemicals as chemotherapeutic agents and antioxidants: Possible solution to the control of antibiotic resistant verocytotoxin producing bacteria. J Medic Plant Res 3(11): 839-848

Engels C, Knodler M, Zhao Y Y, Carle R, Ganzle MG and Schieber A (2009). Antimicrobial activity of gallotannins isolated from mango (Mangifera indica L.) kernels. J Agric Food Chem 57: 7712-7718

Finlay BJ, Esteban G, Clarke KJ, Williams AG, Embley TM, Hirt RR (1994) Some rumen ciliates have endo-symbiotic methanogens. FEMS Microbiol Lett 117: 157-162

Firn R (2010) Nature's Chemicals. Oxford University Press, Oxford. Pp. 74-75

Francis MS, Wolf Watz H and Forsberg A (2002) Regulation of type III secretion systems. Curr. Opi Microbio 5(2): 166-172

Hagerman AE, Riedl KM, Rice RE (1999) Tannins as biological antioxidants. In Plant polyphenols 2: Chemistry, biology, pharmacology, ecology (ed. G.G. Gross, R.W. Hemingway and T. Yoshida), pp. 495–505. Kluwer Academic Publishers/Plenum Press, Dordrecht/New York.

Handique JG, Baruah JB (2002) Polyphenolic compounds: an overview. React Funct Polym 52: 163-188

Hassanpour S, Eshratkhah B, Sadaghian M, Maherisis N, Chaichisemsari M and Kiyaninahand M (2011) Relationship between gastrointestinal parasite infection and faecal protein excretion in Moghani ewes. Int J Anim Vet Adv 3: 167-169

Hegnauer R (1988) Biochemistry, distribution and taxonomomic relevance of higher plant alkaloids. Phytochem 27: 2423

Helander IM, Alakomý HL, Latva-Kala K, Mattýla-Sandholm T, Pol I, Smýd EJ, Gorrýs L G M and Von Wrýght A (1998) Characterization of the action of selected essential oil components on gram-negative bacteria. J Agric Food Chem 46: 3590-3595

Hess HD, Beuret RA, Lotscher M, Hindrichsen IK, Machmuller A, Carulla JE, Lascano CE and Kreuzer M (2004) Ruminal fermentation, methanogenesis and nitrogen utilization of sheep receiving tropical grass hay-concentrate diets offered with Sapindus saponaria fruits and Cratylia argentea foliage. Ani Sci 79: 177-189

Hu, Z.Q., Zhao, W.H. and Shimamura, T. (2004). Different susceptibilities of Staphylococcus and Gram-negative rods to epigallocatechin gallate. J Infect Chemother 10: 55-58

Kahn L P, Diaz-Hernandez A (2000) Tannins with anthelmintic properties. In Tannins in Livestock and Human Nutrition (ed. JD Brooker). ACIAR Proc. No. 92, Australia. Pp. 140-149

Kar A (2007) Pharmacognosy and pharmacobiotechnology (revised-expanded 2nd edition). New Age International Limted Publishers, New Delhi. Pp. 332-600

Madziga H A, Sanni S, Sandabe UK (2010) Phytochemical and elemental analysis of Acalypha wilkesiana leaf. J Amer Sci 6(11): 510-514

Madziga HA, Sanni S and Sandabe UK (2010) Phytochemical and Elemental Analysis of Acalypha wilkesiana Leaf. J Amer Sci 6(11): 510-514

Makkar HPS, and Becker K (1999) Plant toxins and detoxification methods to improve feed quality of tropical seeds - Review. Asian-Aust. J Ani Sci 12: 467-480

Makkar HPS, Sen S, Blummel M and Becker K (1998) Effects of fractions containing saponins from Yucca schidigera, Quillaja saponaria and Acacia auriculoformis on rumen fermentation. J Agri Food Chem 46: 4324-4328

Martinez MJA, Lazaro RM, del Olmo LMB, and Benito PB (2008) Anti-infectious activity in the anthemideae tribe. In: Atta-ur- (Ed.) Stud. Nat Prod Chem 35: 445-516

Maurya R, Singh G, Yadav PP (2008) Antiosteoporotic agents from Natural sources. In: Atta-ur-Rahman (Ed.). Stud Nat Prod Chem 35: 517-545

Merkl R, Hradkova I, Filip V, Smidrkal J(2010) Antimicrobial and antioxidant properties of phenolic acids alkyl esters. Czech J Food Sci 28: 275-279

Min BR, Barry TN, Attwood GT, McNabb WC (2003) The effect of condensed tannins on the nutrition and health of ruminants fed fresh temperate forages: a review. Anim Feed Sci Tech 106: 3-19

Moutsatsou P, (2007) The spectrum of phytoestrogens in nature: our knowledge is expanding. Hormones (Athens) 6: 173-193

Newbold C J, E Hassan S M, Wang J M, Ortega M E and Wallace R J (1997) Influence of foliage from African multipurpose trees on activity of rumen protozoa and bacteria. Br J Nutri 78: 237–249

Pandey VS, Pralomkram W, Kochapakdee S, Saithanoo S (2001). PSU Goat Res Pub., 2 Benzimidazol resistance in Haemonchus contortus from goat in Thailand. pp. 337

Patra AK, Saxena J (2011) Exploitation of dietary tannins to improve rumen metabolism and ruminant nutrition. J Sci Food Agric 91: 24-37

Perchellet EM, Moutaseb HU, Makkar HPS, Perchellet P (1996) Ability of tannins extracted from various tree leaves to inhibit the biomarkers of tumour promotion in mouse skin *in vivo.* Int J Oncol 9: 801-809

Pichersky E and Gang David, R (2000) Genetics and biochemistry of secondary metabolites in plants: an evolutionary perspective. Trends plant Sci 5(10): 439-445

Priolo A, Bella M, Lanza M, Galofaro V, Biondi L, Barbagallo D, Ben Salem H and Pennisi P (2005) Carcass and meat quality of lambs fed fresh sulla (Hedysarum coronarium L.) with or without polyethylene glycol or concentrate. Small Rumin Res 59: 281-288

Priolo A, Waghorn G G, Lanza M, Biondi L and Pennisi P (2000) Polyethylene glycol as a means for reducing the impact of condensed tannins in carob pulp: effects on lamb growth performance and meat quality. J Anim Sci 78: 810-816

Puupponen-Pimia R, Nohynek L, Hartmann-Schmidlin S, Kahkonen M, Heinonen M, Maatta-Riihinen K and Oksman-Caldentey K M (2005) Berry phenolics selectively inhibit the growth of intestinal pathogens. J Appl Microbiol 98: 991-1000

Riedl KM, Carando S, Alessio HM, McCarthy M and Hagerman AE (2002) Antioxidant activity of tannins and tannin-protein complexes: assessment *in vitro* and *in vivo.* American Chem Soc Sym Seri 807: 188-200

Robbins R J (2003) Phenolic acids in foods: an overview of analytical methodology. J Agric Food Chem. 51: 2866-2887

Sarker S D and Nahar L (2007) Chemistry for pharmacy students general, organic and natural product chemistry. England: John Wiley and Sons. pp. 283-359

Scalbert A (1991) Antimicrobial properties of tannins. Phytochem 30: 3875-3883

Schreurs NM, Tavendale MH, Lane G A, Barry TN and McNabb WC (2004) Effect of white colver (Trifolium repens), perennial grass (Lolium perenne) and Lotus corniculatus on *in vitro* skatole and indole formation. Proc. of the 25th bienn. Conf. of the Aust. Soc. Ani. Prod.: animal production in Australia, 4–8 July, 2004, Victoria, Australia, pp. 164-167

Singh B, Bhat TK and Singh B (2003) Potential therapeutic applications of some antinutritional plant secondary metabolites. J Agri Food Chem 51: 5579-5597

Surh YJ (2003) Cancer chemoprevention with dietary phytochemicals. Nat Rev Cancer 3: 768-780

Tavendale MH, Lane, GA, Schreurs NM, Fraser and Meagher LP (2005) The effects of condensed tannins from Dorycnium rectum on skatole and indole ruminal biogenesis for grazing sheep. Aust J Agri Res 56: 1331-1337

Tzounis X, Vulevic J, Kuhnle GG, George T, Leonczak J, Gibson GR, Kwik-Uribe C, Spencer J P (2008) Flavanol monomer-induced changes to the human fecal microfl ora. Br J Nutr 99: 782-792

Van Duynhoven J, Vaughan EE, Jacobs DM, Kemperman RA, van Velzen EJ, Gross G, Roger LC, Possemiers S, Smilde A K, Dore J, Westerhuis J A and Van de Wiele T (2011) Metabolic fate of polyphenols in the human superorganism. Proc Natl Acad Sci. USA 108(Suppl 1): 4531-4538

Vermerris W and Nicholson RL (2006) Phenolic compound biochemistry. Springer, Dordrecht

Voravuthikunchai S P and Kitpipit L (2003) Activities of crude extracts of Thai medicinal plants on methicillin- resistant Staphylococcus aureus. J Clin Microbiol Inf. 9: 236.

Waghorn G C, Shelton I D and McNabb W C (1994) Effects of condensed tannins in Lotus pedunculatus on its nutritive value for sheep. 1. Non-nitrogenous aspects. J Agri Sci Camb. 123: 99-107

Wallace RJ (2004). Antimicrobial properties of plant secondary metabolites. Proc Nutr Soc 63: 621-629

Wallace RJ, McEwan N R, McIntosh F M, Teferedegne B and Newbold C J (2002) Natural products as manipulators of rumen fermentation. Asian-Aus J Ani Sci 15: 1458-1468.

□□□

Chapter 3

Phytobiotics as Conjugated Linoeic Acid Modulator in Dairy Cattle

Sachin Kumar, Prasanta Kumar Choudhury, Srobana Sarkar, Hujaz Tariq and Amrish Kumar Tyagi

Animal Nutrition Division, ICAR-National Dairy Research Institute, Karnal-132001, Haryana, India E-mail: arensachin@gmail.com

ABSTRACT

Conjugated linoleic acid (CLA) is a heterogeneous group of positional and geometric isomers of linoleic acid which has anticarcinogenic, antiatherogenic, antidiabetic, antiadipogenic and immunomodulation properties. Cow's milk is richest natural common source of CLA and its content in milk is highly influenced by type of diet. Feeding strategies based on herbal feed are being explored for manipulating the rumen microbiota. These compounds exert antimicrobial effects on biohy-drogenating species resides in rumen, accumulates biohydrogenation intermediates and enhances CLA content in milk and meat. Many herbs or extracts of herbs such as *Cumin cyminum, Chrysanthemum coronarium, Yucca schidigera, Terminalia chebula, Vicia sativa, Quillaja saponaria,* etc. have been used to modulate CLA contents in ruminant's products. Therefore, supplementation of herbal feed additives can be regarded as a promising strategy for augmenting the CLA content of milk and meat thereby ensuring healthy animal products.

Keywords: Conjugated linoleic acid, Phytobiotics, Milk, Meat, Production.

3.1 Introduction

Milk, meat and their products are vital sources of nutrients for human due to presence of high quality protein, energy and micronutrients. Despite all these essential nutritional components, yet, ruminant products suffer from an adverse health issue associated with high content of saturated fatty acids (SFA). Nevertheless, ruminant fat both in milk and meat contains many specific fatty acids {conjugated linoleic acid (CLA; *cis*-9, *trans*-11 C18:2), vaccenic acid, n-3 and n-6 PUFA} which are associated with their various neutraceutical properties. CLA found mostly in milk fat and ruminant meat, is a functional food component having proven health benefits for human beings. The CLA represent a heterogeneous group of positional and geometric isomers of linoleic acid (Benjamin, 2005). More than 20 different CLA isomers have been identified with varying positions of double bonds in the aliphatic chain (from carbons 6, 8 to 12, 14) and geometry (*trans, trans; trans, cis; cis, trans* and *cis, cis*) (Sehat *et al.*, 1998). Out of these, two physically important isomers, *cis*-9, *trans*-11 is the most prevalent comprising 80-90% of the total CLA in food products from ruminants whereas *trans*-10, *cis*-12 is present in small amounts at 3-5% of total CLA (Parodi, 2003). The predominant form of CLA in ruminant origin food rumenic acid (*cis*-9, *trans*-11 C18:2), can either be synthesized in the animal's tissues using vaccenic acid (*trans*-11 C18:1) as a precursor or directly from microbial biohydrogenation of PUFA in the rumen (Griinari and Bauman, 1999).

Health beneficial effects of CLA include anticarcinogenic, antiatherogenic, antidiabetic and antiadipogenic properties (Kritchevsky, 2000; Belury, 2002) along with bone modelling (Watkins *et al.*, 1999) and immune responses (Cook *et al.*, 2003). Therefore, modifying fatty acid composition to increase CLA content and reduce SFA levels might be a key to enhance the neutraceutical and therapeutic value of ruminant-derived food products. In order to produce CLA enriched foods, several approaches have been accomplished either through optimization of diet formulations or utilization of feed additives which in turn modifies the rumen environment by enhancing or inhibiting specific microbial populations, targeting enzymes involved in biohydrogenation process and enhancing the outflow of PUFA and biohydrogenation intermediates in rumen (Khiaosa-Ard *et al.*, 2009).

Recently, feeding strategies based on herbal feed additives like tropical plants, herbal extracts are being explored for manipulating the rumen microbiota (Christodoulou *et al.*, 2005). These plants as such or their extracts contain a wide array of secondary metabolites which has the potential to modulate fatty acid biohydrogenation (Vasta et al. 2010; Brogna *et al.*, 2011). These compounds exert antimicrobial effects on biohydrogenating species resides in rumen (Durmic *et al.*,

2008), accumulates biohydrogenation intermediates and enhances PUFA and CLA content (Vasta *et al.*, 2008). Furthermore, these native plants are also adapted to the climates and soils, and many have acceptable nutritive value, suggesting that they could be included as a part of sustainable grazing systems or fed in small amounts as rumen modifiers to enhance content of CLA present in milk and meat.

3.2 Fatty Acids

Fatty acids are the building blocks of the fat in our system and in the food we eat. Generally, a fatty acid consists of a straight aliphatic chain of even number of carbon atoms, with hydrogen atoms where as methyl (CH_3) group at one end of the chain and a carboxyl group (COOH) at the other end. These are subdivided according to their chain-length and the number of double bonds. SFA do not contain any double bonds along the chain, and are therefore, "saturated with hydrogen. On the other hand if any of the bonds is double or triple, the acid is unsaturated and is more reactive. Although majority of fatty acids are in a straight chain, few fatty acids have branched chains and others contain ring structures (e.g., prostaglandins). These two carbon atoms in the chain bound to either side of the double bond of a fatty acid can occur either in a *cis* (Z) or *trans* (E) configuration. In a *cis* configuration, the hydrogens on the two carbons of the double bond are on the same plane of the bond whereas, in a *trans* configuration, the two hydrogen atoms are bound to opposite planes of the double bond. Most of the unsaturated fatty acids present naturally are in the *cis* configuration. Desaturases involved in the biosynthesis of unsaturated fatty acids in mammals also produce *cis* double bonds. *Trans* fatty acids are generally the processing results of hydrogenation of oils or fats and/or oil deodorisation. Based on the number of double bonds unsaturated fatty acids can be divided in two groups: monounsaturated fatty acids (MUFA) and poly-unsaturated fatty acids (PUFA). MUFA contain only one double bond, PUFA have 2 to 6 double bonds, generally in the *cis* configuration. The double bonds are generally separated by a single methylene group (methylene-interrupted unsaturation). The shorthand nomenclature of fatty acids includes the number of carbon atoms and double bonds (e.g. C18:1 or 18:1). Each double bond can be either in a *cis* or *trans* conformation or in a different position with respect to the ends of the fatty acid. In the shorthand nomenclature, there are two different ways to make clear where the double bonds are located within the hydrocarbon chain: a) Delta-x or Δx: the double bond is located on the xth carbon-carbon bond, counting from the carboxyl terminus. In case of a molecule having more than one double bond, the notation is for example Δ^9, Δ^{12}. b) Omega-x or ù-x or n-x: a double bond is located on the xth carbon-carbon bond, counting from the ù end (methyl end), determining the metabolic family being n-9, n-6 or n-3 family. Linoleic acid is named in the shorthand nomenclature C18:2 n-6 or C18:2 c9, c12. This compound has 18 carbon atoms, 2 double bonds and there are 6 carbon atoms from the last double bond to the terminal methyl group. According to the International Union of Pure and Applied Chemists (IUPAC) terminology, straight-chain fatty acids are named after the parent hydrocarbons while the final "-e" is changed to "-oic". The exact structure is given by their systematic name "*cis*-9, *cis*-12 octadecadienoic acid.

3.3 Fatty Acids in Milk and Meat

Milk and meat fatty acid composition has both negative and positive implications for the health of consumers. Fatty acid composition of milk and meat of various species have been given in Table 1 and 2, respectively. At present about 2% of total fatty acids in milk are PUFA and about 70% are saturated, but less than 40% of SFA are in categories that are considered to be less healthy. Similarly, intramuscular fat typically consists of SFA (approximately 47%), monounsaturated MUFA (42%) and PUFA (4%) of total fatty acids. Of the total SFA, 30% is represented by stearic acid (C18:0) which is considered to be neutral in its effect on plasma cholesterol in humans. The PUFA within beef contains considerable amounts of n-3 PUFA, particularly "-linolenic (C18:3 n-3) and the longer chain PUFA, eicosapentaenoic acid (EPA; C20:5 n-3) and, docosahexaenoic acid (DHA; C22:6n-3). Though, dietary manipulation can be effective in modification of these values.

Conjugated linoleic acid is a combined term to describe a mixture of geometric and positional isomers of octadecadienoic acid containing a conjugated double bond, i.e, not separated by a methylene group as in case of linoleic acid. Nearly, 28 different CLA isomers have been identified, and a number of these isomers have beneficial biological activity. The most biologically active and abundant isomers of CLA are *cis*-9, *trans*-11 and *trans*-10, *cis*-12 consisting around 80 and 4% of total CLA in ruminant derived food products respectively (Parodi, 2003). The common name of 'rumenic acid' (RA) has been suggested for this isomer because of its exclusive relationship to ruminants (Kramer *et al.*, 1997).

3.4 Conjugated Linoleic Acid

Conjugated linoleic acid is a combined term to describe a mixture of geometric and positional isomers of octadecadienoic acid containing a conjugated double bond, i.e, not separated by a methylene group as in case of linoleic acid. Nearly, 28 different CLA isomers have been identified, and a number of these isomers have beneficial biological activity. The most biologically active and abundant isomers of CLA are *cis*-9, *trans*-11 and *trans*-10, *cis*-12 consisting around 80 and 4% of total CLA in ruminant derived food products respectively (Parodi 2003). The common name of 'rumenic acid' (RA) has been suggested for this isomer because of its exclusive relationship to ruminants (Kramer *et al.*, 1997).

3.4.1 CLA content of Food

CLA is found in milk fat, the tissue fat of ruminant animals and the products derived from them (Table 3). About 90% of CLA is represented by *cis*-9, *tran*-11 isomer or rumenic acid (RA). Cow's milk is richest natural common source of CLA and its content in milk is highly influenced by type of diet. Grazing in high altitude, which is accompanied by a decrease in the proportion of grasses and a corresponding increase in dicotyledonous species, results in higher CLA production as compared to mountain and low lands. Breed, lactation number or age can have little influence on CLA levels (Stanton *et al.*, 2006).

Table 1: Fatty acid composition (g/100 g fatty acids) and content (g/100 g total fatty acids in subcutaneous adipose tissue and muscle) of loin steaks in sheep and cattle

Fatty Acid	Adipose tissue		Muscle	
	Sheep	Cattle	Sheep	Cattle
14:0	4.1	3.7	3.3	2.7
16:0	21.9	26.1	22.2	25.0
16:1 *cis*	2.4	6.2	2.2	4.5
18:0	22.6	12.2	18.1	13.4
18:1 *cis* 9	28.7	35.3	32.5	36.1
18:2 *n* 6	1.3	1.1	2.7	2.4
18:3n 3	1.0	0.5	1.37	0.70
20:4 *n*6	ND	ND	0.64	0.63
20:5 *n*3	ND	ND	0.45	0.28
n6: *n*3	1.4	2.3	1.3	2.1
P:S	0.09	0.05	0.15	0.11
Total	70.6	70.0	4.9	3.8

Adapted from Enser *et al.* (1996)

3.4.2 Biological Activities of CLA

The biological properties of dietary CLA are of substantial concern due to its diverse physiological consequences in animal studies. Dietary CLA is effective in suppressing tumour development during different stages of carcinogenesis (Belury, 2002). The anti-cancerous action of CLA may be due to inhibition of arachidonic acid derivatives (Parodi, 2003), antioxidant mechanisms, pro-oxidant cytotoxicity and inhibition of nucleotide and protein synthesis. Actions of CLA on inhibition of several chemically induced carcinogenesis were observed in case of mammary (Tyagi and Kathirvalen, 2006), epidermal (Belury *et al.*, 1997) and gastrointestinal (Liew *et al.*, 1995).

Table 2: Typical fatty acid composition of bovine, caprine and ovine milk fat

Fatty Acid	Composition (g/100g fatty acids)			
	Buffalo[1]	Cattle[2]	Goat[3]	Sheep[3]
4:0	3.43	3.88	2.64	2.18
6:0	1.92	2.49	2.11	2.39
8:0	1.10	1.39	2.41	2.73
10:0	2.35	3.05	9.35	9.97
10:1*cis*-9	0.25	0.28	0.18	0.24
12:0	2.94	4.16	5.35	5.00
14:0	9.51	11.36	11.99	9.81
14:1*cis*-9	0.59	1.11	0.24	0.18
16:0	29.47	29.36	27.47	28.23
16:1 *cis*-9	0.20	1.94	0.76	1.43
17:0	0.18	0.55	0.90	0.72
17:1 *cis*-9	0.12	0.28	0.40	0.39
18:0	9.36	11.36	6.92	8.88
18:1 *cis*-9	0.20	21.88	16.41	17.17
18:1 *trans*-11	1.45	0.28	0.72	0.78
18:2n-6	1.36	1.94	1.99	3.19
18:3 *n*-3	1.22	0.55	0.96	0.42
20:0	0.20	0.00	0.22	0.15
Summary				
Saturates	62.89	70.08	74.68	74.68
MUFA	25.36	25.76	20.41	20.41
PUFA	2.71	3.32	2.93	2.93

Adapted from [1]Saroj et al. (2017); [2] Black and Paul (1999) and [3]Shingfield *et al.* (2008).

Anti-carcinogenic effect of CLA appears to be dose dependent and most effective at 0.1 to 1% of the diet (Ip *et al.*, 1994). Dietary CLA also reduces the plasma concentration of low density lipoproteins (LDL) and prevents atherosclerosis in mice (Kathirvalen *et al.*, 2008) and hamsters (Valeille *et al.*, 2006) when fed with atherogenic diets. CLA induced alteration of lipid metabolism involves increased lipolysis, fatty acid oxidation (Pariza *et al.*, 2003) and enhanced carnitine palmitoyl transferase activity in several tissues of mice (Park *et al.*, 1997). Anti- inflammatory action of CLA includes modulation of eicosanoid, immunoglobulin production (Sugano *et al.*, 1999) and inhibition of prostaglandin E_2 synthesis from arachidonic acid

(Whigham *et al.*, 2000). Feeding of CLA to rats prone to developing diabetes normalized glucose tolerance and improved hyperinsulinemia as effectively as currently used medications (Houseknecht *et al.*, 1998).

3.5 Biosynthesis of CLA in rumen

3.5.1 Origin of CLA in Milk Fat

In order to find ways of enhancing the outflow of CLA and biohydrogenation intermediates from rumen, it is essential to understand the microbial processes of lipolysis and biohydrogenation of dietary lipids in ruminants. Previously, CLA was considered to be as the first intermediate of unsaturated fatty acids biohydrogenation in the rumen by bacteria *Butyrivibrio fibrisolvens* (Kepler *et al.*, 1966). However, lately CLA has been accepted to have two different origins. The first one is the rumen bio-isomerisation of LA and the second one is desaturation of VA in the tissue, coming from the rumen (Griinari and Bauman, 1999).

Table 3: CLA content of some human food

Products	**Range of CLA (mg/g fat)**
Milk and milk products	
Cow's milk	2-37
Goat's milk	5-10
Sheep's milk	5-29
Human breast milk	2.3-11.2
Cheese	4.5-20
Cultured dairy product*	3.8-10.5
Meat and meat products	
Beef	1.2[a]-14.7
Lamb	5.6-14.9
Fish and marine	0.1-0.9[b]
Vegetable oil product (heating, bleaching and deodorization during refining process) [c]	0.1-0.7

*Yogurt, probiotic yogurt, sour cream, butter milk; [a]perinephric; [b]if ruminant derive ingredient are used in their food; [c]coconut, sunflower, canola, peanut, corn, olive, safflower oils. (Adapted from Parodi, 2006)

3.5.2 Rumen Lipolysis and Biohydrogenation

Fatty acid content of ruminant products is different from the fatty acid composition of the diet as micro-organisms in the rumen alter dietary lipids. Lipid fraction of diets in ruminants is derived primarily from forages and grains. For concentrate-based diets the main dietary lipid is in the form of triglycerides, whereas in forage-based majority of lipid intake is in the form of glycolipids and phospholipids (Harfoot and Hazlewood 1997, Jenkins *et al.*, 2008). Grains are generally rich in C18:1 (Oleic acid) and C18:2 (linoleic acid), whereas green forages, are rich in linolenic acid (C18:3). After consumption, the esterified plant lipids or triglycerides are rapidly and extensively hydrolyzed to free fatty acids by the plants own lipases and microbial lipases (Jenkins 1993). This is the prerequisite step for further bio-hydrogenation of unsaturated fatty acids. The extent of lipolysis is generally high (85-95%) and is predominantly performed by rumen bacteria. These unsaturated free fatty acids are then rapidly bio-hydrogenated by ruminal micro-organisms to saturated end products. Initially released PUFA absorbs onto the surface of plant matter through hydrophobic interactions, so it is believed that plant surface associated micro-organisms are mainly responsible for biohydrogenation. It is noteworthy that biohydrogenation rates are always lower than those of lipolysis and factors that affect lipolysis also impact the biohydrogenation process.

Biohydrogenation involves synthesis of *cis*-9, *trans*-11 C18:2 isomer of CLA in rumen as an intermediate product from linoleic acid by the linoleate acid isomerase of *Butyrivibrio fibrisolvens* (Kepler and Tove, 1967) and other bacterial species. The initial step in rumen biohydrogenation of C18:2*n-6* and C18:3*n-3* typically involves an isomerisation of the *cis*-12 double bond to a *trans*-11 configuration resulting in a conjugated di- or trienoic fatty acid. The next step is a hydrogenation reaction, which results in the conversion of an unsaturated double bond to a saturated single bond. In this step there is reduction of the *cis*-9 double bond by a microbial reductase resulting in C18:1 *t*11 and C18:2 *t*11, *c*15 synthesis of C18:2 *n-6* and C18:3*n-3*, respectively. C18:2 *t*11, *c*15 is further hydrogenated to C18:1 *t*11, C18:1 *c*15 or C18:1 *t*15. The final step in C18:2 *n-6* and C18:3 *n-3* hydrogenation is the conversion of C18:1 *t*11 to C18:0, and is considered rate limiting for complete biohydrogenation of dietary unsaturated fatty acids (Moate *et al.*, 2004). These successive steps represent the predominant biohydrogenation pathway (Fig. 1).

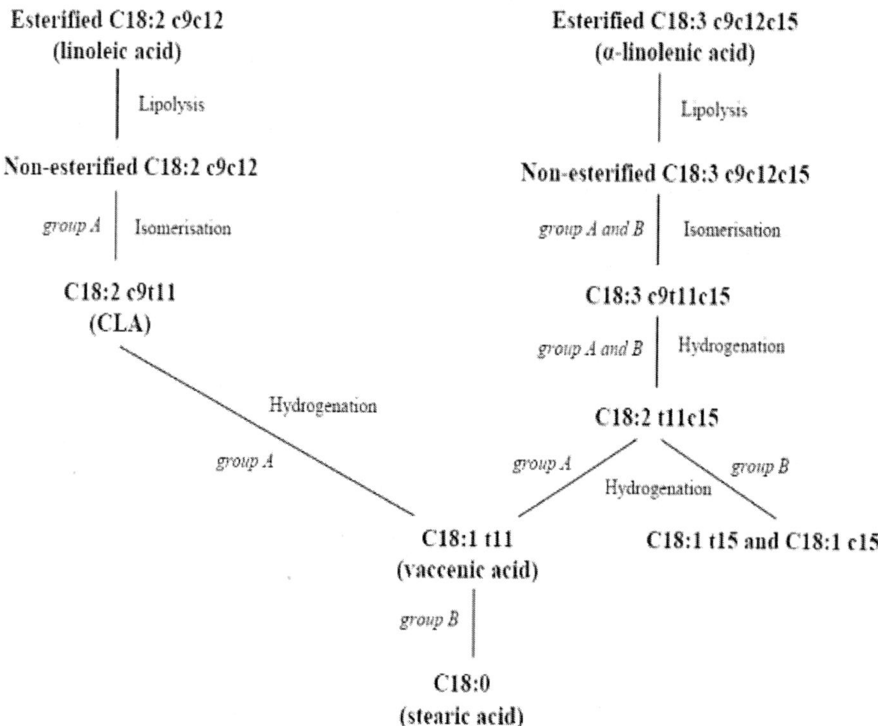

Fig. 1: Biochemical pathways for the biohydrogenation of linoleic and linolenic acids in the rumen (Adapted from Harfoot and Hazlewood, 1997)

3.5.3 Micro-organisms Involved in CLA Synthesis

Rumen bacteria involved in complete biohydrogenation are categorised into two groups (Jenkins *et al.*, 2008). *Group A bacteria:* They hydrogenate linoleic and linolenic acid to *trans*-11 octadeca-enoic acid and other biohydrogenation intermediates but are incapable of hydrogenating octadeca-enoic acid. Ex. *Butyrivibrio, Micrococcus, Ruminococcus* and *Lactobacillus* spp. *Group B bacteria:* They are capable of hydrogenating a wide range of octadecadienoic acids, including *cis*-9 (oleic) and *trans*-11 (*trans*-vaccenic) acids as well as linoleic acid to stearic acid.

More than 250 bacterial strains from 14 genera belonging to the *genera Butyrivibrio, Enterococcus, Pediococcus, Propionibacterium* and *Lactobacillus* are found to produce considerable amounts of CLA from linoleic acid. So far, many species of CLA-producing bacteria have been isolated from the rumen, intestine and starter cultures used in the dairy industry (Kim *et al.*, 2002; Rosberg-Cody *et al.*, 2004). *Butyrivibrio* spp. (*B. fibrisolvens, B. hungatei, B. proteoclasticus, Pseudobutyrivibrio xylanivorans, P. ruminis, B. crossotus*) (Van de Vossenberg *et al.*, 2003; Moon *et al.*, 2008), *Propionibacterium freudenreichi* (Jiang *et al.*, 1998), *Lactobacillus acidophilus* (Ogawa *et al.*, 2001), *Lactobacillus reuteri* (Lee *et al.*, 2003), *Megasphaera elsdenii* (Kim *et al.*, 2002), and *Bifidobacterium breve* (Coakley *et al.*, 2003) have been shown to produce CLA. Formation of CLA in the rumen has mainly associated with group A bacterial activity; however, CLA content of protozoa is also much high as bacteria, suggesting that protozoa may be responsible for a high proportion of CLA (Devillard *et al.*, 2004). However, overall FA biohydrogenation in the rumen is far more complicated as represented in Fig. 2. Pool of reductases and isomerases might generate a wide range of biohydrogenation intermediates (Mosley *et al.*, 2002). Complete *in vivo* biohydrogenation is thought to be a synergistic process involving a consortium of bacteria, each having a share in the conversion of unsaturated to more saturated fatty acids Moreover, under certain dietary conditions, typical pathways of rumen biohydrogenation are altered to produce unique fatty acid intermediates. *Cis*-9, *trans*-11-18:2 is usually the predominant CLA isomer found in the rumen and in milk but many others are also present (Fig. 2). High starch diet or feeding fish or vegetable oil supplements abundances *trans*-10, *cis*-12 isomer. The main supposed primary and secondary biohydrogenation pathways have been outlined by Chilliard *et al.* (2007) and are shown in Fig. 2.

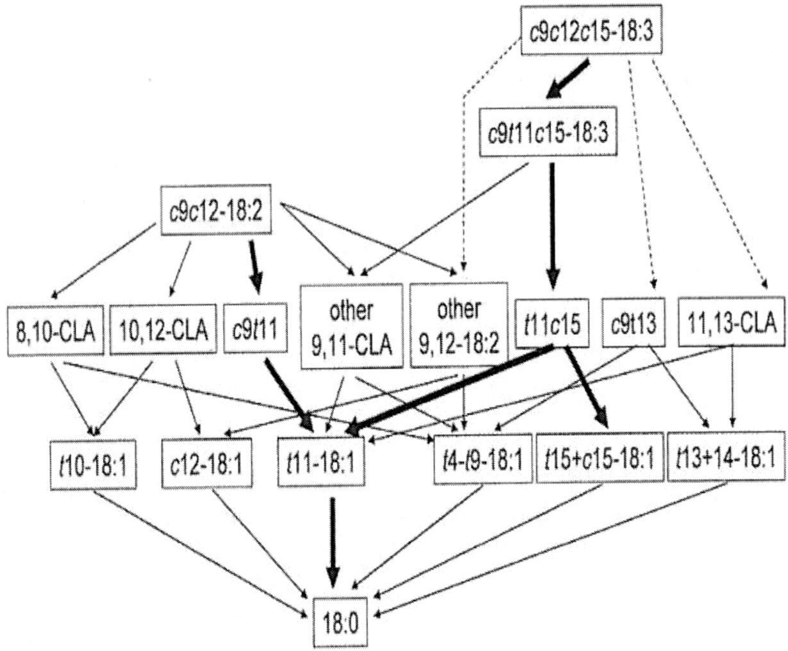

Fig. 2: Main putative rumen primary and secondary biohydrogenation pathways. Thick arrows represent the primary pathways; thin arrows represent other possible secondary pathways. When *cis* or *trans* configurations are not mentioned, it means that the various *cis-cis*, *cis-trans* and *trans-trans* configurations could exist (Adopted from Chilliard et al. , 2007).

3.5.4 Endogenous Synthesis of CLA

A major proportion of CLA in tissue and milk lipids is synthesized endogenously from *trans* vaccenic acid (TVA, *trans*-11 C18:1) by “^{9} desaturase enzyme in tissue as represented in Fig. 3. Griinari *et al.* (2000) examined the potential for endogenous synthesis of CLA by infusing *trans*-vaccenic acid (TVA) abomasally and measuring the changes in milk fat CLA. By day three it resulted in a 31% increase in milk fat CLA indicating that an active pathways for endogenous synthesis existed in the mammary gland. Griinari *et al.* (2000) also showed that the contribution of endogenous synthesis to the overall CLA content in milk fat is around 64% for making it the primary source.

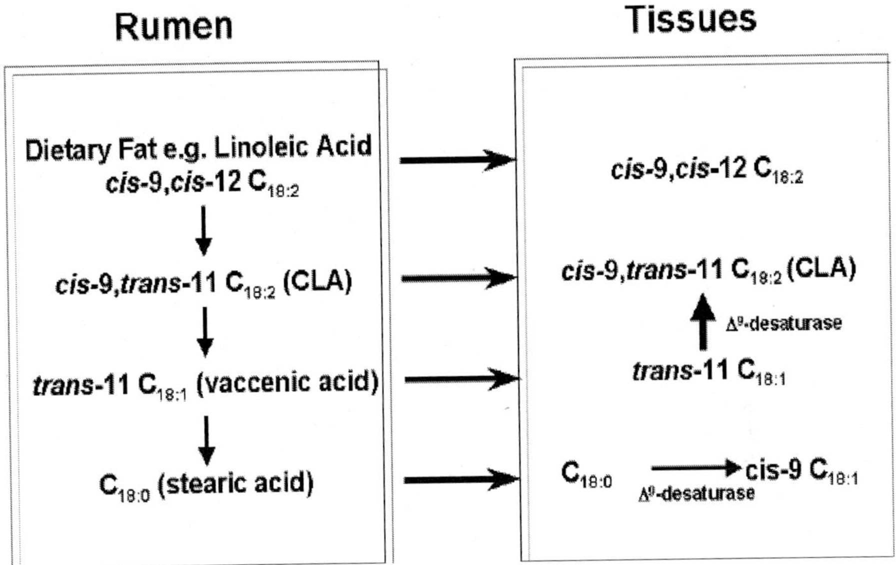

Fig. 3 : Role of rumen biohydrogenation and tissue "9-desaturase in the production of *cis*-9, *trans*-11 conjugated linoleic acid in ruminant fat

3.6 Strategies to Enhance CLA Content of Milk and Meat

Nutrition is the predominant factor affecting ruminant fat and it represents a practical tool to alter the CLA concentration in ruminant fat. A myriad of dietary strategies (Table 4) have been applied for enhancing CLA content of milk and meat which have been broadly divided into four groups on the basis of their mechanism of action:

- The first category includes dietary factors that provide PUFA substrates for ruminal production of CLA and vaccenic acid.
- The second group consists of those dietary factors that affect microbes involved in bio-hydrogenation, either directly or *via* changes in rumen environment.
- The third category includes substances that combine with the lipid substrates and modifies rumen bio-hydrogenation.
- The fourth category is dietary supplementation of CLA or *trans*-11 18:1 fatty acids as such.

CLA in ruminant milk and meat fat as described above is by-product of incomplete biohydrogenation of dietary lipids by rumen bacteria and various studies suggested that, the CLA content could be increased through manipulation of the cow's diet (Dhiman *et al.*, 1999). The *cis*-9, *trans*-11 CLA isomer is an intermediate product of biohydrogenation of linoleic acid by the rumen bacterium, *Butyrivibrio fibrisolvens*. Biohydrogenation in the rumen is affected by the type and amount of fatty acid substrate (Kathirvalen 2007), forage to grain ratio (Tyagi *et al.*, 2007), and nitrogen content of the diet (Gerson *et al.*, 1983). Moreover, changes in substrate supply and extent of biohydrogenation have been found to affect the supply of intermediate and end products of biohydrogenation and thus, influencing the CLA content of milk and meat of ruminants. Increasing the proportion of grazed grass from pasture in the diet of dairy cows linearly increased the CLA content of milk. Cows grazing permanent natural pasture had 500% more CLA compared with cows fed total mixed ration containing conserved forage and grain in a 50:50 ratio. Feeding pasture grass in dry form as hay did not influence milk CLA content (Dhiman *et al.*, 1999). Hydrogenation in the rumen averages 80% for linoleic acid and 92% for linolenic acid. The hydrogenation rate is mainly dependent on the proportion of concentrate in the diet.

When it exceeds 70%, hydrogenation only averages 50 and 65% for these two fatty acids. That phenomenon is related to a collapse in rumen pH (Chilliard and Ferlay, 2004). The addition (53 g/kg dietary dry matter) of peanut oil (high oleic acid), sunflower oil (high linoleic acid) and linseed oil (high linolenic acid) in the diet of lactating cow did not affect on milk fat concentration but CLA concentrations (mg/g of milk fat) were 13.3, 24.4 and 16.7 during peanut oil, sunflower oil and linseed oil treatment, respectively (Kelly *et al.*, 1998). Thus, feeding strategies is the main factor that influences ruminal biohydrogenation, in this text we will mainly emphasize on role of herbal feed additives in enhancing CLA content of milk and meat.

Table 4: Summary of dietary factors that affect concentrations of CLA in ruminant fat

Dietary factor	Content of CLA in milk fat	References
Lipid substrate		
Unsaturated vs saturated fat	Increased by addition of unsaturated fat	Griinari *et al.*, 1999; Malla 2016
Plant oils		
Type of plant oil	Increased with oils high in unsaturated fatty acids	Tesfa *et al.*, 1991; Dhiman *et al.*, 1997
Level of plant oil	Dose-dependent increase	Tesfa *et al.*, 1991; McGuire *et al.*, 1996
Ca salts of plant oils	Increased	Len *et al.*, 2016
High-oil plant seeds		
Raw seeds	No effect	Dhiman *et al.*, 1997
Processed seeds	Increased	Stanton *et al.*, 1997; Lawless *et al.*, 1998
High-oil corn grain and silage	Minimal effect	Dhiman *et al.*, 1996
Animal fat by-products	Minimal effect	Chouinard *et al.*, 1998a
Modifiers of rumen environment		
Forage:concentrate ratio	Variable effect	Chouinard *et al.*, 1998b;
Non-structural carbohydrate level	Minor effect	Chouinard *et al.*, 1998b
Restricted feeding	Variable effect	Timmen and Patton, 1988
Fish oils/fish meal	Increased	Dhiman *et al.*, 1996; Chilliard *et al.*, 1999
Marine algae	Increased	Franklin *et al.*, 1999
Ionophores	Variable effect	Dhiman *et al.*, 1996; Sauer *et al.*, 1998
Dietary buffers	Little effect with sufficient fiber	Chouinard *et al.*, 1998b
Microbial supplementation	Increased	Shivani *et al.*, 2015
Herbs	Increased	Rana *et al.*, 2012; Miri *et al.*, 2015
Combinations		
Pasture	Higher than on conserved forages	Zegarska *et al.*, 1996; Jahreis *et al.*, 1997
Growth stage of forage	Increased with less mature forage	Chouinard *et al.*, 1998b
CLA supplement	Dose dependent increase	Chouinard *et al.*, 1999; Giesy *et al.*, 1999

Adapted from Griinari and Bauman (1999)

When it exceeds 70%, hydrogenation only averages 50 and 65% for these two fatty acids. That phenomenon is related to a collapse in rumen pH (Chilliard and Ferlay, 2004). The addition (53 g/kg dietary dry matter) of peanut oil (high oleic acid), sunflower oil (high linoleic acid) and linseed oil (high linolenic acid) in the diet of lactating cow did not affect on milk fat concentration but CLA concentrations (mg/g of milk fat) were 13.3, 24.4 and 16.7 during peanut oil, sunflower oil and linseed oil treatment, respectively (Kelly *et al.*, 1998). Thus, feeding strategies is the main factor that influences ruminal biohydrogenation, in this text we will mainly emphasize on role of herbal feed additives in enhancing CLA content of milk and meat.

After the ban on antimicrobial feed additives, much interest has turned towards the use of herbal feed additives and their phytochemicals (tannins, saponins and essential oils) for augmenting animal productivity. Herbs and plant extracts used in animal feed are today called as 'phytogenics feed additives' (PFA). These are defined as compounds of plant origin incorporated into animal feed to enhance productivity of livestock through the improvement of digestibility, nutrient absorption and elimination of pathogen residents from the gut. The bioactive components of these feed additives vary widely in their concentration depending on the part of the plant used, such as seeds, leaf, root or bark as well as plant itself. Moreover, different solvent extracts from different active compounds of plants (Table 5). Thus, type of plant extract used influence type of phytochemicals extracted and thereby effect observed in animals.

3.7 Herbal Additives and/or its Secondary Metabolites as CLA Modulators

Phytogenic additives enhance a number of important processes in the animal body and positively affect health of animals as well as animal products by means of their specifically efficacious substances (Karaskova *et al.*, 2015). These plant feed additives are extensively used instead of antibiotic growth promoters. They also act as antibacterial, antioxidant, anticarcinogenic, antifungal, analgesic and insecticidal agents. Majority of these plants have minimum and/or no residual effects in the animal system, hence regarded as safe. Recently, these herbal feed additives are being extensively explored for their rumen manipulating properties. They have the potential to affect rumen fermentation and methane production (Bhatta *et al.*, 2013) lipolysis and biohydrogenation (Wencelova *et al.*, 2015). The major active compounds of herbal plants (essential oils, saponins, flavonoids, tannins and polyphenols) have been tested as extracts with effects on the microbial population (Patra and Saxena, 2009), methanogenesis (Bodas *et al.*, 2008) or lipolysis in the rumen (Jayanegara *et al.*, 2011).

Table 5: Methanol and water extracted phytochemicals

Water	Methanol
Anthocyanin	Anthocyanin
Terpenoids	Terpenoids
Saponins	Saponins
Tannins	Tannins
Starches	Xanthoxyllines
Polypeptides	Totarol
Lectins	Quassinoids
Lactones	
Flavones	
Polyphenols	

Adapted from (Cowan, 1999)

3.7.1 Mode of Action of Herbal feed Additives

The plant secondary compounds in herbal feed additives may alter ruminal biohydrogenation of fatty acids by exerting antimicrobial effect on biohydrogenating microbes in rumen (Durmic *et al.*, 2008), accumulating biohydrogenation intermediates (Vasta *et al.*, 2008) and increasing the activity of various enzymes involved in biohydrogenation process (Miri *et al.*, 2015). These mechanisms either singly or in combination increases the PUFA and CLA content of milk and meat. Furthermore, higher transfer rate of PUFA from feed to milk has been related to protein-bound phenols formed by plant polyphenol oxidase (PPO) that may inhibit the activity of plant lipase (Van Ranst *et al.*, 2009). Cabiddu *et al.* (2010) observed that tannins present in *Vicia sativa* and *Trifolium incarnatum* had a negative relationship with biohydrogenation of C18:3 n-3 and appearance of C18:0 along with a positive correlation to appearance of C18:2 *cis*-9, *trans*-11 fatty acids.

3.7.2 Effect of Herbal feed Additives on CLA Content of Rumen Liquor

In vitro incubation of tropical (Jayanegara *et al.*, 2011) and alpine plants (Jayanegara *et al.*, 2012) along with linseed oil suggested the ability of plant phenolics in modulating FA biohydrogenation, i.e. by decelerating the process right from first step. It was indicated by lower disappearance of C18:3 n-3 and C18:2 n-6 from the incubations of both tropical and alpine plants containing high phenolics in the respective studies. Similarly, Cabiddu *et al.* (2010) observed a negative relationship between tannins present in *Vicia sativa* and *Trifolium incarnatum* with the biohydrogenation of C18:3 n-3, appearance of C18:0 and positively correlated to appearance of C18:2 *cis*-9 *trans*-11 (CLA). Wencelova *et al.* (2015) reported that combination of a medicinal plant (MP) mixture and sunflower oil (SO) increase the concentration of PUFA and *cis*-9, *trans*-11 CLA (g/kg of FA) of rumen liquor. Lourenco *et al.* (2009), found essential oils rich in the monoterpenes limonene and carvone resulted in the ruminal accumulation of *cis*-9, *trans*-11 CLA, suggesting some effects of the latter on the extent of ruminal biohydrogenation *in vitro*. However, Vasta *et al.* (2009a) no change in the CLA concentration of rumen fluid with the inclusion of extracted tannins from carob (CT; *Ceratonia siliqua*), acacia leaves (AT; *Acacia cyanophylla*) and quebracho (QT; *Schinopsis lorentzii*) *in vitro* with cow buffered ruminal fluid. Durmic *et al.* (2008) suggested that the ability of plant extracts to inhibit/ enhance the growth and/or activity of important ruminal biohydrogenating bacteria such as *B. fibrisolvens* and *B. proteoclasticus* were dose dependent. Vasta *et al.* (2010) reported that supplementation of quebracho tannins in the diet of kids (9.57% of DM) significantly increased *trans*-vaccenic acid content in the rumen of kids as compared to control. They also demonstrated that tannin supplementation strongly increased the number of *B. fibrisolvens* (main CLA producing bacteria) in the rumen compared to tannin-free diet as quantified by real time PCR assay.

3.7.3 Effect of Herbal feed Additives on CLA Content of Milk and Meat

The effect of plant additives in enhancing the CLA content of milk and meat is variable (Table 6 and 7). Potential benefits of supplementing *Cumin cyminum* extracts was indicated by 20% increase in CLA content of goat milk when included in their diets (Miri *et al.*, 2015). Apart from increase in CLA content, Cumin supplementation also increased in the content of C18:1 trans-11, MUFA, PUFA and ratio of PUFA to SFA content of milk. *Chrysanthemum coronarium*, another plant also reported to enhance the CLA per cent of milk (Cabiddu *et al.*, 2006). Although, no changes in either CLA content of milk or other fatty acids were observed on feeding *Yucca schidigera* extract (60 g/d; 10% of saponins) to lactating cows (Benchaar and Chouinard, 2009).

Rana *et al.* (2012) reported that supplementation of *Terminalia chebula* (0.59 and 1.79% of DM) in the diet of kids increased vaccenic acid and CLA content in their muscle along with enhanced activity of desaturase enzyme, the main enzyme involved in endogenous synthesis of CLA in tissues. Feeding of vetch (*Vicia sativa*) to lambs along with herbage based diets increased intramuscular "^{9}desaturase protein expression (Vasta *et al.*, 2009a). Dietary supplementation of essential oils from artemisia increased the CLA and PUFA concentration in muscle fatty acid profiles of Barbarine lambs (Vasta *et al.*, 2013). However, Brogna *et al.* (2011) showed no effects of *Quillaja saponaria* on fatty acid composition of lambs.

Table 6: Effect of different plant additives on fatty acid profile of meat from ruminants

Plant additives	Effects	Reference
Sulla (*Hedysarum coronarium*)	Sulla (with or without PEG) ↑ RA, LNA and MUFA and ↓ LA and SFA	Priolo *et al.*, 2005
Carob pulp	↓ RA, VA and SA	Vasta *et al.*, 2007
Carob pulp	Carob ↓ SA, total SFA and n-6/n-3 ratio and ↑ total PUFA, RA, LA and LNA	Gravador *et al.*, 2015
Quebracho tannin extract (*Schinopsis lorentzii*)	↑ VA and RA, ↓ SA in concentrate diet ↓ PUFA and LA in herbage diet ↓ SFA in concentrate and herbage diets	Vasta *et al.*, 2009b
Grape seed extract	Minor effect on fatty acid profile	Jerónimo *et al.*, 2010; Jerónimo *et al.*, 2012
Rockrose (*Cistus ladanifer*)	↑ VA and RA in lambs feed diets supplemented with vegetable oils	Jerónimo *et al.*, 2010; Jerónimo *et al.*, 2012
Rockrose (*Cistus ladanifer*)	20% CL ↑ total trans-MUFA without effect on VA	Francisco *et al.*, 2015
Redberry juniper (*Juniperus inchotii*)	↑ RA and ↓ SA	Whitney *et al.*, 2011
Redberry juniper (*Juniperus inchotii*)	↑ 18:1 trans10 and total 18:1 trans	Whitney and Smith 2015
Sainfoin (*Onobrychis viciifolia*)	↓ SFA and ↑ PUFA, n3 LC-PUFA and PUFA/SFA	Girard *et al.*, 2015
Birdsfoot trefoil (*Lotus corniculatus* L.)	↓ SFA and ↑ PUFA, LNA, LA, n-3 LC-PUFA and PUFA/SFA	Girard *et al.*, 2015
Birdsfoot trefoil (*Lotus corniculatus* L.)	↓ LA and 18:1trans10	Turner *et al.*, 2015
Terminalia chebula	↑ RA and MUFA and ↓ SA and SFA	Rana *et al.*, 2012
Acacia karroo	↑ VA, LNA and n-3 LC-PUFA	Mapiye *et al.*, 2011
High-tannin Sorghum	No effect in meat fatty acid profile	Larraín *et al.*, 2007

(LA-linoleic acid, 18:2 n-6; LNA-linoleic acid, 18:3 n-3; MUFA-sum of monounsaturated fatty acids; n-3 LC-PUFA-sum of n-3 long chain polyunsaturated fatty acids; PUFA-sum of polyunsaturated fatty acids; RA-rumenic acid, 18:2 *cis*-9, *trans*-11; SA-stearic acid, 18:0; SFA-sum of saturated fatty acids; VA-vaccenic acid, 18:1 *trans*-11).

Table 7: Effect of different plant additives on fatty acid profile of meat from ruminants

Plant additives	Effects	Reference
Sulla (*Hedysarum coronarium*)	↓ RA, 18:1 cis-9 and total MUFA ↑ LA, LNA and total PUFA	Piredda *et al.*, 2002; Cabiddu *et al.*, 2005
Sulla (*Hedysarum coronarium*)	↑ RA and VA and ↓ LA and LNA by supplementation with PEG	Cabiddu *et al.*, 2009
Quebracho (*Schinopsis lorentzii*) and chestnut (*Castanea sativa*) tannin extracts	Minor effect on milk fatty acid profile	Toral *et al.*, 2011
Quebracho (*Schinopsis lorentzii*)	Minor effect on milk fatty acid profile	Toral *et al.*, 2013
Quebracho tannins extract (*Schinopsis lorentzii*)	↑ LA, RA and VA ↓ total SFA and SA	Buccioni *et al.*, 2015
Cumin cyminum	↑ LNA and PUFA	Miri (*et al.*, 2015
Quebracho tannins extract (*Schinopsis balansae*)	Without effect in milk fatty acid profile	Benchaar and Chouinard 2009
Quebracho tannins extract (*Schinopsis* spp.)	↑ LNA and total 18:1 trans	Dschaak *et al.*, 2011
Birdsfoot trefoil (*Lotus corniculatus*)	↑ RA, LA and LNA and ↓ VA and SA	Turner *et al.*, 2005

(FA-fatty acids; LA-linoleic acid, 18:2 n-6; LNA -linoleic acid, 18:3 n-3; MUFA-sum of monounsaturated fatty acids; n-3 LC-PUFA-sum of n-3 long chain polyunsaturated fatty acids; PEG-polyethytene glycol; PUFA-sum of polyunsaturated fatty acids; RA-rumenic acid, 18:2 cis-9,trans-11; SA-stearic acid, 18:0; SFA-sum of saturated fatty acids; VA-vaccenic acid, 18:1trans-11).

3.8 Conclusions

Supplementation of herbal feed additives can be regarded as a promising strategy for augmenting the CLA content of milk and meat thereby ensuring healthy animal products. However, the effect of these additives depends on the type and concentration of the secondary metabolites present in them.

References

Belury MA (2002) Inhibition of carcinogenesis by Conjugated Linoleic Acid: Potential mechanisms of action. J Nutr 132: 2995-2998

Belury MA, Moya CSY, Liu KL and Vanden HJP(1997) Dietary Conjugated Linoleic Acid induces peroxisome specific enzyme accumulation and ornithine decarboxylase activity in mouse liver. J Nutr Biochm 8: 579-584

Benchaar C and Chouinard PY (2009) Assessment of the potential of cinnamaldehyde, condensed tannins, and saponins to modify milk fatty acid composition of dairy cows. J Dairy Sci 92: 3392–3396

Benjamin S, Hanhoff T, Börchers T and Spener F(2005) A molecular test system for the screening of human PPAR transactivation by conjugated linoleic acid isomers and their precursor fatty acids. Eur J Lipid Sci Technol 107: 706-715

Bhatta R, Baruah L, Saravanan M, Suresh, KP and Sampath KT (2013) Effect of medicinal and aromatic plants on rumen fermentation, protozoa population and methano-genesis *in vitro*. J. Anim.Physiol. Anim Nutr 97: 446-456

Black AE and Paul AA (1999) McCance & Widdowson's Tables of Food Composition: origins and clarification of the Fifth edition. J Human Nutr Diet 12: 1-5

Bodas R, López S, Fernandez M, García-González R, Rodríguez AB, Wallace RJ and González JS (2008) *In vitro* screening of the potential of numerous plant species as antimethanogenic feed additives for ruminants. Anim. Feed Sci Technol 145(1): 245-258

Brogna DMR, Nasri S, Ben Salem H, Mele M, Serra A, Bella M, Priolo A, Makkar HPS, Vasta V (2011) Effect of dietary saponins from Quillaja saponaria L. on fatty acid composition and cholesterol content in muscle Longissimus dorsi of lambs. Animal 7: 1124-1130

Buccioni A, Pauselli M, Viti C, Minieri S, Pallara G, Roscini, Rapaccini S, Trabalza Murinucci M, Lupi P, Conte G, Mele M(2015) Milk fatty acid composition, rumen microbial population, and animal performance in response to diets rich in linoleic acid supplementation with chestnut or quebracho tannins in dairy ewes. J Dairy Sci 98: 1145-1156

Cabiddu A, Addis M, Pinna G, Spada S, Fiori M, Sitzia M, Pirisi, A, Piredda G and Molle G (2006) The inclusion of a daisy plant (Chrysanthemum coronarium) in dairy sheep diet 1: effect on milk and cheese fatty acid composition with particular reference to C18:2 cis-9, trans-11. Livest Sci 101: 57-67

Cabiddu, A., Decandia, M., Addis, M., Piredda, G., Pirisi, A. and Molle, G. 2005. Managing Mediterranean pastures in order to enhance the level of beneficial fatty acids in sheep milk. Small Rum Res 59: 169-180

Cabiddu A, Molle G, Decandia M, Spada S, Fiori M, Piredda G and Addis M (2009) Responses to condensed tannins of flowering sulla (Hedysarum coronarium L.) grazed by dairy sheep: Part 2: Effects on milk fatty acid profile. Livest Sci 123: 230-240

Cabiddu A, Salis L, Tweed J K S, Molle G, Decandia M and Lee M R F(2010) The influence of plant polyphenols on lipolysis and biohydrogenation in dried forages at different phonological stages: *in vitro* study. J Sci Food Agric 90: 829-835

Chilliard Y and Ferlay A (2004) Dietary lipids and forages interactions on cow and goat milk fatty acid composition and sensory properties. Reprod Nutr Dev 44: 467-492

Chilliard Y, Chardigny JM, Chabrot J, Ollier A, Sebedio and Doreau M(1999) Effects of ruminal or postruminal fish oil supply on conjugated linoleic acid (CLA) content of cow milk fat. Proc Nutr Soc 58: 70A (Abstr.)

Chilliard Y, Glasser F, Ferlay A, Bernard L, Rouel J and Doreau M(2007). Diet, rumen biohydrogenation and nutritional quality of cow and goat milk fat. European J. Lipid Sci. Technol 109: 828-855.

Chouinard P Y, Corneau L, Bauman D E, Butler W R, Chilliard Y and Drackley J K(1998a). Conjugated linoleic acid content of milk from cows fed different sources of dietary fat. J. Dairy Sci 81(Suppl. 1): 233 (Abstr.)

Chouinard P Y, Corneau L, Kelly M L, Griinari JM, Bauman D E (1998b) Effect of dietary manipulation on milk conjugated linoleic acid concentrations. J Dairy Sci 81(Suppl. 1): 233 (Abstr.)

Chouinard PY, Corneau L, Sæbø A, Bauman DE (1999) Milk yield and composition during abomasal infusion of conjugated linoleic acids in dairy cows. J Dairy Sci 82: 2737-2745

Christodoulou V, Bampidis V A, Hucko B, Ploumi K, Iliadis C, Robinson, PH, Mudrik Z (2005) Nutritional value of chickpeas in rations of lactating ewes and growing lambs. Anim. Feed Sci. Technol 118: 229-241.

Coakley M, Ross R P, Nordgren M, Fitzgerald G, Devery D and Stanton C(2003) Conjugated linoleic acid biosynthesis by human-derived Bifidobacterium species. J. Appl. Microbiol. 94: 138-145

Cook M E, Butz D, Li G, Pariza M, Whigham L and Yang M(2003) Conjugated linoleic acid enhances immune responces but protects against the collateral damage of immune events. In advances in Conjugated Linoleic Acid Research. Vol.2 (Ed.J. Sebedio, W.W. Christie and R.Adolf). AOCS Press. Champaign, IL, pp. 283-291

Cowan M M(1999) Plant products as anti-microbial agents. Clin. Microbiol. Rev. 12: 564-582

Devillard E, McIntosh F M, Young K, Castet M, Wallace R J and Newbold C J(2004) CLA composition of rumen bacterial and protozoal populations. Reprodn Nutr Develop 44: 60-65

Dhiman T R, Anand G R, Satter L D and Pariza M (1996) Conjugated linoleic acid content of milk from cows fed different diets. J. Dairy Sci. 79 (Suppl. 1): 137 (Abstr.)

Dhiman T R, Helmink E D, McMahon D J, Fife R L and Pariza M W (1999) Conjugated linoleic acid content of milk and cheese from cows fed extruded oilseeds. J Dairy Sci. 82: 412-419

Dhiman T R, Satter L D, Pariza M W, Galli, M P and Albright K (1997) Conjugated linoleic acid (CLA) content of milk from cows offered diets rich in linoleic and linolenic acid. J. Dairy Sci. 80 (Suppl. 1): 184 (Abstr.)

Dschaak C M, Williams C M, Holt M S, Eun J S, Young A J and Min B R(2011) Effects of supplementing condensed tannin extract on intake, digestion, ruminal fermentation, and milk production of lactating dairy cows. J. Dairy Sci. 94: 2508-2519

Durmic Z, McSweeney C S, Kemp G W, Hutton P, Wallace R J and Vercoe P E(2008) Australian plants with potential to inhibit bacteria and processes involved in ruminal biohydrogenation of fatty acids. Anim. Feed Sci. Technol. 145: 271-284

Enser M, Hallett K, Hewitt B, Fursey G A J and Wood J D(1996) Fatty acid content and composition of English beef, lamb and pork at retail. Meat Sci. 42: 443-456

FranciscoA, Dentinho M T, Alves S P, Portugal P V, Fernandes F, Sengo S, Jerónimo E, Oliveira M A, Costa P, Sequeira A, Bessa R J B, Santos-Silva J (201). Growth performance, carcass and meat quality of lambs supplemented with increasing levels of a tanniferous bush (Cistus ladanifer L.) and vegetable oils. Meat Sci., 100: 275-282

Franklin S T, Martin K R, Baer RJ Schingoethe D J and Hippen A R(1999) Dietary marine algae (Schizochytrium sp.) increases concentrations of conjugated linoleic, docosahexaenoic and transvaccenic acids in milk of dairy cows. J. Nutr. 129: 2048-2052

Gerson T, John A and Sinclair B R(1983) The effect of dietary N on in vitro lipolysis and fatty acid hydrogenation in rumen digesta from sheep fed diets high in starch. J. Agric. Sci. 101: 97-101

Giesy J G, Viswanadha S, Hanson T W, Falen L R, McGuire M A, Skarie C Hand Vinci A (1999) Effects of calcium salts of conjugated linoleic acid (CLA) on estimated energy balance in Holstein cows early in lactation. J. Dairy Sci. 82 (Suppl. 1): 74 (Abstr.)

Girard M, Dohme-Meier F, Silacci P, Ampuero Kragten S, Kreuzer M and Bee (G 2015) Forage legumes rich in condensed tannins may increase n-3 fatty acid levels and sensory quality of lamb meal. J. Sci. Food Agri. DOI: 10.1002/jsfa.7298

Gravador R S, Luciano G, Jongberg S, Bognanno M, Scerra M, Andersen M L, Lund M N, Priolo A (2015) Fatty acids and oxidative stability of meat from lambs fed carob-containing diets. Food Chem. 182: 27-34

Griinari J M and Bauman DE (1999) Biosynthesis of conjugated linoleic acid and its incorporation into meat and milk in ruminants. In: Yurawecz MP, Mossoba MM, Kramer JKG, Pariza MW, Nelson GJ (eds) Advances in Conjugated Linoleic Acid Research AOCS, Illinois, Champaign, pp. 180-200

Griinari J M, Corl B A, Laly S H, Chourinard P Y and Bauman B E(2000) Conjugated Linoleic Acid is synthesized endogenously in lactating dairy cows by delta 9 desaturase. J. Nutri. 130: 2285-2291

Harfoot C G, Hazlewood G P(1997) Lipid metabolism in the rumen. In: Hobson, P.N., Stewart, C.S. (Eds.), The Rumen Microbial Ecosystem, 2nd ed. Blackie Academic & Professional, London, pp. 382–426

Houseknecht K L, Vanden Heuvel J P, Moya-Camarena S Y, Portocarrerro C P, Peck LW, Nickel, KP, Belury M A(1998) Conjugated linoleic acid normalizes impaired glucose tolerance in the Zucker diabetic fatty rat. Biochem. Biophys. Res. Commun. 244: 678-682

Ip C, Chin SF, Scimeca JA, Thompson H J (1994) Conjugated Linoleic acid, a powerful carcinogen from animal fat sources. Cancer 74: 1050-1054

Jahreis G, Fritsche J , Steinhart H (1997) Conjugated linoleic acid in milk fat: high variation depending on production system. Nutr Res 17: 1479-1484

Jayanegara A, Kreuzer M , Leiber F (2012) Ruminal disappearance of polyunsaturated fatty acids and appearance of biohydrogenation products when incubating linseed oil with alpine forage plant species *in vitro*. Livest Sci 147: 104-112

Jayanegara A, Kreuzer M, Wina E, Leiber F (2011) Significance of phenolic compounds in tropical forages for the ruminal bypass of polyunsaturated fatty acids and the appearance of biohydrogenation intermediates as examined *in vitro*. Anim Prod Sci 51: 1127-1136

Jenkins TC (1993) Lipid metabolism in the rumen. J Dairy Sci 76: 3851-3863

Jenkins T C, Wallace RJ, Moate P J and Mosley EE (2008). Recent advances in biohydrogenation of unsaturated fatty acids within the rumen microbial ecosystem. J Anim Sci 86: 397-412

Jerónimo E, Alfaia C MM, Alves S P, Dentinho M TP, Prates JAM, Vasta V, Santos-Silva J, Bessa RJB (2012) Effect of dietary grape seed extract and Cistus ladanifer in combination with vegetable oil supplementation on oxidative stability of lamb meat. Meat Sci 92: 841-847

Jerónimo E, Alves SP, Dentinho M TP, Martins SV, Prates JAM, Santos-Silva J, Bessa, RJB (2010) The effect of grape seed extract and Cistus ladanifer L. and vegetable oil supplementation on fatty acid composition of abomasal digesta and intramuscular fat of lambs. J. Agri. Food Chem. 58: 10710-10721

Jiang J, Bjorck L, Fonden R (1998) Production of conjugated linoleic acid by dairy starter cultures. J Appl Microbiol 85: 95-102

Karaskova K, Suchy P, Strakova E (2015) Current use of phytogenic feed additives in animal nutrition: a review. Czech J Anim Sci 60: 521-530

Kathirvelan C, Tyagi A, Krishnamurthi P (2008) Influence of conjugated Linoleic acid ghee feeding on cancer incidences and histopathological changes in 7, 12 dimethlybenz (a) anthrazene induced mammary gland carcenogenesis in rats. Vet Arhiv 78(6): 511-520

Kathirvelan C (2007) Influence of mudtard oil cake feeding on conjugated linoleic acid content of buffalo milk and its anticarcinogenic potency. PhD. Thesis. Deemed university. NDRI. Karnal, Haryana, India

Kelly M L, Berry J R, Dwyer D A, Griinari J M, Chouinard PY, VanAmburgh M E and Bauman D E (1998) Dietary fatty acid sources affect conjugated linoleic acid concentrations in milk from lactating dairy cows. J Nutr 128: 881–885

Kepler CR, ToveSB (1967) Biohydrogenation of unsaturated fatty acids. J. Biol. Chem. 242: 5686-5692

KeplerCR, Hirons KP, McNeill JJ and Tove SB (1966) Intermediates and products of the biohydrogenation of linoleic acid by Butyrivibrio fibrisolvens. J Biol Chem 241: 1350-1354

Khiaosa-Ard R, Bryner SF, Scheeder MR, Wettstein HR, Leiber F, Kreuzer M, Soliva CR (2009) Evidence for the inhibition of the terminal step of ruminal alpha-linolenic acid biohydrogenation by condensed tannins. J Dairy Sci 92: 177-188

Kim YJ, LiuRH, Rychlik JL, Russell JB (2002) The enrichment of a ruminal bacterium (Megasphaera elsdenii YJ-4) that produces the trans-10, cis-12 isomer of conjugated linoleic acid. J Appl Microbiol 92: 976-982

KramerJK, Fellner V, Dugan ME, Sauer FD, Mossoba MM, Yurawecz MP (1997) Evaluating acid and base catalyst in the methylation of milk and rumen fatty acids with special emphasis on conjugated dienes and total trans fatty acids. Lipids 32: 1219-1228

Kritchevsky D (2000) Antimutagenic and some other effects of Conjugated Linoleic Acid. Br J Nutr 83: 459-465

Larraín RE, Schefer DM, Richards MP, Reed JD (2007) Finishing steers with diet based on corn, high-tannin sorghum or a mix of both: Colour and lipid oxidation in beef. Meat Sci 79: 656-665

Lawless F, Murphy J J, Harrington D Devery R, Stanton C (1998) Elevation of conjugated cis-9, trans-11- octadecadienoic acid in bovine milk because of dietary supplementation. J Dairy Sci 81: 3259-3267

Lee SO, Kim CS, Cho SK, ChoiHJ, Ji G E, Oh DK (2003) Bioconversion of linoleic acid into conjugated linoleic acid during fermentation and by washed cells of Lactobacillus reuteri. Biotechnol Lett 25: 935-938

Len T V, MallaBA, Sharma, A N, Kumar S, Tyagi N, Tyagi AK (2016) Effect of omega-3 and omega-6 polyunsaturated fatty acid enriched diet on plasma IGF-1 and testosterone concentration, puberty and semen quality in male buffalo. Anim Reprod Sci 173: 63-72

Liew C, Schut HA, Chin S F, Pariza MW, Dashwood RH (1995) Protection of conjugated linoleic acids against 2-amino-3-methylimidazo [4, 5-f] quinoline-induced colon carcinogenesis in the F344 rat: a study of inhibitory mechanisms. Carcinog 16: 3037-3043

Lourenco M, Falchero L, Tava A, Fievez V (2009) Alpine vegetation essential oils and their effect on rumen lipid metabolism *in vitro*. In Ruminant physiology: digestion, metabolism, and effects of nutrition on reproduction and welfare (ed. Y Chilliard, F Glasser, Y Faulconnier, F Bocquier, I Veissier and M Doreau), Wageningen Academic Publishers, pp. 88-89

Malla BA (2016) Feeding of n-3 and n-6 PUFA rich oils to augment the reproductive performance in female goats. Ph.D. Thesis submitted to ICAR-National Dairy Research Institute, Karnal, Haryana, India.

Mapiye C, Chimonyo M, Dzama K, Hugo A, Strydom PE, Muchenje V (2011) Fatty acid composition of beef from Ngunisteers supplemented with Acacia Karroo leaf-meal. J Food Comp Anal 24: 523-528

McGuire M A, McGuire MK, Guy MA, Sanchez W K, Shultz TD, Harrison L Y, Bauman, DE, Griinari, JM (1996) Short-term effect of dietary lipid concentration on content of conjugated linoleic acid (CLA) in milk from dairy cattle. J Anim Sci 74 (Suppl. 1):266 (Abstr.)

Miri H V, Ebrahimi SH, Tyagi AK (2015)The effect of cumin (Cuminumcyminum) seed extract on the inhibition of PUFA biohydrogenation in the rumen of lactating goats via changes in the activity of rumen bacteria and linoleate isomerase enzyme. Small Rumin Res 125: 56–63

Miri VH, Ebrahimi SH, Tyagi AK (2015) The effect of cumin (Cuminum cyminum) seed extract on the inhibition of PUFA biohydrogenation in the rumen of lactating goats via changes in the activity of rumen bacteria and linoleate isomerase enzyme. Small Rum Res 125: 56-63

Moate PJ, Chalupa W, Jenkins TC, Boston RC (2004) A model to describe ruminal metabolism and intestinal absorption of long chain fatty acids. Anim Feed Sci Technol 112: 79-105

Moon CD, Pacheco DM, Kelly WJ, Leahy S C, Li D, Kopecny J , Attwood GT (2008) Reclassification of Clostridium proteoclasticum as Butyrivibrio proteoclasticus comb. nov., a butyrate-producing ruminal bacterium. Int J Syst Evol Microbiol 58: 2041-2045

Mosley EE, Powell GL, Riley M B and Jenkins T C(2002) Microbial biohydrogenation of oleic acid to trans isomers *in vitro*. J Lipid Res 43: 290-296

OgawaJ, Matsumura K, Kishino S, Omura Y, Shimizu S (2001) Conjugated linoleic acid accumulation via 10-hydroxy-12-octadecaenoic acid during microaerobic transformation of linoleic acid by Lactobacillus acidophilus. App Environ Microbiol 67(3): 1246-1252

Pariza M W, Park Y Xu X, Ntambi J, Kang K (2003)Speculation on the mechanisms of action of Conjugated Linoleic Acid. In: Advances in Conjugated Linoleic Acid Research. Vol. 2 (Ed. J. Sebedio, W.W. Christie and R. Adolf). AOCS Press, Champaign, IL, pp. 251-266

Park Y, Albright K, Liu W, Storkson J, Cook M, Pariza M (1997) Effect of conjugated linoleic acid on body composition in mice. Lipids 32: 853-858

Parodi PW (2003) Conjugated linoleic acid in food. In: Sebe dio, J.L., Christie,W.W., Adlof, R. (Eds.), Advances in Conjugated Linoleic Acid Research, AOCS Press, Champaign, IL, USA, vol. 2. pp. 101-122

Parodi P W (2006) Nutritional significance of milk lipids. In: Advanced daitu chemistry, 3rd Edition (Eds. P.F. Fox and P.L.H. Mcsweeney), Vol. 2, pp 601-639, Springer, New York

Patra AK, Saxena J (2009) Dietary phytochemicals as rumen modifiers: a review of the effects on microbial populations. Anton van Leeuwen 96: 363-375

Piredda G, Banni S, Carta G, Pirisi A, Addis M, Molle G (2002) Influenza dell'alimentazione al pascolo sui livellidi acido rumenico in latte e formaggio ovino. Progress in Nutrition 4: 231-235

Priolo, A., Bella, M., Lanza, M., Galofaro, V., Biondi, L., Barbagallo, D., Salem, H.B., Pennisi, P. 2005. Carcass and meat quality of lambs fed fresh sulla (Hedysarum coronarium L.) with or without polyethylene glycol or concentrate. Small Rum. Res. 59: 281-288

Rana, M.S., Tyagi, A., Hossain, S.A. and Tyagi, A.K. 2012. Effect of tanniniferous Terminalia chebula extract on rumen biohydrogenation, "9-desaturase activity, CLA content and fatty acid composition in longissimus dorsi muscle of kids. Meat Sci. 90(3): 558-563

Rosberg-Cody, E., Ross, R.P., Hussey, S., Ryan, C.A., Murphy, B.P., Fitzgerald, G.F., Devery, R. and Stanton, C. 2004. Mining the microbiota of the neonatal gastrointestinal tract for conjugated linoleic acid-producing Bifidobacteria. Appl. Environ. Microbiol. 70: 4635-4641

Saroj, Malla, B.A., Tran, L., Sharma, A., Kumar, S. and Tyagi, A. 2017. Seasonal variation in fatty acid profile in the milk of different species under popularly followed feeding system in India. Indian J. Anim. Sci. 87(4): 484-489

Sauer, F.D., Fellner, V., Kinsman, R., Kramer, J.K.G, Jackson, H.A. Lee, A.J. and Chen, S. 1998. Methane output and lactation response in Holstein cattle with monensin or unsaturated fat added to the diet. J. Anim. Sci. 76: 906-914

Sehat, N., Kramer, J.K.G., Mossoba, M.M., Yurawecz, M.P., Roach, J.A.G., Eulitz, K., Morehouse, K.M. and Ku, Y. 1998. Identification of conjugated linoleic acid isomers in cheese by gas chromatography, silver ion high performance liquid chromatography and mass spectral reconstructed ion profiles. Comparison of chromatographic elution sequences. Lipids 33: 963-971

Shingfield, K.J., Chilliard, Y., Toivonen, V., Kairenius P. and Givens, D.I. 2008. Trans fatty acids and bioactive lipids in ruminant milk. Adv. Expt. Med. Biol. 606, 3-65

Shivani, S., Srivastava, A., Shandilya, U.K., Kale, V and Tyagi, A.K. 2015. Dietary supplementation of Butyrivibriofibrisolvens alters fatty acids of milk and rumen fluid in lactating goats. J. Sci. Food Agri. 96: 1716-1722

Stanton, C., Devery, B. and Murphy, A. 2006. Animal feeding strategies for conjugated linoleic acid enrichment of milk, In: Advances in Conjugated Linoleic Acid Research, AOCS Publishing.

Stanton, C., Lawless, F., Kjellmer, G. Harrington, D. Devery, R. Connolly, J.F. and Murphy, J. 1997. Dietary influences on bovine milk cis-9, trans-11-conjugated linoleic acid content. J. Food Sci. 62: 1083-1086

Sugano, M.,Yamasaki, M., Yamada, K. and Huang, Y.S. 1999. Effect of conjugated linoleic acid on polyunsaturated fatty acid metabolism and immune function. In advances in Conjugated Linoleic Acid Research . Vol.2 (Ed.J. Sebedio, W.W. Christie and R.Adolf). AOCS Press. Champaign, IL, pp. 327-339

Tesfa, A.T., Tuori, M. and Syrjälä-Qvist, L. 1991. High rapeseed oil feeding to lactating dairy cows and its effect on milk yield and composition in ruminants. Finn. J. Dairy Sci. 49: 65-81

Timmen, H. and S. Patton. 1988. Milk fat globules: fatty acid composition, size and *in vivo* regulation of fatty liquidity. Lipids 23: 685-689

Toral, P.G., Hervás, G., Belenguer, A., Bichi, E. and Frutos, P. 2013. Effect of the inclusion of quebracho tannins in a diet rich in linoleic acid on milk fatty acid composition in dairy ewes. J. Dairy Sci. 96: 431-439

Toral, P.G., Hervás, G., Bichi, E., Belenguer, A. and Frutos, P. 2011. Tannins as feed additives to modulate ruminal biohydrogenation: Effects on animal performance, milk fatty acid composition and ruminal fermentation in dairy ewes fed diet containing sunflower oil. Anim. Feed Sci. Technol. 164: 199-206

Turner, G.C., Waghorn, S.L. and Thomson, N.A. 2005. Condensed tannins in birdsfoot trefoil (Lotus corniculatus) affect the detailed composition of milk rom dairy cows. Proceedings of the New Zealand Society of Animal Production 65: 283-289

Turner, K.E., Cassida, K.A., Zerby, H.N. and Brown, M.A. 2015. Carcass parameters and meat quality in meat-goat kids finished on chicory, birdsfoot trefoil, or red clover pastures. Meat Sci. 105: 68-74

Tyagi, A.K. and Kathirvelan, C. 2006. Conjogated linoleic acid in milk and its anticarcinogenic potency. Indian Dairyman. 58: 25-29

Tyagi, A.K., Kewalramani, N., Dhiman, T.R., Kaur, H., Singhal, K.K. and Kanawjia, S.K. 2007. Enhancement of CLA content in buffalo milk through green berseem feeding. Anim. Feed Sci. Tech. 132: 15-19

Valeille, K., Gripois, D., Blouquit, M.P., Souidi, M., Riottot, M., Bouthegourd, J.C., Serougne, C. and Martin, J.C. 2006. Lipid atherogenic risk markers can be more favourably influenced by the cis-9,trans-11 octadecadienoic isomer than a Conjugated Linoleic Acid mixture or fish oil in hamsters. Br. J. Nutr. 91: 191-199

Van de Vossenberg, J.L. and Joblin, K.N. 2003. Biohydrogenation of C18 unsaturated fatty acids to stearic acid by a strain of Butyrivibrio hungatei from the bovine rumen. Lett. Appl. Microbiol. 37: 424–428

Van Ranst, G., Fievez, V., Vandewalle, M., De Riek, J. and Van Bockstaele, E. 2009. *In vitro* study of red clover polyphenol oxidase activity, activation, and effect on measured lipase activity and lipolysis. J. Agric. Food Chem. 57: 6611-6617

Vasta, V., Aouadi, D., Brogna, D. M., Scerra, M., Luciano, G., Priolo, A. and Salem, H. B. 2013. Effect of the dietary supplementation of essential oils from rosemary and artemisia on muscle fatty acids and volatile compound profiles in Barbarine lambs. Meat Sci. 95(2): 235-241

Vasta, V., Mele, M., Serra, A., Scerra, M., Luciano, G., Lanza, M. and Priolo, A. 2009b. Metabolic fate of fatty acids involved in ruminal biohydrogenation in sheep fed concentrate or herbage with or without tannins. J. Anim. Sci. 87: 2674-2684

Vasta, V., Nudda, A., Cannas, A., Lanza, M. and Priolo, A. 2008. Alternative feed resources and small ruminants meat and milk quality. A review. Anim. Feed Sci. Tech. 147: 223-246

Vasta, V., Pennisi, P., Lanza, M., Barbagallo, D., Bella, M. and Priolo, A. 2007. Intramuscular fatty acid composition of lambs given a tanniniferous diet with or without polyethylene glycol supplementation. Meat Sci. 76: 739-745

Vasta, V., Priolo, A., Scerra, M., Hallett, K. G., Wood, J. D. and Doran, O. 2009a. Ä 9 desaturase protein expression and fatty acid composition of longissimus dorsi muscle in lambs fed green herbage or concentrate with or without added tannins. Meat Sci. 82(3): 357-364.

Vasta, V., Yanez-Ruiz, D.R., Mele, M., Serra, A., Luciano, G., Lanza, M., Biondi, L. and Priolo, A. 2010. Bacterial and protozoal communities and fatty acid profile in the rumen of sheep fed a diet containing added tannins. Appl. Environ. Microbiol 76: 2549-2555

Watkins, B.A., Li, Y and Seifert, M.F. 1999. Bone metabolism and dietary Conjugated Linoleic Acid. In: (Ed. M.P. Yurawecz, M.M. Mossoba, J.K.G. Kramer, M.W. Pariza and Nelson, G.J.). Advances in Conjugated Linoleic Acid Research. Vol. I. AOCS Press, Champaign, IL, pp. 253-255

Wencelova, M., Varadyova, Z., Mihalikova, K., Cobanova, K., Placha, I., Pristas, P., Jalc, D. and Kisidayova, S. 2015. Rumen fermentation pattern, lipid metabolism and the microbial ommunity of sheep fed a high-concentrate diet supplemented with a mix of medicinal plants. Small Rumin. Res. 125: 64-72

Whigham, L., Cook, M.E. and Atkinson, R.L. 2000. Conjugated linoleic acid: implication for human health. Pharmacol. Res. 42: 503-510

Whitney, T.R. and Smith, S.B. 2015. Substituting redberry juniper for oat hay in lamb feedlot diets: Carcass characteristics, adipose tissue fatty acid composition, and sensory panel traits. Meat Sci 104: 1-7

Whitney, T.R., Lupton, C.J. and Smith, S.B. 2011. Redberry juniper as a roughage source in lamb feedlot rations: Wool and carcass characteristics, meat fatty acid profiles, and sensory panel traits. Meat Sci 89: 160-165

Zegarsk Z, Paszczyk B, Borejszo Z (1996) Trans fatty acids in milk fat. Pol J Food Nutr Sci 5: 89-96.

❑❑❑

Chapter 4

Phytobiotics for Gastrointestinal Health in Farm Animals

Kaushik Pal[1], Melody Lalhriatpuii[2], Amlan Kumar Patra[3]

[1] Krishi Vigyan Kendra, West Bengal University of Animal and Fishery Sciences, West Bengal-743223, India

[2] Department of Animal Nutrition, College of Veterinary Sciences and Animal Husbandry, West Tripura-799008, India

[3] Department of Animal Nutrition, West Bengal University of Animal and Fishery Sciences, Kolkata-700037, India. E-mail: patra_amlan@yahoo.com

ABSTRACT

Herbs are frequently used in animal diets to improve palatability. Essential oils in lower doses may contribute to increased feed intake, improve flavour and palatability and resulting in higher feed consumption by animals. Herbal extracts have revealed significant benefits in the digestive tract of rats, producing laxative effects and preventing flatulence, stimulating digestive secretions and escalating enzymatic activity. Many herbal-derived additives have active ingredients that increase salivary gland secretion and gastric and pancreatic juices. Capsaicin of *Capsicum annum* stimulate salivation and secretion of pancreatic and intestinal enzymes in non-ruminants. Cinnamaldehyde of *Cinnamomum* spp. (cinnamon) increases pancreatic enzymes and increased feed retention time in the stomach owing to reduced gastric motility in pigs. Herbal extracts appear to stimulate mucus secretion in the stomach and intestine. Extracts from sage (*Salvia officinallis*), thyme (*Thymus vulgaris*) and rosemary (*Rosemaryinus officinalis*), and the blend of carvacrol, cinnamaldehyde, and capsaicin has improved feed digestibility in broilers.

Keywords: Esential oil, Flavour, Palatability, Thyme, Rosemary.

4.1 Introduction

Inclusion of feed additives in livestock diet has been a regular practice for the last few decades in food animal production. Feed additives commonly used in animal diets include immunostimulators, antimicrobials, anticoccidials, antifungals, antioxidants, pH control agents, antibiotic growth promoters, hormones and enzymes. Herbal plants are one variety of feed additives which have gained extensive interest in the feed industry in recent years. There are a wide variety of herbs, spices and derivative products, which are mostly essential oils. While numerous reports have confirmed antioxidative, antimicrobial and immune stimulation effectiveness *in vitro*, relevant experimental *in vivo* evidence is still quite inadequate. The exploitation of antibiotics as growth promoters in animal production came into action worldwide. However, the opportunity of developing resistant populations of bacteria and the residue effects of using antibiotics as growth promoters have led the North America (US and Canada) as well to ban on the use of antibiotics in farm animals as feed additives. Herbs and spices are generally well thought-out safe and proved to be helpful against certain ailments. They are also broadly used, particularly, in many Asian, African and other countries. In the past, in view of their positive effects, the use of spices and herbs has been steadily increasing in developed countries also. Compared with synthetic antibiotics or inorganic chemicals, these plant-derived products have confirmed to be natural, less toxic, residue free, and are thought to be ideal growth promoters in animal diets (Hashemi *et al.*, 2008).

All plants generate chemical compounds as a part of their normal metabolic activities. These are randomly divided into primary metabolites, such as sugars and fats, found in all plants, and secondary metabolites or phytochemicals, compounds not essential for basic principle found in a smaller range of plants, some valuable ones found only in a particular genus or species (Patra and Saxena, 2010). Even though there is a worldwide interest in herbal supplementation, there are concerns about use of unproven and unregulated medicines. The scientific community is concerned about the quality, standardization, clinical safety and effectiveness of herbal.

4.2 Herbal feed Additives

Herbal feed additives are defined as herbal-derived compounds that are included into animal diets in order to improve growth performance and the quality of animal products (Kumar and Pawan, 2017). They are classified according to their origins and processes: extracts, spices, essential oils (lipophilic compounds extracted by steam distillation of the ground herbals) and oleoresins (compounds extracted by non-aqueous solvents) (Windisch *et al.*, 2008).

Depending on the chemical distinctiveness of extraction solvents, only certain molecules can be extracted. There are two types of extracts viz. purified and unpurified extracts. Unpurified extracts contain a number of different molecules extracted with certain solvent, which can influence the action of each other, while purified extracts contain only one active component. The purified active molecules extracted from plants can be at times substituted by synthetic naturally identical molecules. Normally, with respect to biological derivation, formulation, chemical depiction, and purity, phytogenics embrace a very wide range of substances and four sub-classes in animal feeding may be categorized: 1) herbs (product from flowering, non-woody and non-persistent plants), 2) botanicals (entire or processed parts of a plant, e.g., root, leaves, bark), 3) essential oils (hydro distilled extracts of volatile plant compounds), and 4) oleoresins (extracts based on non-aqueous solvents) (Windisch *et al.*, 2008). Recent research has established the existence of a synergistic effect between the primary and secondary active principles of herbals. For example, in oregano, carvacrol is present in high concentration (primary active principle) and thymol in a lesser concentration (secondary active principle). The secondary components, which are active principles that are found in small concentrations, act as enhancers of the primary compounds (Kamel, 2000). Nevertheless, antagonistic effects have also been observed among the active principles present in phytogenic compounds, as well as between the various additives used as promoters of animal growth (Costa *et al.*, 2011a). Multiple combinations or various levels of herbal extracts must be measured in order to have control of the equilibrium between synergism and antagonism, as well as animal health and growth in opposition to possible toxicity of the additives, which might result in reduced or improved animal performance (Mellor, 2000).

4.3 Modes of Action of Herbal Extracts

The probable mechanisms of action of herbal extracts in the animal organism for growth promotion consist of changes in the intestinal microbiota (Dorman and Deans, 2000), antimicrobial (Guo *et al.*, 2004a), improved digestibility and nutrient absorption (Alcicek *et al.*, 2004; Oetting *et al.*, 2006a; Kumar *et al.*, 2017; Chowdhury *et al.*, 2018a), improvement of the immune response (Namkung *et al.*, 2004; Guo *et al.*, 2004b; Kumar *et al.*, 2017; Chowdhury *et al.*, 2018b), morphological and histological modifications of the gastrointestinal tract (Utiyama *et al.*, 2006; Kumar *et al.*, 2017, Chowdhury *et al.*, 2018b) and antioxidant activity (Botsoglou *et al.*, 2002) which are given in the Table 1. In animals, the mode of action and place of action of the active components in herbal extracts (phyto-components or phyto-molecules) depend on their structure, metabolism and level of inclusion (Costa *et al.*, 2011b).

4.4 Antimicrobial Activity of Herbs

Functional antimicrobial phytochemicals can be separated into a number of categories such as phenolics and polyphenols, terpenoids and essential oils, alkaloids, and lectins and polypeptides (Cowan, 1999; Windisch *et al.*, 2008; Patra, 2012). The most important mechanism of phytogenic feed additives arises from constructively affecting the ecosystem of gut microflora through controlling potential pathogens. Phytochemicals in phytobiotics are well identified to have antimicrobial ability (Cowan, 1999; Patra, 2012). Phytochemicals exert their antimicrobial activity through different mechanisms; tannins for example, act by iron deprivation, hydrogen bounding or non-specific interactions with vital proteins such as enzymes (Scalbert, 1991; Patra *et al.*, 2012). Chung *et al.* (1993) showed that tannic acid inhibits the growth of gut bacteria such as *Bacteroides fragilis, Clostridium perfringens,* pathogenic *E. coli* and *Enterobacter cloacae*. Alkaloid is known to be a DNA intercalator and an inhibitor of DNA synthesis through topoisomerase inhibition (Karou *et al.*, 2006). The chief mechanism by which saponins exhibit an antimicrobial activity is based on their ability to form complexes with sterols present in the membrane of micro-organisms (Patra and Saxena, 2009). This causes damages in the membrane and the consequent collapse of cells (Morrissey and Osbourn, 1999). Essential oils have long been acknowledged for their anti-microbial properties (Lee *et al.*, 2004), and they have gained much attention for their potential as alternatives to antibiotics in broiler chickens. Some studies with broilers verified *in vivo* antimicrobial efficacy of essential oils against pathogenic bacteria such as *E. coli* and *C. perfringens* (Jamroz *et al.*, 2003, 2005; Mitsch *et al.*, 2004). The exact anti-microbial mechanism of essential oils is poorly understood. However, it has been recommended that their lipophilic property and chemical structure (Dorman and Deans, 2000) can play a role. It was suggested that terpenoids and phenylpropanoids can break through the membranes of the pathogen cells and reach inner part of the cell because of their lipophilicity (Helander *et al.*, 1998). Furthermore, structural properties, such as the presence of functional groups (Farag *et al.*, 1989) and aromaticity (Bowles and Miller, 1993) are also responsible for the antibacterial activity of essential oils.

Herbal extracts and metabolites are known to put forth an *in vitro* antimicrobial effect against many zoonotic and foodborne pathogens (Helander *et al.*, 1998). Studies based on minimum inhibitory concentration (MIC) methods have confirmed that few herbal extracts present similar effects to most commercial antibiotics (Kamel, 2000); but need to be supplemented in greater concentrations to demonstrate their effects (Burt, 2004). Many studies have revealed that herbal extracts and isolated bioactive compounds have a wide spectrum of *in vitro* bactericidal activity. The mechanism by which the majority of herbal extracts wield their antibacterial effect is by acting in the bacterial cell wall structure, denaturing and coagulating proteins (Cowan, 2000). More exclusively, the essential oils act by shifting the permeability of the cytoplasmic membrane to hydrogen (H^+) and potassium (K^+) ions. This change may lead to the disturbance of essential cellular processes such as electron transport, protein translocation, oxidative phosphorylation, and other enzyme-dependent reactions, resulting in the loss of chemiosmotic control.

Table 1: Plants used as gut modulator (Charalambous, 1994; Kamel, 2000)

Plant	Used parts	Phytochemical	Functions
A. Aromatic spices			
Nutmeg	Seed	Sabinene	Digestion stimulant, antidiarrhoeic
Cinnamon	Bark	Cimetaldehyde	Appetite and digestion stimulant, antiseptic
Cloves	Cloves	Eugenol	Appetite and digestion stimulant
Cardamom	Seed	Cineol	Appetite and digestion stimulant
Coriander	Leaves Seed	Linalol	Digestion stimulant
Cumin	Seed	Cuminaldehyde	Digestive, carminative, galactagogue
Anise	Fruit	Anethol	Digestion stimulant
Celery	Fruit, Leaves	Phtalides	Appetite and digestion stimulant
Parsley	Leaves	Apiol	Appetite and digestion stimulant,
Fenugreek	Seed	Trigonelline	Appetite stimulant
B. Pungent spices			
Capsicum	Fruit	Capsaicin	Digestion stimulant
Pepper	Fruit	Piperine	Digestion stimulant
Horsradish	Root	Allyl izotiocianat	Appetite stimulant
Mustard	Seed	Allyl izotiocianat	Digestion stimulant
Ginger	Rizom	Zingerone	Gastric stimulant
Garlic	Bulb	Allicin	Digestion stimulant, antiseptic
C. Herbs			
Rosemary	Leaves	Cineol	Digestion stimulant, antioxidant
Thyme	Whole plant	Thymol	Digestion stimulant, antioxidant
Sage	Leaves	Cineol	Digestion stimulant, carminative
Laurel	Leaves	Cineol	Appetite and digestion stimulant
Mint	Leaves	Menthol	Appetite and digestion stimulant

and, as a result, in bacterial death (Dorman and Deans, 2000). According to these authors, the disruption of bacterial cytoplasmic membrane is unsettled to the lipophilic nature of essential oils that accumulate in the membranes. Gram-negative bacteria have an outer membrane that contains lipopolysaccharides, which form a hydrophilic surface that creates a barrier to the permeability of hydrophobic substances such as essential oils. This could give details about the higher resistance of gram-negative bacteria to the antimicrobial effect of some essential oils, compared with gram-positive bacteria (Oetting *et al.*, 2006b). Additional mechanisms of action may be connected to the inhibition of nutrient absorption, enzymatic inhibition, synthesis of DNA, RNA, and synthesis of proteins by the bacterial cells (Lambert *et al.*, 2001; Luciano and Holley, 2009).

A familiar characteristic of phytogenics is that they are very complex blend of bioactive components. Growth improvement through the use of phytobiotics is probably the result of synergistic effects among complex active molecules obtainable in phytogenics. Some *in vivo* studies with pigs (Li *et al.*, 2012; Yan *et al.*, 2012) have confirmed the antimicrobial potential of herbal extracts to substitute antibiotics in feeds. Nevertheless, the data are incomplete to allow reliable conclusions on the efficiency of many phytogenic feed additives.

4.5 Influence of Herbs on gut Functions

Herbal extracts are frequently used in animal diets to improve palatability and productive performance in particular. On the other hand, studies testing the palatability of diets with the addition of phytogenics are limited. Improved digestive capacity in the small intestine may be considered an indirect side effect of phytogenic stabilizing the microbial eubiosis in the gastrointestinal. Most studies have observed only the effect of phytogenics on feed intake and weight gain during performance tests (Biagi *et al.*, 2006; 2007; Oetting *et al.*, 2006a; Costa *et al.*, 2011b). Schone *et al.* (2006) and Yan *et al.* (2012) reported reduced palatability of the diet in weaned piglets as a result of the inclusion of essential oils. The authors correlated the lower feed intake to the high level of essential oils in this study and to the organoleptic properties of the herbal extract mixture. Essential oils may have strong odours or sharp flavours, if used in high concentrations. On the other hand, essential oils in lower doses may contribute to increased feed intake (Costa *et al.*, 2007), improving flavour and palatability, and resulting in higher feed consumption by pigs. The primary effect of adding herbals to feed for pigs is the motivation of appetite. The aroma of these additives can stimulate the olfactory nerves and taste buds, resulting in a constructive effect on feed intake.

Herbal extracts have revealed significant benefits in the digestive tract of rats, producing laxative effects and preventing flatulence, stimulating digestive secretions (bile and mucus), and escalating enzymatic activity (Platel and Srinivasan, 2004). Many herbal-derived additives have active ingredients that increase salivary gland secretion and gastric and pancreatic juices (Mellor, 2000). Capsaicin, the active constituent of *Capsicum annum* (cayenne pepper), has been shown to be effective in stimulating salivation (producing amylase) (Patel and Srinivasan, 2004) and increasing the secretion of pancreatic and intestinal enzymes in non-ruminants (Costa *et al.*, 2011a). Another active ingredient, cinnamaldehyde, the main component of *Cinnamomum* spp. (cinnamon), showed an inspiring effect on pancreatic enzymes and increased feed retention time in the stomach owing to reduced gastric motility in pigs (Manzanilla *et al.*, 2004). As a result, the increased activity of digestive enzymes increased digestibility of nutrients (Costa *et al.*, 2011a). Herbal extracts encourage gastric secretion (Rafsanjani *et al.*, 2007), which activates pepsin. In addition, they increase the production of pancreatic juice, which leads to increased activity of digestive enzymes (for example trypsin, chymotrypsin, carboxypeptidase and lipase). Although those mechanisms that help to explain the enhancement in feed digestibility generated by the phytogenics have been studied most, other mechanisms might also be involved. Modulation of the gut microbiota and maintenance of intestinal epithelium reliability may be important properties that are exerted by herbal extracts, as happens with other growth promoters.

During the digestion process, oxygen radicals (superoxide radicals) are produced by an incident known as autoxidation. Such reactive oxygen radicals can attack the surface of the intestinal mucosa, impairing the absorption of nutrients. Enzymes such as superoxide dismutase, glutathione S-transferase, and catalase are responsible for converting superoxide radicals into water and molecular oxygen, thus maintaining intestinal health and allowing greater absorption of nutrients by the microvilli (Costa *et al.*, 2007). Herbal extracts appear to stimulate mucus secretion in the stomach and intestine. This effect prevents the adhesion of pathogens and contributes to the stabilization of favourable microbiota, shielding the intestinal villi and, therefore, improving the digestion and absorption of nutrients (Jamroz *et al.*, 2005; 2006). Hernandez *et al.* (2004) showed that extracts from some herbal plants such as sage (*Salvia officinallis*), thyme (*Thymus vulgaris*) and rosemary (*Rosemaryinus officinalis*), and the blend of carvacrol, cinnamaldehyde, and capsaicin improved feed digestibility in broilers. The authors accredited the positive effects of plant extracts on nutrient digestibility to the appetite and digestion-stimulating properties and antimicrobial effects. Consequently, they could make use of multiple functions in the animal body.

4.6 Immunostimulant Function of Herbs

Exploitation of immuno-stimulant properties of herbs is one resolution to improve the immunity of animals and to decrease their susceptibility to infectious diseases. The use of plant yield as immuno-stimulants has a customary history. Modern herb research and new indulgent of the immune system have explained many mechanisms by which these herbs work. Unfortunately, there are a small number of studies which have exposed the mechanism of action of the immuno-stimulatory compounds of herbal plants (Table 2). An understanding of the mechanisms through which phytochemical influences the immune system is essential to appreciate the use of herbal plant as immunostimulator and veterinary medicinal products. Herbs and spices rich in flavonoids, vitamin C and carotenoids improve the activity of the immune system. As a result, phytogenic compounds relieves the host animals from immune defense stress during critical situations to increase the intestinal availability of essential nutrients for absorption, thereby serving animals to grow better within the construction of their genetic potential (Windisch *et al.*, 2008; Hashemi and Davoodi, 2010). The plants containing molecules having immuno-stimulatory properties can improve the activity of lymphocytes, macrophages, and natural killer cells, they increase phagocytosis or stimulate the interpheron synthesis (Craig, 1999). Guo *et al.* (2003) indicated that herbal supplementation (*Lentinus edodes, Tremella fuciformis* and *Astragalus membranaceus*) augmented growth of immune organs such as thymus, bursa and spleen weights in both normal and immune-inhibition-treated chickens and rats. Immuno-active polysaccharides derived from two mushrooms, *Tremella fuciformis* and *Lentinus edodes*, and the herb *Astragalus membranacea* Radix, seem to be potential alternatives for antimicrobial growth and health promoters. These products were well thought-out to play an important role in strengthening the immune system by improving the physical conditions of gut ecosystem and enhancing functions of the defense system of chickens. (Guo *et al.*, 2003).

Table 2: Herbs used to modulate immune system (Source: Tan and Vanitha, 2004)

Species	Plant part	Chemical compound	Chemical identity	Biological activity
Aloe vera	Leaves	Acemannan	Polysaccharide	Selectively stimulates cytokines, activates lymphocytes
Angelica gigas	Roots	Angelan	Polysaccharide	Selectively modulates cytokines
Astragalus membranaceus	Roots	Glucans	Polysaccharide	Increase macrophage
		Soluble extracts	Alkaloids and flavonoids	Selectively stimulates cytokines
Ganoderma lucidum	Fruiting bodies	Water soluble extracts	Glycoproteins	Selectively stimulates cytokines
		GLIS	Proteoglycan	Stimulates lymphocytes
		Water and ethanol soluble extracts	Polysaccharide	Increase natural killer cell count
Panax ginseng	Roots	Panaxadiol, Panaxatriols	Saponins	Stimulates lymphocytes and cytokines
		Ginsan	Acidic Polysaccharide	Stimulates IL-1, IL-12, $TNF_{-\alpha}$ and $IFN_{-\gamma}$
		Rhamnogal acturonan II	Saponins	IL-6 stimulants
Panax ginseng	Leaves	Rhamnogal acturonan II	Saponins	Enhance macrophage actions, Stimulates IL-6 activity
Scutellaria baicalensis	Rhizome	Wogonin	Flavonoid	Stimulates $TNF_{-\alpha}$, activates iNOS
Zingiber officinale	Rhizome	Ethanol soluble extracts	Essential oils	IL-1, IL-6 stimulants

GLIS, Ganoderma lucidum immunomodulating substance; IL, interleukin; TNF, tumour necrosis factor; iNOS, inducible nitric oxide synthetase.

4.7 Nutritional Use of Herbs in Poultry, Pigs and Ruminants

4.7.1 Poultry

Outcome of phytobiotic feed additives on production performance in poultry was reported by Hashemi and Davoodi (2010). No essential oil effects on growth performance were reported by

Botsoglou *et al.* (2002), Zhang *et al.* (2005), Jang *et al.* (2007); while improved growth promoter effect of essential oils were showed at different ages of birds by Jamroz *et al.* (2003), Hernandez *et al.* (2004), Cross *et al.* (2007), Kumar *et al.* (2017), and Chowdhury *et al.* (2018a,b). Several studies on plant extracts are viewing promising results. Çabuk *et al.* (2006) measured production parameters of broilers which were supplemented by a mixture of oregano, laurel, sage, anis and citrus essential oils. The mixture of essential oils significantly enhanced feed conversion, which can be accredited to more effective availability of nutrients due to the changes in intestinal ecosystem including reducing the number of pathogenic micro-organisms.

Lippens *et al.* (2005) tested the efficacy of a mixture of cinnamon, oregano, thyme, cayenne pepper and citrus extracts and a mixture of plant extracts and organic acids in comparison to nutritive antibiotic avilamicin in broiler chickens. Chickens supplemented with plant extracts reached significantly higher body weight than the ones in the control or avilamicin group. Higher body weight was an outcome of increased feed consumption. Feed conversion in group fed plant extracts was 0.4% better than in the group with avilamicin and 2.9% better than in the control group. The authors noticed no synergistic effect between plant extracts and organic acids. It has been noted that growth performance and gut health effects of essential oils was dependent upon the chemical structures of the compounds (Chowdhury *et al.* 2018 a,b). Moreover, plant compounds show better growth performance and gastrointestinal health in the face of challenged pathogenic bacteria (Pathak *et al.,* 2017).

Resistance of coccidia to the currently used coccidiostats represents a serious problem in poultry industry. The use of plant extracts to treat coccidiosis is not a new approach. When searching for the best natural extract to treat coccidiosis, we have to take into account that the extract needs to be at least partially soluble in lipids to go through the cellular membrane, because coccidia are located inside the cells. Two plants of Chinese origin, *Dichroa febrifuga* and *Sophora flavescens* are rich in alkaloids and have been reported to be effective in treating coccidiosis (Youn and Noh, 2001). As infections with *Eimeria tenella* include also lipid peroxidation in the intestine, herbs and spices with strong antioxidant potency may represent a good supportive treatment. In one of the studies, Naidoo *et al.* (2008) found out the capacity of four plants of African origin which would be appropriate to treat coccidiosis: leaves of *Combretum woodii*, leaves and stem of

Artemisia afra, the whole plant and seeds of *Vitis vinifera* and the whole plant of *Tulbaghia violacea*. Extracts of all selected plants improved the feed conversion to the same extent as coccidiostat Toltrazuril. The best effect was seen with *Tulbaghia violacea*, which also partly lowered the shedding of oocysts.

Table 3: Herbal plants and phytogenic compound effects on microflora and immune response of poultry

Herbal plants and their derivatives	Administrative dose	Measured response	Reference
Aloe vera	500 µg injection Intra-muscular	Immunostimulator	Djeraba and Querefr (2000)
Aloe secundiflora	200 mg/kg prior to infection and 400mg/kg post infection	Increase in Antibody titre and IL6 concentration	Waihenya *et al.* (2002)
Astragalus membranaceus extract	2 g/kg	Increase both *Lactobacilli* and *Bifidobacteria*	Guo *et al.* (2004a)
Organo essential oil	2.5 to 6.25 mL/kg	Effect on *E.coli*	Horosava *et al.* (2006)
Agaricus bisporus	20-30 g/kg feed	Increase in ADG, FE, Antibody titre and *Lactobacillus* and *Bifidobacterium* counts	Giannenas *et al.* (2010); Kavyani *et al.* (2012)
Thyme (*Thymus vulgaris*)	0.1% in feed	Improvement in lactic acid bacterial counts, reduced *E.Coli* counts	Rahimi *et al.* (2011)
Euphorbia hirta	7.5 g/kg feed	Lower *E.coli* counts and improved FCR	Hashemi *et al.* (2012)
Thyme or oregano	15 g or 20g/kg	Reduction in colony forming units of *Lactobacillus spp.*, No changes in total plate counts.	Abdel-wareth *et al.* (2012)
Thyme and star anise	250 mg/kg	Reduction in *E. coli* counts and orally challenged *C. perfringens* in small and large intestine.	Cho *et al.* (2014)
Oregano oil and garlic oil	300 mg/kg each in separate group or in combination @150 mg/kg each extract.	Reduction in *Clostridium* counts. No effect on *Streptococcus, Lactobacillus* and *Coliform* counts.	Kirkpinar *et al.* (2011)
Oregano, anis, citrus peel	125 ppm	Longer villi in duodenum, decreased ileum ammonia concentration, no effect on ileum microbiota counts	Hong *et al.* (2012)
Allium cepa L.	10 g and 30 g/kg	Increased *Lactobacillus* spp., reduction in *E. coli* counts	Goodarzi *et al.* (2014)
Black cumin seeds	10-20 g/kg diet	Decreased *Salmonella* spp., Increased villi height	Kumar *et al.* (2017)
Cinnamon oil	300 mg/kg diet	Lowered *E. coli* and *Clostridium*	Chowdhury

4.7.2 Pigs

In the pig production, most problems can be anticipated at the time of weaning. Weaning can be accompanied by infections, especially with enterotoxic *Escherichia coli*. Results from Roselli *et al.* (2007) showed that alicin from garlic protects intestinal cells from increased permeability of membrane in pigs infected with *E. coli*. Garlic also improved the feed intake and daily weight gain of piglets (Janz *et al.*, 2007). Cinnamaldehyde, an active component of cinnamon, possesses antibacterial properties. Namkung *et al.* (2004) found that a mixture of cinnamon, thyme and oregano extracts inhibited the growth of coliform bacteria. A brown algae *Ascophyllum nodosum* could be a good feed supplement with growth promoting activity of pigs infected with *E. coli* (Turner *et al.*, 2002).

Combination of carvacrol, cinnamaldehyde, and capsicum oleoresin beneficially effected gastrointestinal ecosystem and gastric emptying of weaned pigs (Manzanilla *et al.*, 2004). The mixture successfully protected pig's blood lymphocytes against oxidative DNA damage at the concentration of 271.2 mg/ kg of feed. Its effect was equivalent to that of 90.4 mg/kg of vitamin E. The concentration of spice mixture supplemented to pigs in this study was not satisfactory to fully prevent lipid peroxidation induced by high intake of lightly oxidizable polyunsaturated fatty acids (PUFA). Although most studies concerning the effect of herbs and spices in pig production have been conducted on piglets, Allan and Bilkei (2005) carried out an experiment on swine. Swine were fed 1000 ppm of dried oregano leaves and flowers enriched with 500 g/kg of oregano essential oil. Observed valuable effects of oregano supplementation were: lower mortality rate, less culling during lactation period, shorter service interval, more live born and less stillborn piglets.

4.7.3 Ruminants

Microbial ecosystem in the rumen contains complex anaerobic microbial population of bacteria, fungi, protozoa, methanogeneous arhea, and bacterifagi. Plentiful metabolites produced in rumen during microbial fermentation affect the basic digestive and metabolic functions and productivity of the host. Researchers have been probing for new possibilities to modulate the microbial fermentation in the rumen. The main objective of manipulating the rumen fermentation is to increase the effectiveness of digestion and metabolism of nutrients, to increase the productivity of the animals and to suppress the unwanted processes as methanogenesis. In intensive farming systems, the feed additives, including antibiotics, were used to increase the production of milk, meat and wool. The ban on antibiotic use in Europe increased the production costs which triggered the need to search for antibiotic alternatives also in ruminant nutrition.

Table 4: Effect of phytogenic compound on gastro-intestinal microflora of swine

Herbs	Administrative dose	Measured response	Reference
Extract of cinnamon oregano and thyme	7.5 g/kg	Reduction in fecal coliforms. No immunostimulatory (did not afect plasma IL-1β and TNF-α levels) effect	Namkung *et al.* (2004)
Acanthopanax senticosus extract	1 g/kg feed	Increase in *Lactobacillus* counts and decrease in *E. coli* counts	Fang *et al.* (2009)
Astragalus membranaceus polysaccharide	1 g/kg feed	Increase in ileal digestibilities and serum concentrations of amino acids	Yin *et al*. (2009)
Atractylodes macrocephala koid polysaccharide	3 g/kg feed	Improvement in cell-mediated and humoral immune responses, increase in *Lactobacillus* counts and decrease in *E. coli* counts	Li *et al.* (2011)
Bamboo vinegar	0.1% , 0.2%	Increased lymphocyte percentage, reduced fecal *E. coli* numbers, reduced fecal H_2S and NH_3 emission	Yan *et al.* (2012)
Thymol, cinnamaldehyde	50g,100g , and 150g / ton	Reduced occurrence of diarrhoea decreased *E.coli* counts in feces, increased lymphocyte concentration.	Li *et al.* (2012)
Saururus chinensis	1g and 2g/kg	Decreased LDL and HDL. Decreased concentration of NH_3	Ao *et al.* (2011)
Houttuynia cordata and *Taraxacum officinale*	1g/kg 1g/kg	Increased WBC count, increased digestibility of dry matter and nitrogen	Yan *et al.* (2011)

There are abundant studies showing beneficial effects of herbs and spices on feed intake, immune functions and health, rumen fermentation, and productivity of calves, dairy cows, heifers and also beef cattle (Kraszewski *et al.*, 2002; Greathead, 2003; Wawrzynczak *et al.*, 2000; Cardozo *et al.*, 2006). There are some data on the positive effects of plant supplements on the nutrition of ruminants (Patra and

Saxena, 2011). Kudke *et al.* (1999) supplemented calves with powder of *Azadirachta indica* tree. Supplemented calves had higher weight gain than unsupplemented ones. The unsupplemented group had much higher incidence of parasite infections. Gladine *et al.* (2007) tested the antioxidant effect of marigold, grape, rosemary and citrus extracts in sheep. Lipid peroxidation was induced by uninterrupted infusion of linseed oil into the duodenum. The extracts were applied directly into rumen through the rumen cannula. The results showed that all tested plant extracts kept their antioxidant capacity *in vivo* in sheep. The most bioefficient in limiting lipid peroxidation was marigold extract.

4.8 Conclusions

The remuneration of herbal extracts to animals may be correlated to the increase in digestive secretions, improvement of digestion and absorption of nutrients, modification of intestinal microbiota, stimulation of the immune system and antibacterial activities, coccidiostatic, antihelmintic, anti-viral, anti-inflammatory, and antioxidant properties (Costa *et al.*, 2007; 2011a). Realistic use of herbal supplements to diet or extract depends on many factors such as animal species, age, and production purpose. Each herb contains different biological substance, which produces a different outcome due to a different mechanism. In modern years, herbal feed additives have been paid increasing interest as an alternative feeding strategy to replace antibiotic growth promoters. While comparing the effects of various herbs and oils on broiler performance, it can be concluded that the quality as well as the quantity of active chemicals in plant extract determines bird response. Some parameters may affect the goodwill of phytogenic additives such as plant parts and their physical properties, the genetic variation of plant, age of the plant, different dosage used, extraction method, harvest time, and compatibility with the other ingredients which may also explain why difference in body weight gain and difference in feed conversion ratio could happen when different kinds of phytogenics are used in birds diet. In addition, the efficacy of dietary phytogenics can be affected by inherent and irrelevant factors such as nutritional status of animals, infection, diet composition, and environment condition. Even though phytogenics are a group of natural additives, research into their mechanisms of action, compatibility with diet, toxicity and safety assessment needs to be done before they can be well-designed more comprehensively for animal feed.

References

Abdel-Wareth AAA, Kehraus S, Hippenstiel F, Sudekum KH (2012) Effects of thyme and oregano on growth performance of broilers from 4 to 42 days of age and on microbial counts in crop, small intestine and caecum of 42 day, old broilers. Anim Feed Sci Technol 178: 198-202

Alcicek A, Bozkurt M, Çabuk, M (2004) The effect of a mixture of herbal essential oils, an organic acid or a probiotic on broiler performance. S Afr J Anim Sci 34: 217-222

Allan P, Bilkei G (2005) Oregano improves reproductive performance of sows. Theriogenology 63: 716–721

Ao X, Yan L, Meng QW, Zhou T, Wang JP, Kim HJ, Cho JH, Kim IH (2011) Effects of Saururus Chinensis extract supplementation on growth performance, meat quality and slurry noxious gas emission in finishing pigs. Livest Sci 138: 187-192

Biagi G, Piva A, Moschini M, Vezzali E, Roth FX (2006) Effect of gluconic acid on piglet growth performance, intestinal microflora and intestinal wall morphology. J Anim Sci 84: 370-378

Biagi G, Piva A, Moschini M, Vezzali E, Roth FX (2007) Performance, intestinal microflora, and wall morphology of weanling pigs fed sodium butyrate. J Anim Sci 85: 1184-1191

Botsoglou N A, Florou-Paneri P, Christaki E, Fletouris DJ, Spais AB (2002) Effect of dietary oregano essential oil on performance of chickens and on iron-induced lipid oxidation of breast, thigh and abdominal fat tissues. Br Poult Sci 43: 223-230

Bowles BL, Miller AJ (1993) Antibotulinal properties of selected aromatic and aliphatic aldehydes. J Food Prod 56: 788–794

Burt S (2004) Essential oils: their antibacterial properties and potential applications in foods - a review. Int J Food Microbiol 94: 223-253

Çabuk M, Bozkurt M, Alçiçek A, Akbaþ Y, Küçükyýlmaz K (2006) Effect of a herbal essential oil mixture on growth and internal organ weight of broilers from young and old breeder flocks. South African J Anim Sci 36: 135–141

Cardozo, P .W., Calsamiglia, S., Ferret, A. and Kamel, C. 2006. Effects of alfalfa extract, anise, capsicum, and a mixture of cinnamaldehyde and eugenol on ruminal fermentation and protein degradation in beef heifers fed a high-concentrate diet. *J. Anim. Sci.* 84: 2801–2808

Charalambous, G. 1994. Spices, herbs and edible fungi. Amsterdam, Elsevier Science Ltd. p. 764

Cho, J. H., Kim, H. J. and Kim, I. H. 2014. Effects of phytogenic feed additive on growth performance, digestibility, blood metabolites, intestinal microbiota, meat colour and relative organ weight after oral challenge with *Clostridium perfringens* in broilers. Livest. Sci.160: 82-88

Chowdhury, S., Mandal, G. P., Patra, A. K. 2018a. Different essential oils in diets of chickens: 1. Growth performance, nutrient utilization, nitrogen excretion, carcass traits and chemical composition of meat. Anim. Feed Sci. Technol. 236: 86-97

Chowdhury, S., Mandal, G. P., Patra, A. K., Kumar, P., Samanta, I., Pradhan, S., Samanta, A. K. 2018b. Different essential oils in diets of broiler chickens: 2. Gut microbes and morphology, immune response, and some blood profile and antioxidant enzymes. Anim. Feed Sci. Technol. 236: 39-47

Chung, K. T., Stevens, S. E. Jr., Lin, W. F. and Wie, C.I. 1993. Growth inhibition of selected food borne bacteria by tannic acid, propyl gallate and related compounds. Lett. Appl. Microbiol. 17: 29–32

Costa, L. B., Almeida, V. V., Berenchtein, B, Tse, M. L. P., Andrade, C. and Miyada, V. S. 2011a. Phytogenic additives and sodium butyrate as alternatives to antibiotics for weaned piglets. Arch. de Zootec. 60: 733-744

Costa, L. B., Berenchtein, B., Almeida, V. V., Tse, M. L. P., Braz, D. B., Andrade, C., Mourão, G. B. and Miyada, V. S. 2011b. Phytogenic additives and sodium butyrate as growth promoters of weaned piglets. Arch. de Zootec. 60: 687-698

Costa, L. B., Tse, M. L. P. and Miyada, V. S. 2007. Herbal extracts as alternatives to antimicrobial growth promoters for newly weaned piglets. Rev. Bras. de Zootec. 36 (3): 589-595

Cowan, M. M. 1999. Plant products as antimicrobial agents. Clin. Microbiol. Rev. 12: 564–582

Craig, W. J. 1999. Health-promoting properties of common herbs. American J. Clin. Nutri. 70: 491S- 499S

Djeraba, A. and Quere, P. 2000. In vivo macrophage activation in chickens with Acemannan, a complex carbohydrate ex- tracted from Aloe vera. Int. J. Immunopharmacol. 22: 365–372

Dorman, H. J. D. and Deans, S. G. 2000. Antimicrobial agents from herbals: antibacterial activity of herbal volatile oils. J. Appl. Microbiol. 88: 308-316

Fang, J., Yan, F. Y., Kong, X. F., Ruan, Z., Liu, Z. Q., Huang, R. L., Li, T. J., Geng, M. M., Yang, F., Zhang, Y. Z., Li, P., Gong, J., Wu, G. Y., Fan, M. Z., Liu, Y. L., Hou, Y. Q. and Yin, Y. L. 2009. Dietary supplementation with Acanthopanax senticosus extract enhances gut health in weanling piglets. Livest. Sci. 123: 268-275

Farag, R. S., Daw, Z. Y., Hewed, F. M. and El-Baroty, G. S. A. 1989. Antimicrobial activity of some Egyption spice essential oils. J. Food Protect. 52: 665–667

Figen Kirkpinar, Bora Unlu, H. and Guven ozdemir. 2011. Effects of oregano and garlic essential oils on performance, carcase, organ and blood characteristics and intestinal microflora of broilers. Livest. Sci.137(1-3): 219-225

Giannenas, I., Tontis, D., Tsalieb, E., Chronisc, E. F., Doukasb, D. and Kyriazakisa, I. 2010. Influence of dietary mushroom Agaricus bisporus on intestinal morphology and microflora composition in broiler chickens. Res. Vet. Sci. 89: 78-84

Gladine, C., Rock, E., Morand, C., Bauchart, D. and Durand, D. 2007. Bioavailability and antioxidant capacity of plant extracts rich in polyphenols, given as a single acute dose, in sheep made highly susceptible to lipoperoxidation. British J.Nutr. 98: 691–701

Goodarzi M., Nanekarani, S. and Landy, N. 2014. Effect of dietary supplementation with onion (*Allium cepa* L.) on performance, carcass traits and intestinal microflora composition in broiler chickens. Asian pacific J. Trop. Dis. 4: s297-s301

Greathead, H. 2003. Plants and plants extracts for improving animal productivity. Proceedings of the Nutrition Society. 62: 279–290

Guo, F. C., Kwakkel, R. P., Williams, B. A., Parmentier, H. K., Lis, W. K., Yang, Z. Q. and Verstegen, M. W. A. 2004b. Effects of mushroom and herb polysaccharides on cellular and humoral immune responses of *Emeria tenella*-infacted chickens. Poult. Sci. 83: 1124–1132

Guo, F. C., Savelkoul, H. F. J., Kwakkel, R. P., Williams, B. A., Verstegen, M. W. A. 2003. Immunoactive, medicinal properties of mushroom and herb polysaccharides and their potential use in chicken diets. Worlds Poult. Sci. J. 59: 427–440

Guo, F. C., Williams, B. A., Kwakkel, R. P., Li, H. S., Li, X. P., Luo, J. Y., Li, W. K. and Verstegen, M. W. 2004a. Effects of mushroom and herb polysaccharides, as alternatives for an antibiotic, on the caecal microbial ecosystem in broiler chickens. Poult. Sci. 83: 175–182

Hashemi, S. R., Zulkifli, I., Davoodi, H., Zunita, Z. and Ebrahimi, M. 2012. Growth performance, intestinal microflora, plasma fatty acid profile in broiler chickens fed herbal plant (*Euphorbia hirta*) and mix of acidifiers. Anim. Feed Sci. and Technol. 178 (3-4): 167-174

Hashemi, S. R. and Davoodi, H. 2011. Herbal Plants and their derivatives as growth and health promoters in animal. Vet. Res. Commu. 35: 169-180

Hashemi, S. R. and Davoodi, H. 2010. Phytogenics as new class of feed additive in poultry industry. J. Anim. Vet. Adv. 9: 2955–2304

Hashemi, S. R., Zulkifli, I., Hair Bejo, M., Farida, A. and Somchit, M. N. 2008. Acute toxicity study and phytochemical screening of selected herbal aqueous extract in broiler chickens. Int. J. Pharmacol. 4: 352–360

Helander, I. M. , Alakomi, H. L., Latva-Kala, K., Mattila-Sandholm, T., Pol, I., Smid, E.J., Gorris, L. G. M. and Von-Wright, A. 1998. Characterization of the action of selected essential oil components on Gram-negative bacteria. J. Agric. Food Chem. 46: 3590–3595

Hernandez, F., Madrid, J., Garcia, V., Orengo, J. and Megias, M. D. 2004. Influence of two plant extracts on broiler performance, digestibility, and digestive organ size. Poult. Sci. 83: 169–174

Horosava, K., Bujnakova, D. and Kmet, V. 2006. Effect of oregano essential oil on chicken *Lactobacilli* and *E coli*. Folia Microbiol. 51: 278–280

Jamroz, D., Orda, J., Kamel, C., Wiliczkiewicz, A., Wertelecki, T. and Skorupinska, J. 2003. The influence of phytogenic extracts on performance, nutrient digestibility, carcass characteristics, and gut microbial status in broiler chickens. J. Anim. Feed. Sci. 12: 583–596

Jamroz, D., Wertelecki, T., Houszka, M. and Kamel, C. 2006. Influence of diet type on the inclusion of herbal origin active substances on morphological and histochemical characteristics of the stomach and jejunum walls in chicken. J. Anim. Physiol. Anim. Nutr. 90: 255-268

Jamroz, D., Wiliczkiewicz, A., Wertelecki, T., Orda, J. and Skorupinska, J. 2005. Use of active substances of herbal origin in chicken diets based on maize and domestic grains. Br. Poult. Sci. 46: 485-493

Jang, I. S., Ko, Y. H., Kang, S. Y., Lee, C. Y. 2007. Effect of a commercial essential oils on growth performance, digestive enzyme activity and intestinal microflora population in broiler chickens. Anim. Feed Sci. Technol. 134: 304–315

Janz, J. A. M., Morel, P. C. H., Wilkinson, B. H. P. and Purchas, R. W. 2007. Preliminary investigation of the effects of low-level dietary inclusion of fragrant essential oils and oleoresins on pig performance and pork quality. Meat Sci. 75: 350–355

Jia-Chi Hong, Tobias Steiner, Ahmed Aufy and Tu-Fa Lien. 2012. Effects of supplemental essential oils on growth performance, lipid metabolites and immunity, intestinal characteristics, microbiota and carcass traits in broilers. Livest. Sci. 144(3): 253-262

Kamel, C. 2000a. A novel look at a classic approach of herbal extracts. Feed Mix - Int. J. Feed Nutr. Technol. 9(6): 19-24

Karou, D., Savadogo, A., Canini, A., Yameogo, S., Montesano, C., Simpore, J., Colizzi, V. and Traore, A. S. 2006. Antibacterial activity of alkaloids from Sida acuta. Afr. J. Biotechnol. 5: 195–200

Kraszewski, J., Wawrzynczak, S. and Wawrzynski, M. 2002. Effect of herb feeding on cow performance, milk nutritive value and technological suitability of milk for processing. Annals Anim.Sci. 2(1): 147–158

Kudke, R. J., Kalaskar, S. R. and Nimbalkar, R. V. 1999. Neem leaves as feed supplement for livestock. Pashudhan. p. 14: 12

Kumar, P., Patra, A.K. 2017. Beneficial uses of black cumin (Nigella sativa L.) seeds as a feed additive in poultry nutrition. World's Poult. Sci. J. 73: 872-885

Kumar, P., Patra, A. K., Mandal, G. P., Samanta, I., Pradhan, S. 2017. Effect of black cumin seeds on growth performance, nutrient utilization, immunity, gut health and nitrogen excretion in broiler chickens. J. Sci. Food Agric. 97: 3742-3751

Lambert, R. J. W., Skandamis, P. N., Coote, P. J. and Nychas, G. J. E., 2001. A study of the minimum inhibitory concentration and mode of action of oregano essential oil, thymol and carvacrol. J. Appl. Microbiol. 91: 453-462

Lee, K. W., Everts, H., Kappert, H. J., Wouterse, H., Frehner, M. and Beynen, A. C. 2004. Cinnamaldehyde, but notthymol, counteracts the carboxymethyl cellulose-induced growth depression in female broiler chickens. Int. J. Poult. Sci. 3: 608–612

Li, L. L., Yin, F. G., Zhang, B., Peng, H. Z., Li, F. N., Zhu, N. S., Hou, D. X., Yin, Y. L., Luo, J. J., Tang, Z. R. and Liu, G. 2011. Dietary supplementation with Atractylodes macro-phala koidz polysaccharides ameliorate metabolic status and improve immune function in early-weaned pigs. Livest. Sci. 142: 33-41

Li, P., Piao, X., Ru, Y., Han, Xu., Xue, L. and Zhang, H. 2012. Effects of adding essential oils to the diet of weaned pigs on performance, nutrient utilization, immune response and intestinal health. Asian-Aust. J. Anim. Sci. 25: 1617-1626

Li, S. Y., Ru, Y. J., Liu, M., Xu, B., Peron, A. and Shi, X. G. 2012. The effects of essential oils on performance, immunity and gut microbial population in weaner pigs. Livest. Sci. 145: 114-123

Lippens, M., Huyghebaert, G. and Cerchiari, E. 2005. Effect of the use of coated plant extracts and organic acids as alternatives for antimicrobial growth promoters on the performance of broiler chickens. European Poult. Sci. 6: 48–56

Luciano, F. B. and Holley, R. A., 2009. Enzymatic inhibition by allyl isothiocyanate and factors affecting its antimicrobial action against *Escherichia coli* O157:H7. Int. J. Food Microbiol. 131: 240-245

Manzanilla, E. G., Perez, J. F., Martin, M., Kamel, C., Baucells, F. and Gasa, J. 2004. Effect of plant extracts and formic acid on the intestinal equilibrium of early-weaned pigs. J. Anim. Sci. 82: 3210–3218

Mao, X. F., Piao, X. S, Lai, C. H., Li, D. F., Xing, J. J. and Shi, B. L. 2005. Effects of â-glucan obtained from the Chinese herb Astragalus membranaceus and lipopolysaccharide challenge on performance, immunological, adrenal, and somatotropic responses of weanling pigs. J. Anim. Sci. 83: 2775–2782

Mellor, S. 2000. Alternatives to antibiotic. Pig Prog. 16: 18-21

Mitsch, P., Zitterl-Eglseer, K., Köhler, B., Gabler, C., Losa, R., Zimpernik, I. 2004. The effect of two different blends of essential oils components on the proliferation of *Clostridium perfringens* in the intestines of broiler chickens. Poult. Sci. 83: 669–675

Morrissey, J. P. and Osbourn, A. E. 1999. Fungal resistance to plant antibiotics as a mechanism of pathogenesis. Microbiol. Mol. Biol. Rev. 63: 708–724

Naidoo, V., McGaw, L. J., Bisschop, S. P. R., Duncan, N. and Eloff, J. N. 2008. The value of plant extracts with antioxidant activity in attenuating coccidiosis in broiler chickens. Vet. Parasitol. 153: 214–219

Namkung, H., Li, M., Gong, J., Yu, H., Cottrill, M. and De Lange, C. F. M., 2004. Impact of feeding blends of organic acids and herbal extracts on growth performance, gut microbiota and digestive function in newly weaned pigs. Can. J. Anim. Sci. 84: 697-704

Oetting, L. L., Utiyama, C. E., Giani, P. A., Ruiz, U. S. and Miyada, V. S., 2006b. Effects of antimicrobials and herbal extracts on intestinal microbiology and diarrhoea incidence in weaning pigs. Rev. Bras. de Zootec. 35: 2013-2017

Oetting, L. L., Utiyama, C. E., Giani, P. A., Ruiz, U. S. and Miyada, V. S. 2006a. Effects of herbal extracts and antimicrobials on apparent digestibility, performance, organs morphometry and intestinal histology of weaning pigs. Rev. Bras. de Zootec. 35: 1389-1397

Pathak, M., Mandal, G. P., Patra, A. K., Samanta, I., Pradhan, S., Haldar, S. 2017. Effects of dietary supplementation of cinnamaldehyde and formic acid on growth performance, intestinal microbiota and immune response in broiler chickens. Anim. Prod. Sci. 57: 821-827

Patra, A. K., Saxena, J. 2009. The effect and mode of action of saponins on the microbial populations and fermentation in the rumen and ruminant production. Nutr. Res. Rev. 22: 204-219

Patra, A.K., Saxena, J. 2010. A new perspective on the use of plant secondary metabolites to inhibit methanogenesis in the rumen. Phytochemistry 71: 1198-1222

Patra A. K., Min, B. R., Saxena, J. 2012. Dietary tannins on microbial ecology of the gastrointestinal tract in ruminants. In: Dietary Phytochemicals and Microbes (Patra, A. K., ed). Springer, The Netherlands, p. 237-262

Patra AK, Saxena J (2011). Exploitation of dietary tannins to improve rumen metabolism and ruminant nutrition. J Sci Food Agric 91: 24-37

Patra AK (2012). An Overview of Antimicrobial Properties of Different Classes of Phytochemicals. In: Dietary Phytochemicals and Microbes (Ed. Patra, A. K.), Springer, The Netherlands, pp. 1-32

Platel K, Srinivasan, K (2004) Digestive stimulant action of spices: A myth or reality? Indian J Med Res 119: 167-179

Rafsanjani FN, Shahrani M, Ardakani ZV, Ardakani MV (2007) Marjoram increases basal gastric acid and pepsin secretions in rat. Phytother Res 21: 1036-1038

Rahimi S, Teymouri Zadeh Z, Karimi Torshizi MA, Omidbaigi R, Rokni, H (2011). Effect of three herbal extracts on growth performance, immune system, blood factors and intestinal selected bacterial population in broiler chickens. J Agric Sci Technol 13: 527-539

Roselli M, Britti MS, Le Huërou-Luron I, Marfaing H, Zhu WY, Mengheri E (2007). Effect of different plant extracts and natural substances (PENS) against membrane damage induced by enterotoxigenic *Escherichia coli* K88 in pig in-testinal cells. Toxicol 21: 224–229

Scalbert A (1991) Antimicrobial properties of tannins. Phytochem 30: 3875–3883

Schone F, Vetter A, Hartung H, Bergmann H, Biertümpfel A, Richter G, Müller S, Breitschuh G (2006) Effects of essential oils from fennel *(Foeniculi aetheroleum)* and caraway *(Carvi aetheroleum)* in pigs. J Anim Physiol Anim Nutr 90: 500-510

Tan BKH, Vanitha J (2004) Immunomodulatory and antimicrobial effects of some traditional Chinese medicinal herbs: A review. Curr Med Chem 11: 1423-1430

Turner JL, Dritz SS, Higgins JJ, Minton JE (2002) Effects of Ascophyllum nodosum extract on growth performance of an immune function of young pigs challenged with *Salmonella typhimurium*. J Anim Sci 80: 1947–1953

Utiyama CE, Oetting LL, Giani PA, Ruiz US, Miyada VS. 2006. Effects of antimicrobials, prebiotics, probiotics and herbal extracts on intestinal microbiology, diarrhoea incidence and performance of weaning pigs. Rev Bras de Zootec 36: 2359-2367

Waihenya RK, Mtambo MMA, Nkwengalila G, Minga UM (2002) Efficacy of crude extracts of *Aloe secundiflora* against *Salmonella gallinarum* in experimentally infected free-range chickens in Tanzania. J Ethnopharmacol 79: 317-323

Wawrzynczak S, Kraszewski J, Wawrzynski M, Kozlowski J (2000) Effect of herb mixture feeding on rearing perfor-mance of calves. Annal Anim Sci 27: 133–142

Windisch WM, Schedle K, Plitzner C, Kroismayr A (2008) Use of phytogenic products as feed additives for swine and poultry. J Anim Sci 86: 140–148

Yan L, Meng QW, Kim IH (2012) Effect of an herb extract mixture on growth performance, nutrient digestibility, blood characteristics, and fecal microbial shedding in weaning pigs. Livest Sci 145: 189-195

Yan L, Kim IH, Huh K (2012) Influence of bamboo vinegar supplementation on growth performance, apparent total tract digestibility, blood characteristics, meat quality, fecal noxious gas content and fecal microbial concentration in finishing pigs. Livest Sci 144: 240-246

Yan L, Meng QW, Kim IH (2011) The effects of dietary Houttuynia cordata and Taraxacum officinale extract powder on growth performance, nutrient digestibility, blood characteristics and meat quality in finishing pigs. Livest Sci 141: 188-193

Yin FG, Liu YL, Yin YL, Kong XF, Huang RL, Li SJ, Wu GY, Hou Y (2009) Dietary supplementation with Astragalus polysaccharide enhances ileal digestibilities and serum concentrations of amino acids in early weaned piglets. Amino Acids 37: 263-270

Youn, H. J. and Noh, J. W. 2001. Screening of the anticoccidial effects of herb extracts against *Eimeria tenella*. Vet Parasitol 96: 257–263

Zhang KY, Yan F, Keen CA, Waldroup PW (2005) Evaluation of microencapsulated essential oils and organic acids in diets for broiler chickens. Int J Poult Sci 4: 612–619

□□□

Chapter 5

Phytobiotics and Reproductive Performance of Livestock

Nishant Kumar, Punita Kumari, Mohd. Nayeem Ali, Muzaffar Ahmed Naik, Shabir Ahmad Lone and S.S. Lathwal

Animal Reproduction Division, ICAR-National Dairy Research Institute, Karnal-132001, Haryana, India, E-mail: drnishantvet@yahoo.com

ABSTRACT

The success of dairy industry depends on the reproductive performance of its livestock so as to meet the growing demand for milk and milk products. Many attempts have been made for improving reproductive performance of livestock by application of hormones, antibiotics, anti-septics, nutritional supplements, etc. Most of these interventions have serious drawbacks including withdrawal period, residues in milk and meat, cost, availability, development of microbial resistance, etc. Herbal plants have been found effective in modulating reproductive efficiency by influencing estrous cycle, ovulation, embryo devel-opment, pregnancy and post partum physiology. A number of herbs have been found to have remarkable medicinal properties to counter different reproductive disorders. *Asparagus racemosus, Trigonella foenum graecum, Pueraria Tuberosa, Zingiber Officinale, Amaranthus hypochondriacus, Solanum lycopersicum, Sesbania sesban, Lepidium meyenii Walpers and Tribulus terrestris* are some herbs having scientific evidence for their influence on reproductive performance of livestock. This chapter attempts to summarize the effect of herbal feed additive on reproductive performance of female and male animals.

Keywords: Fenugreek, Ginger, Herbs, Maca, Reproduction, Shatavari, Vidarikand.

5.1 Introduction

Fertility improvement is an issue of global and national public health concern. Dairy cattle fertility has been greatly reduced in present situation. During recent times, several developments have taken place in reproductive health management of dairy animals. During last 50 years, considerable research has been conducted in improving reproductive performance and mitigating infertility in dairy cattle and buffaloes by using hormones, antibiotics, antiseptics, nutritional supplements, immunomodulators, etc. Most of these interventions have serious drawbacks like withdrawal period, residues in milk and meat, cost, availability, development of microbial resistance, etc. It is, therefore, necessary to focus on alternative management interventions that are less expensive, safe, widely applicable, and sustainable in the developing world to enhance animal productivity so as to improve the livelihood of animal producers. Traditionally some herbs or their mixtures are used to enhance animal reproductive performance through their flavouring and medicinal properties. Besides they are less expensive and safe than the chemical additives as side effects are rarely observed. Herbs are more compatible with body because of their normal nature and having medicine homologues components together; and usually lack unwanted side effects; therefore, they are most suitable, especially in cases of long consumption as well as in chronic diseases. The traditional use of medicinal plants/herbs to treat different diseases, including fertility related problems is widespread throughout the world as many herbal substances are known to influence male and female reproductive system.

5.2 Phytobiotics and Reproductive Performance of Female

The success of dairy industry depends on the reproductive performance of its livestock so as to meet the growing demand for milk and milk products. Many herbal plants have been claimed to be effective in modulating reproductive efficiency by influencing estrous cycle, ovarian functions, ovulation, embryo development, and pregnancy. A number of herbs are found to have remarkable medicinal properties to counter different reproductive disorders. Some herbs are found to have uterine stimulant activity and stimulate the muscular tissue of the uterus. Some herbs modulate reproductive performance of dairy animals by their antibacterial and anti-inflammatory actions. Most important herbal feed additives reported to influence reproductive performance of female livestock have been described.

5.2.1 Shatavari *(Asparagus racemosus)*

Shatavari (*Asparagus racemosus*) is an important medicinal plant found in tropical and subtropical part of India. This plant belong to Liliaceae family is commonly found at low altitudes, in shades and in tropical climates throughout India, Asia, Australia and Africa. The shatavari root contains saponin (Jadhav and Bhutani, 2006). Besides saponin, root extract of Shatavari contain flavonoids (6.7±3.9 mg/100ml), polyphenol including tannin (88.2±9.3 mg/100ml) and Vitamin-C (42.4 ± 5.1 mg/100ml) (Velavan *et al.*, 2007).

Shatavari is mentioned under six important *Rasayana* in *Ayurveda* (Goel and Sairam, 2002) and considered an important herb for overall health and vitality and as an aphrodisiac. Shatavari tones, cleanses, nourishes and strengthens the female reproductive organs and it nourishes the ovum and increases fertility. Therefore, it is traditionally used for pre-menstrual syndrome and sexual debility (Frawley, 1989), ammenorrhea, dysmenorrhea, dysfunctional uterine bleeding (Chopra and Simon, 2000), menopause and pelvic inflammatory diseases like endometriosis (Prasad *et al.*, 2002) and gonorrhea (Thomsen, 2002). It also supports deeper tissues and builds blood and thus, helps to remove infertility, prepare the womb for conception, prevents miscarriage and acts as a post-partum tonic where it helps to increase lactation and normalize the uterus after parturition and the changing hormones (Tirtha, 1998). Shatavari have been scientifically validated in dairy animals as reproductive system tonic, immuno-modulator, anti-oxidant and anti-stress compound (Kumar *et al.*, 2008). Shatavari is useful for boosting the immune system of both the mother and fetus and considered the best herb for balancing hormone levels and strengthening the reproductive system. It is also described as substances beneficial for maintenance of pregnancy.

Berhane, (2000) reported that when Shatavari was supplemented post-partum @ 100 gm on alternate day to crossbred cows, there was early resumption of estrus in all treated animals and conception rate was 75% as compared to control within 90 days of calving. Similarly, Hegde *et al.* (2002) observed that supplementation of Shatavari root powder 100 gm + 10 gm Aloe dried pulp powder to cows following artificial insemination resulted in improvement in conception rate. Shatavari possess immunomodulatory property and have been reported to shorten the uterine involution period in cattle (Sattar *et al.*, 2007) and buffaloes (Hussein and Badr, 2008). Shatavari stimulate the ovarian function, improves uterine tonicity and helps in early uterine involution which consequently results into early resumption of estrous cycle (Pandey *et al.*, 2005). Jamra (2014) investigated the effect of Shatavari on growth and puberty of Sahiwal heifers. The age of puberty and first service was advanced in Shatavari supplemented group compared to control suggesting that Shatavari could be fed to augment growth and puberty in Sahiwal heifers. Therefore, Shatavari supplementation could serve as potential managemental tool to improve reproductive performance in dairy cows.

5.2.2 Fenugreek *(Trigonella foenum graecum)*

Fenugreek (Methi in Hindi) is a 30-60 cm tall, annual aromatic leguminous plant of Fabaceae family cultivated world wide as a semi-arid crop. Fenugreek is one of the world's oldest medicinal herbs whose immunomodulatory effect (Bilal *et al.*, 2003), anti-inflammatory and anti-neoplastic effect (Sur *et al.*, 2001), antimicrobial effect (Amalraj *et al.*, 2005) and antioxidant effect (Priyanjali *et al.*, 2005) has been reported.

Fenugreek has been reported to influence reproductive performance of animals. Hassan *et al.* (2006) reported that Fenugreek oil stimulates ovarian activity and activating effect on the oviduct has been observed by Balash and Al-Quyem (2003). Hassan *et al.* (2006) studied the effects on the ovarian activity of Swiss albino mice supplemented with different doses of fenugreek oil. Results showed inclusion of fenugreek oil at 0.1 and 0.15 ml/mouse increased the total number of cumulus-oocyte-complex (COC) and improved their quality. It is believed that fenugreek seeds have the potential to enhance animal performance through their active ingredients such as saponins and alkaloids.

In dairy animals, Berhane *et al.* (2000) observed that reproductive performance in terms of onset of estrus and pregnancy rate was improved in dairy cows supplemented with Fenugreek. Rajkumar *et al.* (2008) studied the effect of supplementation of Saraca asoca stem bark and Fenugreek seeds on estrus induction and pregnancy in anoestrus cows and reported that percentage of animals induced in estrus and overall pregnancy rate using fenugreek seeds were higher (83.33 and 80.00 %) as compared to Saraca asoca (66.66 and 50.00 %) at doses of 50 and 100 gm level. Ahmed (2009) investigated the effect of fenugreek seeds as feed additive on reproduction performance of crossbred (Alpine- Beetal crosses) dairy goats and reported that supplementation of Fenugreek seed @ 1 gm per kg body weight reduced postpartum estrus length, improved service period, increased pregnancy rate, and reduced kidding interval. Further studies are required to elucidate the effect of this useful herb on reproductive performance of animals.

5.2.3 Vidarikand (*Pueraria Tuberosa*)

Vidarikand *Pueraria tuberosa*, one of the important plants used in Indian medicine, is commonly known as Vidarikand. It possesses spasmolytic, anti-inflammatory, anti-implantation, anti-hypergl-ycaemic, oestrogenic and contraceptive properties. The tuberous roots of *pueraria tuberosa* are used to relieve symptoms of dysmenorrhoea, dysfunctional uterine bleeding and menopausal syndrome in women (Devaiah and Venkatasubramanian, 2008). Further studies are required to elucidate the effect of this useful herb on reproductive performance of animals.

5.3 Herbal feed Additives and Reproductive Performance of Male

Many herbal plants have been claimed to be effective in modulating fertility of male by influencing spermatogenesis, semen func-tions, semen cryopreservation, etc. In male, few herbs act as aphrodisiacs and improves sexual desire and libido of animals. Most important herbal feed additives reported to influence reproductive performance of male have been described.

5.3.1 Ginger *(Zingiber officinale)*

Ginger *(Zingiber Officinale)* commonly called ginger belongs to the family Zingiberaceae. The plant is a underground stem (rhizome) that has been used in traditional medicine to aid digestion and treat stomach upset, diarrhoea, nausea, and arthritis for centuries (Morakinyo *et al.*, 2008). The important active components of the ginger root are thought to be volatile oils and pungent phenol compounds such as gingerols, shogaols, zingerone, and gingerols (Zancar *et al.*, 2002). It has been reported that Ginger possess anti-oxidant (Sekiwa *et al.*, 2000), aphrododisiac (Moghaddasi and Haddad, 2012) and androgenic activity (Kamtchouing *et al.*, 2002). Morakinyo *et al.* (2008) reported that when aqueous extract of *Zingiber Officinale* were administered orally to two groups of male rats at 500 mg/kg body weight and 1000 mg/kg body weight, there was an increase in testicular weight, sperm count, motility, viability and morphology. There was also a significant increase in serum testosterone concentration and reduced levels of Malonialdehyde production. Similar results have been obtained by Khaki *et al.* (2009) and Saeid *et al.* (2011) who supplemented *Zingiber Officinale* and observed improved sperm viability, motility and serum total testosterones in male rat and poultry, respectively. Hosseini *et al.* (2016) investigated the effects of ginger (Zingiber officinale) on sperm DNA fragmentation (SDF) in infertile men and observed that average positive percentage of SDF in patients receiving ginger was lower after three months of treatment. Studies correlating effect of this useful herbal plant with fertility of dairy animals are lacking and need to be investigated.

5.3.2 Amaranthus *(Amaranthus hypochondriacus)*

Amaranthus is also called Prince-of-Wales-feather. This plant is not only a rich source of vitamins and minerals but is also characterized by a high squalene concentration (Singhal and Kulkarni, 1988). It has been reported that Amaranthus improves semen quantity and quality. Zhang *et al.* (2008) reported that feeding with supplemental squalene at 20 or 40 mg/kg/day significantly improved the reproductive performance in boars as evidenced by reduced mating time, increased semen volume and motility, and increased the size of litter as compared with that in controls. Further studies are required in dairy animals to elucidate and confirm its effect on reproductive performance.

5.3.3 Tomato *(Solanum lycopersicum)*

The skin of the tomato is rich in lycopene ($C_{40}H_{56}$), a red carotenoid pigment with anti-oxidant action. Lycopene has been reported to be present in the testes and seminal plasma of male and is considered to be a part of the non-enzymatic defence system of the semen (Goyal *et al.*, 2006). Gupta and Kumar (2002) reported that dietary lycopene supplementation had positive effects on the concentration and motility of sperm from men suffering from sub-fertility. Its effect on reproductive performance of male domestic animals has to be investigated.

5.3.4 Sesbania *(Sesbania sesban)*

Sesbania *Sesbania sesban* is a well known multipurpose leguminous trees, the leaves of which contain high levels of saponins and tannins. Mekoya *et al.* (2009) supplemented S. sesban to the diet of ram at levels of upto 300 gm/kg and found beneficial effects on the onset of puberty, testicular growth and sperm count. Further research on this herb is warranted for confirmity of these findings.

5.3.5 Maca *(Lepidium meyenii Walpers)*

Maca is a traditional Andean crop of the Brassicaceae family. The below-ground storage organ, the hypocotyl, is the part of the plant assumed to improve fertility. Zheng *et al.* (2000) reported that oral administration of Maca enhanced the sexual function of the mice and rats, as evidenced by an increase in the number of complete intromissions and the number of sperm-positive females in normal mice. Reports are available in male rats and mice which have demonstrated that oral administration of aqueous or ethanolic extracts of Maca hypocotyls improved spermatogenesis (Gonzales *et al.*, 2004). Moreover, an improvement in sperm count was observed in men after four months of treatment (Gonzales *et al.*, 2001). In dairy animals, Matos (1995) reported that Maca supplementation improve sperm count and motility in bulls. Clément *et al.* (2010) performed an extensive experiment and found positive effects for Maca hypocotyl powder on sperm concentration, sperm motility and the DNA fragmentation index in supplemented peri-pubertal breeding bulls. Further research is required to confirm these findings.

5.3.6 Tribulus fruit *(Tribulus terrestris)*

Tribulus fruit *Tribulus terrestris* is a tap rooted herbaceous perennial plant. It is a member of the Zygophyllaceae family, the annual herb found in many tropical and moderate areas of the world (Abeywickrama and Bean, 1991). *Tribulus terrestris*, contains steroidal saponin, and act as a natural testosterone enhancer. *Tribulus terrestris* increases testosterone through increase in luteinizing hormone (LH) as well as it has also been reported that *Tribulus terrestris* is useful as a sexual enhancement herb (Gauthaman *et al.*, 2003). This plant has anti-microbial, anti-bacterial, anti-oxidant and anti-toxic properties which make it useful in the treatment of cardiovascular diseases, diabetes, tumours, articular pains and respiratory diseases

(Firas *et al.*, 2008). *Tribestan* is a component of *Tribulus terrestris* which increases libido in addition to preventing infertility and menopausal disorders (Chemexcil, 1992). Dioscin present in *Tribulus terrestris* increases male sexual ability by increasing free testosterone levels and balancing levels of estrogen, progesterone and pregnenolone. Since this plant contains protodioscin (PTN) and saponin which increases levels of testosterone and Luteinizing hormone (LH), it has been used for the treatment of sexual impotence in the traditional medicines of China and India from long ago (Koumanov *et al.*, 1982). Gauthaman *et al.* (2000) reported that administration of *Tribulus terrestris* to human and animals improves libido and spermatogenesis and increases the levels of testosterone and luteinizing hormone.

In dairy animals, Kistanova *et al.* (2005) added *Tribulus terrestris* extract to forage of rams once daily in dose of 1.5 gm per head for a period of 40 days and observed improvement in semen quality of ram. There was increase in sperm motility, viability and concentration along with improvement in libido and sexual behaviour. Pour *et al.* (2015) investigated effect of adding different levels of aqueous extract of *Tribulus terrestris* in the semen extender on sperm motility of Afshari rams at 5°C and observed improved post thaw semen quality in terms of post thaw motility at 5% level. Further researches are required to elucidate the effect of this important herb on performance of dairy animals.

5.4 Summary and Conclusions

This review attempts to summarize effect of herbal feed additive supplementation on reproductive performance of female and male animals. It can be clearly stated that herbs have remarkable influence on reproductive performance of both male and female animals. However, most of evidence are obtained either from observation or case control trials conducted in man, rats and mice models and few are available in livestock such as cattle, sheep, etc. Based on known findings, we still cannot speculate parallel results arbitrarily to other animals without further investigated. Some studies even did not list the detailed chemical compositions of extracts. Therefore, further studies are required to identify the bioactive substances and their chemical structures in plants extracts and investigate the effects and effective dosage in different animals using *in vivo* and *in vitro* trials. In this way, we can obtain detailed results and exact mechanism of actions of plants derived feed additives in animal reproduction.

References

Abeywickrama K, Bean GA (1991) Toxigenic Aspergillus flavus and aflatoxins in Sri Lankan medicinal plant material. Mycopathologia 113: 187–190

Ahmed MB (2009) Effect of fenugreek (*Trigonella foenumgraecum*) seeds as feed additive on production performance of dairy goats. PhD thesis submitted to Deemed university, National Dairy Research Institute, Karnal, Haryana

Amalraj A, Balasubramanian A, Edwin E, Sheeja E (2005) Anti-microbial effects of fenugreek seeds and leaves. Indian J Natural Product 21: 35-36

Balash KJ, Al-Quyem MA (2003) The effect of fenugreek seeds on the oviduct histology of laying hens. Iraqi J Vet Sci 216: 1-9

Berhane M (2000) Studies on feeding some indigenous galactopoeitic feed supplements on milk production in crossbred cows. M. Sc. Thesis, JNKVV, Jabalpur. pp. 91-93

Bilal BH, Rizwarul H, Suhel P, Suwarna P, Iqbal S, Raisuddin S (2003) Immunomodulatory effects of fenugreek extract in mice. Int Immunopharmacol 3: 257–265

Chemexcil (1992) *Tribulus terrestris L.* (N.O. Zygophyllaceae). Selected medicinal plants of India. A monograph of identity, safety and clinical usage. Bombay Tata Press 323-326

Chopra D, Simon, D. (2000). The Chopra Center. Herbal Handbook. New York, NY: Three Rivers Press: 73-75: 219

Clément C, Urwyler A, Kneubühler J, Witschi U, Kreuzer M (2010) Effect of maca supplementation on bovine sperm quantity and quality followed over two spermatogenic cycles. Theriogenology 74: 173–183

Devaiah KM, Venkatasubramanian P (2008) Development of SCAR marker for authentication of Pueraria tuberose (Roxb. ex. Willd.) DC. Current Science 94: 10

Firas A, Bayati AL, Hassan F (2008) Anti-bacterial and anti-fungal activities of different parts of Tribulus terrestris L. growing in Iraq. J Zhejiang Univ Sc. B 9(2): 154–159

Frawley D (1989) Ayurvedic Healing: A Comprehensive Guide. Salt Lake City, UT: Passage Press 200-211

Gauthaman K, Adaikan PG, Prasad RNV, Goh VHH, Ng SC (2000) Changes in hormonal parameters secondary to intravenous administration of Tribulusterrestris extract in primates. Int J Impot Res 12(2): 6

Gauthaman, K., Ganesan, A. P. and Prasad, R. N. (2003). Sexual effects of puncturevine (*Tribulus terrestris*) extract (protodioscin): an evaluation using a rat model. J Altern Complement Med 9(2): 257-265

Goel RK, Sairam K (2002) Antiulcer drugs from indigenous sources with emphasis on *Musa sapientum*, *Tamrabhasma*, *A. racemosus* and *Zingiber officinale*. Indian J Pharmacol 34(2): 100-110

Goyal A, Delves GH, Chopra M, Lwaleed BA, Cooper AJ (2006) Can lycopene be delivered into semen via prostasomes? *In vitro* incorporation and retention studies. Int J Androl 19: 528–533

Gonzales GF, Gasco M, Cordova A, Chung A, Rubio J, Villegas, L (2004) Effect of *Lepidium meyenii* (Maca) on spermatogenesis in male rats acutely exposed to high altitude (4340 m). J Endocrinol 180: 87–95

Gonzales GF, Cordova A, Gonzales C, Chung A, Vega K, Villena A (2001) *Lepidium meyenii* (Maca) improved semen parameters in adult men. Asian J Androl 3: 301–303

Hafeez B, Haque R, Pervz S, Pandey S, Sayeed I, Raisuddin S (2003) Immunomodulatory effects of fenugreek (*Trigonella foenum graecum*) extract in mice. Int Immunopharmacol 3: 257-265

Hassan AM, Khalil WKB, Ahmed KA (2006) Genetic and pathological study on effect of fenugreek on kinetics of the mice tissue. Vet Medical J 54: 189-204

Hegde GV, Nimbalkar SD, Hegde GS, Naik K (2002) Use of herbal plants for repeatbreeding problem in dairy animals. Indian Vet J 79: 861-862

Hosseini J, Azar MD, Mamaghani M, Hosseinifar H, Gilani MAS, Dadkhah F, and Sepidarkish M (2016) Int J Reprod Biomed 14(8): 533–540

Hussein AA, Badr, AM (2008) Influence of ante-partum administration of immunopotentiators on reproductive efficacy of buffalo and viability of their newborn. Vet Ital 44(2): 373382

Jadhav AN, Bhutani KK (2006) Steroidal saponins from the roots of Asparagus adscendens Roxb and Asparagus racemosus Willd. *Indian* J Chem 45: 1515-1524

Jamra MS, Mehla RK, Singh M, Ali MM, Chouhan N (2014) Effect of the fed shatavari (asparagus racemosus) on body weight and puberty of sahiwal heifers. Int J AgricSc & Vet Med 2(1): 64-67

Khaki A, Fathiazad F, Nouri M, Khaki AA, Ozanci C, Ghafari-Novin M, Hamadeh M (2009) The effects of ginger on spermatogenesis and sperm parameters of rat. Iran J Reprod Med 7: 7-12

Kistanova E, Zlatev H, Karcheva V and Kolev A (2005) Effect of plant Tribulus Terrestris extract on reproductive performance of Rams. Biotechnol Anim 21(1-2): 55-63

Koumanov F, Bozadjieva E, Andreeva M, Platonova E, Ankova V (1982) Clinical trial of Tribestan. Exp Med 4: 211–215

Kumar S, Mehla RK, Dang AK (2008) "Use of Shatavari (*Asparagusracemosus*) as a Galactopoietic and Therapeutic Herb—A Review". Agric. Rev 29(2): 132-138

Matos TW (1995) Efecto de la maca (Lepidium meyenii Walp.) en la presentacióndecelo en vaquillas Holstein en el establo "Chacra Valdivia" Matahuasi-Concepción. Thesis Universidad Nacionaldel Centro delPerú, Huancayo, Peru

Mekoya A, Oosting SJ, Fernandez-Rivera S, Tamminga S, Tegegne A, van der Zijpp A J (2009) Effect of supplementation of *Sesbania sesbanon* reproductive performance of sheep. Live Sci 121: 117–125

Moghaddasi MS, Haddad H (2012) Ginger (*Zingiber officinale*): A review. J Med Plant Res 6(26): 4255-4258

Morakinyo AO, Adeniyi OS, Arikawe AP (2008) Effects of *Zingiber officinale* on reproductive functions in the male rat. Afr J Biomed Res 11: 329- 334

Pandey SK, Sahay A, Pandey RS, Tripathi YB (2005) Effect of Asparagus racemosus rhizome (Shatavari) on mammary gland and genital organs of pregnant rat. Phytother Res 19(8): 721-724

Pour SS, Pirestani A, Alirezai M, Shafiyei K (2015) The effect of adding different levels of aqueous extract of Tribulus terrestris in the extender on sperm motility Afshari rams at 5°C. J Chem Pharm Res 7(4): 957-959

Priyanjali, Saroj D, Mohan GH, Devasagayam TPA (2005) Anti-oxidant properties of germinated fenugreek seeds. Phytother Res 19: 977-983

Rajkumar R, Srivastava SK, Varshney VP, Mahmood S (2008) Effect of medicinal plants Saraca asoca and *Trigonella foenum graecum* in anoestrus cows. Indian Vet J 85: 1281-1283

Reda I, El-Sheshtawy, A.El-Sisy G, El-Nattat WS (2016) Effects of pomegranate juice in Tris-based extender on cattle semen quality after chilling and cryopreservation. Asian Pac J Reprod, 5(4): 335-339

Sattar A, Mirza RH, Hussain SMI (2007) Effect of prepartum treatment of vitamin E and seleniumon postpartum reproductive and productive performance of exotic cows and their calves under subtropical conditions. Pakistan Vet J 27(3): 105-108

Saeid JM, Shanoon AK, Marbut, A (2011) Effects of *Zingiber officinale* Aqueous Extract on semen Characteristic and some Blood Plasma, Semen Plasma Parameters in the Broilers Breeder Male. Int J Poult Sci 10(8): 629-633

Sekiwa Y, Kubota K, Kobayashi A (2000) Isolation of novel glucosides related to gingerdiol from ginger and their anti-oxidative activities. J Agric Food Chem 48: 373-377

Singhal R, Kulkarni P (1988) Review: Amaranths: an underutilized resource. Int J Food Sci 23: 125–139

Sur T, Das M, Gomes A, Vedairomoni JR, Sahu NP, Banerjee S, Sharma RM, Ganguly DK (2001) *Trigonella foenum graecum* (fenugreek) seed extract as anti-neoplastic agent. Phythotherapy Res 15: 257-259

Thomsen M (2002) Shatavari - *Asparagus racemosus*. www. Phytomedicine. com

Tirtha SS (1998) The Ayurvedic Encyclopedia.Bayville, NY: Ayurvedic Holistic Center Press: 102-103

Velavan S, Nagulendran K, Mahesh R, Begum VMH (2007). *In vitro* antioxidant activity of Asparagus racemosus root. Pharmacogn Mag 3(9): 26-33

Zancar KC, Marques MO, Petenate AJ, Meireles MA (2002) Extraction of ginger (*Zingiber officinale Roscoe*) oleoresin with CO_2 and co-solvents: a study of the anti-oxidant action of the extracts. J Supercrit Flu 24: 57-76

Zhang W, Zhang X, Bi D, Wang X, Cai Y, Dai H, Chen, S (2008) Feeding with supplemental squalene enhances the productive performance in boars. Anim Reprod Sci 104: 445–449

Zheng BL, He K, Kim CH, Rogers L, Shao RY, Huang ZY, Lu Y, Yan SJ, Quien C, Zhen QY (2000) Effect of a lipid extract from Lepidium meyenii on sexual behaviour in mice and rats. Urology 55: 598–602.

❑❑❑

Chapter 6

Phytobiotics and Stress Management in Poultry

Bikas Chandra Debnath and Amlan Kumar Patra

Department of Animal Nutrition, West Bengal University of Animal and Fishery Sciences, Belgachiya-700037, Kolkata, India, E-mail: patra_amlan@yahoo.com

ABSTRACT

The livestock and poultry can suffer due to environment, pathological conditions, physiological and managemental conditions. Stress evokes a number of harmful responses that result in lower growth and production, immunosuppression and impairment of general health and feed conversion efficiency. There are various strategies to minimize heat stress in poultry either by changing their environmental condition or by modification of their diets. Nutritional strategy being more viable during heat period is based on diet balancing in order to cover the needs of stressed birds for amino acids (protein), energy and electrolytes. The body requirement of ascorbic acid during heat stress in poultry is greater than the amount synthesized by normal tissues and its administration to broilers during heat stress has been shown to be beneficial to the body. Antioxidants vitamin C and vitamin E are used and are being explored extensively in the poultry diet, because of their antioxidant effect in the neutralization of the free radicals generated during heat stress. Herbs have the potential to mitigate stress in poultry due to their antioxidant activity, therefore, many herbs have been used in poultry to alleviate stress in poultry.

Keywords: Phytobiotics, Stress, Anti-oxidant, Production, Poultry.

6.1 Introduction

The livestock and poultry often expose to several stressful environment and conditions arising from pathological (infectious, systemic, metabolic diseases, etc.), physiological (pregnancy, lactation, etc.), environmental (variation of temperature and climate, etc.) and managemental (transportation, overcrowding, poor ventilation, high intensity of light and poor nutrition) stress. Any factor that disrupts physiological and psychological stability of animals is the stressor, and reaction of stressor is termed as stress (Pande, 2002). Most common causes of stress in poultry include (Rosales, 1994):

- Poor brooding conditions (low temperatures, cold water)
- Contaminated premises (built-up litter, exposure to various disease agents)
- High stocking density (limited feeder and drinker space)
- Temperature (extremes cold and heat)
- Handling, weighing, transportation, vaccination, grading (pain, physical damage)
- Rapid growth (strict nutrient demand)
- Quantitative feed and water restrictions (frustration, hunger)
- Post-vaccinal reactions (reduced feed intake, fever)
- Sexual maturity and onset of egg production (drastic stimulation with feed and light)
- Clinical or subclinical diseases (reduced feed intake fever, pain)
- Harsh caretakers (poor husbandry)
- Feed quality problem (variations in nutrient contents)
- Long or uneven feed distribution (split feeding)
- Poor litter conditions (wet and cold)
- Inadequate ventilation (deterioration of the air quality)

Stress evokes a number of harmful responses that result in lower growth and production, immunosuppression and impairment of general health and feed conversion efficiency (Saxena and Madan, 1997). Variation in feed intake, protein deficiency, starvation, shortage of feeding space leads to stress which ultimately causes immuno-suppression (Rosales, 1994). Animals are exposed to frequent stress factors, and it is, therefore, essential to have an effective management program to lessen their effects on the performance and health. For ameliorating the adverse effects of stress conditions, many different management and nutritional strategies are adopted in farming systems, especially in specialized organized farms. The herbs containing plant bioactive principles have been shown to have several beneficial effects in livestock production (Patra and Saxena, 2010, 2011). The use of herbs that are scientifically established to have adaptogenic, immunomodulatory, free radical scavenging and antioxidant rejuvenating actions has been investigated for stress amelioration in livestock and poultry (Shukla and Srivastava, 1999). This chapter discusses different stressors and their amelioration using herbs and their products.

6.2. Heat stress

Heat stress is a serious problem for poultry and livestock industry in many parts of the world (Rosales, 1994). Animals have known zones of thermal comfort that vary by the species, physiological status, relative humidity, the velocity of ambient air and the degree of solar radiation (NRC, 1981). When the environmental temperature exceeds upper critical temperature of the thermoneutral zone, thermo-regulatory reactions are limited and animal is considered to be heat stressed (Sahin *et al.*, 2009). A summary of effects of stress including heat stress in poultry is given below (Rosales, 1994):

- Increased levels of corticosterone, insulin, or glucagon
- Increased metabolic rate and resting energy expenditure
- Increased reliance on glucose as an energy source
- Elevation of plasma free fatty acids (decreased usage)
- Hypoglycemia (increased glucose utilization)
- Decreased growth and increased muscle degradation
- Release of acute-phase cytokines (monokynes and lymphokynes)
- Impaired growth of cartilage and bone
- Redistribution of trace minerals
- Synthesis of specific stress proteins
- Decreased voluntary feed intake (anorexia)
- Increased body temperature
- Immunosuppression

High ambient temperatures compromise performance and productivity through reducing feed intake and decreasing nutrient utilization, growth rate, egg production, egg quality, and feed efficiency, which lead to economic losses in animal production (Sahin *et al.*, 2009; Mashaly *et al.*, 2004). High temperatures, especially when coupled with high relative humidity, impose severe stress on layer birds (Ajakaiye *et al.*, 2011). In laying hens, heat stress reduces egg production (Mashaly *et al.*, 2004), egg weight (Balnave and Muheereza, 1997), eggshell thickness and strength (Mashaly *et al.*, 2004). Moreover, birds reduce feed intake in high temperatures because of reducing metabolic heat production (Teeter *et al.*, 1985). High temperatures, especially when coupled with high humidity, impose severe stress on layer birds and lead to reduced performance (Ajakaiye *et al.*, 2011). High temperature not only has an adverse effect on laying performance but also can impede disease resistance. Environmental stress may depress the immune function of birds by impeding production of antibodies and effective cell-mediated immunity ([a]ahin *et al.*, 2009). For these reasons, heat stress is a big problem in hot region of the world especially in summer season when animals are kept in conventional, naturally ventilated houses. These adverse environmental conditions lead to oxidative stress associated with increased oxidative damage and lowered plasma concentrations of anti-oxidant vitamins (Sahin *et al.*, 2009).

High environmental temperatures stimulate the hypothalamo hypophyseal adrenocortical axis which increases cortico-steroid secretion in response to stress (Ramnath *et al.*, 2008). Higher levels of circulating corticosteroids have a catabolic effect through increase in the free radicals by altering oxidative metabolism, causing impairment of cellular functions and thus damage to the cell membrane, muscle wasting and retarded growth (Sujatha *et al.*, 2010). During the periods of heat stress, most of the production energy is diverted to thermoregulatory adaptations which results in oxidative stress induced immunosupression, pre-disposing birds to various infectious diseases and high mortality rates (Maini *et al.*, 2007). Therefore, it remains a prime issue to re-evaluate the poultry management in hot weather, so that heat stress is minimized. There are various strategies to minimize heat stress in animals either by changing their environmental conditions or by modification of their diets. Nutritional strategy being more viable during heat period is based on diet balancing in order to cover the needs of stressed birds for amino acids (protein), energy and electrolytes (Balnave, 2004; Daghir, 2009).

6.2.1 Herbs to Ameliorate Heat stress

Antioxidants, lactic acid, probiotic, prebiotic, vitamins and minerals as a nutritional manipulation tools are commonly added to the diets of birds reared under heat stress (ªahin *et al.*, 2009). Ascorbic acid synthesis is decreased at elevated environmental temperature making it an essential dietary supplement during the summer (Sejian *et al.*, 2012). The role of dietary supplements such as natural vitamin C for alleviating the effect of heat stress in poultry either by reduced rectal temperature, increased Hb and PCV %, reduced plasma concentration of cholesterol and overall growth performance has been illustrated by many investigators (Ajakaiye *et al.*, 2011; Ramnath *et al.*, 2008; Sahin and Kucuk, 2003). Its dietary supplementation reduces the respiratory quotient in heat- stressed birds by emphasizing an increase in fatty acid oxidation over the increase in protein-derived gluconeogenesis (McKee *et al.*, 1997). It also improves the growth, feed efficiency, egg production, egg weight, number of eggs hatched, shell quality and livability during heat stress (Rosales, 1994; Sejian *et al.*, 2012). This improved performance is associated with the suppressed stress responses indicated by the reduction in plasma corticosterone level (Mahmoud *et al.*, 2004; Mckee and Hurrison, 1995; Pardue *et al.*, 1985), adrenocorticotropic hormone (Sahin *et al.*, 2003) and increased serum insulin and thyroxine concentrations (Sahin *et al.*, 2002).

6.2.2 Herbs Containing Vitamin C and Flavonoids

The body requirement of ascorbic acid during heat stress is greater than the amount synthesized by normal tissues and its administration to animals during heat stress has been shown to be beneficial to the body (Balogun *et al.*, 1996). Non-enzymatic antioxidants vitamin C and vitamin E are used and are being explored extensively in the poultry diet, because of their anti-oxidant effect in the neutralization of the free radicals generated during heat stress (Ajakaiye *et al.*, 2011; Ramnath *et al.*, 2008; Orban *et al.*, 1993; Zapata and Gernat, 1995). Sticking to the emergency for dietary incorporation of vitamin C, it is being constantly added to poultry diet in synthetic form. However, now-a-days, the poultry industry has focused more attention towards addressing public concern for environmental and food safety (Munj *et al.*, 2010). For this the ascorbic acid in herbal form is being preferred by poultry producers. Natural Vitamin C and bioflavonoids owes its beneficial properties to the constituent herbs *Phyllanthus emblica, Ocimum sanctum, Terminalia chebula and Withania somenifera* (Rindhe *et al.*, 2012). Bioflavonoids are a group of naturally occurring plant compounds, which act primarily as plant pigments and antioxidants. They exhibit a host of biological activities, most notably for their powerful antioxidant properties. Bioflavonoids work with other antioxidants to offer a system of protection. Numerous studies have shown their unique role in protecting Vitamin C from oxidation in the body, thereby allowing the body to reap more benefits from Vitamin C. Its efficacy for improving haematobiochemical profile, thyroid hormone status, growth performance and meat quality attributes (Ajakaiye *et al.*, 2011; Rindhe *et al.*, 2012) has been proved for broiler birds. However its potency in the form of heat stress amelioration for layers and improving the egg production parameters wasn't backed by any scientific validation.

6.2.3 Herbs Containing Essential Oils and Organic Acids

Essential oils extracted from herb and spices are a complex mixture of various compounds, which consist of aromatic and volatile substances (Alçiçek *et al.*, 2003). Two major components of essential oils derived from thyme and oregano are carvacrol and thymol (Bozkurt *et al.*, 2009), and essential oils have some biological properties such as antimicrobial (Patra, 2012), antioxidant (Botsoglou *et al.* 2002), enzymatic (Hernandez *et al.*, 2004), digestion stimulating (Alçiçek *et al.*, 2003). Besides these, essential oils also have anti-heat stress effects and they activate immune system (Çabuk *et al.*, 2006). Organic acids (OA), generated from plants are known to control harmful microorganisms in digestive and respiratory organs of poultry. There are approximately 60 OA classes including lactic, citric, formic and fumaric acids (Park *et al.*, 2009). The most important role of organic acids is to reduce pH in the stomach and gut (Ye°ilbag and Çolpan, 2006). In addition, organic acids improved some immune responses of broilers (Abdel-Fattah *et al.*, 2008). Low gastric pH accelerates the conversion of pepsinogen to pepsin, which enhances the absorption rate of proteins and minerals (Park *et al.*, 2009). Additionally, OA are able to inhibit microorganism growth in the food, and as a result of this function they preserve the microbial balance in the gastrointestinal tract (Ye°ilbag and Çolpan, 2006). Recently, the effects of essential oils in broiler diets have been largely demonstrated (Alçiçek *et al.*, 2003, 2004; Lee *et al.*, 2003). However, it is not well known if the harmful effect of heat stress on productivity and immune function of hens can be overcome by supplementing essential oil and organic acids to diet because the effects of essential oils and OA in laying hen diet have not been studied very much especially in summer season.

6.2.4 Polyherbal Preparations

A number of herbal preparations help the birds to fight stress arising due to various reasons. Adaptogenic herbs like ashwagandha, tulsi, amla, and ginseng, etc. are being used as anti-stress factors for very long years in human and animal medicines with proven results.

A number of Ayurvedic herbal preparations have been extensively used in poultry industry (Ramnath *et al.*, 2008). Polyherbal products containing different immunomodulator (*Withania somnifera*), antistressor (*Phyllanthus emblica, Mangifera indica*) and adaptogenic (*Ocimum sanctum, W. somnifera)* herbs have been used to protect tissues from superoxide radicals and enhance cell survival by stimulating antioxidative enzymatic systems (Sujatha *et al.*, 2010). Supplementation of polyherbal supplement (herbal antistressor vitamin C) has been scientifically well proven to increase body weight gain as well as improve growth and performance of birds during summer (Sahin *et al.*, 2003; Maini *et al.*, 2007; Sujatha *et al.*, 2010). Jadhav *et al.* (2013) reported that the mean egg production (%) recorded in the experimental birds was significantly higher for the polyherbs (containing natural vitamin C and bioflavonoids) supplemented group followed by synthetic vitamin C supplemented group. Lowest egg production was noticed in untreated control group. The vitamin C supplementation in layer birds improved the mean egg production, egg weight and egg shell thickness (Khan and Sardar, 2005). They also recorded the improvement in the mean egg weight of layer birds in polyherbal treated groups. However, synthetic vitamin C supplementation group could not mark its influence over the egg weight as mean egg weight in the untreated control group did not differ significantly from it.

Animals with higher levels of serum cortisol (mg/L) content indicate the effect of high temperature and relative humidity. High ambient temperature induces production and release of corticosteroids (Siegal, 1980), exerts catabolic effects (mobilization of proteins and lipids) through muscle wasting and reduces growth rate (Sujatha *et al.*, 2010; Hayashi *et al.*, 1994, Jadhave *et al.*, 2013). Jadhav *et al.* (2013) conducted trial with the polyherbs and observed that the serum cortisol level (mg/L) significantly reduced in all treated groups as compared to control. The lowered concentration of cortisol signified the amelioration of heat stress in treated birds. The amelioration action was also noted for serum aminotransferases where polyherbal supplementation significantly improved and optimized their levels as compared to control group as well as synthetic vitamin C supplemented group. Similarly, concentrations of blood enzymes (alkaline phosphatise and aminotransferases) were lowered with vitamin C supplementation in all layer birds (Khan and Sardar, 2005).

Supplementation of herbs contacting bioactive compounds has been shown to improve growth performance and feed efficiency in stressed poultry. Jadhav *et al.* (2013) used natural Vitamin C and bioflavonoids containing herbal product containing herbs like *Phyllanthus emblica, Ocimum sanctum, Terminalia chebula and Withania somenifera* in their experiment. Though there was no significant difference observed, polyherbal premix at the rate of 100g/tonne of feed in treatment group had numerically higher body weight (1580 g) than that of control group (1513 g) during heat stress. In another study, broilers under extreme heat stress and receiving vitamin C improved body weight gain and feed conversion ratio (Talebi and Khademi, 2011; Celik and Ozturkcan, 2003). Supplementation of these polyherbs to poultry birds has been proved to increase the body weight of birds (Korde *et al.*, 2011). Jadhav *et al.* (2013) used herbal supplement for natural vitamin C supplementation which had improved feed efficiency in experimental polyherbal group (1.79). This finding was also observed by Korde *et al.* (2011) where supplementation of same polyherbs (consists of *Phyllanthus emblica, Withania somnifera, Magnifera indica, Ocimum sanctum)* premix to the broilers increased live body weight and weight gain and shown a better feed efficiency compared with control birds. However, the feed efficiency in synthetic vitamin C supplemented group (1.86) differed non-significantly from untreated control group (1.92).

6.2.4.1 Egg Production

Many studies have demonstrated that herbs improved egg production in stress conditions. Jadhav *et al.* (2013) observed that the mean egg production (%) was lower in control group (75.9%) than polyherbs with natural vitamin C supplemented group (80.8%). Egg production was also improved over synthetic vitamin C supplemented group (78.2%). Jadhav *et al.* (2013) reported higher mean egg weight due to supplementation of polyherbs with natural vitamin C supplemented group (58.6 g) followed by synthetic vitamin C supplemented group (56.8 g) than untreated control group (55.0 g).

6.2.4.2 Biochemical Analysis

Several studies demonstrated that heat stress causes an increased free radical production (Halliwell and Gutteridge, 1989; Sujatha *et al.*, 2010) and induces production and release of corticosteroids (Siegal, 1980). It exerts catabolic effects (mobilization of proteins and lipids) through muscle wasting and reduces growth rate (Sujatha *et al.*, 2010; Hayashi *et al.*, 1994). It was stated that by decreasing synthesis and secretion of corticosteroids, vitamin C alleviates the negative effects of stress such as heat or cold stress-related depression in performance of poultry (Kutlu and Forbes, 1993). Jadhav *et al.* (2013) and Sujatha *et al.* (2010) reported that polyherbal antistressor premix (which consists of *Phyllanthus emblica, Withania somnifera, Magnifera indica, Ocimum sanctum* @1 kg/tonne of feed) used to minimize heat stress in broilers during summer months decreased serum cortosol levels and aminotransferase enzyme activities.

6.3. Overcrowding

Overcrowding is another important common stressor in poultry, which ultimately results in poor production and growth (Rosales, 1994). Flooring system and stocking density affect the performance of birds by inflicting additional stress on birds, thus deteriorating growth and feed efficiency (Takahashi *et al.*, 1991). Overcrowding also increases the exposure to disease causing organism (Rosales, 1994). With increased environmental temperatures and overcrowding stress, feed utilization efficiency is decreased (Rosales, 1994). Overcrowding stress also alters the biochemical profile of birds which is the 'indicator of stress' (Rosales, 1994).

6.3.1 Herbs to Ameliorate Stress due to Overcrowding

6.3.1.1 Growth and Performance Parameter

The herbs are scientifically proved for their anti-stressor, immunomodulator, adaptogenic and performance enhancing property (Oyagbemi *et al.*, 2008). Pandurang *et al.* (2011) used one polyherbal formulation which consists of *Phyllanthus emblica, Withania somnifera, Magnifera indica, Ocimum sanctum* and many more. Pandurang *et al.* (2011) reported that the average body weight of birds was (1808±7.99 g) significantly lower in experimental group (25% less space) than group (polyherbs +25% less space). Experimental group (50% less space) showed significant decrease in body weight (1750±8.85g) as compared to experimental group (50% less space + polyherbs), (1781±5.99g). Similar results were also reported in other studies (Camci and Erensayin, 2004; Thomas *et al.*, 2004). Singh and Sharma (2003) reported depression in body weight in birds exposed to overcrowding at 0.75 sq.ft./bird and 0.50 sq.ft./bird. The adverse effect of overcrowding stress resulted in poor growth, performance and (feed conversion ratio) FCR of broilers. Singh and Sharma, (2003) revealed that overcrowding resulted in poor FCR and depression in body weight gain. The birds of therapeutic groups (50% less space + polyherbs) showed better FCR (1.45) as compared to positive control group (50% less space) with FCR of 1.68. However, no significant variation in feed intake was evident throughout experiment among the experimental groups. Rajmane (1996) also observed that supplementation of same polyherb (consisting of *Phyllanthus emblica, Withania somnifera, Magnifera indica, Ocimum sanctum)* in stress conditions, help in improving body weight gain and FCR. Results reveal a significant improvement in the body weight and feed conversion in polyherbs administered group in contrast to overcrowding stressed birds owing to the immunomodulating and antistress properties of the constituent herb.

6.3.1.2 Haematological and Biochemical Parameters

The reduction in floor space induced marked increase in stress which is manifested by changes in haematological indices. Birds exposed to overcrowding stress resulted in elevation of serum glucose level (Puvadolpirods and Thaxton, 2000; Olanrewaju *et al.*, 2006). Elevation in haemoglobin (Hb) level was evident in the untreated group (25% less space) and treated group (50% less space) due to overcrowding stress. Haemoconcentration in overcrowding stress is the result of less supply of oxygen to birds resulting in hypoxia, which is a stimulus for erythropoietin secretion and leads to erythropoiesis in stressed birds. The values of Hb concentration of the therapeutic groups on day 15 and 30 significantly reduced compared with the groups with space of 0.75 sq. ft/bird and 0.5 sq. ft/bird. Their findings corroborated with the findings of Dhal *et al.* (1997) and Cheng *et al.* (2000). Similar findings were noticed by Hocking *et al.* (1994); Saxena and Madan (1997), according to whom, overcrowding results in leucocytopenia, eosinopenia and lowers the monocyte and heterophil counts in broiler birds. The evidence of reduction in TLC was concomitant with Saxena and Madan (1997). However, supplementation of polyherbal formulation containing *Phyllanthus emblica, Withania somnifera, Magnifera indica, Ocimum sanctum* and many more in feed to birds under overcrowding stress has led to normalization of haematological values in therapeutic groups at different intervals of study. The normalization in the haematological blood values may be attributed to the efficacy of individual constituent herbs which consist of *Withania somnifera, Ocimum sanctum, Mangifera indica, Phyllanthus emblica and Shilajit* in ameliorating stress and restoring haematobiochemical profile.

6.3.1.3 Pathological Changes

Stress due to overcrowding is known to exert various detrimental effects, which can also be observed as lesions on gross organs, such as liver, kidney, spleen and lungs. For gross pathological studies, organs selected were liver, lung, heart, spleen, kidney and brain. Stress due to overcrowding (50% less space) revealed hepatomegaly, paleness with petechial haemorrhages on liver, while severe congestion was evident on lungs with slight enlargement (Pandurang *et al.,* 2011). The rest of the organs did not reveal any appreciable changes. However, the lesions were found to be normalized in polyherbal treated groups. The gross observations of the present study were in accordance with those of Ghodasara *et al.* (1990) and Takahashi *et al.* (2000). The recovery of the gross pathological lesions after treatment with polyherbal antistressor and immunomodulator product was evident in therapeutic groups. Oyagbemi *et al.* (2008) also reported that polyherbal formulation possesses the hepatoprotective and immunomodulator properties and has ameliorative action in the stressed broiler as evident on histopathological examination.

6.4 Mechanism of Action/Active Principle of Herbs

Many active components of herbs and spices can prevent lipid peroxidation through quenching free radicals or through activation of antioxidant enzymes like superoxide dismutase, catalase, glutathione peroxidase and glutathione reductase. Main molecules responsible for the anti-oxidative properties of herbs and spices are phenolic substances (flavonoids, hydrolysable tannins, proanthocianidins, phenolic acids, phenolic terpenes) and some vitamins (E, C and A). Often used herbs rich in phenolics are rosemary, thyme, oregano, sage, green tea, chamomile, ginko, dandelion and marigold.

Studies have shown that the active agents in the herbs have a strong capability of scavenging superoxide dismutase radicals, hydrogen peroxide and nitric oxide from activated macrophages, reducing iron complex and inhibiting lipid per-oxidation (Gowda *et. al.*, 2009). It has been shown that plant phenoloic components like carbacrol and thymol are responsible for antioxidant activity (Schwarz *et al.* 1996). Apart from these compounds, other phenolics such as caffeic acid, p-cymene-2,3-diol and biphenylic as well as flavonoid compounds have been found to exhibit antioxidant activity (Bolukbasi *et al.*, 2006). Zhang *et al.* (2009) stated that supplementation of ginger at the rate of 5g/kg significantly increased activities of superoxide dismutase and glutathione peroxidase and reduced melonyl dialdehyde concentration in broilers at the age of 21 and 42 days.

6.5 Summary and Conclusions

Heat and overcrowding stress depresses the overall growth and performance of the chicken. Supplementation of herbs containing bioactive compounds such as natural vitamin C, essential oils and bioflavonoids diet improves growth performance, egg production and feed conversion efficiency. Serum biochemical and haematological parameters are improved after the herbal treatment. Simultaneously, herbs improve immune response in supplemented animals. Thus, it may be recommended to use herbal formulation to curb the losses incurred from stress.

References

Abdel-Fattah S A, Ei-Sanhour Y M, Ei-Mednay H N M, Abdul-Azeem F (2008) Thyroid activity of broiler chicks fed supplemental organic acids. Int J Poult Sci 7: 215-222

Ajakaiye J J, Perez-Bello A,Mollineda T A(2011) Impact of heat stress on egg quality in layer hens supplemented with l-ascorbic acid and dl-tocopherol acetate. Veterinarski Archive 81: 119-132

Alçiçek A, Bozkurt M, Çabuk M (2004) The effects of a mixture of herbal essential oil, an organic acid or a probiotic on broiler performance. S Afr J AnimSci 34: 217–222

Alçiçek A, Bozkurt M, Çabuk M (2003) The effects of an essential oil combination derived from selected herbs growing wild in Turkey on broiler performance. S Afr J Anim Sci 33: 89-94

Balnave D (2004) Challenges of accurately defining the nutrient requirements of heat-stressed poultry. Poult Sci 83:5-14

Balnave D, Muheereza SK (1997) Improving eggshell quality at high temperatures with dietary sodium bicarbonate. Poult Sci 76: 558-593

Balogun TF, Afolayan SB, Njoku FC, Dafwang II (1996) Effect of Ascorbic Acid and Acetylsalicylic Acid supplementation of broiler diets on performance during the hot season. Samaru J Agric Educ 5: 80-86

Bölükbasi S C, Erhan MK,Ozkan (2006) Effect of dietary thyme oil and vitamin E on growth, lipid oxidation, meat fatty acid composition and serum lipoproteins of broilers. S Afr J Anim Sci 36: 189-196

Botsoglou NA, Florou-Paneri P, Christaki E, Fletouris DJ, Spais AB (2002) Effect of dietary oregano essential oils on performance of chickens and on iron-induced lipid oxidation of breast, thigh and abdominal fat tissues. Br Poult Sci 43: 223-230

Bozkurt M, Alçiçek A, Çabuk M, Kuçukyilmaz K,Çatli A U(2009) Effect of an herbal essential oils mixture on growth, laying traits, and egg hatching characteristics of broiler breeders. Poult Sci 88: 2368-2374

Cabuk MM, Bozkurt A, Alcicek Y, Akbas Y, Kucukylmaz K (2006) Effect of a herbal essential oils mixture on growth and internal organ weight of broilers from young and old breeder flocks. S Afr J Anim Sci 36: 135-141

Celik L, Ozturkcan O (2003) Effects of dietary supplemental L-carnitine and ascorbic acid on performance, carcass composition and plasma L-carnitine concentration of broiler chicks reared under different temperature. Archives Tier 57: 27-38

Cheng H, Li, Zhao C Ming D,Li, QH(2000) Mechanism of ascites in broiler. I. Effect of low temperature on haematological parameters and broilers incidences. J China Agric Univ 5: 111-116

Daghir NJ (2009) Nutritional strategies to reduce heat stress in broilers and broiler breeders. Loh Inform 44: 6-15

Dhal SK, Misra SC, Misra PK, Dehuri PK, Mohapatra M, Misra, MS (1997) Study on the extent of protection by 'Zeetress' against heat stress on the growth of broiler birds. Indian J Indigenous Med 19: 75-77

Ghodasara DJ, Durrani FR, Imran N, Durrani Z, Zahir-Ud D, Ahmed J, Chand N (1990) Effect of summer stress on pathobiochemical changes in chickens. Pak Vet J 22: 111-115

Gowda KS, Ledouxa D R, Rottinghausa G E, Bermudeja AJ, Chena YC (2009) Antioxidant efficacy of curcuminoids from turmeric (Curcuma longa L.) powder in broiler chickens fed diets containing aflatoxin B1. Br J Nutr 102: 1629-1634

Halliwell BE,Gutteridge JMC (1989) Lipid peroxidation: A radical chain reaction. Pages 188–218 in Free Radicals in Biology and Medicine. 2nd ed. Oxford University Press, New York, NY

Hayashi K, Nagai Y, Ohtsuka A, Tomita Y (1994) Effects of dietary corticosterone and trilostane on growth and skeletal muscle protein turnover in broiler cockerels. Br Poult Sci 35: 789-798

Hernandez F, Madrid J, Garcia V, Orengo J, Megias M D(2004) Influence of two plant extracts on broiler performance, digestibility, and digestive organ size. Poult Sci 83: 169-174

Hocking PM, Maxwell MH, Mitchell MA (1994) Haematology and blood composition at two ambient temperatures in genetically restricted through life. Br Poult Sci 35: 799-807

Jadhav NV, Awati B, Kulkarni S, Waghmare G, Suranagi MD, Ravikanth K, Dandale M, Maini S (2013) Heat stress amelioration and production performance in layers supplemented with herbal liquid anti-stressor product. J Vet Med Anim Health 6: 69-74

Khan SH, Sardar R (2005) Effect of vitamin C supplementation on the performance of Desi, Faoumi and commercial White Leghorn chicken exposed to heat stress. Pak Vet J 25: 136-166

Korde JP, Bahiram KB, Sharma M, Jagtap DG, Shirbhate RN (2011) Effect on growth performance and thyroid hormones in broilers supplemented with AV/LAP/19, ascorbic acid and Ayucee premix during summer. Compendium of Society of Animal Physiologists of India (SAPI), Sustainable Livestock and Poultry Production, VI.P.16: 250

Kutlu HR, Forbes JM (1993) Changes in growth and blood parameters in heat-stressed broiler chicks in response to dietary ascorbic acid. Livest Prod Sci 36: 335–350

Lee KW, Everts H, Kappert H J, Frehner ,Losa R, Beynen G (2003) Effects of dietary essential oils components on growth performance, digestive enzymes and lipid metabolism in female broiler chickens. Br Poult Sci 44: 450-457

Mahmoud KZ, Edens FW, Eisen EJ, Havenstein GB (2004) Ascorbic acid decreases heat shock protein 70 and plasma corticosterone response in broilers (Gallus gallusdomesticus) subjected to cyclic heat stress. Comp Biochem Physiol. B 137: 35-42

Maini S, Rastogi SK, Korde JP, Madan A K, Shukla S K (2007) Evaluation of oxidative stress and its amelioration through certain antioxidants in broilers during summer. J Poult. Sci. 44: 339-347

Mashaly M M, Hendricks GL, Kalama M A, Gehad AE, Abbas AO,Patterson P H(2004) Effect of heat stress on production parameters and immune responses of commercial laying hens. Poult. Sci. 83: 889-894

Mckee JS, Hurrison PC (1995) Effects of supplemental ascorbic acid on the performance of broiler chickens exposed to multiple concurrent stressors. Poult Sci 74: 1772-1785

Mckee JS, Hurrison PC, Riskowski GL (1997) Effects of supplemental ascorbic acid on the energy conversion of broiler chicks during heat stress and feed withdrawal. Poult Sci 76: 1278-1286

Munj CP, Ranade AS, Desai DN, Patil MB, Avari PE, Patil UM, Metkari DV (2010) Synergistic effects of feed additives on performance of broilers. Indian J Poult Sci 45: 292-296

Sejian V, Valtorta S, Gallorda M, Singh AK (2012)Ameliorative measures to counteract environmental stress. In: Environmental Stress and Amelioration in Livestock Production Sejian V, Naqvi S M K, Ezeji T, Lal R(eds.) Springer pp. 153-180

NRC (1981) Effect of Environment on Nutrient Requirements of Domestic Animals. National Academy Press, Washington DC

Orban JI, Roland DA, Cummins K, Lovell RT (1993) Influence of large doses of ascorbic acid on performance, plasma calcium, bone characteristics and egg shell quality in broilers and Leghorn hens. Poult Sci 72: 691-700

Oyagbemi AA, Saba AB, Arowolo ROA (2008) Safety Evaluation of Prolonged Administration of Stresroak in Grower Cockerels. Int J Poult Sci 7: 574-578

Pande CB (2002) Herbal formulation as a promising adaptogenic, antistress and immunomodulatory-A review. Poult Fortune 4: 32-35

Pandurang LT, Kulkarni, GB, Gangane GR, More PR, Ravikanth K, Maini S, Deshmukh VV, Yeotikar PV (2011) Overcrowding Stress Management in Broiler Chicken with Herbal Antistressor. Iranian J Appl Anim Sci 1: 49-55

Pardue SL, Thaxton JP, Brake J (1985) Role of ascorbic acid in chicks exposed to high environmental temperature. J Appl Physiol 58: 1511-1516

Park KW, Rhee AR, Um JS, Paik IK (2009) Effect of dietary avaliable phosphorus and organic acids on the performance and quality of laying hens. J Appl Poult Res 18: 598-604

Patra AK (2012) An Overview of Antimicrobial Properties of Different Classes of Phytochemicals. In: Dietary Phytochemicals and Microbes (Ed. Patra, A. K.), Springer, The Netherlands, pp. 1-32

Patra A K, Saxena J (2011)Exploitation of dietary tannins to improve rumen metabolism and ruminant nutrition. J Sci Food Agric 91: 24-37

Patra A K, Saxena J (2010) A new perspective on the use of plant secondary metabolites to inhibit methanogenesis in the rumen. Phytochemistry 71: 1198-1222

Rajmane BV (1996) Effect of stresroak in stress conditions on broiler performance. BiotechnologijaYogoslavistocarstvu 215-218

Ramnath V, Rekha PS, Sujatha KS (2008) Amelioration of heat stress induced disturbances of antioxidant defense system in chicken by Brahma Rasayana. Evid. Based Complement.Alternat. Med. 5: 77-84

Rindhe S, Ravikanth K, Maini S, Suryawanshi S U, Khose K K,Waghmare R N(2012) Role of polyherbal antistressor product in improving meat quality attributes in broilers. Compendium of International Poultry Science Forum, Atlanta, USA, Jan 23-24, 2012, pp. 4

Rosales AG (1994) Managing Stress in Broiler Breeders: A Review. J Appl Poult Res 3: 199-207

Sahin K, Kucuk O (2003) Heat stress and dietary vitamin supplementation of poultry diets. Nutr Abstr Rev Ser. B Livest Feeds Feeding 73: 41R–50R

Sahin K, Onderci M, Sahin N, Gursu M F,Kucuk O (2003) Dietary vitamin C and folic acid supplementation ameliorates the detrimental effects of heat stress in Japanese quail. J Nutr 133: 1882-1888

[a]ahin K, [a]ahin N, Kucuk O, Hayirli A, Prasad AS (2009) Role of dietary zinc in heat-stressed poultry: A review. Poult Sci 88: 2176-2183

Sahin K, Sahin N, Onderci M, Gursu F, Cikim G (2002) Optimal dietary concentration of chromium for alleviating the effect of heat stress on growth, carcass qualities, and some serum metabolites of broiler chickens. Biol Trace Elem Res 89: 53-64

Saxena MJ, Madan P (1997) Herbals for stress management in pets. Ther Vet 21: 11-14

Schwarz K, ErnstH, Ternes W (1996). Evaluation of antioxidative constituents from thyme. J Sci Food Agric 70: 217-223

Shukla PK, Srivastava PK (1999) Beneficial effect of Stresroak and Livfit Vet supplementation in post infection hydro-pericardium syndrome cases. Indian Vet Med J 23: 335-337

Siegal HS (1980) Physiological stress in birds. Bio-science 30: 529-534

Singh GP, Sharma ML (2003) Effect of stocking density on the performance of commercial broilers. Ann Biol 19: 255-258

Sujatha V, Korde JP, Rastogi SK, Maini S, Ravikanth K, Rekhe DS (2010) Amelioration of heat stress induced disturbances of the antioxidant defence system in broilers. J Vet Med Anim Health 2: 18-28

Takahashi K, Nishimura H, Akiba Y, Horiguchi M (1991) Effect of stocking density and supplemental ascorbic acid on growth, organ weight, mixed function oxidase in hepatic microsomes, lipid metabolism and plasma corticosterone in male broiler chicks. Anim Sci Technol 62: 829-838

Talebi E, Khademi M (2011) Combination effects of ascorbic acid and glucose in drinking water on the broiler performance under acute heat stress. Int J Appl Biol Pharm Technol 2: 92-96

Teeter RG, Smith MO, Owens FN, Arp SC, Sangiagh S, Breazil JE (1985) Chronic heat stress and respiratory alkalosis: Occurrence and treatment in broiler chicks. Poult Sci 64: 1060-1064

Thomas D, Ravindran V, Thomas DV, Camden BJ, Cottam YH, Morel PH, Cook CJ (2004) Influence of stocking density on the performance, carcass characteristics and selected welfare indicators of broiler chicken. *Newzeland Vet J* 52: 76-81

Ye°ilbag D, Çolpan I (2006) Effects of organic acid supplemented diets on growth performance, egg production and quality and on serum parameters in laying hens. Rev Med Vet 157: 280-284

Zapata LF, Gernat, AG (1995) The effect of four levels of ascorbic acid and two levels of calcium on egg shell quality of forced molted White Leghorn hens. Poult Sci 74: 1049-1052

Zhang KY, Yan F, Keen CA, Waldroup PW (2009) Evaluation of microencapsulated essential oils and organic acids in diets for broiler chickens. Int J Poult Sci 4: 612–619.

❑❑❑

Chapter 7

Ethnoveterinary Perspective of Indian Herbal System

Tara Bothra, Neha Sharma, Dinesh Jain, Umesh Kumar Prajapat

College of Veterinary and Animal Sciences, Rajasthan University of Veterinary and Animal Sciences, Bikaner, Rajasthan, India, E-mail.: ddineshvet@gmail.com

ABSTRACT

Ethnoveterinary is a holistic inter-disciplinary study of the local knowledge and the socio-cultural structures and environment associated with animal health care and husbandry. Some of the commonly used herbs in ethnoveterinary practices in India are *Ocimum sanctum, Curcuma longa, Allium sativum, Zingiber officinale, Asparagus racemosus, Withania somnifera, Nigella sativa, Aloe vera, Tinospora cordifolia,* etc. These herbs possess, antibacterial, anti-inflammatory, immunomodulatory activities, etc. These herbs are used to treat mastitis, tympany, internal parasite, retention of placenta, constipation, diarrhoea, skin disease, etc. Limitations of ethnoveterinary are that herbs are not easily quantifiable and standardized due to their complex composition. Besides these, the traditional knowledge of ethnoveterinary practices by various communities not being documented properly is deteriorating due to lack of awareness and incomplete knowledge as being transferred by words of mouth. India has acquired great traditional background in ethnoveterinary medicine and practices. Therefore, it becomes essential to conserve these medicinal plants with miraculous properties, both genetically as well as culturally.

Keywords: Ethnoveterinary, Traditional knowledge, Animal health, Antibacterial, Anti-inflammatory.

7.1 Introduction

Indian system of medicines has a deep root in our cultural inheritance and provide medicare to major sections of our population. India has a very unique distinction of having six recognized traditional medicinal systems-Ayurveda, Siddha, Unani and Yoga, Naturopathy and Homeopathy. These systems are even stated in the ancient Vedas and other scriptures. The Ayurvedic concept emerged and developed between 2500 and 500 BC in India (Subhose *et al.,* 2005). The literal meaning of Ayurveda is "science of life." These ancient systems of medicines mainly use herbs. India has a rich biodiversity in flora and is the largest producer of medicinal plants, out of 20,000 medicinal plants recorded, conventional practitioners use only 7,000 to 7,500 plants for curing different heath problems. The proportion of use of these medicinal plants in different Indian systems of medicine is Ayurveda 2000, Siddha 1300, Unani 1000, Homeopathy 800, Tibetan 500, Modern 200, and folk 4500. Along with this, around 25,000 efficient plant-based formulations are used in traditional and folk medicine.

7.2 Concept and History of Ethnobotanical and Ethnoveterinary Practices

Ethnobotany is defined as the experience of the humans, who observed birds and animals and tested leaves, fruits and tubers for their animals and their capability to heal wounds and satisfy hunger. Indian epics and ancient literature are stated with references to plants (Jain, 2000). Ethnobotanical studies in India initiated long before the term was coined with collection of information by Watt (1889-1896) in association with the compilation of his dictionary, about a century ago. There is tremendous scope for the study of literature for ethnobotanical knowledge in India because of the vast legacy of vedic literature, which dates back to 2000-1000 B.C. Studies on ethnobotany knowledge and practices were instigated by the economic botany section of Botanical Survey of India since 1954.

Ethnoveterinary practices in India were in vogue since time immemorial. In ancient India, the Vedic literature, predominantly Atharvaveda is a repository of traditional medicine together with prescriptions for treatment of animal diseases. Scriptures such as Skanda Purana, Devi Purana, Matsya Purana, Agni Purana, Garuda Purana, Linga Purana, and books written by Charaka, Susruta, Palakapya (1000 BC), and Shalihotra (2350 BC) documented treatment of various animal diseases using medicinal herbs. Ethnoveterinary medicine (EVM) is a holistic inter-disciplinary study of the local knowledge and the socio-cultural structures and environment associated with animal health care and husbandry (McCorkle, 1986). Hence, for optimum productivity of animals along with their sound health, traditional healing practices have been applied for centuries and have been passed down orally from generation-to-generation. It has also appeared as a productive field for the development and transfer of sustainable veterinary alternatives to people everywhere but, especially to third world stock-raisers (De Haan and Bekure, 1991; Schillhorn van veen, 1991).Widespread interest in validating and documenting ethnoveterinary knowledge and practices arose in the early 1980s in India. The three basic elements of EVM are application of natural products, appeal to spiritual forces and manipulation and surgery. Natural products used in EVM are medicinal plants and by-products, edible earth and minerals and parts and products of animals.

Plants are mainly used as ingredients in the preparation of ethnoveterinary medicines. The active principles responsible for the activity of these medicinal plants have diverse structures which fall into four main chemical classes - the phenolics (phenols, flavonoids, quinines, tannins and lignins), terpenoids (monoterpenes, lactones, diterpenes, saponins and others), sulphur compounds (glucosilates, disulphides, acetylenic and thiophenes) and nitrogen compounds (alkaloids, amines, non-protein amino-acids and cyanogenetic glycosides). Certain organic acids and polyacetylenes are also known to exist (Cotton, 1996). The traditional knowledge on ethnoveterinary practices by local healers who are quite experienced in these traditional systems of medicines is important, but their acquaintance are not very well documented and is dwindling fast. It is also pointed out that the knowledge of ethnomedicinal plants is on the edge of irreversible loss and declining due to only oral passage of traditional herbal heritage from one generation to another rather than in writings, in spite of their vital role in furnishing health of human and livestock population. As most of the animal husbandry practices are taken up by rural people and small landholdings, low income, lesser veterinary facilities and a minimal exposure to new products and technology make it hard for the farmers to have high monetary gains from livestock. Therefore, a thorough study and documentation of these herbal medicines and ethnoveterinary practices shall bring an alternative cheap, economic and easily accessible way of augmenting production of animals, thus the income of farmers.

7.3 Common Ethnoveterinary Herbs used in India

Some of the commonly used herbs in ethnoveterinary practices in India by large sections of rural populations are enlisted in Table 1 and their nutritional values are given in Table 2. These herbs or their preparations with others play a very important therapeutic role in various diseases in livestock sector because of their phytoconstituents and active principles (Table 3). Based on the research and studies, these herbal preparations have established their utility and pharmacological properties. There are number of plants, plant extracts and constituents which are well-known as having anti-microbial, antiviral or antifungal activities and are often considered as immune enhancer (Rios and Recio, 2005).

7.3.1 Zingiber officinale

Ginger (*Zingiber officinale*) is a flowering plant whose rhizome or ginger root, is extensively used as a spice or a folk medicine. It is a herbaceous perennial plant which grows annual pseudostems (false stems made of the rolled bases of leaves) about a meter tall bearing narrow leaf blades. The inflorescences bear pale yellow with purple flowers and grow directly from the rhizome on separate shoots (Fig. 1).

Taxonomy

Kingdom	:	Plantae
Clade	:	Angiosperms
Clade	:	Monocots
Clade	:	Commelinids
Order	:	Zingiberales

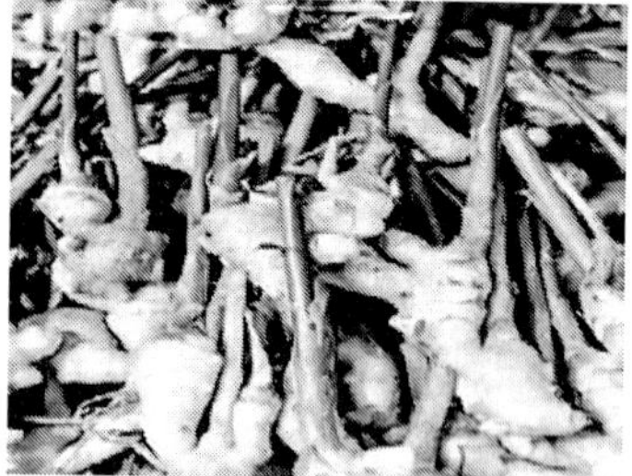

Fig. 1: *Zingiber officinale*

Ginger is in the family Zingiberaceae, to which also belong turmeric (*Curcuma longa*) and cardamom (*Elettaria cardamomum*). Ginger originated in the tropical rainforests from the Indian subcontinent to Southern Asia where ginger plants show considerable genetic variation (Everett, 1982). It has been used in EVM for centuries and has great therapeutic value. *Zingiber officinale* is used by communities of Himalayan region in India to treat heamaturia, eye diseases and indigestion (Tiwari and Pande, 2010). In case of poisoning, rhizomes of ginger are dried and mixed with black salt and given orally to animal. Also, the dried rhizome, commonly called as Sunth, is given during excessive fall of temperature in northern region of India (Sharma *et al.,* 2012).

In some communities of Rajasthan, dried tubers powder of ginger and black pepper is boiled and used to cure stomache in animals. Bolus prepared from the mixture of dried ginger, *Allium sativum* is used to cure pneumonia and paralysis (Galav *et al.,* 2013). Haniadka *et al.* (2013) reported that ginger has protective actions which are mediated through free radical scavenging, antioxidant, cytoprotective, and to adjust the levels of the detoxifying enzymes. *Zingiber officinale* extract exhibits free radical scavenging and reducing power (Mohd Amir, 2011). Xiao-Lan Cheng (2011) studied the antiproliferative effect of steamed ginger at 120pC for 4 hrs. which turned out to be approximately 1.5 and 2-fold higher than that of dried and fresh ginger. The effect of ability of *Zingiber officinale* extract to prevent gastric ulcerations induced by HCl and ethanol (Penna, 2003). *In vivo* antihelmintic activity of *Zingiber officinale* in sheep is also reported (Iqbal *et al.,* 2006).

Table 1: Commonly used Indian herbs in ethnoveterinary medicine

Common Name/ Vernacular Name	Scientific Name	Parts used
Holy basil/ Tulsi	*Ocimum sanctum*	Whole plant, root, leaf, seed
Turmeric/Haldi	*Curcuma longa*	Rhizome
Garlic /Lehsun	*Allium sativum*	Buds
Ginger/Adrak	*Zingiber officinale*	Rhizome
Asparagus /Shatavar	*Asparagus racemosus*	Roots
Indian ginseng/ Ashwagandha	*Withania somnifera*	Root, leaves, seeds
Black cumin/Kalongi	*Nigella sativa*	Seeds
Heart leaved moonseed/Giloy	*Tinospora cordifolia*	Stem
Corriander/Dhaniya	*Coriandrum sativum*	Leaves , seeds
Fenugreek/Methi	*Trigonella foenumgraecum*	Seeds, leaves
Cloves/ Laung	*Syzygium aromaticum*	Clove
Cinnamon	*Cinnamomum cassia*	Bark
Mint/Pudina	*Mentha piperita*	Leaves
Jivanti	*Leptadenia reticulata*	Leaves and Twigs
Bhringraj/False daisy	*Eclpta alba*	Leaves
Indian gooseberry/Amla	*Emblica officianlis*	Fruits
Liquorice/Mulethi	*Glyacerrahezza glabra*	Roots & Rhizomes
Ajwain	*Trachyspermum ammi*	Seeds
Golden apple/Bael	*Agele marmoles*	Fruit
Aloe vera/ Guar-pantha	*Aloe vera*	Leaves

Table 2: Nutritional value (% DM basis) of some commomly used Indian herbs in ethnoveterinary medicine

Name	DM	CP	EE	CF	Ash	Reference
Ocimum sanctum (Dry leaves)	88.56	6.56	2.91	9.50	6.00	Barua *et al.*, 2015
Curcuma longa (Rhizome)	87-94	6-8	5-10	2-7	-	Nelson *et al.*, 2017
Allium sativum (Bulb)	95.45	15.33	0.72	2.10	4.08	Otunola *et al.*, 2010
Zingiber officinale (Rhizome)	93.63	8.58	5.35	3.25	6.30	Otunola *et al.*, 2010
Asparagus racemosus (Roots)	90.00	7.00	0.80	20.40	6.40	Bhardwaj 2009
Withania somnifera (Whole plant)	84.32	6.26	6.89	44.00	6.93	Hameed and Hussain 2015
Nigella sativa (Seeds)	93.00	20.80	34.80	-	3.70	Atta 2003
Tinospora cordifolia (Leaves)	90.36	5.23	1.05	52.50	5.88	Pandey et al.2016
Coriandrum sativum (Leaves)	14.29	4.05	0.95	5.24	1.90	Shahwar *et al.*, 2012
Trigonella foenum-graecum	93.26	24.13	7.07	10.76	3.68	Abbas, 2010

Table 3: Phytochemical constituents of commonly used herbs

Herb	Phytochemical constituents
Ocimum sanctum	Oleanolic acid, rosmarinic acid, ursolic acid, eugenol, carvacrol, linalool, β-caryophyllene (about 8%)
Curcma longa	Diarylheptanoids, curcuminoids such as curcumin, demethoxycurcumin, and bisdemethoxycurcumin, essential oils like turmerone, germacrone, zingiberene and atlantone
Allium sativum	γ-glutamyl-S-alk(en)yl-L-cysteines and S-alk (en)yl-L-cysteinesulfoxides, alliin
Zingiber Officinale	6-gingerol, 6-shogaol and paradol
Asparagus Racemosus	Asparagamine A, steroidal saponins, shatavaroside A, shatavaroside B, filiasparoside C, shatavarins, schidigerasaponin D5 (or asparanin A) and immunosideisoflavone 8-methoxy-5,6,4'-trihydroxy isoflavne 7-*O*-β-D gluco-pyranoside
Withania Somnifera	Tropine, cuscohygrine , steroidal lactones, withanolides and withaferin A
Nigella sativa	Linoleic acid, oleic acid, palmitic acid, and transanethole
Tinospora Cordifolia	Columbin, tinosporaside, palmatine, berberine, jatrorhizine, tembeterine, tinocordifolioside, phenylpropene disaccharides, choline, tinosporal, tinosporic acid and tinosporon
Coriandrum Sativum	Flavonoids include quercitin, kaempferol, rhamnetin, and epigenin
Trigonella foenum-graecum	Flavonoids, alkaloids, coumarins, and saponins; trigonelline and coumarins include cinnamic acid and scopoletin

7.3.1 *Asparagus racemosus*

Asparagus racemosus (shatavar, shatavari, or shatamull) is a species of asparagus common all over Nepal, Sri Lanka, India and the Himalayas. It grows 1–2 m (3 ft 3 in–6 ft 7 in) tall and preferably take root in gravelly, rocky soils high up in piedmont plains, at 1,300–1,400 m (4,300–4,600 ft) elevation. It was botanically described in 1799 (USDA). It has small pine-needle-like phylloclades (photosynthetic branches) that are shiny green and uniform. In the month of July, it produces minute, white flowers, spiky stems, and in September it fruits, generating blackish-purple, globular berries (Fig. 2).

Taxonomy

Kingdom	:	Plantae
Clade	:	Angiosperms
Clade	:	Monocots
Order	:	Asparagales
Family	:	Asparagaceae
Subfamily	:	Asparagoideae
Genus	:	Asparagus
Species	:	*A. racemosus*

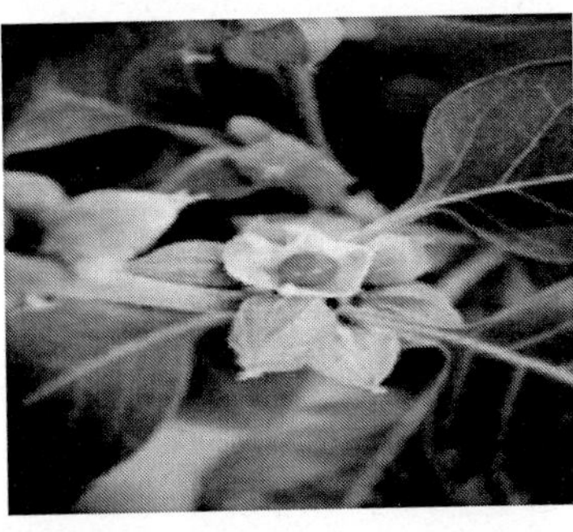

Fig. 2: *Asparagus racemosus*

Asparagus racemosus is well known for its medicinal properties and it is quite popular in traditional and folk medicines. Crushed tuberous roots are mixed with water and given to milch animals to enhance milk yield in Madhya Pradesh (India) (Patil *et al.*, 2015). Decoction of roots is given in sub-Himalayan tracts to cure knee pain (Gaur *et al.*, 2010). As a traditional medicine, 300 grams of root is crushed and mixed in buttermilk and given for a week for treatment of arthritis in cattle in Karnataka (India) (Harsha *et al.*, 2005). Roots of *Asparagus racemosus* were generally used after post-partum for healing and reformation or involution of uterus (Deshmukh *et al.*, 2011). Chauhan *et al.* (1971) reported that Leptaden® tablet containing *Asparagus racemosus* as a major component enhanced the milk production significantly in crossbred cows. Many studies showed the synergistic effect of polyherbal immunomodulator alongwith antibiotic therapy in treatment of subclinical mastitis in cows. Choudhary and Kar (1992) studied mineral composition of *Asparagus racemosus* and found Ca, Mg, K, Fe content to be 0.22, 0.4, 2.5 and 0.005g/100g respectively, whereas,micro-minerals Cu, Zn, Mn, Co and Cr were 5.29, 53.15, 19.98, 22, 1.81μg/g respectively.High concentration of micromineral suggests its role in improving reproductive efficiency and immunopotentiation. Supplementation of *Asparagus racemosus* root powder at 5 and 10% level reduces plasma and hepatic lipid level and also decreases lipid peroxidation (Visavadiya and Narasimhacharya, 2005). The juice, extracted from leaves and fruits is applied in case of animals suffering from diseases of foot. Chloroform/ methanol (1:1) extract of fresh root of *Asparagus racemosus* has been reported to reduce the tumour incidence in female rats treated with DMBA (7,12- dimethylbenz (a) anthracene) (Rao, 1981). This action is thought to be mediated by virtue of mammotropic or lactogenic effect of A. racemosus on normal as well as estrogen-primed animals, which renders the mammary epithelium refractory to the carcinogen.

Taxonomy

Kingdom	:	Plantae
Clade	:	Angiosperms
Clade	:	Eudicots
Order	:	Ranunculales
Family	:	Menispermaceae
Genus	:	Tinospora
Species	:	*T. cordifolia*

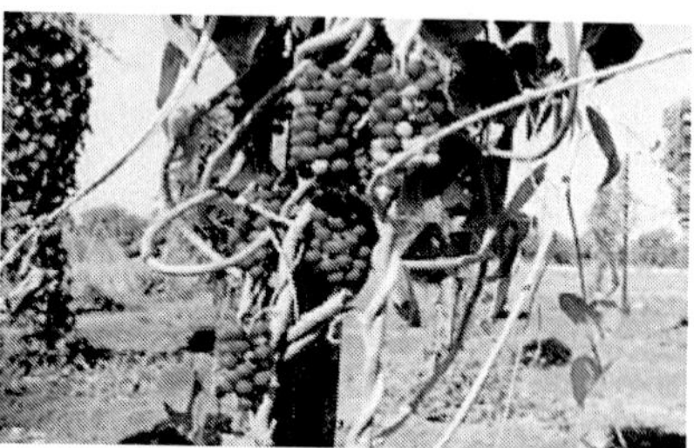

Fig. 3: *Tinospora cordifolia*

7.3.2 Tinospora cordifolia

Tinospora cordifolia, which is known by the common names heart-leaved moonseed, guduchi or giloy, is an herbaceous vine of the family Menispermaceae indigenous to the tropical areas of India, Sri Lanka and Myanmar. It is a large, deciduous shrub with several elongated twining branches. Leaves are simple, alternate, exstipulate, long petioles upto 15 cm long, roundish, pulvinate, both at the base and apex with the basal one longer and twisted partially and half way around. Lamina broadly ovate or ovate cordate, 10–20 cm long or 8–15 cm broad, 7 nerved and deeply cordate at base, membranous, pubescent above, whitish tomentose with a prominent reticulum beneath. Flowers are unisexual with greenish yellow texture on axillary and terminal racemes (Fig. 3).

Tinospora cordifolia is described as adaptogen and immuno-modulator (Dahanukar *et al.*, 1997; Thatte *et al.*, 1994). Stem of *Tinospora cordifolia* is one of the constituents of several ayurvedic and etno-veterinary preparations used in general debility, dyspepsia, fever and urinary diseases. The stem is bitter, stomachic, diuretic (Nayampalli *et al.*, 1988), stimulates bile secretion, allays thirst, burning sensation, and cures jaundice. The stem extract is useful in various skin diseases (Aiyer *et al.*, 1963; Raghunathan *et al.*, 1982). Fresh leaves of *Tinospora cordifolia* are fed to cattle and goat as a galactagogue to increase the flow of milk in Madhya Pradesh (India) (Patil *et al.*, 2015). Solution Tinospora roots with water is given orally to treat debility as a ethnovet practice (Phondani *et al.*, 2010). In Jammu and Kashmir (India), the whole plant is used extensively for increasing the milk yielding capacity of cattle and buffaloes. It removes the general weakness in animals and makes them healthy. Whole plant (200-400gm) is used as galactagogue in West Bengal also (Saha *et al.*, 2013). It is used as aphrodisiac in common ailments of livestock in India (Raikwar and Maurya 2015). Mukherjee *et al.* (2010) used the hydro-methanolic extract standardized dose against bovine subclinical mastitis and concluded that stem of *Tinospora cordifolia* possesses antibacterial and immunomodulatory properties. The alcoholic extract of *Tinospora cordifolia* enhances the differentiation of tumour activaed macrophages to dendritic cell in response to granulocyte, IL-4, TNF (Bishay *et al.*, 2002). This study also revealed that *Tinospora cordifolia* caused significant reduction in serum SGOT, SGPT, ALP, bilirubin and increment in the functional capacities of rat peritoneal macrophages in carbon tetrachloride intoxicated mature rat.

7.3.4 *Allium sativum*

Garlic (*Allium sativum*) is a species in the onion genus, *Allium*. Its close relatives include the onion, leek, chive, shallot and chinese onion. With a long history of human consumption and use, garlic is native to Central Asia and north-eastern Iran. *Allium sativum* is a bulbous plant (Fig. 4). It grows up to 1.2 m (4 ft) in height. It produces hermaphrodite flowers and it is pollinated by bees and other insects. *Allium sativum* was used as a growth promoter in *O. niloticus* (Diab *et al.*, 2002), in which it increased body gain, feed intake, and feed efficiency. It was shown to have broad spectrum activities against bacteria (Gram-positive and Gram-negative) studied *in vitro* as well as *in vivo* and it also possess the greatest anti-helminithic activity which is very popular in ethnoveterinary practices.

Taxonomy

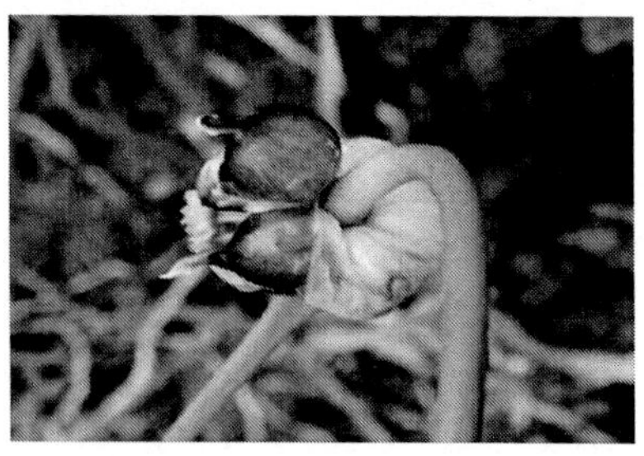

Fig. 4: Allium Sativum

Kingdom : Plantae
Clade : Angiosperms
Clade : Monocots
Order : Asparagales
Family : Amaryllidaceae
Sub-family : Allioideae
Genus : Allium
Species : *A. sativum*

In Rajasthan, paste of onion is prepared by mixing crushed bulbs with two eggs of hen and 1.5 L of milk and given to the animal to treat impaction and lumbago (Galav *et al.,* 2013). Juice of leaves of *Allium sativum* and *Azadirachta indiaca* with water is given orally in case of snakebite as folk medicine in tribal areas (Uttrakhand) (Phondani *et al.,* 2010). Crushed bulbs are mixed with fodder or wheat husks and used by Gujjar communities to get relief from dysentry (Gaur *et al.,* 2010). Cloves are generally being used in food poisoning, arthritis, FMD, tympany, sterility and others in India by animal owners as traditional practice (Tiwari and Pande, 2010). As a part of ethnoveterinary practice by Tharu tribal community in Terai belt of Uttar Pradesh, about 100 g cloves paste is boiled in 500 ml milk and given orally twice a day for 4–5 days to treat fever and cough problems in livestock (Kumar *et al.,* 2012). It has been found in many studies that *Alium sativum* supplementation in cows has improved body weight gain, feed intake and feed conversion efficiency, reduced methane production and also showed antibacterial property. It also possess activities like anti-inflammatory, anti-hyperlipidemic and fibrinolytic (Dixit *et al.,* 2006).

7.3.5 *Curcuma Longa*

Curcuma longa is a rhizomatous herbaceous perennial plant of the family Zingiberaceae. It is native to the Indian Subcontinent and South-east Asia, and requires temperatures between 20 and 30°C and a substantial amount of annual rainfall to thrive. Plants are congregated annually for their rhizomes and propagated from some of those rhizomes in the following season. Turmeric is a perennial herbaceous plant that reaches upto 1 m (3 ft 3 in) tall. It has highly branched, yellow to orange, cylindrical, aromatic rhizomes (Fig. 5). The leaves are alternate and arranged in two rows. The petiole is 50 to 115 cm long. The simple leaf blades are usually 76 to 115 cm long and rarely up to 230 cm (91 in). They have a width of 38 to 45 cm (15–18 in) and are oblong to elliptic, narrowing at the tip. About 34 essential oils are present in turmeric, among which turmerone, germacrone, zingiberene and atlantone are major constituents (Hong *et al.*, 2014; Hu *et al.*, 2014; Bra ga *et al.*, 2003).

Taxonomy

Kingdom	:	Plantae
Clade	:	Angiosperms
Clade	:	Monocots
Clade	:	Commelinids
Order	:	Zingiberales
Family	:	Zingiberaceae
Genus	:	*Curcuma*
Species	:	*C. Longa*

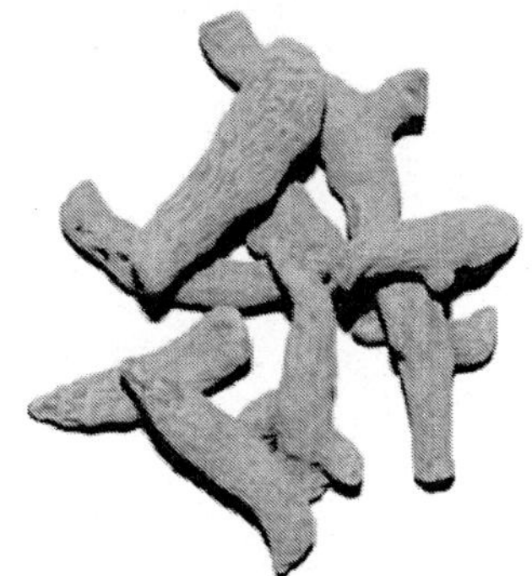

Fig. 5: Curcuma Longa

In Ayurvedic and Siddha practices of Indian medicine system, turmeric has been used as an attempted treatment for a variety of internal disorders, such as indigestion, throat infections or liver ailments, as well as topically, to treat wounds or skin sores. It is very popular among local healers as it is used in FMD, sprains, parasitic infections mouth blisters, mastitis, broken horn and many other diseases of animals in India (Tiwari and Pande, 2010). Rhizome of *Curcuma domestica* is mixed with oil of *Brassica campestris* and rubbed to cure mastitis in Uttrakhand region (India). In these area, rhizomes of *Curcuma domestica* dry over flame, then grind and mixed with oil of *Brassica compestris* and used externally to the infected part to cure yolk galls (Phondani *et al.*, 2010). For the treatment of FMD, 300 g of rhizome of turmeric crushed with 100 g of coriander plant is used by local healers of Karnataka (Harsha, 2005). In Jammu and Kashmir (India), grinded rhizome of *Curcuma longa* with butter is given orally to ox for curing blood in excreta; in powdered form, it is mixed with milk and fed to the animal suffering from fever during summers (Sharma *et al.*, 2012). Bulmus *et al.* (2013) studied the protective effects of curcumin on anti-oxidant status, body weight gain, and reproductive parameters in male rats exposed to subchronic 2,3,7,8-

tetrachlorodibenzo-p-dioxin. Curcumin exhibits a wide spectrum of biological activities, including anti-inflammatory, antioxidant, anticoagulant, antifertility, antidiabetic, antibacterial, antifungal, antiviral, antibrotic, antivenom, antiulcer, hypotensive, hypocholesterolemic, cardioprotective, anticarcinogenic and antimutagenic activities (Chattopadhyay *et al.*, 2004; Kurup and Barrios, 2008). Thus, *Curcuma longa* comprises a vast range of medicinal uses in ethno-veterinary practices.

7.3.6 *Ocimum sanctum*

Taxonomy

Kingdom	:	Plantae
Clade	:	Angiosperms
Clade	:	Eudicots
Clade	:	Asterids
Order	:	Lamiales
Family	:	Lamiaceae
Genus	:	Ocimum
Species	:	*O. sanctum*

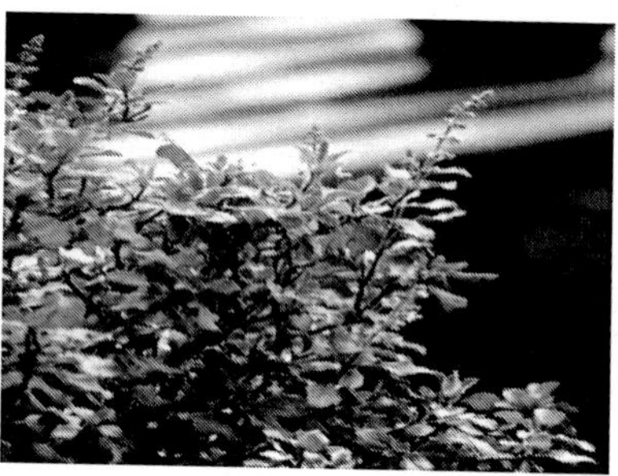

Fig. 6: *Ocimum sanctum*

Ocimum sanctum, commonly known as holy basil, tulasi or tulsi, is an aromatic perennial plant in the family Lamiaceae. It is native to the Indian sub-continent and widespread as a cultivated plant throughout the South-east Asian tropics (Warrier, 1995). *Ocimum sanctum* is cultivated for religious and traditional medicine purposes, and also for its essential oil. *Ocimum sanctum* is an erect, many-branched subshrub, 30–60 cm (12–24 in) tall with hairy stems. Leaves are green or purple; they are simple, petioled, with an ovate, upto 5 cm (2.0 in)-long blade which generally has a slightly toothed margin; they are strongly scented and have a decussate phyllotaxy (Fig 6). The purplish flowers are placed in close whorls on elongate racemes. It has several properties like adaptogen, antioxidant, hypoglycemic, immunomodulator, radio-protector (Umadevi, 2006). As a traditional medicine, it is also being used in cough problems. Leaves of *Ocimum sanctum* is used as folk medicines in constipation and to treat wound especially in Himalayan region in livestock (Tiwari and Pande, 2010). Leaves along with other ingredients are given orally to cattle during bloat and decoction of whole plant mixed with honey is applied in the eye to remove redness or extreme infection as a traditional medicine in northern state of India (Sharma *et al.*, 2012). In Rajasthan, paste of about 10 g leaves of *Ocimum sanctum* is applied over the skin to cure scabies (Galav *et al.*, 2013). Singh *et al.* (2005) reported *Ocimum sanctum* fixed oil showed good antibacterial activity against *Staphylococcus aureus, Bacillus pumilus and Pseudomonas aeroginosa.* The aqueous extract of *Ocimum sanctum* treatment reduced the total bacterial count, increased neutrophil and lymphocyte counts with enhanced phagocytic activity and phagocytic index, lysosomal enzymes contents of milk polymorphonuclear cells (Reena *et al.*, 2005).

7.3.7 *Trigonella foenum-graecum*

Taxonomy

Kingdom	:	Plantae
Clade	:	Angiosperms
Clade	:	Eudicots
Clade	:	Rosids
Order	:	Fabales
Family	:	Fabaceae
Genus	:	Trigonella
Species	:	*T. foenum-graecum*

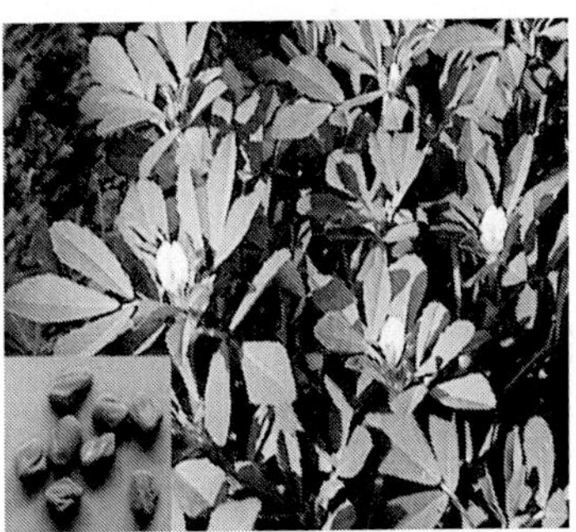

Fig. 7: *Trigonella foenum-graecum*

Fenugreek (*Trigonella foenum-graecum*) is an annual plant in the family Fabaceae, with leaves having three small obovate to oblong leaflets (Fig. 7). It is cultivated worldwide as a semi-arid crop. The seeds of *Trigonella foenum-graecum* are reported to possess hypoglycemic properties in both animal and human subjects. Leaves of fenugreek along with other herbs are traditionally used by various communities of Uttrakhand to treat pneumonia (Phondani *et al.*, 2010). The seeds are also fed to cows and buffaloes after abortion in Jammu and Kashmir (Sharma *et al.*, 2012). For bloat related problems in ruminants, a decoction prepared from the seeds (50-75gm) is fed orally in tribal region of West Bengal (India). Fresh leaves and seeds of fenugreek mixed with fodder are fed to animals suffering from rheumatism. Seeds mixed with jaggery are fed to enhance lactation in rural areas of Gujarat (Jadeja *et al.*, 2006).

There are several medicinal uses of *Trigonella foenum-graecum* as anti ulcer, wound healing, CNS stimulant, immunomodulatory, anti-oxidant, antidiabetic, anti-inflammatory, anti-pyretic and anti-neoplastic drugs.

7.3.8 *Coriandrum sativum*

Coriander (*Coriandrum sativum*), also known as cilantro or Chinese parsley, is an annual herb in the family Apiaceae. All parts of the plant are edible, but the fresh leaves and dried seeds are most traditionally used. Coriander is native to regions from Southern Europe and Northern Africa to south-western Asia. It is a soft plant growing to 50 cm (20 in) tall. The leaves are broadly lobed at the base of the plant, and slender and feathery higher on the flowering stems with variable shapes. (Fig 8).The flowers are borne in small umbels, asymmetrical, white or very pale pink in colour, with the petals pointing away from the center of the umbel longer (5–6 mm or 0.20–0.24 in) than those pointing toward it (only 1–3 mm or 0.039–0.118 in long). The fruit of *Coriandrum sativum* is a globular, dry schizocarp 3–5 mm (0.12–0.20 in) in diameter. Oil contains carvone, geraniol, limonene, borneol, camphor, elemol, and linalool. It has prominent roles as appetizer, stomachic and carminative.

Taxonomy

Kingdom	:	Plantae
Clade	:	Angiosperms
Clade	:	Eudicots
Clade	:	Asterids
Order	:	Apiales
Family	:	Apiaceae
Genus	:	Coriandrum
Species	:	*C. sativum*

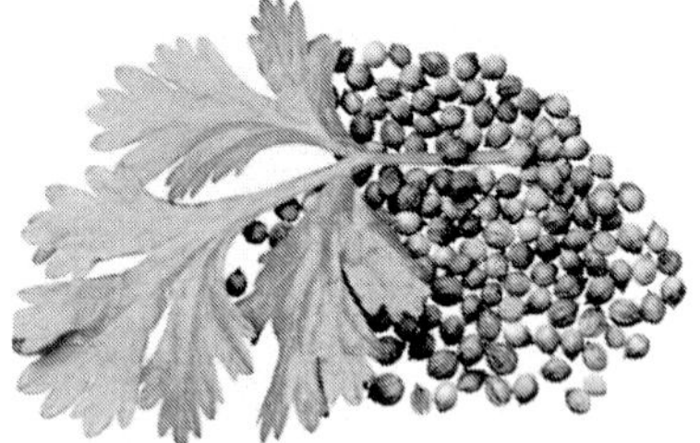

Fig. 8: Coriandrum sativum

It is used as traditional medicine in diarrhoea, constipation, fever, indigestion (Tiwari and Pande, 2010). Some communities of Alaknanda belt use coriander seeds powder mixed with water in case of poisoining (Phondani *et al.*, 2010). To increase the rate of conception, about 100 g fruit powder is given orally twice a day for two days to cattle after mating (Kumar *et al.*, 2012).

One preliminary study showed coriander essential oil inhibiting Gram-positive and Gram-negative bacteria, including *Staphylococcus aureus, Enterococcus faecalis, Pseudomonas aeruginosa,* and *Escherichia coli* (Brennan, 2015). Although seeds of Coriandrum sativum generally have lower content of vitamins, they do provide considerable amounts of dietary fiber, calcium, selenium, iron, magnesium and manganese. Coriander seeds contain an essential oil upto 1%, the main component is linalool, which has potential antibacterial (Burt, 2004; Cantore *et al.,* 2004), antioxidant (Wangensteen *et al.,* 2004), hypolipidemic (Chithra and Leelamma, 2000) and antidiabetic (Gallagher *et al.,* 2003) properities. Like stated before it has appetizing and stimulatory effects in the digestion process (Cabuk *et al.,* 2003). Guler *et al.* (2005) reported that coriander seeds could be considered a potential natural growth promoter for poultry, and showed the best responses at a 2% level of inclusion.

7.3.9 *Withania somnifera*

Withania somnifera, known commonly as ashwagandha, Indian ginseng, winter cherry or poison gooseberry, is a plant in the Solanaceae or nightshade family. This species is a short, tender perennial shrub growing 35–75 cm (14–30 in) tall. Leaves are dull green, elliptic, usually upto 10–12 cm (4 to 5 in) long. The flowers are green, small and bell-shaped (Fig. 9). The ripe fruit is orange-red in color. Withania somnifera is cultivated in many drier regions of India, such as Mandsaur District of Madhya Pradesh, Punjab, Sindh, Gujarat, Kerala and Rajasthan (Mirjalili *et al.,* 2009). It is also found in countries like Nepal, China and Yemen.

Taxonomy

Kingdom	:	Plantae
Clade	:	Angiosperms
Clade	:	Eudicots
Clade	:	Asterids
Order	:	Solanales
Family	:	Solanaceae
Genus	:	Withania
Species	:	*W. somnifera*

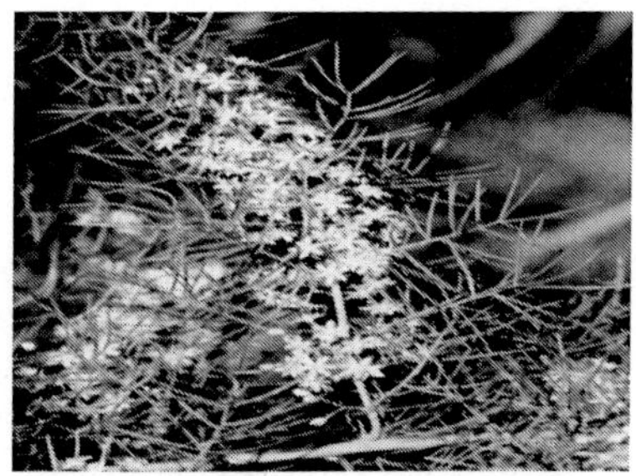

Fig. 9: *Withania somnifera*

Studies indicate ashwagandha possesses anti-inflammatory, antitumour, antistress, immunomodulatory, hemopoetic, antioxidant and rejuvenating properties. It has also hepatoprotective and analgesic action. It also appears to exert a positive effect on the endocrine, cardiopulmonary, and central nervous systems, therefore being used widely for a long period in ethnovet practices. As a part of folk medicine, Gujjar communities of Himalayan region use infusion of roots of *Withania somnifera* to treat ear infections in animals (Gaur *et al.*, 2010). One kg tubers of *Withania somnifera* along with 2L sesamum oil is given to the cattle to treat lumbadgo (Galav *et al.*, 2013). Toxicity studies reveal that *Withania somnifera* appears to be a safe compound and it has adaptogenic properties (Dadkar, 1987). Oral administration of powdered root (suspended in 2% of gum acacia) at the rate 1g/kg body weight in rats caused considerable reduction in Freud's complete adjuvent induced inflammation through significant reduction in acute phase plasma inflammatory proteins viz. 2 glycoprotein ,major acute phase protein 1-protein (Anbalagan and Sadique, 1981). These anti-inflammatory property of *Withania somnifera* might be due to inhibition of cyclo-oxygenase enzyme (Al-Hindwani *et al.*, 1992).

7.3.10 *Nigella sativa*

Nigella sativa (also known as black cumin, nigella and kalonji) is an annual flowering plant in the family Ranunculaceae, native to south and south-west Asia. *Nigella sativa* grows to 20–30 cm (7.9–11.8 in) tall, with linear (but not thread-like) leaves. The flowers are delicate, and usually coloured pale blue and white, with five to ten petals (Fig 10). The fruit is a large and inflated capsule composed of three to seven united follicles, each consisting of numerous seeds.

Taxonomy

Kingdom	:	Plantae
Clade	:	Angiosperms
Clade	:	Eudicots
Order	:	Ranunculales
Family	:	Ranunculaceae
Genus	:	*Nigella*
Species	:	*N. sativa*

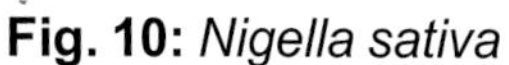

Fig. 10: *Nigella sativa*

Nigella sativa possess anti-inflammatory and immunomodulatory activities. The antioxidant action of N. sativa may explain its claimed usefulness in folk medicine. After parturition, fresh rice mixed with ghee and *Nigella sativa* powder given regularly for early recovery in ganjam district of Odisha (Mishra and Patro, 2010). Some local communities of West Bengal (India) use seeds of *Nigella sativa* (boiled with particulated rice grain) and given orally in cows after 1st parturition to prevent cows from mastitis (Mandal and Rahaman, 2016). *Nigella sativa* oil has been shown to possess anticestodal and antinematodal properties comparable to those of piperazine (Agrawal *et al.,* 1979). In southern Punjab (Pakistan) local healers use Black cumin seeds (50-100gm) in jaggery as an antihelmentic in ruminants (Jabbar *et al.,* 2006). Ozugurlu *et al.* (2005) reported that *Nigella sativa* protect the brain and medulla spinal is tissue against oxidative stress induced by experimental autoimmune encephalomyelitis. In addition, *Nigella sativa* display its antioxidant and regulatory effects via inflammatory cells rather than the host tissue. This antioxidant property would explain its action against CCl_4 hepatotoxicity (Nagi *et al.,* 1999), liver brosis and cirrhosis (Türkdogan *et al.,* 2000), and hepatic damage induced by Schistosoma mansoni infection (Mahmoud *et al.,* 2002). Parhizkar *et al.* (2011) reported the estrogenic activity of *Nigella sativa* in ovariectomized rats using vaginal cornification assay.

7.4 Indigenous Ethnoveterinary Traditional and Folk Practices

Besides above described medicinal plants, there are many other herbs which have been used in large number of ethnoveterinary practices all around the world. Either it is a breeding or feeding practice, some ailment or accidental wound, their use is quite versatile. Ethnoveterinary practices and traditional knowledge in different regions are summarized by Balakrishnan, 2009 (Table 4), Tanaji, 2016 (Table 5) and Kumar and Singh, 2012 (Table 7).

In some areas, dropping of pigeon was fed to the cattle to bring them in heat (Samal *et al.,* 2003). The droppings are said to have estrogens required for inducing heat in animals. Also, fried salt with cucumber leaves (*Cucumis sativus*) was fed to the animal for inducing heat. Saha *et al.* (2014) stated that juice prepared from the bark powder of *Holarrhena antidysenterica* (kurchi) and 6-10 slices of Carica papaya fruits (pepe) with water, was fed orally thrice a day to induce lactation. Another preparation prepared from the whole plant (2-5 plants) of

Amaranthus spinosus along with the roots (50gm) of *Glycosmis pentaphyla* was used to induce lactation.Wangi (*Solanum melongena*) fruits was fed as fodder to the animals to treat FMD (Wath and Jambu, 2014). Das and Tripathi (2009) reported that Soot (uchhali), common salt and chilli paste were mixed with water and used topically on affected areas in FMD. Along with this, the bark of *Ficus religiosa*, badi tree, *Allium sativum* and *Acacia catechu* were boiled or fried together and fried materials was mixed with water to wash oral cavity and hoof in animals suffering from FMD. Documented Ethnoveterinary practices for the treatment of FMD practised in Pollachi Taluk of Coimbatore District is given in Table 6 (Rajkumar *et al.*, 2014). In case of tympany, Kanwar and Yadav (2005) reported that a mixture of kneaded wheat flour, *Boerhaavia diffusa, Trachyspermum ammi Sprague, Trigonella foenum-graeum, Allium cepa , Femia assafsetida , Allium sativum ,Curcuma domestica Valeton* and jaggery were mixed together and fed to animal for early relief. Paste of *Dendrobium amoenum* and *Parthenocissus semicordata* was mixed together and plastered around fractured bone (Shah *et al.*, 2008). Wood of *Debregeasia salicifolia* was used as splints in bandaged kept till complete recovery. Similarly, in case of eye infection, Kumar and Bharti (2012) stated that roots of *Trachyspermum ammi* was used and Malla and Chhetri (2012) reported that *Cynoglossum zeylanicum* leaf juice was used to treat conjunctivitis. Deshmukh *et al.* (2011) reported that *Crotalaria verrucosa* leaf extract was given to the animal for treating hemorrhagic septicemia. Farmers treat fever by providing adequate quantity of fig leaves thrice a day in the first stage and then rubbing of fig leaves in the tongue of animals (Saha *et al.*, 2010). Fresh paste of *Enicostema littorale* leaves were applied against infectious skin wound due to parasites and maggots (Mistry *et al.*, 2003). Paste made from root and bark of Syzygium jambolanum is applied topically for wound healing (Mishra, 2013). Pranjale and Dube (2016) reported that 1 inch rhizome of *Gloriosa superba* with wheat flour was fed to treat maggoted wound. The whole *Cissampelos pareira* plant was fed to animals with fodder to cure dysentary and blood tinged diarrhoea. Animals were fed with tamarind leaves and mustard (*Brassica juncea*) seeds with some water for consecutive three days in the morning in empty stomach to control bleeding dysentery (Saha *et al.*, 2010). Also Fruits of *Cucumis cailosus* were crushed and mixed with sugar, oil and water and fed to animals suffering from diarrhoea. Sometimes, fruits and seeds of *Cyamopsis tatragooloba* were given along with fodder by some communities to cure diarrhoea (Gulav *et al.*, 2010). In case of indigestion, leaves and inflorescence of *Cannabis sativa* is used by various communities.

Satapathy (2010) stated that leaf pulp of *Aloe vera* (L.) was applied on the swollen portion of the udder of cows or buffaloes against mastitis. Fumigation is an age old method used to repel insects in animal shed is still performed by local rural people by using leaves of *Artimisia vulgaris* L. and *Pogostemon benghalensis* (Burm.f.) (Kulkarni, 2015). *Chloroxylon swietenia* was also used to control flies and insects due to fumigation.

Table 4: Extensively used traditional treatment methods in dairy cattle (Balakrishnan, 2009)

Ailments	Traditional Applications
Mastitis	Applying turmeric on udder
Foot and mouth ucers	Allowing animals to walk in hot sand and applying sand to wounds externally; applying linseed oil and turmeric externally; applying kerosene if the wounds are infested with maggots.
Tympany	Drenching linseed oil along with a mixture of ginger, turmeric and asafetida; keeping the animal's mouth open by tying a piece of wood into it.
Retention of Placenta	Feeding bamboo leaves or a mixture of oil, bran and bajra (finger millet) grain
Diarrhoea.	Drenching about 1 kg fruit pulp extract of Aegle marmelos and mango seed kernal for 2-3 days

Table 5: Ethnoveterinary methods used in India (Tanaji 2016)

Ailments	Traditional Applications
Retention of Placenta	20-30gm paste of Gunj seeds
Cystic ovaries / Nymphomania	100-200gm of Waghnaki (*Leptadenia reticulata*) leaves were mixed with 200 ml of Sesame (*Sesamum indicum*) seed oil
To induce heat	750-950gm of sprouted cereals like Matki (*Vigna aconitifolia*) were mixed with Gul (*Saccharum officinale*) 100 gm of Bhendi (*Thespesia populnea*) was fed with one raw egg for 5-6 days
Prevent Abortion	50 ml juice of Amarvel (*Cuscuta reflexa*) leaves
Prolapse	2-3 whole plants of Lajalu *(Mimosa pudica)* in vaginal prolapsed 200-250gm dry powder of Bhuiphoda (*Pisolithus tinctorius*) i.e wild edible mushroom was directly applied on the whole uterine prolapse portion Paste of crushed whole Amarvel (*Cuscuta reflexa*) plant in uterine prolpase 4-5 crushed flowers of Moha (*Madhuca longifolia*) in uterine prolpase
Performance booster	1-2 whole plant of Ran-bhendi or Jungali-Bhendi (*Abelomoschus manihot*) were fed to dairy animals for maintaining good health and as performance booster.
Increased milk production	Whole plant of Amarvel (*Cuscuta chinensis*) Whole plant of Shatawari (*Asparagus racemosus*) 500-750gm of Shevga (*Moringa oleifera*) leaves 100-150gm of Gulvel (*Tinospora cordifolia*) leaves
Ruminal disorders	Feeding of 100-150gm Gulnashi (*Gymnema sylvestre*)

Wound	Paste prepared by properly crushing and mixing 50-60gm bark of Hirda (*Terminalia chebula*) + 100-150gm bark of Dhamni (*Grewia tiliaefolia*) + handful of Aavla (*Emblica officinalis*) leaves were applied on wound for twice a day for 1-2 days 20-30gm leaves of Kurmudi (*Tridax procumbens*) were crushed and applied on wound twice a day 50-60gm dry leaves each of Bamani (*Colebrookea oppositifolia*), Kurmudi (*Tridax procumbens*) and Aavla (*Emblica officinalis*) 10-15ml Bilayat *(Argemone mexicana)* leaf juice extract was mixed with 10-15ml of Bilayat seed oil 100-150gm crushed leaves of Kala-dhotra (Datura metel) were mixed with 15- 20ml of groundnut oil 400-500gm paste of the whole branch along with leaves of shevga *(Moringa oleifera)* 10-15gm grilled pulp of Bel *(Aegle marmelos)* was tightly applied on wound for1-2 days 50-60gm powder of Ghaneri *(Lantana camara)* leaves were applied on wound for 4-5 days
Tympany	90-100gm of Ajwain seeds (*Trachyspermum amami*) were roasted on low flame, powdered and 150-170gm of soda bicarb was added and mix it in 1 litre of water. 100-110gm of Cumin (*Cuminum cynimum*) seed powder and 50-60gm of black salt were mixed in 1-2 litres of water and given orally twice a day for 1-2 days
Anorexia	Branches of Mogli erand (*Jatropha curcas*)
Indigestion	50-60gm of Cumin (*Cuminum cynimum*) seed powder and 10 gm of black salt were mixed with 1 litre of water and given orally for 3-4 days
Snake bite	150-170gm roots of Mungusmungali (*Corallocarpus epigaeus*) 1 tsp of fresh juice of Rui (*Calotropis procera*) roots were fed to animal for 2-3 days. In addition to it, 40-50gm of Rui leaves were fed to animal. Also, 8-10 drops of fresh latex of Rui was applied over the snakebite
Swelling	Massage of affected area with Karanj (*Pongamia pinnata*) oil for 2-3 days 40-50gm of Khandvel (*Marsdenia volubili*) leaves were mixed with 10-15gm of turmeric powder and 50-60ml of groundnut oil. This ground paste was applied twice a day on affected shoulder of animal (usually bull) for 2-3 days 20-30 gm pulp of Korpad (*Aloe vera*) leaf was mixed with 15 -20gm of turmeric powder and paste prepared was applied on affected swellings areas and massage was given to that area twice a day for 2-3 days
Pain	5-10ml of Karanj (*Pongamia pinnata*) oil was applied on affected area of animals and then 4-5 warm leaves of Panphuti (*Bryophyllum Pinnatum*) were tightly bandage all over the surrounding area for 2-3 days 20-25gm of Bilayat (*Argemone mexicana*) seed paste were mixed with 10-15ml of sesame oil and was applied over joints to relieve pain 100gm of powder of Jungli limbara (*Ailanthus excels*) was mixed with 50 gm crushed fruits pulp of Bel (*Aegle marmelos*) in stomach pain
Ear infection	50-100gm leaves of Panfuti (*Bryophyllum Pinnatum*) were boiled in water and mixed with 5 ml of of Karanj oil and poured few drops in ear
Diarrhoea	Bolus prepared by mixing 50gm bark powder of Ran-bhendi (*Abelomoschus ficulneus* L) with sorghum flour 100-150gm leaf paste of Shisav *(Dalbergia sissoo)* was ground and

	given daily for 2-3 days 50-60gm supporting root paste of Vad (*Ficus benghalensis*) tree were mixed in 1litre of butter milk 100-150gm bark paste of Jambhul (*Syzyium cumini*) was mixed with 50-60gm paste of jambhul seeds
Dysentry	250-300ml decoction of Palas (*Butea monosperma*) leaves 100 gm bark of Jungli limbara (*Ailanthus excels*) was crushed and its juice was given orally Whole bulb of Jungli kela (*Musa acuminata*) was crushed and mixed with 250-300gm of sorghum flour
Skin infection	100gm paste of Sagwan (*Tectona grandis*) leaves and 50 gm paste of Sagwan bark were mixed together and applied all over the skin 50-60gm of Tulsi (*Ocimum tenuiflorum*) leaves and 100-120gm Neem leaves (*Azadirachta indica*) were mixed and paste prepared was applied all over body 100-200gm of Nirgudi (*Vitex negundo*) leaves were used to wash the affected animals
Foot and Mouth diseases (FMD)	100gm of partially grilled Bibba (*Semecarpus anacardium*) seeds were crushed and the paste prepared was directly applied on the FMD lesions 100gm paste of Lal khair (*Acacia chundra*) bark was mixed with 20-25 gm of turmeric (*Curcuma longa*) powder and was applied 100-150gm paste of Vedibabul (*Acacia nilotica*) leaves and pods were mixed with 50-60ml of coconut oil and this paste was externally applied 80-100gm fruit pulp of Bel (*Aegle marmelos*) was externally applied 10-15ml fresh Rui (*Calotropis procera*) latex was mixed with 40-50ml of groundnut oil and this mixture was applied on FMD wounds
Haemorrhagic septicemia (HS)	100gm bark each of Bel (*Aegle marmelos*) tree , chinch (*Tamarindus indica*) tree and Shisav (*Dalbergia sissoo*) tree were burnt together. To it, 40-50ml of honey was added drop by drop and animal was allowed to inhale the smoke to cure hemorrhagic septicemia 10ml juice of fresh latex of Nivdung (*Euphorbia neriifolia*) and 10ml groundnut oil were mixed with 1 tea spoon of turmeric powder and tamarind pulp Paste prepared after mixing 1-2 leaves of Khajrya aalu (*Colocasia gigantea*) with 100-200gm bark of old mango tree (*Mangifera indica*), 50-60gm of Chinch leaves (*Tamrindus indica*), 100-150gm bark of Palas tree (*Butea monosperma*) and 2 teaspoons of turmeric powder was applied on the affected tongue and neck area twice a day for 2-3 days
Poisoning	Fresh 2-3 tsp of Bilayat (*Argemone mexicana*) latex were mixed with 200-250gm Sorghum floor and round bolus was given to animals for 1-2 days
Cough / Respiratory disorders	50-100gm of leaves of Bhui ringani (*Solanum surattense*) were boiled in hot water and 50ml of Neem (*Azadirachta indica*) oil and 50ml of honey was added and given orally 50-60gm of Adulsa (*Adhatoda vasica*) leaves and 40-50gm of tulsi (*Ocimum tenuiflorum*) leaves were crushed and mixed in 50-60ml honey 100-150gm paste of Nilgiri (*Eucalyptus globulus*) leaves were mixed with 100-150ml of honey and this mixture was fed to animal
Eye infection	Fresh 250-300gm leaves of Neem (*Azadirachta indica*) and 40-50gm turmeric (*Curcuma longa*) powder were boiled in water and applied

Tail Gangrene	100 gm grilled Bibba (*Semecarpus anacardium*) seeds were crushed and mixed with 30-40 ml of Karanj (*Pongamia pinnata*) oil
Fracture	100-200gm paste of stem and bark of Arjun (*Terminalia arjuna*) was applied over bone fracture Whole stems with leaves of Hadjod (*Cissus quadrangulaus*) were crushed together and prepared paste were applied on fractured bone
Fever	150-200ml roots decoction of Arjun (*Terminalia arjuna*) was given to animal twice a day for 2-3 days

Table 6: Documented ethnoveterinary practices for the treatment of Foot and Mouth Disease (Rajkumar *et al.*, 2014)

Common Name	Binomial Name	Animals Treated	Quantity and Frequency of Administration
Sirumalai banana	*Musa paradisiaca*	Cattle	Five fruits of Sirumalai banana with Amanakku oil 25 ml is effective to treat FMD when it is given orally for three days
Amanakku oil	*Ricinus communis*		
Sirumalai banana and pig fat	*Musa paradisiaca and Lard*	Cattle	Mixture of five fruits of Sirumalai banana and 100gm pig fat (Lard) is effective to treat FMD when it is given orally once a day for five days
Chiryanangai	*Andrographis paniculata*	Cattle	Paste of leaves of Chiryanangai, Periyanangi, Seeragam and bulb of Allium cepa is given orally to cattle for three days
Periyanangi	*Peristrophe paniculata*	Cattle	
Seeragam	*Cuminum Cyminum*	Cattle	
Onion	*Allium cepa*	Cattle	
Kambu	*Pennisetum Typhoides*	Cattle	Kambu ground with water daily during recovery stage
Ellu oil	*Sesamum indicum*	Affected Animals (Cattle and Goat)	An infusion of dry fish (150 gm with 5 L of water) mixed with Ellu oil (100ml),Amanakku oil (100ml) and neem oil (100 ml) is applied externally for a week
Neem oil	*Azadirachta Indica*		
Amanakku oil	*Ricinus communis*		
Oduvanelai	*Cleistanthus collinus*	Sheep and Goat	A paste of handfull leaves of Oduvanelai, Thumbai and a spoon of calcium carbonate powder given orally once a day for five days
Thumbai	*Leucas aspera*		
Neem with few pieces of bones	*Azadirachta indica*	Cattle (Shed)	Fumigation is also done by burning the leaves of neem with few pieces of bones for three days

Table 7: Summary of Indigenous practices for livestock and animal healthcare (Kumar and Singh, 2011)

Disease	Disease Traditional Treatment
Diarrhoea	(a) Decoction of barks of Kendu and Bankulthi (b) Tawayan + Methi + Saunf + Sonth and rock salt with molasses
Constipation	(a) Shoot of Kathal + leaves of Jashtimadhu along with jaggery given orally (b) Leaves of Kadam + bark of Mango tree
Stomach pain	(a) Leaves of Tabenada + Tobacco are given orally
Internal parasite	(a) Leaves and bark of Farhar with molasses (b) Fruit of Baibidan with molasses (c) Blood of duck
Ectoparasite	(a) Tobacco shoot with kerosene oil (b) Leaves of Karanj or Karanj oil (c) Dung ash with leaves of Saripha
H.S.	(a) Hunmgata + Golki are mixed and half is given orally and rest half is pasted
Bloat	(a) Ajwain + Hing + Black salt (b) Onion + Ginger + Hing
Fever or cold	(a) Salam lutur leaves + leaves of Pitusing + Lahsun are mixed and are given orally (b) Application of mustard oil with Lahsun (c) Leaves of Har Shingar and honey (d) Bhui-champa + Kalmeg + Pepper + Gol mirch
Foot and mouth disease	(i) Foot lesion : (a) Making the animal walk in canal/river water (b) Application of lard (c) Leaves of kokarota + leaves of Borkunda are mixed and pasted (ii) Mouth lesion : (a) Application of fitkiri on affected part (b) Rubbing and feeding of arhar leaves
Fracture	(a) Powdered root or paste of the stem of Harjaura (b) Harjaura + Pechki + Sajiwan
Skin disease	(a) Oil expressed from seeds of Karanj is applied on the skin
Rinder pest	(a) A mixture of root of Solam lutur (*Clerodendrom serratum*), leaves of Asaria (*Coparis honida*) and leaves of Bhajisay with gud (gruel) are given orally
Falling tail	(a) Tendrel of Bar (*Zizyhus injba*) + Rola (*Termindlia chebula*) + Junapa are mixed and are pasted on the tail

7.5 Limitations of Herbal Medicines

Herbs are not easily quantifiable and standardized due to their complex composition. The composition of plants may be affected by the location, soil type, weather conditions, altitude, season during which the plant is grown, harvesting procedure and storage conditions in various regions. There are various constituents which are photo labile, thermo labile, thus less stable. Possibility of synergistic or antagonistic effects as well as the variety and environmental growth conditions, harvesting time and state of maturity, method and duration of conservation and storing, extraction method of the plant or microbial contamination are some important factors which may substantially concern the use of herbal medicines in various species of animals. Besides these, the traditional knowledge of ethnoveterinary practices by various communities not being documented properly is deteriorating due to lack of awareness and incomplete knowledge as being transferred by words of mouth.

7.6 Conclusions

India has acquired great traditional background in ethno-veterinary medicine and practices. Ethno veterinary practices have immense contemporary relevance in various aspects. There are enormous opportunities for the development of drugs or treatments on the ethnobotanical leads. Therefore, it becomes essential to conserve these medicinal plants with miraculous properties, both genetically as well as culturally. To determine a remedy's efficacy, it is necessary to follow such studies closely along with the local way of preparation and application. The government & non-governmental organizations must work in this direction and the rich inheritance of this knowledge should be documented and standardized properly as to benefit maximum livestock raisers. Other than this, they must also provide some monitory assistance to the traditional healers, so that we may conserve these rich traditions of animal care for our future generations.

References

Abbas RJ (2010) Effect of using Fenugreek, Parsley and Sweet basil seeds as feed additives on performance of broiler chickens. Int J of Poult Sci 9(3): 278-282

Agrawal R, Kharya MD, Srivastava R (1979) Antimicrobial and antihelminthic activities of the essential oil of Nigella sativa Linn. Indian J Exp Biol 17: 1264–1265

Aiyer KN, Kolammal M (1963) Pharmacognosy of Ayurvedic Drugs, Series 1. 1st ed. Trivendrum: The Central Research Institute.

Al-Hindwani MK, Al-Khafagi S,Abdul Nabi M (1992) Anti-granuloma activity of iraqi Withania somnifera. J Ethnopharmocol. 37: 113

Anbalagan K, Sadique J (1981) Influence of an Indian medicine (Ashwagandha) on acute phase reactants in inflammation. Indian J Exp Biol. 19: 245-249

Atta MB (2003) Some characteristics of nigella (Nigella sativa L.) seed cultivated in Egypt and its lipid profile Food Chemistry 83: 63–68

Balakrishnan V (2009) Ethnoveterinary studies among farmers in Dindigul district, Tamil Nadu, India: Global J Pharmacol 3(1): 15-23

Barua CC, Bora M, Saikia BN, Hazarika M Ishwar, Barua C (2015) Quantitative analysis of proximate and mineral composition of a few important medicinal plants of north-east region. International Journal of Applied Biology and Pharmaceutical Technology 6 (3): 188-193

Bhardwaj RK (2009) Study on the efficacy of Shatavari and Ashwagandha root powder supplementation on production, reproduction and carcass traits of Japanese quails. Govind ballabh pant university of agriculture & technology. Ph.D thesis

Bishayi BR, Ghose S, Sengupta M (2002) Hepatoprotective and immunomodulatory properties of Tinospora cordifolia in CCl_4 intoxicated mature albino rats. J of Toxicol Sci. 27(3): 139-46

Braga ME, Leal PF, Carvalho JE, Meireles MA (2003) Comparison of yield, composition, and antioxidant activity of turmeric (Curcuma longa L.) extracts obtained using various techniques". J Agric Food Chem 51(22): 6604–11

Brennan E (2015) Effective intercropping for biological control of Aphids in transplanted organic lettuce organic. http://articles.extension.org/pages/72642

Bulmus FG, Sakin F, Turk G, Sonmez M, Servi K (2013) Protective effects of curcumin on antioxidant status, body weight gain, and reproductive parameters in male rats exposed to subchronic 2,3,7,8-tetrachlorodibenzo-p-dioxin. Toxicological Environment Chem 95(6): 1019-1029

Burt S (2004) Essential oils: Their antibacterial properties and potential applications in foods: A review. Int J Food Microbial 94: 223–253

Cabuk M, Alcicek A, Bozkurt M, Imre N (2003) Antimicrobial properties of the essential oils isolated from aromatic plants and using possibility as alternative feed additives. II. National Animal Nutrition Congress; Kanya, Turkey. 18–20 September pp. 184–187

Cantore PL, Iacobellis NS, De Marco A, Capasso F, Senatore F (2004) Antibacterial activity of Coriandrum sativum L. and Foeniculum vulgare Miller var. vulgare (Miller) essential oils. J Agric Food Chem 52: 7862–7866

Chattopadhyay I, Biswas K, Bandopadhyay U, Banerjee R (2004) Turmeric and Curcumin: Biological Actions and Medicinal Applications. Current Sci 87: 44–53

Chauhan RA S, Nair N R, Mittal VP, Rangan R (1971) Observation on galactagogue effect of 'Leptaden' in she buffaloes and cows. Jawahar Lal Nehru Krishi Vishwavidyalaya. 5(1): 51

Chithra V, Leelamma S (2000) Coriandrum sativum–effect on lipid metabolism in 1, 2-dimethyl hydrazine induced colon cancer. J Ethnopharmacol 71: 457–463

Choudhary BK, Kar A (1992) Mineral contents of Asparagus racemosus. Indian Drugs 29(13): 623

Cotton CM (1996) Ethnobotany: principles and applications. John Wiley & Sons.

Dadkar VN, Ranadive NU, Dhar HL (1987) Evaluation of antistress (adaptogen) activity of Withania somnifera (Ashwagandha). Ind J Clin Biochem 2: 101-108

Dahanukar SA, Rege NN, Thatte U (1997) Adaptogens. In Medicinal plants, their bioactivity, screening and evaluation. Proceedings of the International Workshop, CDRI, Lucknow (India), December 2-5, pp. 143-163

Das SK, Tripathi H (2009) Ethnoveterinary practices and socio-cultural values associated with animal husbandry in rural Sunderbans, West Bengal. Indian J Tradit Knowle. 8: 201–205

De Haan S, Bekure A (1991) Animal Health Services in Sub-Saharan Africa: Initial Experiences with Alternative Approaches. World Bank, Washington

Deshmukh DC, RR, Rathod VN, Pardeshi VN (2011). Ethnoveterinary medicine from Jalna district of Maharashtra state. Indian J Tradi Knowledge 10(2): 344-348

Diab AS, El-Nagar GO, Abd-El-Hady YM (2002) Evaluation of nigella sativa (black seeds; baraka), Allium sativum (garlic) and biogen as feed additives on growth performance and immunostimulants of O. niloticus fingerlings. Suez Canal Vet Med J. pp 745-75.

Dixit PP, Londhe JS, Ghaskadbi SK, Devasagayam TPA (2006) Anti-diabetic and related beneficial properties of Indian medicinal plants. In Herbal Drugs: A twenty First century Perspective. (Sharma, R.K. and Arora, R. Eds). Jaypee Brothers, New Delhi, pp. 377-395

Everett TH (1982) The New York botanical garden illustrated encyclopedia of horticulture, Vol 10. Taylor & Francis. pp. 3591.

Galav P, Jain A, Katewa SS (2013) Traditional veterinary medicines used by livestock owners of Rajasthan, India. Indian J Traditional Knowledge 12(1): 47-55

Gallagher AM, Flatt PR, Duffy G, Abdel-Wahab YH (2003) The effects of traditional antidiabetic plants on *in vitro* glucose diffusion. Nutr Res 23: 413–424

Gaur RD, Sharma J, Painuli RM (2010). Plant used in traditional healthcare of livestock by Gujjar community of Sub-Himalayan tracts , Uttarakhand, India. Indian Journal of Natural Products and Resources 1(2): 243-248

Guler T, Ertas On, Ciftci M, Dalkilic B (2005) The effect of coriander seed (Coriandrum sativum L.) as diet ingredient on the performance of Japanese quail. South African J Anim Sci. 35(4): 261-267

Hameed I, Hussain F (2015) Proximate and elemental analysis of five selected medicinal plants of family Solanaceae. Pak J Pharm Sci 28(4): 1203-1215

Haniadka R, Saxena A, Shivashankara AR, Fayad R, Nazreth N, Francis A, Arora R, Balinga MS (2013) Ginger protects the liver against the toxic effects of xenobiotic compounds: Preclinical observations. J Nutr Food Sci. 3: 5

Harsha VH, Shripathi V, Hedge VR (2005) Ethnoveterinary practices in Uttara Kannada district of Karnataka. Indian J Traditional Knowledge 4(3): 253-258

Hong SL, Lee GS, Rahman SN, Ahmed Hamdi OA, Awang K, Aznam Nugroho N, Abd Malek SN (2014) Essential oil content of the rhizome of curcuma purpurascens bl. (temu tis) and its antiproliferative effect on selected human carcinoma cell lines". Scientific World J. 397-430.

Hu Y, Kong W, Yang X, Xie L, Wen J, Yang M (2014) "GC-MS combined with chemometric techniques for the quality control and original discrimination of Curcumae longae rhizome: Analysis of essential oils". J Separation Sci 37(4): 404-11

Iqbal Z, Lateef M, Akhtar MS, Ghayur MN, Gilani AH(2006) *In vivo* antihelminthic activity of ginger against gastrointestinal nematodes of sheep. J of Ethnopharmacol 106(2): 285-287

Jabbar A, Raza MA, Iqbal Z, Khan MN (2006) An inventory of the ethnobotanicals used as antihelminthics in the southern Punjab (Pakistan). J of Ethnopharmacol. 108(2006): 152–154

Jadeja BA, Odedra NK, Solanki KM, Baraiya NM (2006) Indigenous animal healthcare practices in district Porbandar, Gujarat 5(2): 253-258

Jain SK (2000) Plants in Indian ethnoveterinary medicine:status and prospectus. Ind J Vet Medicine 20: 1-11

Kanwar P, Yadav D (2005) Indigenous animal healthcare practices of Kangra district, Himachal Pradesh. Indian J Trad Knowledge. 4(2): 164-168

Kulkarni S, Kulkarni DK, Deo AD, Pande AB, Bhagat RL(2014)Use of Ethno-Veterinary medicines (EVM) from Vidarbha Region (MS) India. Bio-science Discovery. 5(2): 180-186

Kumar A, Pandey VC, Tewari DD (2012). Documentation and determination of consensus about phytotherapeutic veterinary practices among the Tharu tribal community of Uttar Pradesh, India. Trop Anim Health Prod 44: 863–872

Kumar A, Singh BB (2011) Indigenous Livestock Practices of Tribal Farmers. Indian Res J Ext Edu 11(1): 113-116

Kurup VP, Barrios CS (2008) Immunomodulatory Effects of Curcumin in Allergy (Review). Molecular Nutrition & Food Research 52: 1031–1036

Mahmoud MR, El-Abhar HS, Saleh S (2002) The effects of Nigella sativa oil against the liver damage induced by Schistosoma mansoni in mice. J Ethnopharmacol 79: 1–11

Malla B, Chhetri RB (2012) Ethnoveterinary practices of some plant species by thnic people of Parbat district, Nepal. J Sci Engineering Technol 8(1): 44-50

Mandal SK, Rahaman CH (2016) Documentation and Consensus Analysis of Traditional Knowledge about Ethnoveterinary Medicinal Plants of Birbhum District, West Bengal (India) International J Livestock 6(1): 43-56

McCorkle CM (1986) An introduction to ethnoveterinary and development. J Ethnobiol 6(1): 129-49

Mirjalili MH, Moyano E, Bonfill M, Cusido R M, Palazon J (2009) Steroidal Lactones from Withania somnifera, an Ancient Plant for Novel Medicine. Molecules 14(7): 2373–2393

Mishra D (2011) Ethnoveterinary Practices and use of herbal medicines for treatment of skin diseases in cattle: A study in Polsara Block, Ganjam District, Odisha, India. Vety World 4(6): 250-253

Mishra D, Patro L (2010) Ethnoveterinary practices among the rural people of Ganjam district (Odisha) India: a case study on some common veterinary ailments. The Bioscan 3: 739-746

Mishra, D (2013). Cattle wounds and ethnoveterinary medicine: a study in Polasara block, Ganjam district, Orissa, India. Indian J Tradit Knowl 12: 62-65

Mistry N, Silori CS, Gupta L, Dixit AM (2003) Indigenous knowledge on animal healthcare practices in district Kachchh, Gujarat. Indian J Traditional Knowledge 2(3): 240-254

Mohd. Amir, Ahsanullah Khan, Mohd Mujeeb, Ajaz Ahmad, Sheeba Usmani, Mohd. Akhtar (2011) Phytochemical Analysis and *in vitro* Antioxidant Activity of Zingiber officinale. Free Rad Antiox. 1(4): 75-81

Mukherjee R, De UK, Ram GC (2010) Evaluation of mammary gland immunity and therapeutic potential of *Tinospora cordifolia* against bovine sub-clinical mastitis. Trop Anim Health Prod 42(4): 645-651

Nagi MN, Alam K, Badary OA (1999) Thymoquinone protects against carbon tetrachloride hepatotoxicity in mice via an antioxidant mechanism. Biochem Mol Biol Int 47: 143–159

Nayampalli SS, Ainapure SS, Samant BD, Kudtarkar RG, Desai NK, Gupta KC (1988) A comparative study of diuretic effects of Tinospora cordifolia and hydrochloro-thiazide in rats and a preliminary phase I study in human volunteers. J Postgrad Med 34: 233-236

Nelson KM, Dahlin JL, Bisson J (2017) The essential medicinal chemistry of Curcumin: Miniperspective". J Medicinal Chem 60(5): 1620–1637

Otunola GA, Oloyede OB, Oladiji AT, Afolayan AJ (2010) Comparative analysis of the chemical composition of three spices – Allium sativum L. Zingiber officinale Rosc and Capsicum frutescens L. commonly consumed in Nigeria. Afr J of Biotechnol 9(41): 6927-6931

Ozugurlu F, Sahin S, Idiz N, Akyol O, Illhan A, Yigitoglu R, Isik B (2005) The effect of Nigella sativa oil against experimental allergic encephalomyelitis via nitric oxide and other oxidative stress parameters. Cell Mol Biol 51(3): 337-342

Parhizkar S, Latiff LA, Rahman SA, Dollah MA (2011) Preventive effect of *Nigella sativa* on metabolic syndrome in menopause induced rats. J Medicinal Plants Res 5(8): 1478-1484

Patil US, Deshmukh OS (2015) Plants used In Ethnoveterinary medicines by tribal peoples in Betul district, Madhya Pradesh, India. International J Sci Res 4(10): 9-16

Penna SC, Medeiros MV, Aimbire FSC, Faria-Neto HCC, Sertie JAA, Lopes RAB (2003) Anti-inflammatory effect of the hydralcoholic extract of Zingiber officinale rhizomes on rat paw and skin edema. Phytomedicine 10: 381–385.

Phondani PC, Maikhuri RK, Kala CP (2010) Ethnoveterinary uses of medicinal plants among traditional herbal healers in Alaknanda catchment of Uttarakhand, India. Afr J Trad 7(3): 195-206

Pranjale A, Dube KG (2016) Ethno-Veterinary Traditional Knowledge of Some Plants Used in Wardha district (Maharashtra). Intern J Sci Res 5(5): 1279-1283

Raghunathan K, Mittra R (1982) Pharmacognosy of Indigenous Drugs. New Delhi: Central Council for Research in Ayurveda & Siddha

Raikwar A, Maurya P (2015) Ethnoveterinary medicine: in present Perspective Int J Agric Sci Vet Med 3(1): 44-49

Rajkumar NV, Kavithaa NV, Sree Lakshmi CM (2014) Ethnoveterinary practices in Coimbatore district during foot and mouth disease outbreak. Inter J Sci Environ Technol 3(4): 1480-1483

Rao AR (1981) Inhibitory action of Asparagus racemosus on DMBA-induced mammary carcinogoenesis in rats. Int J Cancer 28: 607-10.

Reena M, Dash PK, Ram GC (2005) Immunotherapeutic potential of *Ocimum sanctum* (L) in bovine subclinical mastitis. Res V Sci 79(1):37-42

Rios JL, Recio MC (2005) Medicinal Plants and Anti-microbial Activity. J Ethnopharmacol 100(12): 80-84

Saha A, Mukhopadhyay, SB, Gupta DD (2010) Inventory of indigenous healthcare practices of dairy animals. Indian J Traditional Knowledge 9(2): 326-332

Saha MR, Sarker DD, Sen A (2014) Ethnoveterinary practices among tribal community of Malda district of West Bengal, India. Indian J Traditional Knowledge 13(2): 359-367

Satapathy KB (2010) Ethnoveterinary practices in Jajpur district of Odisha. Indian J Trad Knowledge 9(2): 338-343

Schillhorn van veen TW (1991) The present and future veterinary practitioners in the tropics. Vet Quarterly 15: 41–47

Shah R, Pande PC, Tiwari L (2008) Folklore biomedicine for some veterinary diseases in western part of Almora district. Indian J Traditional Knowledge 7(2): 355-359

Shahwar MK, El-Ghorab AH, Anjum FM, Butt MS, Hussain S, Nadeem M (2012) Characterization of coriander (coriandrum sativum l.) seeds and leaves: volatile and non volatile extracts. Int J Food Properties15: 736–747

Sharma R, Manhas RK, Magotra R (2012) Ethnoveterinary remedies of diseases among milk yielding animals in Kathua, Jammu and Kashmir. J Ethnopharmacol 141(2012): 265–272

Singh S, Malhotra M, Majumdar DK (2005) Antibacterial activity of Ocimum sanctum L. fixed oil. Indian J of Exp Bio 43(9): 835-837

Subhose V, Srinivas P, Narayana A (2005) Basic principles of pharmaceutical science in Ayurveda. Bulletin of the Indian Institute of History of Medicine 35(2): 83–92

Tanaji NV (2016) Study of indigenous technical knowledge (itks) on dairy husbandry practices followed by tribal dairy farmers in Palghar district of Maharashtra, Bombay Veterinary College, Mumbai, MVSc thesis

Thatte UM, Rao SG, Dahanukar SA (1994) Tinospora cordifolia induces colony stimulating activity in serum. J Postgrad Med 40: 202-203

Tiwari L, Pande PC (2010) Ethnoveterinary medicine in Indian perspectives: Reference to Uttarakhand, Himalaya. Indian J Tradit Knowl 9(3): 611-17

Turkdogan MK, Agaoglu Z, Yener Z, Sekeroglu R, Akkan HA, Avci ME (2000) The role of antioxidant vitamins (C and E), selenium and Nigella sativa in the prevention of liver brosis and cirrhosis in rabbits, new hopes. Dtscch Tierarzt Wschr 108: 71–73

Uma Devi P (2006) Development of a radioprotective drug from Ocimum sanctum. In: Herbal Drugs: A twenty First century Perspective. (Sharma, R.K. and Arora, R. Eds). pp. 291-300

Vishvadiya NP, Narasimhacharya AVRL (2005) Hypolipidemic and antioxidant activities of Asparagus racemosus in hypercholesteremic rats. Indian J Pharmacol 37: 376-380

Wangensteen H, Samuelsen AB, Malterud KE (2004) Antioxidant activity in extracts from coriander. Food Chem 88: 293–297

Warrier PK (1995) Indian Medicinal Plants, Orient Longman. p. 168

Wath M, Jambu S (2014) Documentation of Ethnoveterinary practices among the Kolams of Yavatmal District. Biolife 2(2): 14-16

Xiao-Lan Cheng, Qun Liu, Yong-Bo Peng, Lian-Wen Qi (2011) Ping Li Steamed ginger (Zingiber officinale): Changed chemical profile and increased anti-cancer potential. Food Chem 129: 1785–1792.

❑❑❑

Part II:

Phytobiotics for Animal Production and Health

Chapter 8

Turmeric (*Curcuma longa*)

Pankaj Kumar Singh and Kaushalendra Kumar

Department of Animal Nutrition, Bihar Animal Sciences University, Patna, India, E-mail: vetpank@gmail.com

ABSTRACT

Turmeric (*Curcuma longa* L.) is a rhizomatous herbaceous perennial plant of the ginger family, Zingiberaceae. Turmeric rhizome powder contains 6.3% protein, 5.1% fat, 3.5% minerals, 69.4% carbohydrates, and 13.1% moisture. Turmeric rhizome powder posses antioxidant, antibacterial, anti-inflammatory, antihypertensive and hypo-cholesterolemic properties due to presence of phytochemicals *viz.* curcumin, demethoxycurcumin, tetrahydro-curcumin, curcuminoids, arturmerone, zingiberene, turmerone and curlone, etc. Turmeric powder is well known to have a property as a safe, natural and residue free phytobiotics. Turmeric preparations have many useful applications in production and health of livestock and poultry. Turmeric has growth promoting effect in poultry due to its antioxidant, antimicrobial and anti-inflammatory effect. Turmeric has been used in poultry ration as feed additive to improve growth performance and egg production without affecting carcass quality. Phytochemicals in turmeric are known to be natural, less toxic, residue free, and are thought to be ideal as feed additives in animal diets.

Keywords: Turmeric, Curcumin, Antioxidant, Antibacterial, Phytobiotics, Production.

8.1 Introduction

Turmeric (*Curcuma longa*) is a perennial herb of Zingiberaceae family that is widely used and cultivated in the tropical and sub tropical regions of the world (Govindarajan and Stahl, 1980). This medicinal plant possesses rhizomes and underground root-like stems that had been originally used as a food additive in curries to improve the storage condition, appearance, flavour, palatability and preservation of food (Jayaprakasha *et al.*, 2005). The Indian people used to call turmeric as kitchen queen. Turmeric rhizome powder posses antioxidant, antibacterial, anti-inflammatory, antihypertensive and hypo-cholesterolemic properties (Chattopadhyay *et al.*, 2004) due to presence of phytochemicals *viz.* curcumin, demethoxycurcumin, tetrahydro-curcumin, curcuminoids, arturmerone, zingiberene, turmerone and curlone (Burt, 2004). Curcumin contains powerful anti-inflammatory, anti-diabetic, antioxidant, and even anti-cancer properties that render it a powerful, disease-fighting medicine in addition to being a culinary spice. It fights harmful bacteria, bad cholesterol, and disease-causing inflammation. When compared with the synthetic antibiotics, phytochemicals in turmeric are known to be natural, less toxic, residue free, and are thought to be ideal as feed additives in animal diets (Wang *et al.*, 1998). The World Health Organization declared turmeric and its yellow colouring agent (curcumin) as safe to be used in human food and animal feed (WHO, 1987). In human and animal studies so far turmeric is considered to have low toxicity (Alia *et al.*, 2006), therefore, this yellow additive is believed to be secure and ideal for poultry. Turmeric powder is well known to have a property as a safe, natural & residue free phytobiotics.

8.2 Taxonomic Position of Turmeric

Chattopadhyay *et al.* (2004) described taxonomic position of turmeric as follows:

Kingdom	:	Plantae
Class	:	Liliopsida
Subclass	:	Commelinids
Order	:	Zingiberales
Family	:	Zingiberaceae
Genus	:	*Curcuma*
Species	:	*longa*

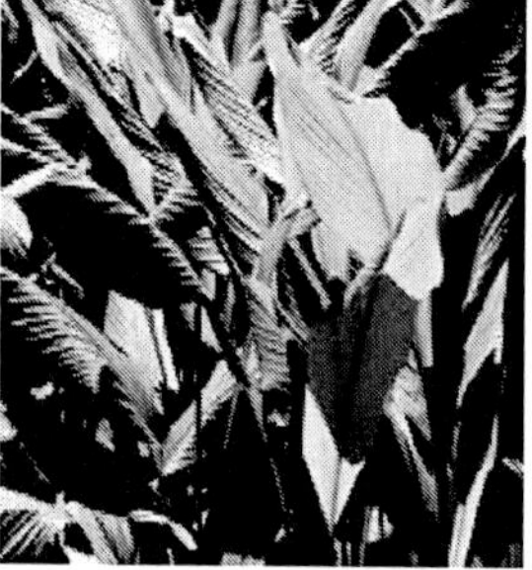

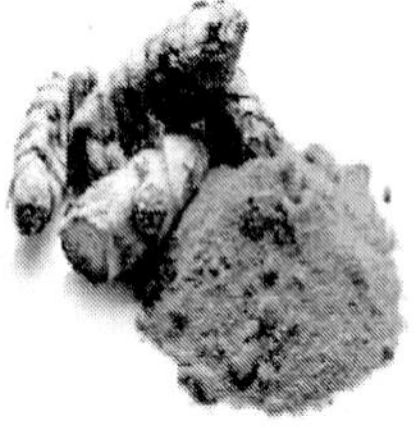

8.3 Morphology of Plant

Turmeric plant possesses underground rhizomes like ginger plant. It is a perennial, leafy and erect herbaceous plant. Turmeric is usually grown as annual crop. It needs warm and slightly humid atmosphere.

It requires temperature between 20-30°C and also a significant amount of rainfall to bloom. It is 60-90 cm in height. The colours of flower are yellow, grouped together in a dense spike like structure and 10-15 cm in length. The blade of leaf is thin, ovate, sheath like long petiole and entire margined. The Leaves are oblong, broad and narrowed towards base. They are slight green, 35-40 cm long and 8-14 cm wide. The plant has no fruits above the ground. The rhizomes of turmeric possess finger like projections and segmented skin. The central rhizome is mostly thickened like a tuber and has numerous roots. The roots are terminates in many elliptical tubers. The turmeric rhizomes are branched and fleshy. The primary rhizome is ovate and mostly pear shaped, known as "bulb" and the secondary one are cylindrical (Ahmad *et al.,* 2010). The rhizomes colour is yellow and a orange line is present inside the rhizomes. But externally rhizomes are brownish and scaly. The rhizomes are mostly 2.6-7 cm in length and 2-2.4 cm in width. It was used as household therapy for inflammation of wounds, digestive.

8.4 Chemical Composition of Turmeric

Turmeric rhizome powder contains 6.3% protein, 5.1% fat, 3.5% minerals, 69.4% carbohydrates, and 13.1% moisture (Chattopadhyay *et al.,* 2004). The main bioactive substances of turmeric are curcumin, demethoxycurcumin and bidemethoxy curcumin which is present to the extent of 2-5 % of the total spice in turmeric powder. Phyto-chemicals of turmeric rhizomes consist of volatiles and non-volatiles constituents. The major active substances in the non-volatile components are the colouring agents and are a rich source of phenolic compounds, such as curcumin (Roughley and Whiting, 1973), demethoxycurcumin, bisdemethoxycurcumin, and colourless metabolites tetrahydro-curcumin (Huang *et al.,* 1995). The major active substances in volatile oil are curcuminoids (Toennesen, 1992), ar-turmerone (Ferreira *et al.,* 1992), zingiberene (Smith and Robinson, 1981), turmerone (Baik *et al.,* 1993), and curlone (Kiso *et al.,* 1983). The particular aroma of turmeric rhizome is due to the aromatic volatile oil like turmerone (25%), curdione (11.58%) and ar-turmerone (8.5%) whereas phenolic compound like curcumin impart yellow colour to the rhizomes of *Curcuma longa.* Curcumin (diferuloylmethane) is the main yellow bioactive component that has a wide spectrum of biological actions, including anti-inflammatory (Ammon *et al.,* 1993; Holt *et al.,* 2005), antioxidant (Sugiyama *et al.,* 1996; Iqbal *et al.,* 2003), antibacterial (Negi *et al.*, 1999; Mandroli and Bhat, 2013) and hypolipidaemic (Ramirez-Tortosa *et al.*, 1999), antifungal, anti-protozoal, antiviral, antihypertensive, and hypocholesteremic activities (Chattopadhyay *et al.*, 2004). Curcumin and curcuminoids also posses anti-nematocidal (Kiuchi *et al.*, 1993), anti-coccidians (Abbas *et al.*, 2010), and imunomodulatory (Kumari *et al.*, 2007; Yarru *et al.*, 2009) properties. Additionally, it has been suggested that curcumin possess hepatoprotective, antitumour, antiviral and anticancer activity (Polasa *et al.*, 1991). On the other hand, there were reports to show that turmeric had the ability to stimulate the digestive enzymes such as intestinal lipase, sucrose, and maltase activities (Patel and Srinivasan, 1996) as well as the secretion of pancreatic lipase, amylase, trypsin, and chimotrypsin enzymes (Patel and Srinivasan, 2000). Therefore, turmeric is used in gastrointestinal and respiratory disorders (Anwarul *et al.*, 2006).

8.5 Biological Activities of Turmeric and its Constituents

The biological activities of the compounds present in turmeric powder have been widely studied. The most important activities for poultry production are those mentioned below.

8.5.1 *Antioxidant properties*

Turmeric and its component show great antioxidant activity as compared to vitamins E and C. Curcuminoids have powerful antioxidant activity, which has been evaluated both in *in vitro* and *in vivo* tests. Curcuminoids hinder the biosynthesis of leukotriene through lipoxygenase pathway and it also decreases the formation of prostaglandin. The aqueous extracts of fresh rhizomes exhibited greater antioxidant potential as compared to dry rhizomes. There was considerable loss of antioxidant potential of turmeric rhizomes, when they are turned into dry powder. The antioxidant activity of curcumin is linked to the presence of phenolic groups in the molecule, and this activity can be related to anti-inflammatory, hepato- and cardio-protective effects of curcumin. Furthermore, it has been demonstrated that curcumin can be successfully used, along with standard drugs, as an adjuvant in a drug therapy of oxidative stress-induced diseases (Amalraj *et al.*, 2017).

8.5.2 *Anti-inflammatory Activity*

Turmeric shows high anti-inflammatory properties as it encompasses many natural cyclo-oxygenase inhibitors. The curcumin of turmeric powder has potent anti-inflammatory properties. The action of cur-cumin against inflammation is affected by several molecular pathways, i.e. by reducing immune response, increasing xenobiotic metabolism, amelioration of inflammation by decreasing neutrophil migration and improving barrier remodelling. Overall, curcumin is a highly pleiotropic molecule, able to interact with numerous molecular targets leading to inflammation (Jurenka, 2009). The inhibition of inflammatory cytokines is a typical action of several anti-inflamatory drugs – the one of the mechanisms which is affected by curcumin. It has been demonstrated in *in vitro* studies that curcumin regulates the activation of some transcription factors, such as activating protein-1 (AP-1) and nuclear factor kappa B (NF-êB) in stimulated monocytes and alveolar macrophages, thus blocks the expression of genes encoding cytokines (Jobin *et al.,* 1999). On the other hand, in the *in vivo* studies it has been shown that curcumin also inhibits arachidonic acid metabolism and inflammation in mouse skin epidermis *via* down-regulation of the cyclooxygenase and lipoxygenase pathways (Huang *et al.,* 1991).

8.5.3 *Antibacterial Property*

Curcumin extracts have been proved very effective for retarding the growth of pathogenic bacterial strains. Turmeric was investigated for its antimicrobial and antioxidant properties by using sensitive microbiological and chemical assays. The mechanism behind the antimicrobial action of different spices involves the hydrogen bonding of various phenolic compounds to the membrane proteins, membrane damage, disruption of the electron transport chain and cell wall distruction (Odhav *et al.,* 2002). Growth of both gram negative and gram positive bacteria were retarded by using concentrations of 20 to 90 µg/mL of turmeric extracts (Aly *et al.,* 2011).

Turmeric extracts and essential oil of turmeric obstruct the growth of various pathogenic bacteria, fungi and parasites. In a study of chicks infested with *caecal parasite* and with *Eimera maxima* revealed that diets with 1% turmeric demonstrated a decrease in intestinal lesion marks and improved net weight gain (Dujic *et al.,* 2009). In a study, antibacterial activity of ethanol and hexane extracts of turmeric and curcuminoids (isolated from ethyl acetate extract of *Curcuma longa*) was observed against 24 strains of pathogenic bacteria that were isolated from chicken and shrimp. Ethanolic extract exhibited the highest antibacterial activity with the MIC of 3.91 to 130 ppt. The methanol and hexane extracts of *C. longa* showed anti-microbial activity against 13 different bacterial strains. Hexane extracts and curcuminoids displayed the MIC values of 120 to 1000 ppt and 3.90 to 500 ppt, individually (Lawhavinit *et al.,* 2010). Turmeric oil a byproduct of curcumin was also found active against *B. coagulans, Staph. aureus, B. subtilis, P. aeruginosa* and *E. coli* (Moghadamtousi *et al.,* 2014).

In a study, dried rhizome of turmeric and Oleo resins of *Boswellia serrata* were evaluated for their antimicrobial activities against gram negative (*Escherichia coli* and *Salmonella typhi*) and gram positive (*Staphylococcus aureus, Bacillus subtilis*) micro-organisms. Both of the extracts showed considerable anti-microbial activities. Turmeric oil and its ether extracts were effective against *Bacillus coagulans, Bacillus subtilis, Bacillus cereus, Staphylococcus aureus, Pseudomonas aeruginosa* and *Escherichia coli* (Chandarana *et al.,* 2005].

8.5.4 *Antiviral Activity*

Curcumin has been revealed to possess high antiviral activities. It inhibits the activities of Epstein-Barr virus in Raji DR-LUC cells. Epstein-Barr virus inducers like 12-0- tetradecanoylphorbol-13-acetate, transforming growth factor-beta and sodium butyrate raise the level of BZLF1 in cells at 12-48 h of treatment, which is efficiently obstructed by curcumin. Most significantly, curcumin also demonstrates anti-HIV activity by constraining the HIV-1 integrase which is needed for replication of virus. It also obstructs HIV gene expressions induced by UV light. Consequently, curcumin and its different analogues may possibly be used as a novel drug therapy against HIV (Chattopadhyay *et al.,* 2004). The *in vitro* activity of curcumin against influenza viruses was evaluated by Chen *et al.* (2010) with promising results. It was found that curcumin interrupts virus-cell links hindering the multiplication of the influenza virus and exerts a direct effect on viral particle infectivity.

8.5.5 *Antifungal Activity*

Turmeric oil proved effective activity against seven different fungi which are responsible for spoilage of stored agriculture commodities. More than 70% growth inhibition was found in *Aspergillus parasiticus, Fusarium moniliforme, Penicillium digitatum* and *Aspergillus flavus* (Jayaprakasha *et al.*, 2001). Due to traditional use of turmeric powder in food products, several researches have done to study the antifungal aspects of turmeric and curcumin. The study of adding turmeric in the plant tissue culture exhibited that turmeric at the concentration of 0.8 to 1.0 g/L had substantial inhibitory action against different fungal contaminations. Regarding the antifungal activities of *Curcuma longa* the most noteworthy effect was recorded against *Paracoccidioides brasiliensis* and *Aspergillus parasiticus,* species, although curcumin shown fungicide effect against several fungi. The methanolic extract of *Curcuma longa* revealed antifungal activity against *Candida albicans* and *Cryptococcus neoformans* with MIC values of 126 and 258mg/mL, respectively (Moghadamtous *et al.*, 2014). Zhang *et al.* (2012) tested the action of curcuminoids on *Candida albicans* growth with the use of microcalorimetry. Structural activity relationship confirmed that the existence of the methoxyl group might enhance lipophilicity of the mother nucleus, which made easier for the molecule to enter into the cell membrane of fungi inhibiting its growth.

8.5.6 *Anti-coccidial Effects*

Coccidiosis is one of the most detrimental and lethal management diseases of poultry. It causes high mortality in affected flocks. Abbas *et al.* (2010) found maximum coccidiostatic effect with Turmeric added at 3% levels in the diet as compared to other infected groups receiving Turmeric containing rations, which were comparable with using a standard coccidiostat i.e., salinomycin sodium. In the same study, the peak excretion of oocysts was delayed about 1 or 2 days relative to the control infected group. Lee *et al.* (2010) reported that faecal oocyst shedding from birds experimentally infected with E. acervulina was significantly decreased, when broiler chickens were fed with a diet containing C. longa. Khalafalla *et al.* (2011) reported that curcumin at concentrations of 25, 50, 100, 200 and 400 μM showed considerable effects on Emeria tenella sporozoite morphology and viability in a dose-dependent manner after incubation over 3, 6, 18 and 24 hours. In the same experiment, in comparison to the untreated control, sporozoite infectivity was reduced at curcumin concentrations of 100 and 200μM by 41.6% and 72.8%, respectively. Allen *et al.* (1998) reported that mid small intestinal lesion scores induced by Emeria maxima were reduced in broilers fed with 1% dietary turmeric during infection. Khalafalla *et al.* (2011) suggested that the ability of curcumin (diferuloylmethane) to kill extra cellular stages of *E. tenella* could be due to its cytotoxic damage affecting parasite viability, morphology and hence, activity. Allen *et al.* (1998) proposed the anticoccidial activity of turmeric is due to its antioxidant properties.

8.5.7 *Immunomodulatory Properties*

The polar fraction of *C. longa* has been tested for immunomodulatory activities on human peripheral blood mononuclear cells. This extract exhibited stimulatory effects on the proliferation of such cells, evaluated by the (methyl- 3H)-thymidine incorporation assay. It was concluded that curcuminoids and polysaccharides can be used as potentially adjuvant supplement for cancer patients whose immune system was suppressed by chemotherapy (Yue *et al.*, 2010a). Furthermore, α-turmerone and ar-turmerone have shown stimulatory effects on peripheral blood mononuclear cells proliferation and cytokine production (Yue *et al.*, 2010b). It has been shown that curcumin can modulate the immune system. Mucosal CD4 (+) T and B cells increases in animals treated with curcumin, suggesting that it modulates lymphocyte-mediated immune functions (Churchill *et al.*, 2000). Al-Sultan (2003) reported that the higher levels of Turmeric inclusion (0.5 and 1.0%) increased both erythrocytic and total leukocytic count in broilers, which may be due to curcumin, an active compound in Curcuma longa (Antony *et al.*, 1999). Kumari *et al.* (2001) recorded significant high antibody titres in broiler chicks fed with C. longa at the level of 1g/kg. Kurkure *et al.* (2001) reported that Turmeric restored the reduced humoral response caused by aflatoxin induced immuno-suppression, suggesting humoral immunestimulatory potential. Sawale *et al.* (2009) recorded increased haemagglutination titre in laying hens treated with herbomineral toxin binder containing turmeric.

8.6 Effect of Turmeric Supplementation in Poultry

Turmeric acts as an antioxidant, antimutagenic, anti-inflammatory and antimicrobial agent and protects liver against a variety of toxicants. These significant biological properties of turmeric powder make it a potential substitute for in-feed antibiotics in livestock diets. The literature on the effects of supplementation turmeric powder on growth performance, carcass characteristics, nutrient utilization, serum bio-chemical parameters and sensory properties in broiler chicken and egg production and egg quality in laying hens have been reviewed as under.

8.6.1 *Growth Performances*

Turmeric has growth promoting effect due to its antioxidant, anti-microbial and anti-inflammatory effect. Al-Sultan (2003) reported that dietary supplementation of 5.0 g/kg turmeric meal in the diets of broiler chickens improved body weight gain and reduced feed intake, resulted in a better feed conversion ratio. Turmeric administration in broiler was actually hoped to be able to enhance the nutrients metabolism (Al-Sultan and Gameel, 2004) that later on could be improve feed efficiency of broilers. Similar results were found by Durrani *et al.* (2006) that 5.0 g/kg supplementation significantly improved body weight gain and reduced feed consumption of broiler chickens and a better feed conversion ratio. In this study, turmeric meal supplementation also improved carcass quality, reduced fat percentage, increased dressing percentage, as well as improved the weight of breast, thigh and giblet. Namagirilakshmi (2005) observed that the cost of feed to produce one kg live broiler chicken was lowest in 0.50 % turmeric supplemented groups in comparison to control. Kumar *et al.* (2005) also observed a significant ($P<0.05$) increase in weight gain in broiler fed with turmeric (1g/kg of diet) over those of the control group. Kumari *et al.* (2007) reported that turmeric meal supplementation at the rate of 1.0 g/kg improved growth performance of 42-d old Vencob broiler chickens. Mehala and Moorthi, (2008) expressed similar opinion and reported that inclusion of turmeric at 0.1 % level improved feed efficiency. Whereas, Zainali *et al.* (2008) reported that dietary supplementation of 10.0 g/kg turmeric meal increased the body weight gain of (Ross x Ross) broiler chickens reared under the heat stress condition.

A feeding study was conducted by Gowda *et al.* (2008) to evaluate the efficacy of turmeric (*Curcuma longa*) powder (TMP), containing 1.48% of curcumin and a hydrated sodium calcium aluminosilicate (HSCAS) to ameliorate the adverse effects of aflatoxin B_1 (AFB_1) in broiler chicks and found that the addition of TMP to the AFB_1 diet significantly ($P < 0.05$) improved the weight gain of chicks. Gowda *et al.* (2009) reported that feeding broiler chickens with diets containing

74 ppm curcuminoids from turmeric meal ameliorated the growth-depression effect of aflatoxin B_1. Similarly, Yarru *et al.* (2009) reported positive effects of 5.0 g/kg turmeric meal supplementation in birds exposed to aflatoxin. Basavaraj *et al.* (2010) performed an experiment to study the effect of dietary supplementation of *Curcuma longa* on the voluntary feed intake and growth performance of broiler rabbits under summer stress by feeding turmeric rhizome powder at varying level and reported that the weekly mean body weight gain, feed conversion efficiency, and digestibility of nutrients did not show significant difference due to the supplementation of turmeric rhizome powder in the diets of rabbits. Lee *et al.* (2010) noted that turmeric meal supplementation alleviated growth-depression effect of Eimeria infection.

Galib *et al.* (2011) conducted an experiment to determine the performance of broilers fed diets supplemented with mixture of turmeric *(Curcuma longa*) and cumin (*Cuminum cyminum)* in which five levels of mixture of turmeric and cumin at the rate of 0.0, 0.25, 0.50, 0.75 and 1% were incorporated in the basal diets for 6 weeks to the five groups of total 300 days old broiler chicks and revealed that the inclusion of mixture of turmeric and cumin at the level of 0.75 and 1% in the diets improved body weight gain, feed intake and feed conversion ratio. Nouzarian *et al.* (2011) studied the effect of turmeric powder supplementation (3.3, 6.6 and 10 g/kg) on carcass traits in male broiler chickens and results obtained showed that broilers fed turmeric supplemented diets exhibited better feed efficiency over the grower and entire experimental periods in comparison with control group ($P<0.05$). Sugiharto *et al.* (2011) studied the effect of turmeric extract (200, 400, 600 and 800 mg/ kg live body weight), on blood parameters, feed efficiency and abdominal fat content in broilers and observed that haemoglobin values of broilers given turmeric extract 800 mg/ kg live body weight was significantly higher ($P<0.05$) at week 3 and week 4 but not at week 5, compared to broilers given turmeric extract with lower doses or control group. Raghdad (2012) studied the effect of turmeric (0.25, 0.50, 1.00 and 1.5%) on broiler performance and physiological traits in which 250 days-old broiler chicks for 42 days. Results revealed that inclusion of turmeric at the level of 0.50% in the diet improved body weight and feed conversion ratio, whereas there was a significant difference in feed consumption. In an another study using Arbor Acre broiler chickens, Rajput *et al.* (2013) showed that supplementation on 0.2 g/kg pure curcumin (phytochemicals derived from turmeric) increased the body weight gain and reduced the FCR of broiler chickens. Improvement on the growth performance due to supplementation of turmeric meal in those studies might be attributed to the beneficial properties of phytochemicals in turmeric that posses antimicrobial, antifungal, and antioxidant activities in broiler chickens that may improve the bird utilisation of dietary nutrients (Osawa *et al.*, 1995; Al-Sultan, 2003; Radwan *et al.*, 2008). On the other hand, there were reports to show that turmeric had the ability to stimulate the digestive system, such as stimulate the intestinal lipase, sucrose, and maltase activities (Patel and Srinivasan, 1996) as well as the secretion of pancreatic lipase, amylase, trypsin, and chimotrypsin enzymes (Platel and Srinivasan, 2000). Rajput et al. (2013) showed that dietary supplementation of pure curcumin at the rate of 0.2 g/kg in a corn-soybean based diets increased villus length and width in the duodenum, jejunum, and caeca of 42 days old broiler chickens. Besides this, positive effect of turmeric is attributed due to its antioxidant activity of turmeric (Osawa *et al.*, 1995; Sugiyama *et al.*, 1996) through stimulation of protein synthesis in the gut by enzymatic system.

8.6.2 Nutrients Utilization

Turmeric also has beneficial effects on nutrients utilization in broiler chickens. Samarasinghe *et al.* (2003) demonstrated that incorporation of man nanoligosaccharides and turmeric (1g/kg feed) significantly increased energy metabolizability and net protein utilization (NPU), whereas at higher levels (2g/kg and 3g/kg) of turmeric reduced the NPU and energy metabolizability in broiler chicken. Maneewan *et al.* (2012) investigated the effects of dietary turmeric on nutrient digestibility in nursery pigs by adding 0.00%, 0.05%, 0.10% and 0.20% turmeric in the feed of 48 nursery pigs divided into four groups with four replicates each and found out that nutrient digestibility of dry matter and energy did not differ significantly among the groups. Digestibility of crude protein, crude fibre ,crude fat , ash and the biological value of protein increased with increasing level of dietary turmeric, and were higher in 0.10% and 0.20% turmeric supplemented groups as compared to control. Rajput *et al.* (2013) studied the effect of dietary supplementation of curcumin on growth performance and nutrients utilization of broiler chicks. For the study, four hundred and eighty days-old Arbor Acre boiler chicks were allocated into four groups with 6 replicates of 20 birds per cage. Birds were fed a corn-soyabean based basal diet supplemented with cucurmin at 0, 100, 150 and 200 mg/kg for 42 days. The results revealed that dietary supplementation of cucurmin at the level of 200mg/kg significantly improved live body weight gain and feed efficiency at marketable age while there was no significant difference on feed intake as compared to control. Cucurmin significantly improved utilization of apparent metabolizable energy and decreased abdominal fat at 42 days in broiler chicken.

8.6.3 Serum Biochemical and Haematological Parameters

Turmeric also has beneficial effects on blood parameters in broiler chickens. It was found that higher levels of turmeric inclusion @1.0%) significant increased both erythrocytic and total leukocytic count in broiler chicken (Antony *et al.,* 1999; Al-Sultan, 2003). Curcumin has also been reported to be able to enhance the concentration of catalase (Reddy and Lokesh, 1994), as well as the expression of hepatic superoxide dismutase (Cheng *et al.,* 2005) and glutathione peroxidase (Yarru *et al.,* 2009), the enzymes that known to have a close relationship with the antioxidant status of the body. These results were consistent with the result in Dias *et al.* (2006) study and showed beneficial properties of phytochemicals in turmeric as antioxidant and hepato-protective agents in poultry (Maheshwari *et al.,* 2006; Shukla and Singh, 2007). Kermanshahi and Riasi (2006) showed that 0.5 to1.5 g/kg turmeric meal supplementation decreased level of triglyceride, total cholesterol, HDL-cholesterol, and increased level of low-density lipoproteincholesterol (LDL-cholesterol) in the blood of Hy-Line W-36 laying hens. Emadi *et al.* (2007) reported that 2.5 g/kg turmeric meal supplementation in the diet increased the total cholesterol and HDL-cholesterol, while 5.0 g/kg supplementation increased haemoglobin and reduced LDL-cholesterol, very low-density lipoproteincholesterol (VLDL-cholesterol), and red blood cells of male Ross broiler chickens at 42 days of age. Emadi and Kermanshahi (2007) reported that supplementation of turmeric meal in the diets reduced the concentrations of alkaline phosphatase (ALP), alanine aminotransferase (ALT), aspartate aminotransferase (AST), and lactate dehydrogenase (LDH) in the blood of broiler chickens.

Broiler birds, when given feed mixed with powdered rhizome of turmeric at the rate of 1g/ kg for 42 days of age, showed significant decrease in serum uric acid and albumin as compared to control, whereas significant increase was recorded in the serum total protein and globulin. Haematological parameters, level of serum glucose, alkaline phosphatase, aspartate amino transferase and calcium showed no significant variation between the treatments (Kumari *et al.*, 2007). Fat metabolism studies using male Wanjiang Yellow (Zhongze *et al.*, 2008) and Arbor Acres (Zhongze, 2009) broiler chickens showed that dietary supplementation of turmeric meal at the rate of 0.35 g/kg consistently stimulated the activity of hormone sensitive lipase (HSL) and increased the content of high-density lipoprotein (HDL) in the serum. Dietary supplementation of turmeric meal also reduced the total cholesterol concentration, total triglycerides, as well as the very low-density lipoprotein (VLDL) content in the blood serum. Other study using (Ross x Ross) male broiler chickens (Gowda *et al.*, 2009) showed that dietary inclusion of 222 mg/kg curcuminoids from turmeric ameliorated the adverse effects of aflatoxin B_1 on serum chemistry in terms of total protein, albumin and glutamyltransferase activity. In that study, the depression in antioxidant functions caused by aflatoxin B_1 was also mitigated by 222 mg/kg curcuminoids inclusion in the diets.

Al- Noori *et al.* (2011) carried out an experiment to determine the effects of turmeric powder on some blood parameter of broiler chickens in which turmeric powder was supplemented to the basal diet at 0.0 (Control), 0.5 and 1.0% (groups 2 and 3), respectively, and the feeding trial lasted for 6 weeks. They observed that addition of turmeric powder significantly increased Hb, PCV, total protein and globulin compared with the control. Sugiharto *et al.* (2011) reported a significant increase in erythrocyte following 600 mg/kg live body weight turmeric meal supplementation in the drinking water of broiler chickens. However, Basavaraj *et al.* (2011) did not find significant ($P>0.05$) effect on the concentration of erythrocytes in the blood of broilers due supplementation of turmeric extract. Malekizadeh *et al.* (2012) demonstrated that adding of turmeric rhizome powder at 3% level to the diets of laying hen significantly ($P<0.05$) decreased total serum cholesterol, ALT, AST and blood uric acid. Riasi *et al.* (2012) also reported that turmeric has a strong property to change the serum lipid profile in laying hens. Dietary supplementation of 0.5 g/kg turmeric meal in the study reduced the serum triglyceride, total and LDL-cholesterol and increased the serum HDL-cholesterol of Hy-Line W-38 laying hens. In other studies using broiler chickens, dietary supplementation of turmeric meal reduced ALT (Akbarian *et al.*, 2012) and alkaline phosphatase (ALP) activities in the blood serum (Emadi and Kermanshahi, 2007), which can be indication of better function of liver. Raghdad (2012) reported that the inclusion of turmeric powder at the level of 0.5% in the diets of broilers had no significant difference in PCV, RBC, Hb and WBC. Hussein (2013) reported that addition of turmeric powder at the rate of 7 g/kg of broiler diet reduced serum concentration of cholesterol and triglycerides. Nayaka *et al.*, (2013) reported that feeding of neem alone or its combination with turmeric and vitamin E significantly increased PCV values in broiler chicken as compared to control.

8.6.4 Carcass Characteristics

Dietary supplementation with turmeric may have beneficial effects on the carcass traits of broiler chickens as it contains beneficial phytochemicals, like curcumin, ar-turmerone, methylcurcumin, and other active compounds. Using a higher level of supplementation (5.0 g/kg), Durrani *et al.* (2006) showed beneficial effects of dietary turmeric meal supplementation to reduce fat content, increase carcass quality and dressing percentage, as well as to increase the breast, thigh, and giblet weight of broiler chickens. Dietary supplementation of turmeric meal had favourable effect to reduce the cost per chick ratio. However, some studies did not find any significant effect of turmeric supplementation at the rate of 1.0 g/kg (Rahmatnejad *et al.*, 2009) or 2.0 g/kg (El-Hakim *et al.*, 2009) on carcass production.

Dietary supplementation of curcumin meal at the rate of 0.35 g/kg reduced the abdominal fat content, subcutaneous fat thickness, intermuscular fat width, and liver fatness of male Wanjiang Yellow (Zhongze *et al.*, 2008) chickens. In another study, Zhongze (2009) reported that percentage of abdominal and liver fat weight as well as subcutaneous fat thickness of Arbor Acres and Wangjiang Yellow broiler chickens were reduced following 0.25 to 0.35 g/kg curcumin supplementation. Samarasinghe *et al.* (2003) noted that 3.0 g/kg turmeric rhizome meal supplementation reduced the fat content and improved carcass quality of broiler chickens. Sultan (2003) revealed that incorporation of turmeric powder at the levels of 0.25, 0.5%, and 1% of broiler diet does not induce any abnormal flavour, colour or smell. He reported that the higher bursa and thymus weight indices were detected in birds received diet containing 0.5% turmeric, while the higher spleen weight index was observed in birds received feed contained 1.0% turmeric powder. Using a higher level of supplementation (5.0 g/kg), Durrani *et al.* (2006) showed beneficial effects of dietary turmeric meal supplementation to reduce fat content, increase carcass quality and dressing percentage, as well as to increase the breast, thigh, and giblet weight of broiler chickens. Emadi and Kermanshahi (2006) observed that the dietary inclusion of turmeric rhizome powder (0.5 and 0.75%) in broiler diets had significantly (p<0.05) decreased the abdominal fat pad size. Similarly, Samarasinghe *et al.* (2003) stated that supplementation of turmeric (3g/kg and 1g/kg feed) markedly reduced fat content to 1.2 and 0.6 % of body weight as compared to 1.91 and 1.22 %, respectively in the control group. Nouzarian *et al.* (2011) studied the effects of turmeric rhizome powder supplementation (3.3, 6.6 and 10 g/ kg) on carcass traits in male broiler chickens. A significant decrease in abdominal fat pad and liver relative weight was observed in chickens fed the supplemented diets. Issa and Omar (2012) investigated the effect of feeding garlic powder on carcass cuts of broilers. Results of this study showed that garlic powder had no significant effects on broilers weight gain, feed intake (FI), feed conversion ratio (FCR), carcass cuts, visceral organs. Reddy *et al.* (2012) showed that inclusion of turmeric powder in the broiler diets at the level of 0.25% and 0.5 % did not influence carcass traits.

Hussein (2013) investigated the effect of dietary level of turmeric (*Cucurma longa*) powder (0, 5, 7, and 9 g/kg diet) on carcass traits and meat quality in broilers. Results indicated that TP supplementation at 7 g/kg of diet significantly (P<0.05) increased liver, gizzard and proventriculus weight and significantly (P> 0.05) decreased abdominal fat compared with the control.

8.6.5 Egg Production and Egg Quality

Turmeric has positive effects on egg production and egg quality of poultry. Kermanshahi and Riasi (2006) conducted a study to evaluate the effect of turmeric (0.0, 0.05, 0.10, 0.15, and 0.20 %) and enzyme (0.0, and 0.05%) on blood parameters of laying hens and revealed that increasing dietary levels of turmeric powder with or without a dietary enzyme significantly (P<0.05) decreased serum triglyceride, total cholesterol and LDL-cholesterol. In a study, Radwan *et al.* (2008) investigated that 5.0 g/kg dietary supplementation of turmeric meal significantly reduced feed conversion ratio, improved body weight gain, as well as increased egg production, egg weight, and egg mass of laying hens. Nadia *et al.* (2008) determined the effect of dietary thyme, rosemary, oregano and turmeric on production performance of laying hens. The results indicated that the addition of 1.0% thyme, rosemary, or oregano or 0.5% turmeric powder to laying hens resulted in the best performance in terms of egg production, egg mass and feed conversion ratio (feed intake/egg mass). Lagana *et al.* (2011) reported that inclusion of turmeric (1%) and annatto (1%) powder improved egg production and yolk colour. Riasi *et al.* (2012) studied the effects of different levels of turmeric rhizome powder (0.0, 0.5, 1, 1.5, and 2 g/ kg) on production performance, egg quality and some serum metabolites of laying hens (Hy-Line W-36) in their second laying cycle. Results showed adding turmeric powder to the diet had no significant effect on egg specific gravity, egg shell thickness, egg shell weight and egg shell weight to egg weight ratio. However, the diets supplemented with 0.5 to 2 g/ kg of turmeric powder markedly decreased ($P<0.05$) feed conversion ratio, serum triglyceride, total and LDL cholesterol.

Park *et al.* (2012) investigated the dietary effects of turmeric powder (0.10, 0.25 or 0.50%) on laying performances, egg qualities and its transfer into eggs. The observed significantly higher egg production, Roche colour fan number due to turmeric supplementation but there were no differences in feed intakes, egg and eggshell. The cholesterol levels of egg yolk were not influenced by dietary turmeric powder. Saraswati *et al.* (2013) conducted an experiment to study the effect of turmeric powder (54 mg/quail/day) supplementation on egg production in Japanese quails. They concluded that turmeric supplementation could be used to increase total number of egg production in Japanese quails improving liver function and increased follicular growth and development.

8.7 Summary and Coclusions

Turmeric (*Curcuma longa*) is a perennial herb of Zingiberaceae family that is widely used and cultivated in the tropical and sub-tropical regions of the world. Turmeric rhizome powder posses antioxidant, antibacterial, anti-inflammatory, antihypertensive and hypo-cholesterolemic properties due to presence of phytochemicals *viz.* curcumin, demethoxycurcumin, tetrahydro-curcumin, curcuminoids, arturmerone, zingiberene, turmerone and curlone. Curcumin contains powerful anti-inflammatory, anti-diabetic, antioxidant, and even anti-cancer properties that render it a powerful, disease-fighting medicine in addition to being a culinary spice. Turmeric has been used in poultry ration as feed additive to improve groth performance and egg production without affecting carcass quality. When compared with the synthetic antibiotics, phytochemicals in turmeric are known to be natural, less toxic, residue free, and are thought to be ideal as feed additives in animal diets.

References

Abbas RZ, Iqbal Z, Khan MN, Zafar MA, Zia MA (2010) Anticoccidial activity of Curcuma longa L. in broilers. Braz Arch Biol Technol 53: 63-67

Akbarian A, Golian A, Kermanshahi H, Gilani A, Moradi S (2012) Influence of turmeric rhizome and black pepper on blood constituents and performance of broiler chickens. Afr J Biotech 11(34): 806-811

Al-Noori MA, Hossain AB, Al-Maahidy AHA, Rawi SJA (2011) The effect of dietary Curcuma longa (turmeric) powder supplementation on some blood parameters and carcass traits of broiler chickens. Al-Anbar J Vety Sci 4: 69-74

Alia BH, Marrif H, Noureldayemc SA, Bakheitd AO, Blunden G (2006). Biological properties of curcumin: A review. Natural Product Commun 1: 509-21

Allen PC, Danforth HD, Augustine PC (1998) Dietary modulation of avian coccidiosis. International J Parasitol 28: 1131-1140

Al-Sultan SI, Gameel AA (2004) Histopathological changes in the livers of broiler chicken supplemented with turmeric (Curcuma longa). International J Poult Sci 3: 333-36

Al-Sultan SI (2003) The effect of curcuma longa (tumeric) on overall performance of broiler chickens. International J Poult Sci 2: 351-53

Ammon HPT, Safayhi H, Mack T, Sabieraj, J. 1993. Mechanism of anti-inflammatory actions of curcumine and boswellic acids. J Ethnopharmacol 38: 105-112

Antony S, Kuttan R, Kuttan G (1999) Immunomodulatory activity of curcumin. Immunol Investigations 28: 291-303

Anwarul HG, Abdul J, Muhammad N, Kashif M (2006) Pharmacological basis for the use of turmeric in gastrointestinal and respiratory disorders. Life Sci 76: 3089-3105

Baik KU, Jung SH, Ahn BZ (1993) Recognition of pharmacophore of ar-turmerone for its anticancer activity. Archives Pharmacol Res. 16: 254-256

Basavaraj M, Nagabhushana V, Prakash N, Mallikarjunappa S, Appannavar MM, Wagmare, P (2010) Effect of dietary supplementation of Curcuma longa on the voluntary feed intake, nutrient digestibility and growth performance of broiler rabbits under summer stress. Vety World. 3(8): 369-372

Basavaraj M, Nagabhushana V, Prakash N, Appannavar MM, Wagmare P, Mallikarjunappa S (2011) Effect of dietary supplementation of Curcuma longa on the biochemical profile and meat characteristics of broiler rabbits under summer stress. Vety World. 4(1): 15-18

Burt S (2004) Essential oils: Their antibacterial properties and potential applications in foods: A review. International J Food Microbial. 94: 223-253

Chattopadhyay I, Biswas K, Bandyopadhyay U, Banerjee RK (2004) Turmeric and curcumin: Biological actions and medicinal applications. Current Sci 87: 44-53

Chen YJ, Kim I J, Choi J H, Yoo, J S, Wang Q, Wang Y, Huang Y (2008) Evaluation of dietary l-carnitine or garlic powder on growth performance, dry matter and nitrogen digestibilities, blood profiles and meat quality in finishing pigs. *Anim Feed Sci Technol* 141 (1): 141-152

Churchill M, Chadburn A, Bilinski RT, Bertagonlli MM (2000) Inhibition of intestinal tumors by curcumin is associated with changes in the intestinal immune cell profile. J Surgical Research 89: 169-175

Dias MC, Spinardi-Barbisan ALT, Rodrigues MAM, De Camargo JLV, Teran E, Barbisan LF (2006). Lack of chemo-preventive effects of ginger on colon carcinogenesis induced by 1, 2-dimethylhydrazine in rats. Food Chem Toxicol 44: 877-884

Durrani FR, Ismail M, Sultan A, Suhail SM, Chand N, Durrani Z (2006) Effect of different levels of feed added turmeric (Curcuma longa) on the performance of broiler chicks. J Agric Biol Sci 1: 9-11

El-Hakim ASA, Cherian G, Ali MN (2009) Use of organic acid, herbs and their combination to improve the utilization of commercial low protein broiler diets. International J Poult Sci 8: 14-20

Emadi M, Kermanshahi H (2007) Effect of turmeric rhizome powder on the activity of some blood enzymes in broiler chickens. International J Poult Sci 6(1): 48-51

Ferreira, L.A.F., Henriques, O.B., Andreoni, A.A.S. Vital, G.R.F., Campos, M.M.C., Habermehl, G.G. and DeMoraes, V.L.G. 1992. Antivenom and bio- logical effects of ar-turmerone isolated from Curcuma longa (Zingiberaceae). Toxicol 30: 1211-1218

Galib AM A, Akhil MM, Raghad AA (2011) Modification of productive performance and physiological aspects of broilers on the addition of a mixture of cumin and turmeric to the diet. Res Option Animal Vet Sci 1(1): 31-34

Govindarajan VS, Stahl WH (1980) Turmeric - Chemistry, technology and quality. Critical Rev Food Sci Nutr 12: 199-301

Gowda NKS, Ledoux DR, Rottinghaus GE, Bermudez AJ and Chen YC (2009) Efficacy of turmeric (Curcuma longa), containing a known level of curcumin, and a hydrated sodium calcium aluminosilicate to ameliorate the adverse effects of aflatoxin in broiler chicks. Poult Sci 87(6): 1125-1130

Holt PR, Katz S, Kirshoff R (2005) Curcumin therapy in inflammatory bowel disease: a pilot study. Digestive Dis Sci 50: 2191-2193

Huang M, T, Ma W, Lu YP, Chang RL, Fisher C, Manchand PS, Newmark HL, Conney AH, You M (1995) Effects of curcumin, demethoxycurcumin, bisdemethoxycurcumin and tetrahydrocurcumin on 12-O-tetradecanoylphorbol-13-acetate induced tumour promotion. Carcinogenesis 16: 2493-2497

Hussein SN (2013) Effect of turmeric (Curcuma longa) powder on growth performance, carcass traits, meat quality and serum biochemical parameters in broilers. J Advance Biomedical Pathobiology Res 3(2): 25-32.

Iqbal M, Sharma SM, Fujisawa M, Okada SU (2003) Dietary supplementation of curcumin enhances antioxidant and phase ii metabolizing enzymes male mice: possible role in protection against chemical carcinogenesis and toxicity. J Pharma Toxicol 92: 33-38

Issa KJ, Omar JM (2012) Effect of garlic powder on performance and lipid profile of broilers. Open J Anim Sci 2(2): 62-68

Jayaprakasha GK, Jagan Mohan Rao L, Sakariah KK (2005) Chemistry and biological activities of C. longa. Trends Food Sci Technol 16: 533-548

Johnson AM, Rohifs E M, Silverman LM (1999) Protein. In: The Textbook of Clinical Chemistry. W.B. Saunders Philadelphia

Kermanshahi H, Riasi A (2006) Effect of turmeric rhizome powder (Curcuma longa) and soluble NSP degrading enzyme on some blood parameters of laying hens. International J Poult Sci 5(5): 494-498

Khalafalla R E, Müller U, Shahiduzzaman M, Dyachenko, V, Desouky AY, Alber G, Daugschies A (2011). Effects of curcumin (diferuloylmethane) on Eimeria tenella sporozoites in vitro. Parasitol Res 108: 879-886

Kiuchi F, Goto Y, Sugimoto N, Akao N, Kondo K Tsuda Y (1993) Nematocidal activity of turmeric: Synergistic action of curcuminoids. Chem Pharmaceutical Bulletin 41: 1640-1643

Kumar J, Singh Y, Verma PK, Nazki AR (2010) Effect of dietary supplementation of Emblica officinal is on biochemical indices inVanaraja chicks. Ind J Anim Sci 80(1): 78-80

Kumari P, Gupta MK, Ranjan R, Singh KK, Yadava R (2001) Curcuma longa as feed additive in broiler birds and its patho-physiological effects. Indian J Exp Biol 45: 272-277

Kurkure NV, Paswar SP, Kongole SM, Ganorkar AG, Bhandarkar AG, Kalorey DR (2001) Ameliorative effect of Turmeric (*Curcuma longa*) in induced aflatoxicosis in cockerels. Indian J Vety Pathol 10: 35

Lagana C, Pizzolante CC, Salanha ESPB, Moraes JE (2011). Turmeric root and Annato Seed in second cycle layer diet: performance and egg quality. Braz J Poult Sci 13(3): 171-176

Lee K, Lillehoj HS, Siragusa GR (2010) Direct-fed microbials and their impact on the intestinal microflora and immune system of chickens. J Poult Sci 47: 106-114

Maheshwari RK, Singh AK, Gaddipati J, Srimal RC (2006) Multiple biological activities of curcumin: a short review. Life Sci 78: 2081-2087

Malekizadeh M, Moeini MM, Ghazi S (2012) The effects of different levels of ginger (Zingiber officinale Rosc) and turmeric (Curcuma longa) rhizomes powder on some blood metabolites and production performance characteristics of laying hens. J Agric Sci Technol 14: 127-134

Mandroli PS, Bhat K (2013) An *in-vitro* evaluation of antibacterial activity of curcumin against common endodontic bacteria. Journal of Applied Pharmam Sci 3(10): 106-108

Maneewan C, Yamaochi K E, Mekbungwan A (2012) Effect of turmeric on growth performance, nutrient digestibility, haematological values, and intestinal histology in nursery pigs. J Swine Health Prod 20(5): 231-240

Mehala C, Moorthy M (2008) Production performance of broilers fed with aloe vera, Curcuma longa (turmeric). International J Poult Sci 7: 852-856

Nadia RL, Hassan RA, Qota EM, Fayek HM (2008) Effect of natural antioxidant on oxidative stability of eggs and productive and reproductive performance of laying hens. International Journal Poultry Science. 7(2): 134-150

Nayaka HB, Umakantha B, Ruban SW, Murthy SNN, Narayanaswamy HD (2013) Performance and hematological parameters of broilers fed neem, turmeric, vitamin E and their combinations. Journal of Food and Agriculture. 25(6): 483-488

Negi PS, Jayaprakasha GK, Jagan L, Rao Mohan Sakariah KK (1999) Antibacterial activity of turmeric oil: a by-product from curcumin. Journal of Agriculture and Food Chemistry. 47: 4297-4300

Nouzarian R, Tabeidian SA, Toghyani A, Ghalamkari G, Toghyani M (2011) Effect of turmeric powder on performance, carcass traits, humoral immune responses, and serum metabolites in broiler chickens.Journal of Animal and Feed Science. 20: 389-400

Odhav B, Juglal, R Govinden (2002). Response of broiler chicks in terms of performance and meat quality to garlic (*Allium sativum*) supplemation. Afr J Agric Res 4(5): 511-517

Osawa TY, Sugiyama M Inayoshi, Kawakishi S (1995) Antioxidative activity of tetrahydro curcuminoids. Bio-sci Biotechnol Biochem 59: 1609-1612

Park SS, Kim JM, Kim EJ, Kim HS, An BK, Kang CW (2012). Effects of Dietary Turmeric Powder on Laying Performance and Egg Qualities in Laying Hens. Korean J Poult Sci 39(1): 27-32

Platel K, Srinivasan K (2000) Influence of dietary spices and their active principles on pancreatic digestive enzymes in albino rats. Food Nahrung 44: 42-46

Polasa K, Raghuram TC, Krishna TP (1991) Turmeric (Curcuma longa L.) induced reduction in urinary mutagens. Food Chem Toxicol 29: 699-706

Radwan NL, Hassan RA, Qota EM, Fayek HM (2008) Effect of natural antioxidant on oxidative stability of eggs and productive and reproductive performance of laying hens. International J Poult Sci 7: 134-150

Raghdad A (2012) Use of turmeric (Curcuma longa) on the performance and some physiological traits on the broiler diets. Iraqi JVet Med 36(1): 51-57

Rahmatnejad E, Roshanfekr H, Ashayerizadeh O, Mamooee M, Ashayerizadeh, A. (2009) Evaluation the effect of several non-antibiotic additives on growth performance of broiler chickens. J Anim Vet Adv 8: 1670-1673

Rajput N, Muhammad N, Yaan R, Zhong X, Wang T (2013) Effect of dietary supplementation of curcumin on growth performance, intestinal morphology and nutrients utilization of broiler chicks. J Poult Sci 50: 44-52

Ramirez-Tortosa MC, Mesa MD, Aguilera MC, Quiles JL, Baro L (1999) Oral administration of a turmeric extract inhibits LDL oxidation and has hypocholesterolemic effects in rabbits with experimental atherosclerosis. Atherosclerosis. 147: 371-378

Reddy AC, Lokesh B R (1994) Effect of dietary turmeric (Curcuma longa) on iron-induced lipid peroxidation in the rat liver. Food Chem Toxicol 32: 279-283

Riasi A, Kermanshahi H, Mahdavi AH (2012) Production performance, egg quality and some serum metabolites of older commercial laying hens fed different levels of turmeric rhizome (Curcuma longa) powder. J Medicinal Plants Res 6(11): 2141-2145

Roughley PJ, Whiting DA (1973) Experiments in the bio-synthesis of curcumin. J Chem Society Perkin Transactions. 20: 2379-2388

Samarasinghe K, Wenk Silva KFST, Gunasekera JM (2003) Turmeric (*Curcuma longa*) root powder and manna oligosaccharides as alternatives to antibiotics in broiler chicken diets. Asian-Austr J Anim Sci 16(10): 1495-1500

Saraswati TR, Manalu W, Ekastuli DR, Kisumorini N (2013) Increased egg production of Japanese quails (*Contunix japonica*) by improving liver function through turmeric powder supplementation. International J Poult Sci 12(10): 601-614

Shukla Y, Singh M (2007) Cancer preventive properties of ginger: A brief review. Food Chem Toxicol 45: 683-690

Smith RM, Robinson JM (1981) The essential oil of ginger from Fiji. Phytochem. 20: 203-206

Sugiharto I, Widiastuti E, Prabowa N S (2011) Effect of turmeric extract on blood parameters, feed efficiency and abdominal fat content in broilers. J Indonesian Trop Anim Agric 36(1): 21-26

Sugiyama Y, Kawakishi S, Osawa T (1996) Involvement of the beta-diketone moiety in the antioxidative mechanism of tetrahydro-curcumin. Biochem Pharama 52: 519-525.

Sultan SI (2003). The effect of Curcuma longa (turmeric) on overall performance of broiler chickens. Int J Poult Sci 2: 351-353

Toennesen HH (1992) Chemistry of curcumin and curcuminoids. In Phenolic Compounds in Food and their Effect of Health, Vol. 1 : Analysis, Occurrence and Chemistry. ACS Symposium Series No. 506, eds. Ho C-T, Lee C, and Huang M-T, pp. 143-153. American Chemical Society, Washington DC

Wang R, Li D Bourne (1998) Can 2000 years of herbal medicine history help us solve problems in the year 2000? In: Biotechnology in the Feed Industry. Proceedings of Alltech's 14th Annual Symposium, ed. Lyons TP and Jacques KA. pp. 273-291

WHO (1987) Principles for the safety assessment of food additives and contaminants in (IPCS), in co-operation with the Joint WHO/FAO Expert Committee on Food Additives (JECFA), Geneva, Switzerland. No. 70

Yarru LP, Settivari RS, Gowda NK, Antoniou E, Rottinghaus GE (2009) Effects of turmeric (Curcuma longa) on the expression of hepatic genes associated with biotransformation, antioxidant, and immune systems in broiler chicks fed aflatoxin. Poult Sci 88(12): 2620-2627

Zainali A, Riasi A, Kermanshahi H, Ziaei H (2008) Effect of selenium and (or) turmeric rhizome powder on growth performance of broiler chickens reared under heat stress condition. 1st Mediterranean Summit of WPSA, Advances and Challenges in Poultry Science. Greece. pp. 790-792

Zhongze H (2009) Effect of curcumin on fat deposition and its mechanism in different breeds chickens. Anhui Agric Sci Bull 5: 107-115.

❑❑❑

Chapter 9

Garlic (*Allium sativum*)

Lipismita Samal

Post-Graduate Department of Poultry Science, College of Veterinary Science and Animal Husbandry, Orissa University of Agriculture and Technology, Bhubaneshwar-751003, India, E-mail: lipismitasamal@gmail.com

ABSTRACT

Garlic has been revered for its formidable prophylactic and therapeutic medicinal properties in many cultures since antiquity. This reverence has escalated further as a result of the emergence of data indicating its potent antioxidant action, its ability to modulate immunological responsiveness, stimulation of prostanoid synthesis, lowering of cholesterol, anti-bacterial, anti-viral, anti-fungal, anti-parasitic and cardio-protective effects. It is an herbal remedy to prevent and treat a variety of metabolic diseases, such as atherosclerosis, thrombosis, hypertension, dementia, cancer and diabetes. In addition to these proclaimed beneficial effects, some garlic preparations also possess anti-inflammatory, hepato-protective, enhanced foreign compound detoxification, radio-protection, restoration of physical strength, resistance to various stresses, anti-aging and hormone-like properties. Garlic supplementation inhibits methane production in ruminants, improves gastrointestinal tract development and live weight in pigs, and improves meat quality in broilers and egg quality in layers. These effects of garlic likely arise from a wide variety of components e.g. steroid saponins, organosulphur compounds and their precursors possibly working synergistically. The chemistry of garlic is quite complex. It contains at least 33 sulphur compounds, several enzymes, 17 amino acids and trace minerals. The toxic components are sulfoxides and aliphatic sulfides. The complex chemistry of garlic makes it plausible that variations in processing can yield quite different preparations, i.e. essential oil, garlic oil macerate, dehydrated garlic powder, garlic extract and by-products.

Keywords: Garlic, Organosulphur compounds, Steroid saponins, Sulfoxides, Sulfides.

9.1. Introduction

Garlic has been widely used as both food and medicine in many cultures since antiquity. Its use in gastrointestinal medicine is noted in the Hippocratic writings, by Galen and Dioscorides. Investigations have shown that garlic plays an important pharmacological role as an anti-bacterial, anti-viral and anti-fungal agent (Amagase *et al.*, 2001). It has been known as an herbal remedy to prevent and treat a variety of heart diseases and metabolic diseases, such as atherosclerosis, thrombosis, hypertension, dementia, cancer and diabetes (Agrawal 1996; Konjufca *et al.*, 1997; Amagase *et al.*, 2001). In addition to these proclaimed beneficial effects, some garlic preparations also appear to possess anti-inflammatory, hepato-protective, immune-modulatory, antioxidant, anti-tumour, enhanced foreign compound detoxification, radio-protection, restoration of physical strength, resistance to various stresses, anti-aging and hormone-like properties (Reuter *et al.*, 1996).

The health benefits of garlic likely arise from a wide variety of components e.g. steroid saponins (monodesmosidic spirostanol saponins, eruboside-B, isoeruboside-B, proto-isoeruboside-B, etc.) and organosulphur compounds (fat soluble, diallyldisulfide; water-soluble, S-allyl methylcysteine; etc.) and their precursors (alliin, diallyl sulfide and diallyl trisulfide) possibly working synergistically. The organosulphur compounds and their precursors may be altered during processing (Amagase *et al.*, 2001). These compounds provide garlic its characteristic odour and flavour. The enzyme allinase that is responsible for converting alliin to allicin is inactive. The enzyme allinase sequestered within garlic cell vacuoles plays a key role in reaction of the chemical substrate and can be changed by temperature, duration of drying, use of polar and non-polar extraction solvents and period of maceration before final extraction. When garlic is chopped or crushed, the allinase enzyme present in garlic is activated and acts on alliin (present in whole garlic) to produce allicin (Fenwick and Hanley, 1985; Fenelli *et al.*, 1998). Traditionally, allicin was thought to be the potentially active component of garlic; however, pharma-cokinetic studies showed that its half-life *in vivo* may be too short to account for the activity seen *in vitro*. Increasingly, attention is being focused on the smaller metabolic breakdown products of this molecule.

9.2 Taxonomy

Garlic (*Allium sativum* L.) belongs to the family *Liliaceae*, which is a genus of 500 species.

Domain	:	Eukarya
Kingdom	:	Plantae
Phylum	:	Magnoliophyta
Class	:	Lilopsida
Order	:	Liliale
Family	:	Liliaceae
Genus	:	*Allium*
Species	:	*Sativa*

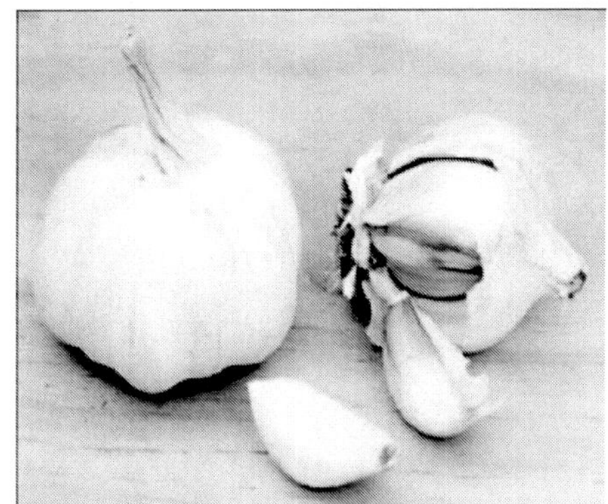

9.3 Chemistry of Garlic

The chemistry of garlic is quite complex. It contains at least 33 sulphur compounds (aliin, allicin, ajoene, allylpropyl disulfide, diallyl trisulfide, S-allyl-cysteine, Vinyldithiines, S-allylmercaptocystein and others), several enzymes (allinase, peroxidases, myrosinase, and others), 17 amino acids (arginine and others) and trace minerals such as selenium, germanium, tellurium and other trace minerals. The toxic components in garlic are sulfoxides and aliphatic sulfides, specifically allyl and propyl di-, tri- and tetra-sulfides.

Processed garlic contains a variety of sulphur-containing compounds other than those found naturally in intact garlic cloves, depending on the conditions applied (Fenwick and Hanley, 1985; Lawson, 1993). Additional constituents of intact garlic include steroidal glycosides (Matsuura *et al.*, 1988), lectins (Kaku *et al.*, 1992), prostaglandins, fructan, pectin, essential oil, adenosine, vitamins B_1, B_2, B_6, C and E, biotin, nicotinic acid, fatty acids, glycolipids, phospholipids, anthocyanins, flavonoids, phenolics and essential amino acids (Fenwick and Hanley, 1985). The primary sulphur-containing constituents in whole intact garlic are the ^-glutamyl-*S*-alk(en)yl-L-cysteines and *S*-alk-(en)yl-L-cysteine sulfoxides, including alliin. The ^-glutamyl peptides are biosynthetic intermediates for corresponding cysteine sulfoxides (Lancaster and Shaw, 1989). Whole garlic typically contains; 1% alliin, together with (1)-*S*-methyl-L-cysteine sulfoxide (methiin), (1)-*S*-(trans-1-propenyl)-L-cysteine sulfoxide, *S*-(2-Carboxypropyl) glutathione, ^-glutamyl-*S*-allyl-L-cysteine, ^-glutamyl-*S*-(trans-1-propenyl)-L-cysteine and ^-glutamyl-*S*-allyl-mercapto-L-cysteine (Fenwick and Hanley, 1985). During storage of garlic bulbs at cool temperatures, alliin accumulates naturally. On average, a garlic bulb contains upto 0.9% ^-glutamyl-cysteine and up to 1.8% alliin. Garlic is famous for its characteristic odour, arising from allicin and other oil-soluble sulphur components. Typical volatiles in crushed garlic and garlic essential oil include diallyl sulfide, diallyl disulfide, diallyl trisulfide, methyl allyl disulfide, methyl allyl trisulfide, 2-vinyl-1,3- dithiin, 3-vinyl-1,2-dithiin and *E*, *Z*-ajoene (Fenwick and Hanley, 1985).

When garlic is attacked by a microbe, crushed, cut or chewed, or when it is dehydrated, pulverized and then exposed to water, the vacuolar enzyme, alliinase (a cysteine sulfoxide lyase), rapidly lyses the odourless amino acid alliin (cysteine sulfoxides) to form the cytotoxic and odiferous alkyl alkane-thiosulfinates that are the source of the characteristic odour of garlic. The transiently formed compound, allicin, an oily, odorous, colourless liquid, comprises 70–80% of the thiosulfinates. Thiosulfinates and other secondary metabolites of garlic, including ^-glutamyl peptides, scordinins, steroids, terpenoids, flavonoids and other phenols, may be responsible for the range of therapeutic effects reported for garlic. Allicin is highly unstable thiosulfinate compound that decomposes to sulphides, including ajoene and dithiins. Allicin and ajoene are potent cardiac and smooth muscle relaxants, vasodilators, and hypotensive agents. Although freshly crushed garlic may contain limited amount of allicin, no commercially available processed garlic preparations contain allicin.

9.4 Different Garlic Preparations

The complex chemistry of garlic makes it plausible that variations in processing can yield quite different preparations, i.e. essential oil, garlic oil macerate, dehydrated garlic powder, garlic extract and by-products.

9.4.1 *Essential Oil*

Garlic essential oil is obtained by steam distillation of garlic. The essential oil content of garlic cloves is 0.2–0.5% and consists of a variety of sulphides, such as diallyl disulfide and diallyl trisulfide (Block, 1985). Whole garlic cloves, ground in water, are heat-distilled or extracted in an organic solvent (e.g., hexane) to obtain the oil fraction. Water-soluble compounds are totally eliminated by this process. Allicin is also completely eliminated from the oil.

9.4.2 *Dehydrated Garlic Powder*

Garlic cloves are sliced or crushed, dried and pulverized into powder. Garlic powder is thought to retain the same ingredients as raw garlic; however, the proportions and amounts of various constituents differ significantly (Iberl *et al.,* 1990a). The main sulphur compound in both raw garlic and garlic powder is alliin. Garlic cloves contain approximately 0.8% alliin. More than half of the alliin is lost during dehydration and a pure dehydration process would result into 2–2.5 mg/g alliin content in the powder.

9.4.3 *Garlic oil Macerate*

Oil macerate products are made of encapsulated mixtures of whole garlic cloves ground into vegetable oil. During the manufacturing process, some alliin is converted to allicin. Because allicin is unstable and decomposes quickly, oil macerate preparations contain allicin-decomposed compounds such as dithiins, ajoene, sulfides and residual amounts of alliin (Block 1985; Iberl *et al.,* 1990b).

9.4.4 *Garlic Extract*

The irritating, acidic and oxidizing compounds in raw garlic can be eliminated or modified by extraction. For garlic extract, whole or sliced garlic cloves are soaked in extracting solution (e.g., purified water and diluted alcohol) for varying periods. After separation of the solution, the extract is generally concentrated and used. Powdered forms of the extract are also available. Aged garlic extract (AGE) is prepared by aging upto 20 months. During this aging process, the odorous, harsh and irritating compounds in garlic are converted naturally into stable and safe sulphur compounds. AGE is a complex mixture of allin, cycloalliin, S-allyl-L-cysteine, S-methyl-L-cysteine, S-ethyl-cysteine, S-1-proponyl-L-cysteine, S-allylmercapto-L-cysteine, *N*a-fructosyl-arginine, β-chlorogenin, L-arginine, L-cysteine, and L-methionine. AGE reduces the parameters associated with cardiovascular disease, including the inhibition of platelet aggregation. In some cultures, garlic is soaked or extracted with alcohol, wine, milk or vinegar before use.

9.4.5 *Garlic By-products*

The garlic industry produces by-products such as husk and stems that are wasted with no further use. Garlic bulbs yield approximately 760 g of cloves and 240 g of outer and inner husks per kg (Qureshi *et al.*, 1983b), which may possess substantive nutritional value such as polyphenols and flavonoids. Garlic husk had even higher total phenolics than garlic bulb.

9.5 Biological Activities of Garlic in Livestock and Poultry

9.5.1 *Methane Mitigating Effects*

Organosulphur compounds of garlic seem to have a great potential for suppressing rumen-derived CH_4 due to their effect on methanogens. Another effect is the increase in the propionate-to-acetate ratio resulting in lower amounts of H_2 available for methanogenesis. Clear CH_4 mitigating effects were found in many *in vitro* studies when supplementing garlic extracts (e.g., Cardozo *et al.*, 2005; Chaves *et al.*, 2008), ground garlic bulbs (Kongmun *et al.*, 2010) or essential oils derived from garlic and other herbs (Busquet *et al.*, 2005; Patra and Yu, 2012). When used at low doses, garlic, garlic oil and its organosulphur compounds consistently decreased methane production *in vitro* without negatively affecting feed fermentation (Busquet *et al.*, 2005), but no effects of garlic oil or its compounds on methanogenesis have been observed in lactating cows (van Zijderveld *et al.*, 2011), sheep (Patra *et al.*, 2011) or fattening bulls (Staerfl *et al.*, 2012). The lack of response *in vivo* is partly attributed to the adaptation of microbes (Bodas *et al.*, 2012), but also to the use of lower doses compared to those in the in vitro experiments. The strong CH_4 mitigating effect of garlic bulbs compared to the control was found in several studies (e.g. Cardozo *et al.*, 2005; Kongmun *et al.*, 2010). Chaves *et al.* (2008) added 100 and 250 mg/l of garlic oil to mixed ruminal microbes which decreased CH_4 formation by about 70%. Cardozo *et al.* (2005) found a decrease in acetate proportion with garlic oil at unchanged propionate proportions but this was associated with a decrease in total short-chain fatty acids concentration. However, propionate proportion was decreased with a garlic extract at an unchanged acetate proportion in the study of Chaves *et al.* (2008). The hydrogen could also be utilized to reduce sulphate to sulphides, which might be relevant as garlic is rich in sulphur containing compounds. Entire garlic bulbs so far have only been researched with respect to their efficiency in mitigating CH_4 when added to a rice straw-concentrate diet *in vitro* (Kongmun *et al.,* 2010). Calsamiglia et al. (2007) observed that garlic oil may increase propionate production; reduce acetate and methane production in the rumen. Patra *et al.* (2006) observed methane reduction with dietary supplementation with ethanol and methanol extract of garlic. There was a tendency towards an increase in the diversity of methanogens in comparison to *Methanosphaera stadtmanae, Methanobrevibacter smithii* and some uncultured groups with garlic supplementation (Ohene-Adjei *et al.,* 2008).

9.5.2 *Inhibition of Carcinogenesis*

Consumption of garlic, fresh garlic extracts, aged garlic, garlic oil and its associated sulphur components reduced carcinogen induced mammary, colon, oesophageal, lung, breast, uterine, oesophagus, fore stomach, skin and liver tumours in laboratory animals, including prostate cancer (Amagase and Milner, 1993). Selenium-enriched garlic is each more effective cancer chemopreventive agent in various animal models than regular garlic. The ability of garlic and related allyl sulphur compounds to block tumours in different organs suggests general mechanisms that are not tissue specific. This protection may arise from several mechanisms including the following: blockage of *N*-nitroso compound (NOC) formation, suppression in the bioactivation of several carcinogens, enhanced DNA repair, reduced cell proliferation and/or induction of apoptosis. Molecular investigations support existing clinical and epidemiological data that garlic-derived allylsulfides reduce cancer risk. It is also apparent that the allyl sulphur compounds in garlic do not function in isolation but are influenced by several components of the diet. Various allylsulfides can diminish progression of cancer cells at either the G1/S or G2/M phase. Allylsulfide derivatives modify redox-sensitive signal pathways and cause growth inhibition, mitotic arrest and apoptosis induction. â-elimination reactions with cysteine S-conjugates in garlic may modify cancer-cell growth by targeting redox-sensitive signal proteins at sulfhydryl sites, thereby regulating cell proliferation and/or apoptotic responses. Several animal model studies demonstrate that allylsulfides, in particular diallylsulfide, diallyltrisulfide, allylmethylsulfide and ajoene specifically modulate the activities of cytochrome P450 mixed-function oxidases and thus, inhibit tumours induced by a wide variety of carcinogens. Concurrent with selective modification of phase I P450 enzymes, organosulfides facilitate detoxification of carcinogens through up regulation of phase II-conjugating enzymes such as glutathione S-transferases, epoxide hydrolase, quinone reductase, and UDP-glucuronosyltransferase. Considerable information points to the ability of garlic to suppress the formation of NOC carcinogens (Dion *et al.*, 1997). Exposure to these potential carcinogens can occur through either ingestion or inhalation of preformed nitrosamines or by the ingestion of their precursors. A reduction in nitrosamines may occur as a result of the enhanced formation of nitrosothiols after ingestion of garlic.

9.5.3 *Anti-bacterial Activity*

Historically, garlic has been used worldwide to fight bacterial infections. Louis Pasteur was the first to describe the anti-bacterial effect of garlic juice. There is extensive literature on the anti-bacterial effects of fresh garlic juice, aqueous and alcoholic extracts, lyophilized powders, steam distilled oil and other commercial preparations of garlic. Garlic exhibits a broad antibiotic spectrum against both gram-positive and gram-negative bacteria. It has been reported to inhibit *Aerobacter, Aeromonas, Bacillus, Citrella, Citrobacter, Clostridium, Enterobacter, Escherichia, Klebsiella, Lactobacillus, Leuconostoc, Micrococcus, Mycobacterium, Proteus, Providencia, Pseudomonas, Salmonella, Serratia, Shigella, Staphylococcus, Streptococcus* and *Vibrio*. Enterotoxic coli strains and other pathogenic intestinal bacteria, which are responsible for diarrhoea in animals, are more easily inhibited by garlic than the normal intestinal microbiota (Caldwell and Danzer, 1988). Garlic is active even against organisms that have become resistant to antibiotics. The combination of garlic extracts with antibiotics leads to partial or total synergism (Didry *et al.*, 1992). Raw juice of garlic was found to be effective against many common pathogenic intestinal bacteria, which are responsible for diarrhoea in animals; garlic is effective even against those strains that have become resistant to antibiotics (Singh and Shukla, 1984); the combination of garlic with antibiotics leads to partial or total synergism; complete lack of resistance has been found; even toxin production by microorganisms is prevented by garlic. A garlic oil preparation showed good anti-tuberculosis activity in guinea pigs with an intra-peritoneal dose of 0.5 mg/kg (Jain, 1993). *Helicobacter pylori* is susceptible to garlic extract at a fairly moderate concentration (Sivam *et al.*, 1997). *H. pylori is* a bacterium implicated in the etiology of stomach cancer and ulcers (Fuchs and Mayer, 1995). Even some antibiotic-resistant *H. pylori* strains are susceptible to garlic.

Thiosulfinates play an important role in the antibiotic activity of garlic. Hughes and Lawson (1991) showed that the antimicrobial activity of garlic is completely abolished when the thiosulfinates (e.g., allicin) are removed from the extract. Also, upon reduction of allicin to diallyl disulfide, the anti-bacterial activity is greatly reduced (Reuter *et al.*, 1996). Feldberg *et al.* (1988) showed that allicin exhibits its anti-microbial activity mainly by immediate and total inhibition of RNA synthesis, although DNA and protein syntheses are also partially inhibited, suggesting that RNA is the primary target of allicin action. The structural differences of bacteria affect their susceptibility to garlic constituents. The cell membrane of *Escherichia coli* contains 20% lipid, whereas that of *Staphylococcus aureus* contains only 2% lipid. The lipid content of the membranes will have an effect on the permeability of allicin and other garlic constituents. Differential inhibitory effects against *Escherichia coli* and *Lactobacillus casei*, whereby a 10-fold greater sensitivity was evident in the former (Rees *et al.*, 1993) have been observed because of the different membrane structures in gram-positive and gram-negative bacteria.

9.5.4 *Anti-protozoal Activity*

Anti-protozoal studies of garlic on *Entamoeba histolytica* and *Giardia intestinalis* (Harris *et al.*, 2000) include a wide range of ultra-structural lesions affecting cytoplasmic membranes, organelles and cytoskeletal organization. The microaerophilic flagellate parasitic protozoon, *G. intestinalis* is the most commonly diagnosed cause of waterborne diarrhoea. Kaempferol and quercetin compounds of garlic have been shown to have anti-giardial activity *in vitro*.

9.5.5 *Anti-fungal Activity*

Monodesmosidic spirostanol saponins of garlic have significant anti-fungal activity. Eruboside-B was found to be active against *Candida albicans* with a mean inhibitory concentration of 25 mg/mL. The anti-fungal activity of eruboside-B is comparable to that reported for allicin or ajoene (Yoshida *et al.*, 1987). The anti-candidal effects of garlic also include a wide range of ultra-structural lesions affecting cytoplasmic membranes, organelles and cytoskeletal organization.

9.5.6 *Anti-parasitic Activity*

Garlic can be used as a prophylactic and therapeutic treatment against *Schistosoma mansoni*. Garlic treatment significantly evoked a reduction in the egg and worm burden. Garlic also resulted in various ultra-structural alterations in the tegument of the surviving worms including tubercular disruption, oedema, blebbing, ulcers and vacuolization of other tegumental structures.

9.5.7 *Cholesterol-lowering Effects*

It has been reported that steam-distilled garlic oil, the ether fraction of garlic, alliin and its enzymatic transformation products i.e. allicin and diallyl disulfide, might be responsible for the cholesterol-lowering effects of garlic in animals (Adamu *et al.,* 1982; Abo-Doma *et al.,* 1991). Koch (1993) indicated that the cholesterol-lowering effect of garlic preparations may be due to its saponin content. Several studies reported that the crude glycoside fraction from methanolic raw-garlic extracts, which mainly contains spirostanol saponins produced by the conversion of furostanol saponins via â-glucosidase, lowered total plasma cholesterol and low-density lipoprotein (LDL) cholesterol without changing high-density lipoprotein (HDL) cholesterol levels in a hypercholesterolemic animal model. Garlic supplementation in the diet depressed the hepatic activities of several lipogenic and cholesterogenic enzymes, including malic enzyme, fatty acid synthase, glucose-6 phosphate dehydrogenase, acetyl-CoA synthetase, 3-hydroxy-3-methylglutaryl-CoA (HMG-CoA) reductase and cholesterol 7á-hydroxylase (Qureshi *et al.,* 1983a; 1983b; 1987) and it is possible that additional enzymes in the cholesterol synthesis pathway are also inhibited. Water-soluble organosulphur compounds may be the major principles of garlic responsible for the inhibition of cholesterol synthesis and reduction in plasma cholesterol level.

There have been reports on the beneficial effects of garlic extract and oil in controlling hyperlipidemia in animals. Because hyperlipidemia is a major etiopathological factor for atherosclerosis, garlic may play an important role in the prevention of atherosclerosis. Compounds containing an allyl-disulfide or allyl-sulfhydryl group are most likely responsible for the inhibition of cholesterol synthesis by garlic and that this inhibition is likely mediated at sterol 4á-methyl oxidase. Garlic has beneficial effects on risk factors associated with cardiovascular disease, including modulation of plasma lipid levels. Confirming these reports, previous studies with rabbits and rats treated with garlic also reported a modulation of plasma lipids, caused by a decrease in concentrations of plasma cholesterol and triglycerides and markers of cholesterol synthesis and absorption. The magnitude of hypocholesterolemic properties of garlic leads to lowering of 80% in cholesterol-fed rabbits. Garlic was fed in these various studies as the raw clove, steamed or fried cloves, as garlic pearls, powder, as juice or extract or as the essential oil. Serum cholesterol levels fall when chickens as well as other species are fed garlic supplemented diets. When fed in conjunction with cholesterol, garlic decreased the incorporation of acetate into cholesterol and increased faecal bile acid and neutral sterol excretion. Both actions are consistent with the lowering of serum cholesterol. Garlic paste (3.8%), solvent-extracted fractions (petroleum ether, methanol and water in sequence), or garlic oil equivalent reduced the amount of serum cholesterol by 18 and 23% in broilers and 12-wk-old Leghorn pullets, respectively, when diets were fed for 4 wk (Qureshi *et al.*, 1983b). The dietary garlic paste was effective in reducing the amount of cholesterol in laying hens and egg yolk (Chowdhury *et al.*, 2002). Sklan *et al.* (1992) observed depressed hepatic cholesterol concentration in chickens when 2% garlic was fed for 14 d. In another study conducted on 5-wk-old male broilers, Qureshi *et al.* (1983a) observed inhibition of the key enzymes involved in cholesterol and lipid synthesis upon supplementation with polar fractions of garlic powder (garlic equivalent to 1, 2, 4, 6, and 8% fresh garlic paste) for 3 wk. Konjufca *et al.* (1997) reported that feeding 3% garlic powder resulted in a decrease of plasma cholesterol and breast and thigh muscle cholesterol in broilers. In the study of Yalcin *et al.* (2006), supplementation of diets with 5 and 10 g/kg of garlic powder increased egg weight and decreased egg yolk cholesterol and serum triglyceride without adverse effects on performance and egg traits of laying hens. However, decreased yolk and serum cholesterol levels in laying hens fed 3% garlic powder for 8 months were not observed by Birrenkott *et al.* (2000).

9.5.8 *Pro-circulatory Effects*

Isoeruboside-B of garlic inhibited blood coagulation and had a fibrinolysis-promoting effect whereas proto-isoeruboside-B was found to promote only fibrinolysis. Reports have shown that garlic extract may affect the RBC count adversely during the acute phase by inducing hemolytic anaemia. These are thought to be caused by oxidant stress due to compounds such as allicin contained in garlic extract. Lee *et al.* (2000) studied whether dogs given garlic extract developed haemolytic anemia. Garlic extract was administered intragastrically @ 1.25 ml/kg BW (5 g whole garlic/kg) once a day for 7 days. Compared with initial values, erythrocyte count, haematocrit and hemoglobin concentration decreased to a minimum value on days 9 to 11. Heinz body formation, an increase in erythrocyte-reduced glutathione concentration and eccentrocytes were also detected, however, no dog developed hemolytic anemia. Eccentrocytosis appears to be a major diagnostic feature of garlic-induced haemolysis in dogs (Lee *et al.*, 2000; Yamato *et al.*, 2005). Garlic is toxic for horses; a daily dose of >0.2 g/kg causes Heinz body anemia in them (Pearson *et al.*, 2005).

9.5.9 *Inhibition of Platelet Aggregation*

The AGE has inhibitory effect on platelet aggregation. The mechanisms involved appear to be multiple in nature and may involve membrane fluidity changes, inhibition of phospholipase C, inhibition of calcium mobilization, increase in nitric oxide and cAMP production and inhibition of TXA2, all of which will lead to an inhibition of platelet aggregation. The AGE may be further evaluated as a potential therapeutic agent to ameliorate complications of sickle-cell anaemia.

9.5.10 *Anti-oxidant Activity*

The AGE exhibits anti-oxidative activities, whereas raw or heated garlic stimulates oxidation (Imai *et al.*, 1994). Garlic and garlic extracts have been shown to have antioxidant activity in various meat types as well as in egg-type chicken (Chowdhury *et al.*, 2002; Yin and Cheng 2003; Sallam *et al.*, 2004; Tang and Cronin 2007). Polyphenol compounds found in garlic husk could be an antioxidant source. Nuutila *et al.* (2002) reported that garlic husk had 7 times greater total polyphenols than garlic bulb and the non-edible garlic husk had 1.5 times greater radical scavenging activity than the edible part. Thus, the addition of garlic husk to broiler diets could significantly affect chicken meat quality (Kim *et al.*, 2009). Induction of glutathione peroxidase and an increase in the ratio of glutathione (GSH) to glutathione disulfide (GSSG) may contribute to the protective effects of organosulphur compounds in diminishing oxidative stress within cells. Tetrahydro-*â*-Carboline Derivatives (THâCs), which are formed during the natural aging process, are potent antioxidants in AGE and thus may be useful for the prevention of diseases associated with oxidative damage (Ichikawa *et al.*, 2006).

9.5.11 *Meat Quality*

A major problem in the meat industry is a reduction in the acceptability and nutritional quality of meat as well as changes in flavour due to the process of lipid oxidation. Therefore, changes and improvements in eating habits of people have led to an interest in the development of new convenience meat products with natural flavour and taste. As a result, an approach for overcoming the lipid oxidation problem of the meat industry is to use dietary garlic and α-tocopherol supplementation in animals (Cannon *et al.*, 1995; Konjufca *et al.*, 1997; Lewis *et al.*, 2003; Kim *et al.*, 2005). Increasing the levels of garlic powder or providing a combination of garlic powder and α-tocopherol led to decreased serum cholesterol levels, shear force, thiobarbituric acid reactive substances (TBARS) values, saturated fatty acid (SFA), and total SFA and increased unsaturated fatty acid (USFA), total USFA, total USFA: total SFA ratios, indicating that synthetic enzyme activity or lipid oxidation should be reduced or delayed. Supplementing broiler chicken diets with garlic can produce chicken meat with favourable lipid profiles and can enhance eating quality because sensory panels found that thigh meat from chickens fed a garlic-supplemented diet had better texture and flavour. In addition, the different levels of garlic powder or a combination of garlic powder and á-tocopherol did bring about colour stability in thigh muscle. However, broiler growth, water holding capacity (WHC) and shear force were not significantly affected by the levels of garlic powder and á-tocopherol, which were important for practical application. These results suggest that applying 5% garlic powder or 3% garlic powder plus 200 IU of α-tocopherol to diets was effective for enhancing lipid and colour stability thereby improving the meat quality of chickens (Choi *et al.*, 2010). Moreover, meat from broilers fed garlic-supplemented diets had greater protein content and lower fat content compared with broilers fed a control diet (Kim *et al.*, 2009).

9.5.12 *Egg Quality*

Garlic was reported to enhance performance of laying hens and improve egg quality when supplemented in diet (Lim *et al.*, 2006; Yalcin *et al.*, 2006; Khan *et al.*, 2007). Egg weight and albumen quality of fresh eggs were significantly improved by dietary garlic powder, although with a strong garlic flavour in eggs at high dietary levels (Olobatoke and Mulugeta, 2011). The authors have suggested that moderate addition of GP (upto 3%) to layer diets is beneficial in improving egg weight and albumen quality of eggs without compromising hen performance or consumer taste and preference.

9.5.13 *Immune Enhancement*

Feeding garlic extract maintain immune function and prevent psychologically induced damage. It has also been reported that fresh dietary garlic improve the immune-stimulatory effect during Ehrlisch ascites tumour cell challenge in mice and Newcastle disease, avian influenza and bursal disease challenge in broilers (Jafari *et al.,* 2010). Dietary fermented garlic has potential as an immunity enhancer in growing pigs (Wang *et al.,* 2011).

9.5.14 *Reproductive Functions*

Garlic supplementation enhances protein anabolism and suppresses protein catabolism by the stimulation of steroid hormones, leading to greater testis testosterone content (due to the stimulation of LH secretion from the pituitary gland by the increased plasma noradrenaline concentration) and lower plasma corticosterone concentration in rats fed a high protein diet (Oi *et al.,* 2001). The pharmacologic activities of 4 garlic preparations, raw garlic juice (RGJ), heated garlic juice (HGJ), dehydrated garlic powder (DGP) and aged garlic extract (AGE) were investigated. The study used three animal models, i.e., testicular hypogonadism (hypospermatogensis and impotence) induced by warm water treatment, intoxication of acetaldehyde and growth of inoculated tumour cells. RGJ was found to be effective only in recovery of testicular function. The efficacy of HGJ was observed in three models; however, it did not improve impotence. DGP was effective in recovery of spermatogenesis and stimulated acetaldehyde detoxification. Significant beneficial effects of AGE were found in all three models. Although all four garlic preparations significantly enhanced natural killer (NK) and killer cell activities of the spleen cells of tumour-bearing mice, only AGE and HGJ inhibited the growth of inoculated tumour cells. Among the four garlic preparations studied, AGE was the most useful garlic preparation (Kasuga *et al.,* 2001).

9.5.15 *Growth Performance*

Bampidis *et al.* (2005) found no differences in final BW, feed conversion ratio (kg of DM intake/kg of BW gain), DM intake and carcass yield in lambs fed 60 kg/t garlic bulb or 100 kg/t garlic husk.

However, exogenous supplementation of fermented garlic by *Weissella koreensis* in growing pigs improved average daily gain without any influence on the appetite and had a beneficial effect on the immune response during an inflammatory challenge (Wang *et al.,* 2011). Feeding garlic extract to sows has been found to improve the gastrointestinal tract development and BW of newborn piglets (Tatara *et al.,* 2005).

9.5.16 *Food Preservation*

Garlic inhibits the growth of micro-organisms as well as their toxin production. More research must be done to assess the value of garlic as an alternative to chemical food preservatives, especially in foods in which the garlic flavour would be an added bonus. There is also potential use for garlic by itself or in combination with other herbs and spices to extend the shelf life of raw meat products.

9.6 Adverse Reactions

Some adverse effects may be associated with raw garlic and garlic powder e.g. stomach disorders and diarrhoea (Desai *et al.,* 1990; Nakagawa *et al.,* 1980); decrease in serum protein and calcium (Shashikanth *et al.,* 1986); anemia (Nakagawa *et al.,* 1980); bronchial asthma; contact dermatitis (Burden *et al.,* 1994) and inhibition of spermatogenesis and a decrease in intestinal flora (Dixit and Joshi 1982). Freshly crushed garlic is chemically unstable and has been shown to cause undesirable side effects, such as stomach disorders (Desai *et al.,* 1990; Nakagawa *et al.,* 1980) and allergic reactions (Lybarger *et al.,* 1982). Imada (1990) reported allicin as one of the major irritants in raw garlic. Many adverse reactions to garlic can be attributed to an excess of oil-soluble organosulphur constituents. The lipid-lowering effects of some oil-soluble sulphur compounds in hepatocytes coincide with cytotoxicity, as revealed by increased lactate dehydrogenase release from cells. Water-soluble sulphur compounds, on the other hand, although effective at reducing cholesterol, were not cytotoxic. Topically applied diallyl sulfide is the most allergenic (Papageorgiou *et al.,* 1983). When garlic is extracted for a certain period, its toxicity is greatly reduced Imada (1990).

9.7 Conclusions

Garlic has long been revered for its formidable prophylactic and therapeutic medicinal properties in the folklore of many cultures over the centuries. This reverence has escalated in recent years as a result of the emergence of data indicating its potent antioxidant action, its ability to modulate immunological responsiveness, stimulation of prostanoid synthesis, antithrombotic activity, lowering of cholesterol, anti-cancer and cardio-protective effects. For preventive purposes, daily, long-term ingestion of garlic products is necessary. Thus, the safety of products should be considered seriously. Because some garlic preparations may cause undesirable effects, including gastrointestinal problems, one should be cautious about their safety as well as their effectiveness, when choosing a preparation. The efficacy and safety of these preparations in preparing dietary supplements based on garlic are also contingent on the processing methods employed.

References

Abo-Doma MH, Said MM, Shahat NE, Riad RF, Nassar AR (1991) Effect of onion and garlic oils as well as some of their sulphur constituents on lipid metabolism in albino rats. J Drug Res 20: 1–11

Adamu I, Joseph PK, Augusti KT (1982) Hypolipidemic action of onion and garlic unsaturated oils in sucrose fed rats over a two month period. Experientia 38: 899–901

Agrawal PK (1996) A systematic NMR approach for the determination of the molecular structure of steroid saponins. In: Waller GR, Yamasaki K (eds) Saponins used in food and agriculture. vol. 405, pp.299–316. Plenum Press, New York. USA

Amagase H, Milner J. (1993) Impact of various sources of garlic and their constituents on 7,12-dimethylbenz[a]anthracene binding to mammary cell DNA. Carcinogenesis 14: 1627–1631

Amagase H, Petesch BL, Matsuura H, Kasuga S, Itakura Y (2001) Intake of garlic and its bioactive components. J Nutr 131: 955S–62S

Bampidis VA, Christodoulou V, Christaki E, Florou-Paneri P, Spais AB (2005) Effect of dietary garlic bulb and garlic husk supplementation on performance and carcass characteristics of growing lambs. Anim Feed Sci Technol 121: 273–283

Birrenkott G, Brockenfett GE, Owens M, Halpin E (2000) Yolk and blood cholesterol levels and organoleptic assessment of eggs from hens fed a garlic supplement diet. Poult Sci 79 (Suppl. 1): 75 (Abstr.)

Block E (1985) The chemistry of garlic and onions. Sci Am 252: 114–119

Bodas R, Prieto N, García-González R, Andrés S Giráldez FJ, López S (2012). Manipulation of rumen fermentation and methane production with plant secondary metabolites. Anim Feed Sci Tech 176: 78–93

Burden AD, Wilkinson SM, Beck MH, Chalmers RJG (1994) Garlic induced systemic contact dermatitis. Contact Dermatitis 30: 299–300

Busquet M, Calsamiglia S, Ferret S, Kamel C (2005) Screening for the effects of natural plant extracts and secondary plant metabolites on rumen microbial fermentation in continuous culture. Anim Feed Sci Tech 123: 597–613

Caldwell DR, Danzer CJ (1988) Effects of allyl sulphides on the growth of predominant gut anaerobes. Curr Microbiol 16: 237–241

Calsamiglia S, Busquet M, Cardozo PW, Castillejos L, Ferret A (2007) Invited Review: Essential oils as modifiers of rumen microbial fermentation. J Dairy Sci 90: 2580–2595

Cardozo PW, Calsamiglia S, Ferret A, Kamel C (2005) Screening for the effects of natural plant extracts at different pH on *in vitro* rumen microbial fermentation of a high-concentrate diet for beef cattle. J Anim Sci 83: 2572–2579

Chaves AV, He ML, Yang WZ, Hristov AN, McAllister TA, Benchaar C (2008) Effects of essential oils on proteolytic, deaminative and methanogenic activities of mixed ruminal bacteria. Can J Anim Sci 89: 97–104

Choi IH, Park WY, Kim YJ (2010) Effects of dietary garlic powder and á-tocopherol supplementation on performance, serum cholesterol levels, and meat quality of chicken. Poult Sci 89: 1724–1731

Chowdhury SR, Chowdhury SD, Smith TK (2002) Effects of dietary garlic on cholesterol metabolism in laying hens. Poult Sci 81: 1856–1862

Desai HG, Kalro RH, Choksi AP (1990) Effect of ginger and garlic on DNA content of gastric aspirate. Indian J Med Res 92: 139–141

Didry N, Dubreuil L, Pinkas M (1992) Antimicrobial activity of naphthaquinones and Allium extracts combined with antibiotics. Pharm Acta Helv 67: 148–151

Dion ME, Agler M, Milner JA (1997) S-allyl cysteine inhibits nitroso-morpholine formation and bioactivation. Nutr Cancer 28: 1–6

Dixit VP, Joshi S (1982) Effects of chronic administration of garlic (*Allium sativum* Linn.) on testicular function. Indian J Exp Biol 20: 534–536

Feldberg RS, Chang SC, Kotik AN, Nadler M, Neuwirth Z, Sundstrom DC, Thompson NH (1988) *In vitro* mechanism of inhibition of bacterial growth by allicin. Anti-microb Agents Chemother 32: 1763–1768

Fenelli SL, Castro GD, Toranzo EG, Castro JA (1998) Mechanism of the preventive properties of some garlic compounds in the carbon tetrachloride promoted oxidative stress. Diallyl sulfide. Res Commun Mol Pathol Pharmacol 110: 163–169

Fenwick GR, Hanley AB (1985) The genus Allium-part 3. Medicinal effects. CRC Crit Rev Food Sci Nutr 1: 1–74

Freeman F, Kodera Y (1995) Garlic chemistry: Stability of S-(2-propenyl)2-propene-1-sulfinothioate (allicin) in blood, solvents, and simulated physiological fluids. J Agric Food Chem 43: 2332–2338

Fuchs CS, Mayer RJ (1995) Gastric carcinoma. N Engl J Med 333: 32–41

Hughes BG, Lawson LD (1991) Antimicrobial effects of *Allium sativum* L. (garlic), *Allium ampeloprasum* (elephant garlic), and *Allium cepa* (onion), garlic compounds and commercial garlic supplement products. Phytother Res 5: 154–158

Iberl B, Winkler G, Knobloch K (1990a) Products of allicin transformation: ajoenes and dithiins, characterization and their determination by HPLC. Planta Med 56: 202–211

Iberl B, Winkler G, Muller B, Knobloch K (1990b) Quantitative determination of allicin and alliin from garlic by HPLC. Planta Med 56: 320–326

Ichikawa M, Yoshida J, Ide N, Sasaoka T, Yamaguchi H, Ono K (2006) Tetrahydro-â-carboline derivatives in aged garlic extract show antioxidant properties. J Nutr 136: 726S–731S

Imada O (1990) Toxicity aspects of garlic. In: First World Congress on the Health Significance of Garlic and Garlic Constituents. Nutrition International, Irvine, CA, pp. 47

Imai J, Ide N, Nagae S, Moriguchi T, Matsuura H, Itakura Y (1994) Antioxidant and radical scavenging effects of aged garlic extract and its constituents. Planta Med 60: 417–420

Jafari RA, Razi-Jalali M, Kiani R (2010) Effect of fresh dietary garlic powder on some of the serum biochemical parameters in broiler chicks. Comp Clin Pathol doi:10.1007/s00580-010-0989-2

Jain RC (1993) Anti-tubercular activity of garlic oil. Indian Drugs 30: 73–75

Kaku H, Goldstein IJ, Van Damme EJM, Peumans W (1992) New mannose-specific lectins from garlic (*Allium sativum*) and ramsons (*Allium ursinum*) bulbs. Carbohydr Res 229: 347–353

Kasuga S, Uda N, Kyo E, Ushijima M, Morihara N, Itakura Y (2001) Pharmacologic activities of aged garlic extract in comparison with other garlic preparations. J Nutr 131: 1080S–1084S

Khan SH, Rozina S, Mohammad AA (2007) Effects of dietary garlic on performance and serum and egg yolk cholesterol concentration in laying hens. Asian J Poult Sci 1:22–27

Kim YJ, Jin SK, Yang HS (2009) Effect of dietary garlic bulb and husk on the physicochemical properties of chicken meat. Poult Sci 88: 398–405

Koch HP (1993) Saponine in knoblauch und ku¨ chenzwiebel. Dtsch Apoth Zgt 133: 3733–3743

Kongmun P, Wanapat M, Pakdee P, Navanukraw C (2010) Effect of coconut oil and garlic powder on *in vitro* fermentation using gas production technique. Livest Sci 127: 38–44

Konjufca VH, Pesti GM, Bakalli RI (1997) Modulation of cholesterol levels in broiler meat by dietary garlic and copper. Poult Sci 76: 1264–1271

Lancaster JE, Shaw ML (1989) g-Glutamyl peptides in the biosynthesis of S-alk(en)yl-L-cysteine sulfoxides (flavor precursors) in Allium. Phytochem 28: 455–460

Lawson LD (1993) Bioactive organosulfur compounds of garlic and garlic products. In: ACS Symposium Series 534, Human Medicinal Agents From Plants (Kinghorn AD, Balandrin MF eds.), pp. 306–330 American Chemical Society, Washington DC

Lee KW, Yamato O, Tajima M, Kuraoka M, Omae S, Maede Y (2000) Haematologic changes associated with the appearance of eccentrocytes after intragastric administration of garlic extract to dogs. Am J Vet Res 61(11): 1446–1450

Lim KS, You SJ, An BK, Kang CW (2006) Effects of dietary garlic powder and copper on cholesterol content and quality characteristics of chicken eggs. Asian-Australas J Anim Sci 19: 582–586

Nakagawa S, Masamoto K, Sumiyoshi H, Kunihiro K, Fuwa T (1980) Effect of raw garlic juice and aged garlic extract on growth of young rats and their organs after peroral administration. J Toxicol Sci 5: 91–112

Nuutila AM, Puupponen-Pimia R, Aarmi M, Oksman-Caldentey KM (2002) Comparison of antioxidant activities of onion and garlic extracts by inhibition of lipid peroxidation and radical scavenging activity. Food Chem 81: 485–493

Ohene-Adjei S, Chaves AV, McAllister TA, Benchaar C, Teather RM, Forster RJ (2008) Evidence of increased diversity of methanogenic archaea with plant extract supplementation. Microbial Ecol 56: 234–242

Oi Y, Imafuku M, Shishido C, Kominato Y, Nishimura S, Iwai K (2001) Garlic supplementation increases testicular testosterone and decreases plasma corticosterone in rats fed a high protein diet. J Nutr 131: 2150–2156

Olobatoke RY, Mulugeta SD (2011) Effect of dietary garlic powder on layer performance, fecal bacterial load, and egg quality. Poult Sci 90: 665–670

Papageorgiou C, Corbet JP, Menezes-Brandao F, Pecegueiro M, Benzra C (1983) Allergic contact dermatitis to garlic (*Allium sativum* L.) Identification of the allergens: the role of mono-, di- and trisulphides present in garlic. Arch Dermatol Res 275: 229–234

Patra AK, Kamra DN, Bhar R, Kumar R, Agarwal N (2011) Effect of *Terminalia chebula* and *Allium sativum* on *in vivo* methane emission by sheep. J Anim Physiol Anim Nutr 95: 187–191

Patra AK, Kamra DN, Agarwal N (2006) Effect of plant extracts on *in vitro* methanogenesis enzyme activities and fermentation of feed in the rumen liquor of buffalo. Anim Feed Sci Tech 128: 276–291

Patra AK, Yu Z (2012) Effects of essential oils on methane production and fermentation by and abundance and diversity of rumen microbial populations. Appl Environ Microbiol 78: 4271–4280

Pearson W, Boermans HJ, Bettger WJ, McBride BW, Lindinger MI (2005) Association of maximum voluntary dietary intake of freeze-dried garlic with Heinz body anaemia in horses. Am J Vet Res 66(3): 457–465

Qureshi AA, Din ZZ, Abuimeileh N, Burger WC, Ahmad Y, Elson CE (1983b) Suppression of avian hepatic lipid metabolism by solvent extracts of garlic: Impact on serum lipids. J Nutr 113: 1746–1755

Qureshi AA, Abuimeileh N, Din ZZ, Elson CE, Burger WC (1983a) Inhibition of cholesterol and fatty acid biosynthesis in liver enzymes and chicken hepatocytes by polar fractions of garlic. Lipids 18: 343–348

Qureshi AA, Crenshaw TD, Abuirmeileh N, Peterson DM, Elson CE (1987) Influence of minor plant constituents on porcine hepatic lipid metabolism: impact on serum lipids. Atherosclerosis 64: 109–115

Rees LP, Minney SF, Plummer NT, Slater JH, Skyrme DA (1993) A quantitative assessment of the antimicrobial activity of garlic (*Allium sativum*). World J Micrbiol Biotechnol 9: 303–307

Reuter HD, Koch HP, Lawson DL (1996) Therapeutic effects and applications of garlic and its preparations. In: Garlic: The Science and Therapeutic Applications of Allium sativum L. and Related Species, 2nd ed. (Koch HP, Lawson DL, eds.), pp. 135–212. William & Wilkins, Baltimore, MD.

Sallam KI, Ishioroshi M, Samejima K (2004) Antioxidant and antimicrobial effects of garlic in chicken sausage. Lebensm Wiss Technol 37: 849–855

Shashikanth KN, Basappa SC, Murthy VS (1986) Effect of feeding raw and boiled garlic (*Allium sativum* L.) extracts on the growth, caecal microflora, and serum proteins of albino rats. Nutr Rep Int 33: 313–319

Singh KV, Shukla NP (1984) Activity on multiple resistant bacteria of garlic (*Allium sativum*) extract. Fitoterapia 55: 313–315

Sivam GP, Lampe JW, Ulness B, Swanzy SR, Potter JD (1997) *Helicobacter pylori-in vitro* susceptibility to garlic (*Allium sativum*) extract. Nutr Cancer 27: 118–121

Sklan D, Bermer YN, Rabinowitch HD (1992) The effect of dietary onion and garlic on hepatic lipid concentrations and activity of antioxidative enzymes in chicks. J Nutr Biochem 3: 322–325

Staerfl SM, Amelchanka SL, Kälber T, Soliva CR, Kreuzer M, Zeitz JO (2012) Effect of feeding dried high-sugar ryegrass ('AberMagic') on methane and urinary nitrogen emissions of primiparous cows. Livest Sci 150: 293–301

Tang X, Cronin DA (2007) The effects of brined onion extracts on lipid oxidation and sensory quality in refrigerated cooked turkey breast rolls during storage. Food Chem 100: 712–718

Tatara MR, Œliwa E, Dudek K, Mosiewicz J, Studziñske T (2005) Effect of aged garlic extract and allicin administration to sows during pregnancy and lactation on body weight gain and gastrointestinal tract development of piglets. Bull Vet Inst Pulawy 49: 349–355

Van Zijderveld SM, Gerrits WJJ, Dijkstra J, Newbold JR, Hulshof RBA, Perdok HB (2011) Persistency of methane mitigation by dietary nitrate supplementation in dairy cows. J Dairy Sci 94: 4028–4038

Wang JP, Yoo JS, Jang HD, Lee JH, Cho JH, Kim IH (2011) Effect of dietary fermented garlic by *Weissella koreensis* powder on growth performance, blood characteristics, and immune response of growing pigs challenged with *Escherichia coli* lipopolysaccharide. J Anim Sci 89: 2123–2131

Yalcin S, Onbasilar I, Sehu A, Yalcin S (2007) The effects of dietary garlic powder on the performance, egg traits and blood serum cholesterol of laying quails. Asian-Australas J Anim Sci 20: 944–947

Yamato O, Kasai E, Katsura T, Takahashi S, Shiota T, Tajima M, Yamasaki M, Maede Y (2005) Heinz body hemolytic anemia with eccentrocytosis from ingestion of Chinese chive (*Allium tuberosum*) and garlic (*Allium sativum*) in a dog. J Am Anim Hosp Assoc 41(1): 68–73

Yin M, Cheng W (2003) Antioxidant and antimicrobial effects of four garlic-derived organosulphur compounds in ground beef. Meat Sci 63: 23–28

Yoshida S, Kasuga S, Hayashi N, Ushiroguchi T, Matsuura H, Nakagawa S (1987) Antifungal activity of ajoene derived from garlic. Appl Environ Microbiol 53: 615–617.

□□□

Chapter 10

Black Cumin (*Nigella sativa*)

Pankaj Kumar Singh

Department of Animal Nutrition, Bihar Animal Sciences University, Patna, India, E-mail: vetpank@gmail.com

ABSTRACT

Black cumin (*Nigella sativa*) locally is a small and valuable annual flowering plant. The seed of black cumin is a good source of nutritionally essential components and contains active compounds *viz.* thymoquinone, thymohydroquinone, dithymoquinone, p-cymene, carvacrol, 4-terpineol, nigillidine and nigillicine, etc. Black cumin seed possess antioxidant, anti-microbial, anti-fungal, anti-parasitic, anti-diabetic, diuretic, anti-neoplastic activity. It has been widely used as antihypertensive, liver tonics, diuretics, digestive, anti-diarrhoeal, appetite stimulant, analgesics, anti-bacterial and in skin disorders. Black cumin seed has been used in poultry feed to improve growth performance, feed intake, feed efficiency, immunity, carcass traits, egg quality, etc. Black cumin seed is miraculous herb having great nutritional potential and many therapeutic properties.

Keywords: Black cumin, Thymoquinone, Anti bacterial, Antioxidant, Poultry.

10.1 Introduction

Black cumin (*Nigella sativa*Linn.) locally known as *Kalonji, Kalika, Kunchika, Ajai* is a small and valuable annual flowering plant belongs to Ranunculaceae family. The seeds of black cumin are black in colour and mainly used in confectionaries, breads, cakes and other baking products (Guler *et al.*, 2006). Seeds and oil have a long history of folklore usage in various systems of medicines and food. The seeds of black cumin are used in folkloric (herbal) medicine all over the world in the treatment and prevention of a number of diseases and conditions that include asthama, diarrhoea and dyslipidaemia. The seeds and their oil have been used as a drug in the Indian traditional Unani and Ayurveda for centuries in the treatment of ailments including infectious diseases (Ahmad *et al.*, 2013). In Islamic literature, it is considered as one of the greatest forms of healing medicine and recommended as prophetic medicine in *Tibb-e-Nwab* Nabwi (Prophetic Medicine). It has been widely used as antihypertensive, liver tonics, diuretics, digestive, anti-diarrheal, appetite stimulant, analgesics, anti-bacterial and in skin disorders. Extensive studies on Black cumin have been carried out by various researchers and a wide spectrum of its pharmacological actions have been explored which may include antidiabetic, anticancer, immunomodulator, analgesic, antimicrobial, anti-inflammatory, spasmolytic, bronchodilator, hepato-protective, renal protective, gastro-protective, antioxidant properties, etc. Due to its miraculous power of healing, black cumin has got the place among the top ranked evidence based herbal medicines. This is also revealed that most of the therapeutic properties of this plant are due to the presence of thymoquinone which is major bioactive component of the essential oil.

10.2 Taxonomy and Morphology of Black Cumin

Taxonomic classification of black cumin is as follows:

Kingdom	:	Plantae
Subkingdom	:	Tracheobionta
Superdivision	:	Spermatophyta
Division	:	Magnoliophyta
Class	:	Magnoliopsida
Subclass	:	Magnoliidae
Order	:	Ranunculales
Family	:	Ranunculaceae
Genus	:	*Nigella*
Species	:	*Sativa*

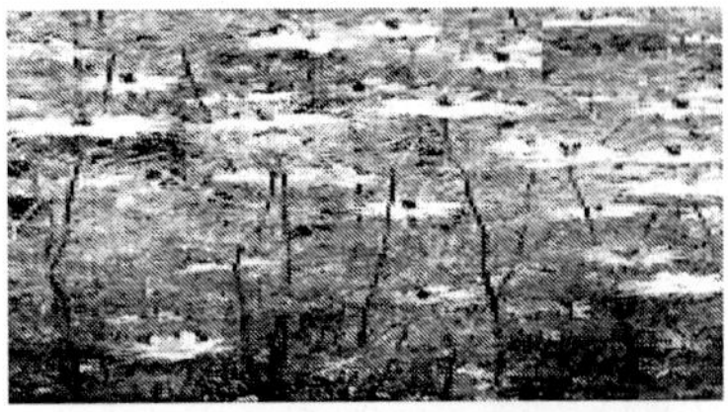

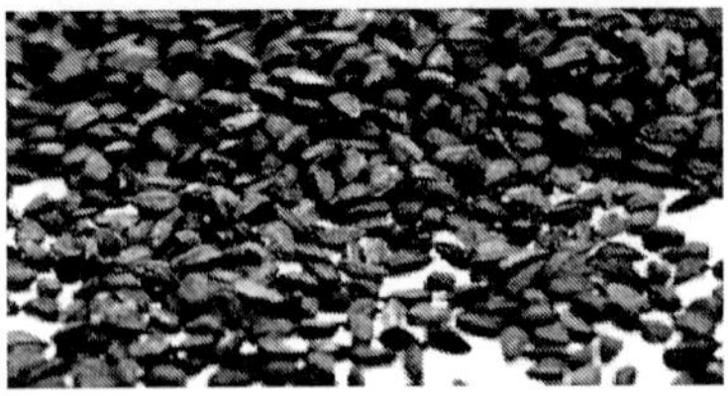

Nigella *sativa* is an annual flowering plant which grows to 20-90 cm tall, with finely divided leaves, the leaf segments narrowly linear to threadlike. The flowers are delicate, and usually coloured white, yellow, pink, pale blue or pale purple, with 5-10 petals. The fruit is a large and inflated capsule composed of 3-7 united follicles, each containing numerous seeds. Seeds are small dicotyledonous, trigonus, angular, regulose-tubercular, 2-3.5mm, 1-2 mm, black externally and white inside, odor slightly aromatic and taste bitter. Microscopically, transverse section of seed shows single layered epidermis consisting of elliptical, thick walled cells, covered externally by a papillose cuticle and filled with dark brown contents. Epidermis is followed by 2-4 layers of thick walled tangentially elongated parenchymatous cells, followed by a reddish brown pigmented layer composed of thick walled, rectangular elongated cells. Inner to the pigment layer, is present a layer composed of thick walled rectangular elongated or nearly columnar, elongated cells. Endosperm consists of thin walled, rectangular or polygonal cells mostly filled with oil globules. The powder microscopy of seed powder shows brownish black, parencymatous cells and oil globules (Khan *et al.*, 1979).

10.3 Chemical Composition of Black Seeds

Many active compounds have been isolated, identified and reported so far in different varieties of black seeds. The most important active compounds are thymoquinone (30%-48%), thymohydro-quinone, dithymoquinone, p-cymene (7%-15%), carvacrol (6%-12%), 4-terpineol (2%-7%), t-anethol (1%-4%), sesquiterpene longifolene (1%-8%) α-pinene and thymol, etc. Black seeds also contain some other compounds in trace amounts. Seeds contain two different types of alkaloids; i.e. isoquinoline alkaloids e.g. nigellicimine and nigelliciminеN-oxide, and pyrazol alkaloids or indazole ring bearing alkaloids which include nigellidine and nigellicine. Moreover, Black cumin seeds also contain alpha-hederin, a water soluble pentacyclic triterpene and saponin, a potential anticancer agent. Some other compounds e.g. carvone, limonene, citronellol were also found in trace amounts. Most of the pharmacological properties of Black cumin are mainly attributed to quinine constituents, of which thymoquinone is the most abundant. On storage, TQ yields dithymoquinone and higher oligocondensation products. The seeds of Black cumin contain protein (26.7%), fat (28.5%), carbohydrates (24.9%), crude fibre (8.4%) and total ash (4.8 %). The seeds are also containing good amount of various vitamins and minerals like Cu, P, Zn and Fe, etc. The seeds contain carotene which is converted by the liver to vitamin A. Root and shoot are reported to contain vanillic acid. The seeds reported to contain a fatty oil rich in unsaturated fatty acids, mainly linoleic acid (50-60%), oleic acid (20%), eicodadienoic acid (3%) and dihomolinoleic acid (10%).

10.4 Nutritional Composition of Black Cumin

Black cumin is a good source of nutritionally essential components. The seeds contain moisture, oil, proteins, ash and total carbohydrates contents are in range of 3.8-7.0%, 22.0-40.3%, 20.8-31.2%, 3.7-4.7% and 24.9-40.0%, respectively (Takruri and Dameh, 1998; Haq *et al.*, 1999; Soliman *et al.*, 1999; Atta, 2003; Salem, 2005). Black cumin fixed oil is important in many aspects as it is rich in unsaturated fatty acids *viz.* linoleic and oleic acids 47.0-60.0 and 18.9-25.7%, respectively. Additionally, it also contains some minor quantities of linolenic, arachidic and eicosenoic acids (Atta, 2003; Ramadan and Mörsel, 2004; Ashraf *et al.*, 2006; Cheikh-Rouhou *et al.*, 2007). Polyunsaturated fatty acids constitute the bulk of the oil ranging from 48-70%, while monounsaturated and saturated fatty acids are comparatively in lesser proportions (Nickavar *et al.*, 2003; Ramadan and Mörsel, 2003; Atta, 2003). The seeds have also been found to contain minerals; e.g. Fe, Na, Cu, Zn, P, Ca and vitamins like ascorbic acid, thiamine, niacin, pyridoxine and folic acid (Ashraf *et al.*, 2006; Cheikh-Rouhou *et al.*, 2007).

Black cumin seeds contain several bioactive molecules that include thymoquinone, thymol, alkaloids (nigellicines and nigelledine) and saponins (└-hederin), tocopherols, trans-retinols, and selenium (Sultan *et al.*, 2009). The most important active compounds in *Nigella sativa*are thymoquinone (30%-80%), thymohydroquinone, dithymoquinone, p-cymene (7%-15%), carvacrol (6%-12%), 4-terpineol (2%-7%), t-anethol (1%-4%), sesquiterpenelongifolene (1%-8%), └-pinene and thymole etc. Seeds contain n-oxide, and pyrazol alkaloids or indazole ring bearing alkaloids which include nigillidine and nigillicine (Nickavar *et al.*, 2003; Mozzafari *et al.*, 2000).

10.5 Pharmaceutical Properties of Black Cumin

Black cumin possess antioxidant (Ahmad *et al.*, 2013), anti-microbial (El-Kamali *et al.*, 1998; Nair *et al.*, 2005), anti-fungal, anti-parasitic (Mahmoud *et al.*, 2002), anti-diabetic (Al-Hader *et al.*, 1993), diuretic (Zaoui *et al.*, 2000) anti-neoplastic activity (El-Tahir *et al.*, 1993; El-Daly, 1998) and various other pharmacological activities (Mahfouz and El-Dakhakhny, 1960 and El-Dakhakhny, 1963). *Nigella sativa*is found to posses antibacterial activity against gram positive and gram negative bacteria e.g. Staphylococcus *aureus, Pseudomonas aeruginosa, Shigella dysentriae, S. sonnei, S. boydii, Vibrio cholera* and *Escherichia coli* (Ferdous *et al.*, 1992).

10.5.1 *Anti-bacterial Activity*

Black cumin oil acts as a more efficient remedy against certain types of bacteria including those which most strongly resist antibiotic drugs (Clark, 2014). Antibacterial and antifungal effects of *Nigella sativa*extracts against *S. aureus, P. aeroginosa* and *C. albicans* was established. A study showed that the extract destroyed non-fatal subcutaneous *staphylococcal* infection in mice (Paradise, 2005). Black cumin is found effective against multidrug resistant strains of *P. aeruginosa* and *S. aureus* because it is rich in 3 key natural chemicals: thymoquinone, thymohydroquinone and thymol (Salman *et al.*, 2008). Extract of black cumin also possesses anti-bacterial activity against clinical isolates of MRSA (methicillin resistant *Staphylococcus aureus* (Renter, 2013).

10.5. 2 *Anti-inflammatory Activity*

Extract of black cumin contains anti-inflammatory, analgesic and antioxidant effects. Ultimately, the researchers concluded that black cumin seed extract is a justified treatment for rheumatism and related inflammatory diseases (Paradise, 2005). Thymoquinone acts as an anti-inflammatory agent. It was discovered that the agents possessed anti-oxidant activity and inhibited eicosanoid generation in cells. Black cumin has now become a viable option to treat and/or heal people afflicted with auto-immune diseases.

10.5.3 *Anti-oxidant Activity*

Thymoquinone, the major bioactive compound of *Nigella sativa*is considered as potent antioxidant (Badary *et al.*, 2003), anti-carcinogenic and anti-mutagenic agent (Khader *et al.*, 2010). Much of the biological activities of the seeds have been shown to be due to thymoquinone. Badary *et al.* (2003) documented the Black cumin as an excellent superoxide anion scavenger. The addition of black cumin ethanolic extracts to the corn oil prevented the oxidative damage of triglycerides (Bassim *et al.*, 1998). The anti-oxidative properties are related to the inhibition of eicosanide generation, thromboxane B_2 and leukotriene B_4 because of inhibition of cyclooxigenase and 5-lipooxigenase, respectively. The antioxidant potential by capturing free radicals became evident when Black cumin oil was given to pentylenetatrazol induced seizure kindled mice (Ilhan *et al.*, 2005). These effects of black seeds might be due to the active constituents like thymoquinone, carvacole, anethole and 4-terepinol (Guler et al., 2007). Methanolic extracts of black cumin showed that phenolic compounds such as syringic acid, hydroxybenzoic and pcumaric acids possess significant antioxidant properties under *in vitro* system (Mariod *et al.,* 2009). Diet treated with 0.5 and 1% black seeds resulted in significantly decreased erythrocyte malondialdehyde (MDA) concentration, production of lipid peroxidases and increased glutathione (GSH) concentration compared to control group in chicken. The scientist concluded that Black cumin exhibits protective properties on the injury produced by oxidative stress by inhibiting free radical production and by regulation of glutathione preventing oxidative stress. Black seeds might decrease the production of hydrogen peroxide (H_2O_2), hydroxyl (OH) and superoxide (O_2) radicals that are produced as a result of aerobic respiration (Tuluce *et al.,* 2009). In rat and mouse models, many researchers have indicated the antioxidant effects of Black cumin. Nagi *et al.* (1994)] showed that the mice treated with carbon tetrachloride (CCl_4) were protected by antioxidant mechanisms of black cumin oil.

10.5.4 *ImmunmodulatorActivity*

Black cumin develops the immune system through boosting the body's immune cell production, cancer and HIV prevention and bone marrow and natural interferon production: The seeds improve the immune system by stimulating the production of bone marrow and cells of the immune system. It increases the production of interferon, protects normal cells from the damaging effects of harmful invaders and helps destroy tumour cells.

Black cumin's immune-building properties and active compounds have been proven to help fight a large number of diseases and auto-immune disorders through the boosting of the body's immune cell production, bone marrow, and natural interferon. Even for people in the best state of health, consuming black cumin regularly has greatly increased their vitality and well-being (Clark, 2014).

10.5.5 *AntidiabaticActivity*

*Nigella sativa*has traditionally been used to treat diabetes as well as hypertension. Several research studies have confirmed that black seed oil helps in stabilizing blood sugar levels in diabetics while also stimulating pancreatic function. Black seed oil can help prevent both type-1 and type-2 diabetes by causing partial regeneration of pancreatic beta-cells, increasing the serum insulin, and decreasing elevated glucose. It was shown that anti-diabetic effect of black cumin appeared to be rooted in the ability of the seed to improve insulin sensitivity. Researchers also found that just 2 g daily of black seed could result in reduced fasting blood sugar levels, along with decreased insulin resistance, and increased beta-cell function in the pancreas. The water and alcohol extracts of black cumin at low doses also have a blood-sugar lowering effect (Bamosa *et al.*, 2010). Studies disclose that oxidative stress may decrease the efficiency of pancreatic L cells, which control the production and release of insulin. As such, oxidative stress is thought to play a role in the development of diabetes. Black cumin decreases oxidative stress and may preserve the integrity of pancreatic β cells (Shafiq *et al.*, 2014). When diabetic people consumed two grams of black cumin per day for three months, it led to reductions in fasting blood sugar and HbA1c and increased the functionality of pancreatic β cells, which suggests black cumin may be a "beneficial adjuvant therapy in type 2 diabetes" (Shafiq *et al.*, 2014).

10.5.6 *Anti-tumour Agent*

Black cumin oil has been extensively researched as a possible cancer treatment. Black seed provides powerful benefits for various inflammatory cancers such as liver, melanoma, skin, pancreatic, cervical, breast, bone, stomach, lymphoma, prostate, colon, and brain. A study concluded that black seed oil has carcino preventive and chemopreventive potential, which means that it could possibly be used to prevent cancer and lessen the need for chemotherapy in the early stage of cancer (McCarthy, 2015). Alpha (α)-hederin, a pentacyclictriterpene saponin isolated from the seeds of *Black cumin*, was also reported to have potent *in vivo* antitumor activity. Numerous studies show that thymoquinone can help to induce cell death or apoptosis in a number of cancerous cells including leukemia, breast cancer, pancreatic cancer and cervical cancer. There is a growing body of research that shows thymoquinone reduces the size and the growth of tumours in rats. It has been reported that black seed stimulates bone marrow and immune cells, and raises the interferon production, protects normal cells against cell destroying effects of viruses, destroys tumour cells and raises the number of anti-bodies producing B cells. All these functions make the black seed oil an ideal natural product for the prevention and treatment of cancer. Black cumin helps stimulate the activity of neutrophil granulocytes – the most abundant type of white blood cell in the body. These neutrophils target cancer cells before they multiply, and help eliminate them before they can develop into harmful tumours (Clark, 2014).

Many studies were performed on lab animals (mice and rats) regarding the anti-cancerous effects of Black cumin. *In-vitro* studies indicated that the Black cumin possess marked growth inhibiting properties of two leukemic cell lines and five solid tumour cell lines (Iddamaldeniya *et al.,* 2003). Ethanol extracts of Black cumin were capable of inhibiting ehrilich ascites tumour growth by reducing cell count as well as inhibit tumour development (Musa *et al.,* 2004). Different extracts of Black cumin produced different levels of cytotoxic effects on different cell lines when tested *in-vitro,* for example essential oil produced the most cytotoxic effects against the P815 cell line as compared to ethanol acetate and butanolic extracts. Whereas against the BSR line of cells, ethyl acetate extracts showed more cytotoxicity. Butanolic extract showed the greatest cytotoxic effects, when ICO1 cell line was used. When treatment of solid tumour in mice was carried out with essential oil it was noted that the tumour growth significantly arrested as compared to PBS treated mice, suggesting that the cytotoxic activity of the extract particularly from day 0 to 12 of treatment and remained constant from day 12 to 30 indicated inhibition of cell growth. Furthermore, it was observed that the administration of the essential oil into the tumor site prevented the incidence of liver metastasis and improved the mouse livability (Mbarek *et al.,* 2007).

10.6 Effect of Back Cumin on Poultry Production

10.6.1 *Growth Performance*

Black seeds contain mixture of essential fatty acids, particularly oleic, linoleic and linolenic acids that cannot be synthesized in the body. There are fifteen amino acids of the proteins of black cumin out of which eight are essential (Takruri and Dameh, 1998). Therefore, black cumin affects growth performance of poultry. Different studies on the effect of black cumin seed on broiler performance have been carried out. El-Ghammry *et al.* (2002) and Hassan *et al.* (2004) reported an increased body weight by incorporating grounded black cumin seed in broiler feed. Improved average daily weight gain and better feed conversion ratio in broilers was achieved with fed 1% black cumin seed in broiler diet (Singh *et al.,* 2017). Feed conversion ratio was improved by using 4g/kg black seed (Toghyani *et al.*, 2010). The growth performance of poultry is thought to be due to high nutritive value as well as pharmacologically active substances present in the seeds. Jamroz and Kamel (2002) reported a stimulating effect of black seed on digestive system, resulting in better absorption and performance. Addition of black cumin in feed increased bile flow rate results in increased emulsification that activates the pancreatic lipases which then aid in fat digestion and absorption of fat soluble vitamins. Black seed oil and thymoquinone have hepatoprotective effects (Mahmoud *et al.*, 2002; Mansour *et al.*, 2002) therefore, these seeds have been traditionally used in a wide range of gastrointestinal disorders. The increased performance might also be due to antimicrobial effects of the active ingredients of black seed. Antimicrobial activities of Black cumin inhibit Shigella dysenteriae, Vibrio cholera, Shigella sonne, Escherichia coli (Ferdous *et al.*, 1992), Bacillus pumilus, Bacillus suptilus, Staphylococcus lutea (El-Kamali *et al.*, 1998). Shigella flrxneri (Chowdhury *et al.*, 1998). Staphylococcus aureus and Pseudomonas aeruginos (Sokmen *et al.*, 1999).

10.6.2 *Feed Intake and Efficiency*

Feed efficiency is the prime factor to assess feed quality. Research regarding the effect of Black cumin on feed efficiency is neutral as well as positive. Feed efficiency was improved by incorporating black seeds in the broiler rations (Halle *et al.*, 1999; Al-homidan *et al.*, 2002) (Guler *et al.*, 2006) reported no significant change in dietary intake of broiler by consuming feed containing black cumin and antibiotics. In another research it was found that diets with 4% grounded black cumin resulted in less feed intake but better FE as compared to control diet (Durrani *et al.*, 2007). However, controversy results were reported by (Abbas *et al.*, 2010).as poor FE was observed in broiler chicks fed diet supplemented with 1 and 2 % black seeds. Feed intake remained unaltered by feeding diet having 1, 2 and 3% black cumin seeds (Aydin *et al.*, 2008).

10.6.3 *Carcass Traits*

Dietary black cumin seed also affects carcass traits of broiler chickens (Guler *et al.*, 2006) and (Toghyani *et al.*, 2010) and (Singh *et al.*, 2017) reported an increased carcass yield, liver, abdominal fat, breast, thigh, wing and neck weights in broilers by feeding diet having 1% black cumin. However, non-significant values were obtained regarding heart weight. Al-Beitawi *et al.* (2008) found no improvement in carcass characteristics by feeding different levels of crushed as well as uncrushed Black cumin seed in broilers, however, breast percentage significantly increased (Ismail *et al.,* 2011) This increase breast weight indicated that Black cumin might have a good effect on protein metabolism. The greater ash percentage of the meat in the same study might be due to enhanced availability of minerals in black seeds. Fat percentage, breast meat colour, shear force value and electrical conductivity revealed non-significant effects. Cooking losses were significantly greater in Black cumin seeds treated birds' meat. Broilers fed diet containing 1% whole grounded Black cumin resulted in a significant decrease of dressing percentage as compared to the control, however, there were non-significant effects regarding liver, gizzard, heart, and abdominal fat percentage by supplementation of whole Black cumin seeds (Abbas *et al.,* 2010). Hermes *et al.* (2011) showed no significant effect on giblet and abdominal fat percentage in broilers. The bone percentage was greater in the control group as compared to black cumin treated groups. Birds treated with Black cumin oil (0.5, 1%) or seeds (1, 2%) represented higher meat protein and lower fat percentage on dry matter basis. Non-significant values were obtained regarding tenderness and meat pH.

10.6.4 *Egg Production and Quality*

Different scientists documented contradictory results regarding the effect of Black cumin on egg production in layers. Egg production markedly increased by using 1% black cumin seed (Singh, 2016), 1.5% powdered black cumin (Akhtar *et al.,* 2003) and 3% black seeds Aydin *et al.,* 2008) in layer diet. However, (El Bagir *et al.,* 2006) reported that supplementation of 1 and 3% black cumin in diet resulted in reduced egg production by approximately 9 and 16%, respectively without effecting egg length and width. The reduction in egg production might be due to the 10% increased final body weight of layers as energy from the black cumin oil extract was used to increase the weight gain rather than egg production. The dropped egg production might also be due to decrease in cholesterol (Akhtar *et al.,* 2003). It was observed that decrease in egg yolk cholesterol upto 30% by the addition of synthetic HMG-CoA reductase inhibitor in the diet resulted in reduced egg production by 20 % without effecting egg weight. So, it can be inferred that cholesterol is needed for egg production and there may be a certain limit for cholesterol level, below which egg formation or production may be completely stopped. Egg weight increased from 54 to 58g by supplementation of 1.5% Black cumin in layers (Akhtar *et al.*, 2003) and 1% black cumin extract increased egg weight as well as egg shell weight and thickness in quails (Denli *et al.*, 2004). Shell thickness and strength increased with 2 and 3% black seed in layer diets as compared to low levels i.e. 1% and without black cumin (Aydin *et al.*, 2008). reported that dietary supplementation of Black cumin oil had no significant effect on egg weight, egg production, ratio of yolk, albumen and shell. The addition of 3 ml/kg Black cumin oil in layer diet decreased the Haugh unit of the egg. Diet containing 3% Black cumin seeds decreased the egg-yolk total lipids, cholesterol, phospholipids as well as triacylglycerols by 34, 45, 11 and 20%, respectively. The decrease in egg yolk cholesterol is highly desirable as efforts are being made to decrease the total cholesterol consumption in human diets because of its damaging effects on the health. The mechanism by which black cumin decreases the egg yolk cholesterol is not fully understood. However, speculations are made that the decrease in cholesterol can be related to the decreased in serum cholesterol by the black seeds. It is further assumed that seeds may inhibit the de-novo synthesis of cholesterol (EL-Bagir *et al.*, 2006). Albumin quality of eggs was improved by addition of black cumin in the diet (Akhtar *et al.*, 2003 and EL-Sheikh *et al.*, 1998).Non-significant results were observed regarding yolk index by supplementing diet with black cumin (EL-Sheikh *et al.*, 1998).

10.6.5 *Blood Biochemistry*

Dietary Black cumin also affects blood biochemistry in poultry. The cholesterol level of eggs was markedly decreased from 227 to 199 mg/egg yolk, when diet supplemented with 1.5% Black cumin (Akhtar *et al.*, 2003). The study conducted by El-Bagir *et al.* (2006) indicated that addition of 1 or 3% black cumin in the diets of 68 weeks old layers resulted in a dose dependent decrease of serum phospholipids and cholesterol, whereas a general decline in serum lipids was observed. The addition of 3% Black cumin reduced the serum cholesterol and serum phospholipids by 23 and 30% respectively. The feeding of 3% crushed and non-crushed Black cumin seeds reduced plasma cholesterol, triglycerides concentration and increased the plasma High Density Lipoprotein (HDL) concentrations compared to 1.5, 2 and 2.5% crushed Black cumin seeds AL-Beitawi *et al.* (2009). The reduction in the triglycerides and cholesterol level might be due to the active ingredients such as thymoquinone and compounds like monoun-saturated fatty acids that lower the cholesterol synthesis by hepatocytes and decrease the fractional absorption of cholesterol from small intestine (Brunton *et al.,* 1998). Studies conducted on broiler chicks have shown that replacing bacitracin methylene disalicylate by grounded black cumin seeds decreased serum cholesterol and triglycerides levels while HDL concentration increased (Chowdhury *et al.,* 2002). The decrease in serum cholesterol levels might be due to enhanced bile production as reported by El-Dakhakhny *et al.* (2000) and (EL-Kaiaty *et al.,* 2002) documented decrease in serum glucose levels up to 16% by adding the black cumin in the diet. EL-Ghammry *et al.* (2002) found that by the incorporation of 4 g/kg black seeds, total plasma protein, albumin as well as globulin values were close to control birds. However, the addition of 2% Black cumin seeds in broiler diet resulted in increased total plasma protein AL-Beitawi *et al.* (2008). The research on rats indicated a significant increase in RBC, WBC, PCV and Hb of Trypanosoma brucei infected rats when treated with black seed oil as compared to control rats.

10.6.6 *Bird's Immunity*

Black cumin bears an excellent potential as alternative to antibiotics and vaccines to improve immunity and to reduce mortality in poultry. Mortality was decreased from 16.67 to 4.17% by supplementation of layer diet with 1.5% Black cumin Akhtar *et al.* (2003) and from 3.5% in the control group to 2% in the group fed diet containing 1% powdered Black cumin seeds in broilers. The volatile oils in Black cumin exhibit 67 constituents capable of inducing beneficial and pharmacological effects against bacteria such as Staphylococcus and *E. coli*. Active components of black seed possessing antibacterial, antioxidant, and anti-inflammatory activities induced positive effects on the immunity and organs involved. Antibody titer against Newcastle Disease (ND) and Infectious Bursal Disease (IBD) improved significantly by replacing bacitracin methylene disalicylate with grounded Black cumin seed in broiler diets; however, antibody titer against Infectious Bronchitis (IB) was not affected significantly. The improvement in ND and IBD titer is attributed to Black cumin oil components such as thymoquinone, carvacrol, nigellimine, thymol and nigellicine treatments (Al-Beitawi *et al.,* 2009). Increase in the lymphoid organ weight was observed, when broilers fed diet supplemented with 0.2 and 0.4 % black seeds. However, incorporation of Black cumin seeds failed to induce any significant impact on antibody titers against Influenza and ND virus at 18 and 28 days of age. It was also noticed that heterophil to lymphocyte and albumin to globulin ratios were not statistically affected by the treatments (Al-Beitawi *et al.,* 2009). Hermes *et al.* (2009) found that broilers under heat stress condition behaved well with reduced mortality in Black cumin treated groups as compared to control group. The reduced mortality rate was attributed to the antimicrobial effects, which helped the birds to overcome bacterial diseases, increased immunity and promote health. Controversy results regarding mortality were reported by Ismail (2011) who observed no effect on mortality, when black cumin was added in the broiler diet.

10.6.7 *Reproductive Performance*

In a study carried out on male broiler breeder birds (45 weeks old) fed diet containing 0.5% and 1% Black cumin oil and seeds showed that the addition of either seed or oil resulted in best semen characteristics which were studied in the traits. The treated groups amazingly showed an increase ejaculation volume, sperm mass motility, progressive motility, count, and total sperm output as well as viability percentage. On the other hand, breeders exhibited a decrease in time of ejaculation and sperm abnormalities. In the second part of this study inclusion of Black cumin in the diet of cocks significantly improved the fertility and hatchability of the treated cock groups, as compared to on non-black cumin diets.

10.7 Conclusions

Black cumin seed is miraculous herb having many therapeutic properties due to the presence of thymoquinone and other bio-active components. Use of Black cumin in poultry diet is beneficial regarding therapeutic and nutritional purposes. Being a good source of different nutrients it boosts up the growth rate, enhance the egg production, egg quality, dressing percentage and is effective against pathogenic organisms.

References

Abbas RZ, Iqbal Z, Khan MN, Zafar MA, Zia MA (2010) Anticoccidial activity of Curcuma longa L. in broilers. Braz Arch Biol Technol 53: 63-67.

Ahmad A, Husain A, Mohd. Mujeeb M, Khan SA, Abul Kalam Najmi AK, Siddique NA, Zoheir A, Damanhouri, Anwar F (2013) A review on therapeutic potential of Nigella sativa: A miracle herb. Asian Pacific J Tropical Biomedicine 3(5): 337-352

Akhtar MS, Nasir Z, Abid, AR (2003) Effect of feeding powdered *Nigella sativa*L. seeds on poultry egg production and their suitability for human consumption. Veterinarsk Arhiv. 73: 181-190

AL-Beitawi NA El-Ghousein SS, Nofal AH (2009) Replacing bacitracin methylene disalicylate by crushed *Nigella sativa*seeds in broiler rations and its effects on growth, blood constituents and immunity. Livestock Sci 125: 304-307

Al-Beitawi N, El-Ghousein, SS (2008) Effect of feeding different levels of *Nigella sativa*seeds (black cumin) on performance, blood constituents and carcass characteristics of broiler chicks. International J Poult Sci 7: 715-721

Ashraf M, Ali Q, Iqbal Z (2006) Effect of nitrogen application rate on the content and composition of oil, essential oil and minerals in black cumin (*Nigella sativaL.*) seeds. J Sci Food Agric 86: 871-876

Atta MB (2003) Some characteristics of nigella (*Nigella sativaL.*) seed cultivated in Egypt and its lipid profile. Food Chem 83: 63-68

Aydl n R, Bal MA, O zugur AK, Toprak HHC, Kamalak A, Karaman M (2006) Effects of black seed (*Nigella sativa*L.) supplementation on feed efficiency, egg yield parameters and shell quality in chickens. Pakistan J Biol Sci 9: 243–247

Badary OA, Taha RA, Gamal-el-Din AM, Abdel-Wahab MH (2003) Thymoquinone is a potent superoxide anion scavenger. Drug Chem Toxicol 26: 87-98

Bamosa AO, Kaatabi H, Lebdaa FM, Elq AM, Al-Sultanb A (2010) Effect of *Nigella sativa*seeds on the glycemic control of patients with type 2 diabetes mellitus. Indian J Physiol Pharmacol 54: 344–354

Bassim-Atta M, Imaizumi (1998) Antioxidant activity of Nigella (*Nigella sativaL.*) seeds extracts. J Japan Oil Chem Soc 47: 475-480

Brunton LL (1999) Agents affecting gastrointestinal water flux and motility, digestants, and bile acids. In: Gilman AG, Rall TW, Nies AS, Taylor P, eds. Goodman and Gilman's The Pharmacological Basis of Therapeutics. 8th ed. Elmsford, NY: Pergamon Press 1990:923

Chowdhury SR, Chowdhury SD, Smith TK, (2002) Effects of dietary garlic on cholesterol metabolism in laying hens. Poult Sci 81: 1856–62

Clark I (2014) Black cumin seed oil: Your ultimate life http://www.activationproducts. com/marine-phytoplankton-supplement/blackcumin-healing/

Denli M, Okan F, Uluocak AN (2004) Effect of dietary supplementation of herb essential oils on the growth performance, carcass and intestinal characteristics of quail (*Coturnix coturnix japonica*).South African J Anim Sci 34: 174-179

Durrani FR, Chand N, Zaka K, Sultan A, Khattak FM, Durrani Z (2007) Effect of different levels of feed added black seed (*Nigella sativaL*) on the performance of broiler chicks. Pakistan J Biol Sci 10: 4164- 4167

El-Bagir NM, Hama AY, Hamed RM, Abd El-Rahim AG, Beynen AC (2006) Lipid composition of egg yolk and serum in laying hens fed diets containing Black cumin (*Nigella sativa*). International J Poult Sci 5: 574-578

El-Dakhakhny M, Barakat M, El-Halim MA, Aly S (2000) Effects of *Nigella sativa*oil on gastric secretion and ethanol induced ulcer in rats. J Ethnopharmacol 72: 299–304

El-Dakhakhny M (1963) Studies on the chemical constitution of Egyptian *Nigella sativa*L. Seeds II. The essential oil. Plant Med 11: 465-470

El-Daly ES (1998) Protective effect of cysteine and vitamin E, Crocus sativus and *Nigella sativa*extracts on cispla.tin-induced toxicity in rats. J Pharmacol Belgium 53: 87-95

EL-Ghammry AA, EL-Mallah GM, EL-Yamny AT (2002) The effect of incorporation yeast culture, *Nigella sativa*seeds and fresh garlic in broiler diets on their performance. Egypt Poult Sci 22: 445–459

El-Kaiaty AM, Soliman AZM, Hassan MSH (2002) Combine effect of garlic, fenugreek and black seed on some productive and physiological response of laying hens. Egypt Poult Sci 22: 147–174

El-Kamali HH, Ahmed AH, Mohammed AAM, (1998) Antibacterial properties of essential oils from *Nigella sativa*seeds, *Cymbopogon citratus* leaves and *Pulicaria undulata* aerial parts. Fitoterapia 69: 77-79

Elkin RG (2006) Reducing shell egg cholesterol content. I. Overview, genetic approaches, and nutritional strategies. World Poult Sci J 62: 665-687

El-Sheikh AMA, Amin AE, Khadiga AA (1998) The effect of feeding different levels of *Nigella sativa*seeds on layer performance and egg quality characteristics. Sudan J Vet Sci Anim Husb 37: 121-128

El-Tahir KEH, Ashour MM, Al-Harbi MM (1993) The respiratory effects of the volatile oil of the black seed (*Nigella sativa*) in guinea-pigs: Elucidation of the mechanism(s) of action. J Pharmacol 24: 1115-1122

Ferdous AJ, Islam SN, Ahsan M, Hasan CM, Ahmad ZU (1992) In vitro antibacterial activity of the volatile oil of *Nigella sativa*seeds against multiple drug-resistant isolates of Shigella species and isolates of Vibrio cholerae and Escherichia coli. Phytother Res 6: 137-40

Guler T, Dalkilic B, Ertas ON, Ciftci M (2006) The effect of dietary black cumin seeds (*Nigella sativa*L.) on the performance of broilers. Asian Australasian J Anim Sci 19(3): 425-430

Halle I, Thomann R, Flachowsky G, Schubert R, Flachowsky G, Bitsch R, Jahreis G (1999) Effect of ethereal (essential) oil and oil seeds on the growth of broilers. Vitamine und Zusatzstoffe in der ernahrung von Mensch und Tier. 7: 469-472

Haq A, Lobo PL, Al-Tufail M, Rama NR, Al-Sedairy ST (1999) Immunomodulatory effect of *Nigella sativa*proteins fractionated by ion exchange chromatography. International Journal of. Immunopharmacol 21: 283-285

Hassan II, Askar AA, Gehan El-Shourbagy A (2004) Influence of some medicinal plants on performance, physiological and meat quality traits of broiler chicks. Egyptian Poult Sci 24: 247-266

Hermes IH, Faten AM, Attia KA, Ibrahim EL-Nesr SS (2009) Effect of dietary *Nigella sativa*l. On productive performance and Nutrients Utilization of broiler chicks raised under summer conditions of Egypt. Egypt Poult Sci J 29: 145-172

Hermes IH, Attia FM, Ibrahim KA, El-Nesr SS (2011) Physiological responses of broiler chickens to dietary different forms and levels of *Nigella sativa*L., during Egyptian summer season. J Agric Vety Sci 4 (9): 17-33

Iddamaldeniya SS, Wickramsinghe N, Thabrew I, Ratnatunge N, Thammitiyagodage MG (2003) Protection against diethy-lnitrosamineinduced hepatocarcinogenesis by an indigenous medicine comprised of *Nigella sativa, Hemidesmus indicus* and *Smilax glabra*: a preliminary study. J. Carcinog 3(188): 3-6

Ilhan A, Gurel A, Armutcu F, kamisli S, Iraz M (2005) Antiepileptogenic and antioxidant effects of *Nigella sativa*oil against pentylenetetrazol-induced killing in mice. Neuropharmacol 49: 456-464

Ismail ZSH (2011) Effects of dietary Black cumin growth seeds (*Nigella sativa* L.) or its extract on performance and total coliform bacteria count on broiler chicks. Egypt. Poult Sci 31: 139-148

Jamroz D, Kamel C (2002) Plant extracts enhance broiler performance. In non-ruminant nutrition; antimicrobial agents and plant extracts on immunity, health and performance. J Anim Sci 80: 41

Khader M, Bresgen N, Eckl PM (2010) Antimutagenic effects of ethanolic extracts from selected Palestinian medicinal plants. J Ethnopharmacol 27: 319–324

Khan SH, Ansari J, Haq AU, Abbas G, (2012) Black cumin seeds as phytogenic product in broiler diets and its effects on performance, blood constituents, immunity and caecal microbial population. Italian J Anim Sci 11: 438-444

Mahfouz M, EL-Dakhakhny M (1960) Chemical and pharmacological properties of the new anti-asthmatic drug, Nigellone. Egyptian Pharmacol Bulletin 24: 411-424

Mahmoud KZ, Gharaibeh SM, Zakaria HA, Qatramiz AM (2010) Garlic (Allium sativum) supplementation: influence on egg production, quality, and yolk cholesterol level in layer hens. Asian-Australasian J Anim Sci 23 (11): 1503-1509

Mansour MA, Nagi MN, El-Khatib AS, Al-Bekairi AM (2002) Effects of thymoquinone on antioxidant enzyme activities, lipid peroxidation and DT-diaphorase in different tissues of mice: A possible mechanism of action. Cell Biochem. Funct 20: 143-151

Mariod AA, Ibrahim RM, Ismail M, Ismail N (2009) Antioxidant activity and phenolic content of phenolic rich fractions obtained from cumin (*Nigella sativa*) seed cake. Food Chem 116: 306-312

Mbarek LA, Mouse HA, Elabbadi N, Bensalah M, Gamouh A (2007) Anti-tumor properties of blackseed (*Nigella sativa* L.) extracts. Braz J Med Biol Res 40: 839-847

McCarthy K (2015) Black Seed Oil & Cancer. http://www.livestrong .com/ article/502091-black-seed-oil-cancer/accessed on April 2017

Mozzafari FS, Ghorbanli M, Babai A, Farzami Scpehr M (2000) The effect of water stress on the seed oil of *Nigella sativa* L. J Essential Oil Res 12: 36-38

Musa D, Dilsiz N, Ulakoglu G, Ulakoglu G, Bitiren M (2004) Antitumor activity of an ethanol extract of *Nigella sativa*seeds. Biologia 59: 735–740

Nagi MN, Alam K, Badary OA, Al-Shabanah OA, AL-Sawaf HA, AL-bekairi AM(1999). Thymoquinone protects against carbon tetrachloride hepatotoxicity in mice via an antioxidant mechanism. Biochem Mol Biol Int 47: 153-159

Paradise L (2005) Black cumin seed extract. http://www.encyclopedia.com/doc/1G2-3435100100.html Accessed on July 2017

Ramadan MF, Morsel JT (2003) Analysis of glycolipids from Black cumin (*Nigella sativa* L.), coriander (*Coriandrum sativum* L.) and niger (*Guizotia abyssinica cass.*) oilseeds. Food Chem 80: 197–204

Renter E (2013) 10 Health Benefits of Black Seed (*Nigella sativa*)- Part 1 http://naturalsociety.com/10-health-benefits-of-black-cumin-seednigella-sativa/

Salem ML (2005) Immunomodulatory and therapeutic properties of the *Nigella sativa*L. Seed. Intern J Immunopharmacol 5: 13-14

Salman MT, Khan RA, Shukla I (2008) Antimicrobial activity of *Nigella sativa*seed oil against multi-drug resistant bacteria from clinical isolates. Net Prod Radiance, 7(1): 10-14

Singh, J, Sethi APS, Sikka SS, Chatli MK, Kumar P (2017) Effect of sun dried whole bulb garlic powder on growth, carcass characteristics and meat quality of commercial broilers. Indian J Anim Sci 85(1): 67-71

Soliman AZM, Ghazalah AA, El-Samra SH, Atta AM, Abdo ZMA (1999) The synergistic effect of either black seed or garlic with fat on broiler performance and immunity. Proceedings of the 7th Scientific Conference on Animal Nutrition (Ruminants, Poultry and Fish) El-Aris, Egypt 2 (Special Issue)

Sultan MT, Butt MS, Anjum FM, Jamil A, Akhtar S, Nasir M (2009) Nutritional profile of indigenous cultivar of Black cumin seeds and antioxidant potential of its fixed and essential oil. Pakistan J Botany 41: 32-40

Takruri HRH, Dameh MAF, (1998) Study of the nutritional value of Black cumin seeds (*Nigella sativa*). J Sci Food Agric 76: 404-410

Toghyani M, Toghyani M, Gheisari A, Ghalamkari G, Mohammadrezaei M (2010) Growth performance, serum bio-chemistry and blood haematology of broiler chicks fed different levels of black seed (Nigella sativa) and peppermint (Mentha piperita). Livestock Sci 129: 173-178

Tuluce YH, Ozkol B, Sogut I, Celik M (2009) Effects of *Nigella sativa*on lipid peroxidation and reduced glutathione levels in erythrocytes of broiler chickens. Cell Membra Free Radi Res 1: 1-3

Zaoui A, Cherrah Y, Lacaille-Dubois MA, Settaf A, Amarouch H, Hassar M (2000) Diuretic and hypotensive effects of *Nigella sativa*in the spontaneously hypertensive rat. Therapie 55: 379-382.

□□□

Chapter 11

Clove (*Syzygium aromaticum*)

Guru Prasad Mandal and Bikas Chandra Debnath

Department of Animal Nutrition, West Bengal University of Animal and Fishery Sciences, 37 & 68, K.B.Sarani, Belgachhia, Kolkata-700037, India, E-mail: gpmandal1@gmail.com

ABSTRACT

Clove (*Syzygium aromaticum*) is one of the most valuable herb which have been used for centuries as food preservative and for many medicinal purposes. Clove represents one of the richest sources of phenolic compounds such as eugenol, eugenol acetate and gallic acid. Volatile compounds that are present in lower concentrations in its essential oil are β-pinene, limonene, farnesol, benzaldehyde, 2-heptanone and ethyl hexanoate. Clove oil has antioxidant, antimicrobial, antiparasitic, anti-inflammatory, analgesic, cytotoxic, immunostimulant and antidepressant effect. The essential oils present in clove have been suggested to improve growth performance, gut function, nutrients digestibility and carcass traits in poultry and pig. Clove as feed additive has effect on rumen fermentation, methane production, milk yield and milk quality in ruminants.

Keywords: *Syzygium aromaticum*, Eugenol, Antioxidant, Antimicrobial, Immunostimulant, Livestock.

11.1 Introduction

Use of herbal feed additives has increased manifolds due to development of microbial resistance to the antibiotics. They play a significant role in livestock and poultry production, health and nutrition. Antibiotic growth promoters (AGPs) for animal diets have been banned in the European Union since 2006. Strictness of the FDA guidelines has also increased possibility of banning antibiotics in the USA in near future. More countries are too expected to follow the same guidelines. To meet the market demands for alternatives to AGPs in animal production, scientific screening program is being carried out extensively with essential oil of various spices in order to establish their potential antibacterial activity (Pruthi, 1980). Essential oil of various spices is important aromatic components which contribute to natural preservation of foods. The antibacterial properties of essential oil of spices are well documented and recognized (Kalemba and Kunicka, 2003) both *in vitro* (Ouwehand *et al.*, 2010) and *in vivo* (Tiihonen *et al.*, 2010). The stimulation of endogenous enzymes by hot spices is a well known effect (Blumberger and Glatzel, 1963). Apart from antibacterial action, now-a-days many reports confirm the antifungal, antiviral and anti-carcinogenic properties of spices.

Among various spices, clove (*Syzygium aromaticum*) is one of the most valuable which have been used for centuries as food preservative and for many medicinal purposes. Clove represents one of the richest sources of phenolic compounds such as eugenol, eugenol acetate and gallic acid and posses' great potential for pharmaceutical, cosmetic, food and agricultural applications. Clove in particular has attracted an attention due to the potent antioxidant and antimicrobial activities present in it (Shan *et al.*, 2005). A new application of clove as larvicidal agent is an interesting strategy to combat dengue (*Aedes aegypti L.*) which is a serious health problem in the tropical countries (Sritabutra *et al.*, 2011) including India. Clove is used in traditional medicine in many countries of Asia, also as an anthelmintic. Clove oil is largely responsible for the ability to keep food from spoiling. Cloves are the richest plant source of eugenol, which is a very powerful fat-soluble antioxidant, inhibits the accumulation of fat peroxide products in red blood cells and maintains the activities of the body's antioxidant enzymes at normal levels. Small amount of eugenol is actually required for a significant protective effect because it can be directly incorporated into cell membranes, which prevents lipid peroxidation in the cells.

Syzygium aromaticum (synonym: Eugeniacariophylata. Family: *Mirtaceae*) is commonly known as clove. Clove is native of Indonesia but presently it is cultivated in tropical and subtropical countries including India. It is a median size tree with a height of 8-12 meter. Cloves are the immature unopened flower buds. The tree starts giving flower buds after 4 years of plantation. Flower buds, is the commercialized part of this tree. Flower buds are collected in the maturation phase before flowering. The collection is done either manually or chemically-mediated using a natural phytohormone which liberates ethylene in the vegetal tissue, producing precocious maturation (Filho *et al.*, 2013). Cloves are normally green or pink, when they are picked. They need to be dried until they become brown before they can be stored and sold. They resemble tiny nails of about 1.5cm long and have a diameter of about 0.5cm. The dried flower buds are highly appreciated as a spice worldwide. Cloves are used in cuisines all over the world not only as feed additives in the food but also in pharmaceutical, tobacco and cosmetics industries. Eugenol can be extracted from clove as an essential oil, which have the 'essence' of the plant that gives it its taste and smell. Eugenol has a boiling point of 254°C and can be steam distilled from freshly ground clove.

11.2 Chemistry of Clove

Essential oil of clove is rich in eugenol and b-caryophilene (Kung *et al.*, 2008). Clove is a very good source of phenolic compounds. These compounds are mainly flavonoids, hidroxibenzoic acids, hidroxicinamic acids and hidroxiphenyl propens. Eugenol is the main bioactive compound of the clove. This organic molecule consists of a six carbon ring of alternating double bonds. It is considered a phenylpropene molecule, which contains a modified benzene ring (6 carbon atoms with hydrogen normally attached to each) with an allyl group. Two oxygen atoms are singly bonded to carbons in the ring, one of the oxygen atoms is single bonded to another carbon with three hydrogen atoms and the other is bonded only to hydrogen. Another carbon atom is singly bonded to a remaining carbon in the ring, which is bonded to two other carbons, each of which are also bonded to hydrogen atoms. The concentration of eugenol is 938.17 to 1,465.00 ppm on as such basis (Nevew *et al.*, 1993). Phenolic acids found in clove are gallic acid, hydrolizable tannins caffeic, ferulic, elagic and salicylic acids. The concentration of hydrolizable tannin is very high (237.58 ppm on as such basis) (Shan *et al.*, 2005). However, concentration of gallic acid is 78.35ppm on as such basis. Flavonoids like kaempferol, quercetin and its derivates (glycosilated) are also found in clove in lower concentrations. The concentrations of essential oil in the clove flower buds may rise upto 18%. Patra *et al.* (2009) reported that eugenol contains in clove oils is 78%. However, Jirovetz *et al.* (2006) reported presence of 89% essential oil, eugenol in clove. The rest is eugenol acetate and â-cariofileno which ranges from 5-15%. Apart from this, another important compound found in the essential oil is α-humulen (about 2.1%). Volatile compounds that are present in lower concentrations in its essential oil are β-pinene, limonene, farnesol, benzaldehyde, 2-heptanone and ethyl hexanoate.

11.3 Taxonomy of Clove

Kingdom	:	Plantae
(unranked)	:	Angiosperms
(unranked)	:	Eudicots
(unranked)	:	Rosids
Order	:	Myrtales
Family	:	Myrtaceae
Genus	:	*Syzygium*
Species	:	*Aromaticum*

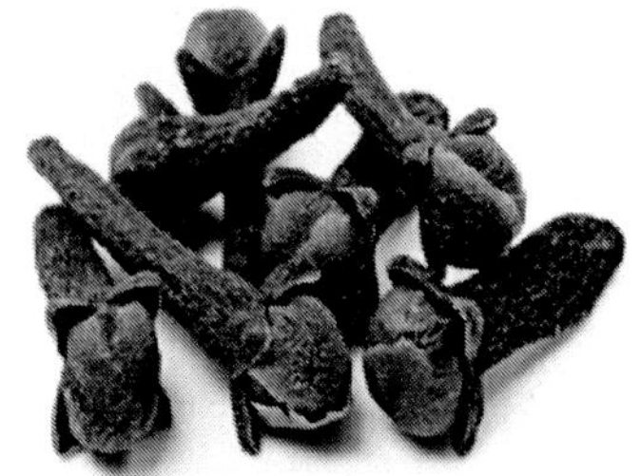

11.4 Biological Activity of Clove

Clove oil is a natural antibacterial, antiviral and antifungal agent (Valero and Salmeron, 2003; Singh *et al.*, 2002; Pina Vaz *et al.*, 2004), antiparasitic (Kim *et al.*, 2004). Apart from these, clove oil has anti-oxidant, anti-inflammatory, analgesic, cytotoxic, immunostimulant and antidepressant effect.

11.4.1 *Antibacterial Property*

Antimicrobial potentiality of clove was established, when its essential oil extracts killed many Gram positive and Gram negative organisms (Gislene *et al.*, 2000). As mentioned above, the most efficient source of eugenol is cloves. Due to eugenol supplementation in poultry feed, there was increased population of beneficial micro-organisms like lactobacillus (Agostini *et al.*, 2012) and decreased population of harmful bacteria like *Escherichia coli* in intestine of layers (Ordonez *et al.*, 2008). Eugenol has shown to be an effective antibacterial agent, such as against *Salmonella typhi*. Eugenol can break down bacterial cell membranes (Devi *et al.*, 2010). Its antibacterial properties are being developed in nanoemulsion delivery studies to use eugenol as a food preservative against *Staphylococcus aureus* in fruit juices and shown to be effective against microbial spoilage (Ghosh *et al.*, 2014). Though the modes of action of the extracts are not clear, their antimicrobial agents include thymol, terpenes, eugenol, flavones, glycosides of phenolic monoterpenoids and aliphatic alcohols among other elements (Hammer *et al.*, 1999). These substances either alone or in combination may result in a broad spectrum of antimicrobial activity exhibited for both bacteria and fungi. Clove oils possess antimicrobial activity against *S. aureus*, *E. coli*, *P. aeruginosa* as well as against *S. pyogenes*,

Corynebacterium, Salmonella, Bacteroides and *C. albicans* at various dilutions of the extracts, whereas clove water extract showed inhibitions with all the organisms tested except with *S. pyogenes, B. fragilis* and *C. albicans*. Eugenol reduced *Salmonella Typhimurium* DT104, *E. coli* O157:H7, and other coliforms with little inhibition towards beneficial bacteria (Si *et al.*, 2006). Eugenol could be a potential antimicrobial against *Salmonella enteritidis* in chickens, when supplemented in the feed. Eugenol at 1% in feed significantly reduced *Salmonella enteritidis* populations in market age broilers, when supplemented for 5 days before slaughter. Dental caries and periodontitis in human beings are caused by *Streptococcus mutans*. Strong bactericidal activity of clove oil (@0.1mg/ml) was observed against these bacteria (Moon, Kim and Cha, 2011). Clove oil synergistically acts with antibiotic (Ampicillin) and reduces 4-8 folds the concentration needed to inhibit or kill the bacteria. Formulations containing eugenol encapsulated in a non-ionic surfactant were tested against four strains of two important food borne pathogens, *E. coli* O157:H7 and *Listeria monocytogenes*, results reinforces the employment of eugenol to inhibit the growth of these micro-organisms in surfaces in contact with food (Perrz-Conesa *et al.*, 2006). Pure clove oil was tested against *Staphylococcus epidermidis, Staphylococcus aureus, Bacillus subtilis, E.coli, Proteus vulgaris, Pseudomonas aeruginosa* and results showed minimum inhibitory concentrations between 0.062% and 0.500% (v/v) which is promising as an anti-infectious agents as well as food preservative (Fu *et al.*, 2007). Eugenol at 2 μg/mL inhibited the growth of 31 strains of Helicobacter pylori, after 9 h of incubation, being more potent that amoxicillin and without developing resistance. The activity and stability of those compounds was checked at low pH values since Helicobacter pylori resides in the low pH of stomach (Ali *et al.*, 2005).

11.4.2 *Antifungal Activity*

Clove bud oil has a broad spectrum antifungal activity. The important species are *Cadida albicans, Aspergillus flavus*, and *Aspergillus niger* and dermatophytes (fungal skin infection-causing species). Among them, the dermatophytes are the most susceptible as minimum concentration needed to inhibit Candida is 0.16 μl/ml (Pinto *et al.*, 2009). The eugenol is the main compound responsible for the antifungal activity. It causes membrane disruption and deformation of macromolecules leading to lysis of the spores and micelles (Devi *et al.*, 2010).

11.4.3 *Antiviral Property*

Clove has antiviral activity. Eugeniin, a compound isolated from the clove is responsible for this antiviral activity. Eugeniin was found to be effective against herpes virus @5 μg/ml. Eugeniin inhibits the viral DNA polymerase synthesis which leads to the reduction of the viral DNA synthesis (Kurokawa *et al.*, 1998). When antiviral drug acyclovir was administered along with the aqueous extracts of clove, a strong antiherpes simplex virus type 1 (HSV-1) activity was observed. This non-toxic synergic activity was found stronger in the brain than in the skin of mice (Kurokawa *et al.*, 1995). Replication of the hepatitis C virus was also inhibited (≥90% inhibition at 100 μg/ml) by the clove extract.

11.4.5 *Anti-parasitic Activity*

Intestinal protozoa are susceptible to the clove oil. The oil is very much potential for prevention as well as anti-giardial therapy (Machado *et al.*, 2011). Clove oil can effectively inhibit the growth of *Giardia lamblia,* a protozoon that is a significant problem in children in many countries. Three hours of exposure to clove oil is sufficient to eliminate the protozoa from the intestine. Clove oil was also found to be effective against Chaga's disease, caused by a protozoa *Trypansoma cruzi*. The study of Evans *et al.* (2001) showed that a mixture of essential oil containing 1% clove oil reduced the coccidial oocyst in broiler chicks as compared to those fed non-supplemented diet.

11.4.6 *Anti-oxidant Agent*

Clove has a high content of polyphenols and antioxidant compounds. A high correlation also exists between polyphenols content and antioxidant activity (Shan *et al.*, 2005). The potentiality of clove is very high as radical scavenger and as a commercial source of polyphenols. The antioxidant activity (*in vitro*) of clove is comparable with synthetic food preservative compound, butylated hydroxytoluene (BHT) (Bamdad *et al.*, 2006). The antioxidant activity of clove oil compared with synthetic antioxidants as measured by scavenging of the DPPH (1-1-Diphenyl-2-Picryl-Hydroxyl) radical decreased in the following order: clove oil>BHT>α-tocopherol> butylated hydroxyanisole>Trolox (Gülçin *et al.*, 2012). The antioxidant activity of aqueous extracts of clove has inhibition capacity upto 95%, when tested as metal quelants, superoxide radical capture and scavenging of the DPPH radical. The powerful antioxidant activity of clove extracts may be attributed to the strong hydrogen donating ability, metal chelating ability and scavanging of free radicals, hydrogen peroxide and superoxide (Gülçin *et al.*, 2004). Polyphenols of clove has multifunctional activities as reducing agents, hydrogen atom donators, and single oxygen scavengers. Eugenol allows the donation of a hydrogen atom and subsequent stabilization of the phenoxil radical generated forming stable compounds that do not start or propagate oxidation.

11.4.7 *Anti-nociceptive Agent*

Cloves have been used extensively since the 13th century as a relief for toothache, join pain and visceral pain. Eugenol is the main compound responsible for this pain relieving activity. Activation of calcium and chloride channels in ganglion cells is caused by the eugenol. The eugenol inhibits ATP induced P_2X currents in trigeminal ganglion thereby affecting sodium and calcium channels which contributed to the analgesic effect of clove (Li *et al.*, 2008). Another probable reason is that an inhibition of prostaglandins and other inflammatory mediators such as leukotrienes as the mechanisms of analgesic action and eugenol also blocks pain receptors, thus preventing the brain from receiving pain signals (Hosseini, Asl and Rakhshandeh, 2011).

11.4.8 *Cytotoxic (anti-cancer) Agent*

Eugenol can act as an anti-cancer potential substance through interference of several cell-signaling pathways. Free radicals (formed during cellular metabolism) activates such signal pathways which results in the expression of gens that suppress apoptosis and induce cellular transformation, proliferation, invasion, metastasis among others (Aggarwal and Sisodia, 2006). The eugenol has anti-oxidative, cytotoxic and genotoxic effects which have the ability to modulate resistance against the damaging effects of H_2O_2 on DNA of different strains of human cells. The eugenol suppressed the growth of the malignant melanoma, decreased size of tumours and inhibited melanoma invasion and metastasis by the inhibition of the two transition factors of the E_2F_1 transcriptional activity (Ghosh *et al.*, 2005). In the absence of oxidative stress, eugenol acts as an antioxidant at low concentrations but acts as a prooxidant at high concentrations. In the presence of oxidative stress eugenol increased ROS levels at low concentrations (5-10μmol/L), but decreased them at high concentrations (500 μmol/L) concluding that the cytotoxicity of eugenol occurs in a ROS-independent manner in the presence of oxidative stress.

11.4.9 *Anti-inflammatory Activity*

Clove and eugenol possesses anti-inflammatory activity (Daniel *et al.*, 2009). In rats, injections of eugenol significantly reduced paw oedema (swelling) compared to untreated controls.

11.4.10 *Anti-allergic Activity*

Anti-allergic activity of clove may be useful for treatment of hay fever or asthama. Tracheal smooth muscle normally contracts in allergic reactions such as asthama. In such condition, clove and eugenol were both found to possess tracheal smooth muscle relaxant property (Reiter and Brandt, 1985). Clove oil was found inhibit artificially-induced systemic anaphylaxis and IgE antibody-mediated passive cutaneous anaphylaxis reactions. The levels of histamine in the blood are significantly reduced due to inhibition of release of histamine from mast cells (Kim *et al.*, 1998).

11.4.11 *Immunostimulant Activity*

Cell-mediated responses are important for defending against viruses and intracellular bacteria and fungi. Clove oil helps in activating this response to protect against these organisms. Clove and eugenol caused an increase in delayed-type of hypersensitivity reactions stimulating a cell-mediated response. There was increase in 71% of the white blood cell count in non-and immuno-suppressed mice when fed clove oil @ 200mg/kg for a period of 7 days (Carrasco *et al.*, 2010).

11.4.12 *Antidepressant Activity*

Clove oils have an antidepressant activity due to the action of eugenol. Eugenol's activity was comparable to imipramine, an antidepressant drug (Irie *et al.*, 2004). An oral administration of 200mg/kg clove oil to mice exerted significant anti-depressant effects. Long term oral administration of 50-200mg/kg clove oil to mice exposed to chronic unpredictable mild stress also significantly increased the protein levels of hippocampal p-ERK, p-CREB, and brain-derived neurotrophic factor, which are usually decreased in depression (Liu *et al.*, 2015).

11.5 Toxicity and Pharmacokinetics

An oral dose of clove essential oil, lower than 1500 mg/kg is generally recognized as safe. When eugenol was administrated orally, the mean half lives of 14.0 h and 18.3 h, respectively was noticed for plasma and blood. Kreydiyyeh *et al.* (2000) used eugenol, at the concentration of 850 ppm, and concluded that these levels impaired the absorption of alanine by rat jejunum. The authors reported that eugenol inhibits the activity of Na-K- ATPase which is located in enterocyte and consequently impair transport process in the intestine.

11.6 Clove oil as Feed Additives in Ruminants

11.6.1 *Rumen fFermentation*

Total volatile fatty acid (TVFA) was increased by clove oil supplementation indicating an improved digestibility (Morsy *et al.*, 2012). Clove oil or other essential oils supplementation decreased acetate production while increased propionate and butyrate production (Cardozo *et al.*, 2006; Findino *et al.*, 2008 and Morsy *et al.*, 2012). Clove oil facilitates growth of *Butyrivibrio fibrisolvens*, a major butyrate producer in rumen (Bryant and Small, 1956). It was also reported that clove oil inhibit hyper ammonia producing bacteria in the rumen by reducing deaminase activity thereby reduces rumen ammonia production. Clove oil reduces number of ruminal protozoa. Ruminal protozoa has proteolytic and deamination activity. As ruminal protozoa number is decreased due to clove oil supplementation then proteolytic and deamination activity is also reduced which leads to reduced ammonical N concentration in rumen (Cardozo *et al.*, 2006; Castillejos *et al.*, 2008 and Morsy *et al.*, 2012). However, the *in vitro* study of Benchaar *et al.* (2008) did not reveal such effect, when eugenol was added @8oo mg/L along with cinnamon leaf oil @250mg/L.

11.6.2 *In-vitro Digestibility*

Clove oil supplementation (@300 ppm) significantly increased *in vitro* true DM disappearance (IVTDMD), *in vitro* NDF disappearance (IVNDFD), and estimated energy contents (TDN, ME and NEL) values compared to control (Rofiq, 2014). The inclusion of clove oil @300 ppm had no effect on *in vitro* rumen gas production using Hohenheim gas technique (HGT) after 96 hour fermentation (Rofiq *et al.*, 2012) indicated no negative effect on digestibility of insoluble fraction of TMR, however, clove oil at 0.25 ml and 0.50 ml level of extract could inhibit enzyme CMCase, xylanase and acetylesterase (Patra, 2010). Generally, main action mechanism of clove oils as rumen manipulator is its antimicrobial effects. Cell membrane disruption would be happen when essential oil active with micro-organism cell membrane including electron transport, ion gradients, protein translocation, phosphorilation and other enzyme-dependent reactions (Dorman and Deans, 2000).

11.6.3 *Rumen Methane Production*

Patra and Yu (2012) tested clove oil *in vitro* at 3 different doses (0.25, 0.50 and 1.0g/L) and revealed that clove oil linearly ($P < 0.01$) reduced methane production, with a reduction by 34.4%, at 1.0 g/L compared with the control. In another study, Shabestari *et al.* (2011) evaluated the effects of clove methanol extract (@ 0.5 and 1ml) on methane production under *in vitro* condition and observed that if incubation time is lengthened for a period of 12 hours, then methane production could be reduced.

11.6.4 *Dry matter Intake*

Previous studies showed that dry matter intake was not affected due to clove oil or any other essential oil supplementation (Benchaar *et al.*, 2008, Santos, 2010, Tager and Krause, 2011 and Morsy *et al.*, 2012). In early lactation period, when the animals are in negative energy balance, then the supplementation of clove oil will be helpful as the oil can provide an additional energy to the animal. It helps in improving performance of the animal without much loss of body reserves (Tedeschi *et al.*, 2003).

11.6.5 *Milk yield and Composition*

Milk yield and milk lactose component in dairy cattle was not significantly affected by clove oil (Benchaar *et al.*, 2007; Tassoul and Shaver, 2009 and Morsy *et al.*, 2012). However, feed efficiency (milk yield/DMI) improved due to addition of clove oil and other essential oil (Tassoul and Shaver, 2009 and Morsy *et al.*, 2012). A higher content of milk protein with low level of NPN in the milk on clove oil supplementation was reported (Morsy *et al.*, 2012). The reason behind is that there was a reduction of ruminal ammonical nitrogen and increased synthesis of microbial protein. Ruminal acetate production is also reduced due supplementation of clove oil. This resulted in lower milk fat percentage in lactating animals (Morsy *et al.*, 2012). In contrast, Santos *et al.* (2010) revealed that supplementation of essential oil containing eugenol produced higher milk fat percentage without affecting the milk yield or other components. Benchaar *et al.* (2007) and Tassoul and Shaver (2009) observed no effect on milk components on essential oil supplementation. *In vivo* experiments using used blend oils containing eugenol @ 0.5 g/day/cow had no effected on dry matter intake and milk yield, but increased in fat percentage in milk (Santos *et al.*, 2010). However, oral infusion of clove oil in goats had no significant ($P>0.05$) effect on milk production, fat corrected milk 4%, and live weight change (Rofique and Gorgulu, 2012). Milk component were also not affected ($P>0.05$) by clove oil. Average value of milk composition such as total solid (TS) solid non-fat (SNF), fat, protein, casein and lactose were same between treatments on clove oil supplementation.

11.6.6 *Milk and Meat Fatty Acid Profile*

Supplementation of clove oil will lead to a change in the TVA profile in the rumen. Hence, there will also be a change in the milk fatty acid profile. Clove essential oil supplementation leads to higher content of 18:0, C18:1N9C and C18:3N3 omega 3 fatty acid (FA) and C18:3N6 than the control diet. N6:N3 ratio was decreased with clove oil supplementation as compared to control which gives a positive healthy effect (Benchhar *et al.*, 2007 and Morsy *et al.*, 2012). Due to supplementation of clove oil there was increased proportion of saturated fatty acid and decreased proportion of saturated FA indicating healthy milk for the milk consumers (Morsy *et al.*, 2012). Addition of clove (2.5 g/kg DM) decreased ($P<0.01$) the proportion of total saturated FA, but increased the proportion of total polyunsaturated FA (PUFA; $P<0.032$) in both muscle and adipose tissues of goat .Proportions of total CLA and cis-9, trans-11 CLA tended ($P<0.10$) to increase in muscle and adipose tissues owing to the inclusion of clove in the diet (Mandal *et al.*, 2014).

11.6.7 *Biochemical Parameters*

It is reported that supplementation of clove oil leads to increased serum total protein, albumin and globulin. This increase in serum level may be due to reduction of ammonical N production which ultimately leads to increased production of microbial protein. There is a significant reduction in blood cholesterol level observed due to clove oil supplementation. The quality of fatty acid present in clove may help in reducing blood cholesterol concentration. Clove oil supplementation does not affect the liver function also as indicated by normal SGOT and SGPT level (Morsy *et al.*, 2012). Mandal *et al.* (2014) reported that serum concentration of glucose, total protein, cholesterol and triglyceride in goat was not affected by supplementation of clove (2.5 g/kg DM) in the diet.

11.7 Clove as Feed Additive in Pigs

Piglets fed on diets containing clove oil @5ml/kg had average daily gain (ADG) similar to that of control, but improved feed conversion ratio and lowered incidence of diarrhea (Tartrakoon *et al.*, 2003). However, Marcin *et al.* (2006) revealed that the average daily weight gains of piglets supplemented with of clove oil (22ml/100kg body wt.) was increased by 43.79 gm per day compared with control. Clove oil supplementation decreased enterobacteriaceae number and amylolytic activity in faeces.

11.8 Clove as Feed Additive in Poultry

The recent trend toward reduction of antibiotics growth promoter (AGP) in poultry diet has compelled the researchers to explore the utility of other non-therapeutic alternatives. In this context, phytogenic feed additive like clove oil (200-600 pm) was found to improve feed intake, weight gain and FCR of broiler chickens (Dalkilic and Guler, 2009; Istabel and Santos, 2009; Mukhter, 2011; Tedesco, 2001). The improved performance in broiler could be due to the positive effects of clove oil on the digestive system and presence of high concentration of manganese, trace minerals necessary for protein and carbohydrate metabolism, the synthesis of fatty acids and cholesterol (Cabuk *et al.*, 2003). The greater efficiency in the utilization of feed by the clove extract might have resulted in enhanced growth. There is evidence to suggest that herbs, spices, and various plant extracts have appetite and digestion stimulating properties and antimicrobial effects (Kamel,

2001). Clove extract contain different molecules (mainly eugenol) that have intrinsic bio-activities on animal physiology and metabolism. The mechanisms by which these products influence the gut microflora and growth performance of poultry are not known properly. As antibiotics, plant extracts could control and limit the growth and colonization of numerous pathogenic and nonpathogenic species of bacteria in the gut. Mher *et al.* (2014) observed that at starter period, broiler chicks refuse to consume feed but they have been acclimatized to the especial aroma of the clove containing diets after some days. They found that from 23-42 d and 0-42 days of experiment, feed intake and body weight gain were significantly increased in broilers fed 450 ppm clove essential oil compared to control group. Results also showed that clove essential oil at the level of 450 ppm increased BWG and improved FCR in finisher period ($P<0.05$).

Supplementation of clove showed increased dressing percentage and breast weight in Japanese quail without any effect on other cut up parts and organ weight, which suggests a better growth than the control (Tariq *et al.*, 2015). They observed numerically higher CP and lower EE in drumstick meat in comparison to breast and thigh meat, when clove powder was supplemented @5g/kg feed in quail's diet. Proximate composition with respect to moisture%, CP, EE, and total ash contents estimated in drumstick, thigh, and breast muscle did not vary due to clove powder supplementation. However, Mehr *et al.* (2014) showed that different levels of clove essential oil (150, 300 and 450ppm) had no significant effect on dressing percentage, abdominal fat and internal organs percentage (liver, heart and gizzard) ($P>0.05$) in broilers.

Clove oil at 450 ppm in feed of had significantly decreased the level of cholesterol on 21 days of age ($P<0.05$). The main components of this essential oil inhibits hepatic 3-hydroxy-3 methylglutaryl coenzyme A (HMG-COA) reductase activity, which is a key regulatory enzyme in cholesterol synthesis (Mehr *et al.*, 2014).

11.9 Summary and Conclusions

Clove can be used as natural non-antibiotic growth promoter which contains eugenol with antibacterial, antiviral, antifungal and anti-parasitic properties. Additionally it has anti-oxidant, anti-inflammatory, analgesic, cytotoxic, immunostimulant and antidepressant effect. The essential oils present in clove have been suggested to improve growth performance, gut function, nutrients digestibility and carcass traits. However, further research is still essential to determine the optimal dietary inclusion level and the mode of action of clove oil to achieve optimal digestion, growth and performance. Its application in livestock and poultry animal production has been limited, largely owing to their inconsistent efficacy and lack of full understanding the modes of action. A better understanding the effects of clove on the gastrointestinal ecosystem (gut microbiota, gut physiology and immunology) and the mechanisms behind will possibly allow the best use of clove for sustainable animal production. Economically effectiveness is also important because cost-effectiveness in substituting antibiotics with spices/herbs is another most challenging one, which remains critical for ensuring the long-term sustainable animal production. Finally, the potential risks in the use of clove as phytogenic feed additives for livestock and poultry production need to be evaluated even though phytogenic compounds are generally recognized as safe (GRAS).

References

Aggarwal BB, Sisodia S (2006) Molecular targets of dietary agents for prevention and therapy of cancer. Biochem Pharmachol 71(10): 1397-1421

Agostini PS, Sola-Oriol D, Nofrarý M, Barroeta AC, Gasa J, Manzanilla EG (2012) Role of in-feed clove supplementation on growth performance, intestinal microbiology, and morphology in broiler chicken. Livest. Sci., 147(1-3): 113-118

Ali SM, Khan AA, Ahmed I, Musaddiq M, Ahmed KS, Polasa H (2005) Antimicrobial activities of eugenol and cinnamaldehyde against the human gastric pathogen Helicobacter pylori. Ann Clin Microbial Antimicrob. 4: 20-26

Bamdad F, Kadivar M, Keramat J (2006) Evaluation of phenolic content and antioxidant activity of Iranian caraway in comparison with clove and BHT using model systems and vegetable oil. Int J Food Sci Technol 41(Suppl 1): S20-S27

Benchaar C, Calsamigilia S, Chaves AV, Fraser GR, Colombotto D, McAllister TA (2008) A review of plant derived essential oils in ruminant nutrition and production. Anim. Feed Sci Technol 145: 209-228

Benchaar C, Petit HV, Berthiaume R, Ouellet DR, Chiquette J, Chouinard PV (2007) Effects of essential oils on digestion, ruminal fermentation, ruminal microbial populations, milk production and milk composition in dairy cows fed alfalfa silage or corn silage. J Dairy Sci 90: 886-897

Blumberger W, Glatzel H (1963) Contributions to the physiology of spices and seasonings. I. Effect of spices on saliva quantity and composition. Dtsch. Z. Verdau.- Stoffwechselkr. 23: 97-118

Bryant MP, Small N (1956) The anaerobic monotrichus butyric acid producing curved rod-shaped bacteria in rumen. J Bacteriol 72: 16-21

Çabuk M, Alçiçek A, Bozkurt M, Imre N (2003) Antimicrobial properties of the essential oils isolated from aromatic plants and using possibility as alternative feed additives. II. National Animal Nutrition Congress, 18-20 September, pp. 184-187

Cardozo PW, Calsamiglia S, Ferret A, Kamel C (2006) Effect of alfalfa extract, anise, capsicum and a mixture of cinnamaldehyde and eugenol on rumen fermentation and protein degradation in beef heifer fed a high concentrate diet. J Anim Sci 84: 2801-2808

Carrasco FR (2009) Immuno-modulatory activity of Zingiber officinale Roscoe, Salvia officinalis L. and Syzygium aromaticum L. essential oils: evidence for humour- and cell-mediated responses. J Pharmacy Pharmacol 61(7): 961-967

Castillejos LS, Calsamiglia S, Martyn J, Wijlen HT (2008) *In vitro* evaluation of effects of ten essential oils at three doses on ruminal fermentation of high concentrate feedlot-type diets. Anim Feed Sci Technol 145: 259-270

Dalkilic B, Güler T (2009) The effects of dietary clove extract on carcass characteristics, digestive organ size and total coliform counts of small intestine in broilers. Fýrat Üniv Saðlýk Bilimleri Dergisi 23(3): 153-159

Daniel AN (2009) Anti-inflammatory and antinociceptive activities A of eugenol essential oil in experimental animal models. Revista Brasileira de Farmacognosia 19(1): 34-41

Devi KP, Nisha SA, Sakthive R, Pandian SK (2010) Eugenol (an essential oil of clove) acts as an antibacterial agent against Salmonella typhi by disrupting the cellular membrane. J Ethnopharmacol 130(1): 107–115

Dorman HJD, Deans SG (2000) Antimicrobial agents from plants: antibacterial activity of plant volatile oils. J Appl Microbiol 88: 308-316

Evans, JW, Plunkett MS, Banfield MJ (2001) Effect of an essential oil blend on coccidiosis in broiler in broiler chicks. Poult Sci 80:258 (Abstract)

Fandino I, Calsamiglia S, Ferret A, Blanch M (2008) Anise and capsicum as alternative to monensin to modify rumen fermentation in beef heifers fed on a high concentrate diet. Anim Feed Sci Technol 145: 409-417

Filho GA, Cesar JO, Ramos JV (2013) [Cravo from India]. Itabuna: CEPLAC. 2013. [Online] Available from: http://www.ceplac.gov.br /radar.htm [Accessed on 21st April, 2013]. Portuguese

Fu Y, Zu Y, Chen L, Shi X, Wang Z, Sun S (2007) Antimicrobial activity of clove and rosemary essential oils alone and in combination. Phytother Res. 21(10): 989-994

Geda AK, (1995) Antibacterial activity of essential oils and their combinations. Fett Wiss Technol 97(12): 458-461

Ghosh R, Nadiminty N, Fitzpatrick JE, Alworth WL, Slaga TJ, Kumar AP (2005) Eugenol causes melanoma growth suppression through inhibition of E2F1 transcriptional activity. J Biol Chem 280(7): 5812-5819

Ghosh V, Mukherjee A, Chandrasekaran N (2014) Eugenol-loaded antimicrobial nanoemulsion preserves fruit juice against, microbial spoilage. Colloids and Surfaces B: Biointerfaces 114: 392–397

Gislene GF, Paulo C, Giuliana L (2000) Antibacterial Activity of Plant Extracts and Phytochemicals on Antibiotic Resistant Bacteria. Braz J Microbial 31: 314–325

Gülçin I, Elmasta° M, Aboul-Enein HY (2012) Antioxidant activity of clove oil-A powerful antioxidant source. Arab J Chem 5(4): 489-499

Gülçin Ì, Þatb ÝG, Beydemira Þ, Elmastaþc M, Küfrevioglu, ÖÝ (2004) Comparison of antioxidant activity of clove (Eugenia caryophylata Thunb) buds and lavender (Lavandula stoechas L.). Food Chem 8(3): 393-400

Hammer KA, Carson CF, Riley TV (1999) Antimicrobial activity of essential oils and other plant extracts. J Appl Microbial 86(6): 985-990

Hosseini M, Asl MK, Rakhshandeh H (2011) Analgesic effect of clove essential oil in mice. Avicenna J Phytomedicine 1(1): 1-6

Irie Y (2004) Eugenol exhibits antidepressant-like activity in mice and induces expression of metallothionein-III in the hippocampus. Brain Res 1011(2): 243-246

Istabel B, Santos Y, (2009) Effects of dietary organic acids and essential oils on growth performance and carcass characteristics of broiler chickens. J Appl Poult Res 18: 472-476

Jirovetz L, Buchbauer G, Stoilova I, Stoyanova A, Krastanov A, Schmidt E (2006) Chemical composition and antioxidant properties of clove leaf essential oil. J Agric Food Chem 54(17): 6303-6307

Kalemba D, Kunicka A (2003) Antibacterial and anti-fungal properties of essential oils. Current Med Chem 10: 813–829

Kamel C (2001) Tracing modes of action and the roles of plant extracts in non-ruminants. Pp. 135-150 in Recent Advances in Animal Nutrition. P.C. Garnsworthy and J. Wiseman, Eds. Nottingham Univ. Press, Nottingham, UK

Kim MH (1998) Effect of Syzygium aromaticum extract on immediate hypersensitivity in rats. Journal of Ethnopharmacol 60(2): 125-131

Kim SI, JH Yi, JH Tak,. Ahn YJ (2004) Acaricidal Activity of plant essential oils against Dermanyssus gallinae (Acari: Dermanyssidae). Vet Parasitol 120: 297-304

Kreydiyyeh SI, Usta J, Copti R (2000) Effect of cinnamon, clove and some of their constituents on the Na+K+-ATPase activity and alanine absorption in the rat jejunum. Food and Chemical Toxicology 38: 755-762

Kung L, Williams P, Schmidt RJ, Hu W (2008) A Blend of Essentials Oils Used as an Additive to Alter Sillage Fermentation or Used as a feed Additive for Lactating Dairy Cows. J Dairy Sci 91: 4793-4800

Kurokawa M, Hozumi T, Basnet P, Nakano M, Kadota S, Namba T, (1998) Purification and characterization of eugeniin as an antiherpesvirus compound from Geum japonicum and Syzygium aromaticum. J Pharmacol Exp Ther 284(2): 728-735

Kurokawa M, Nagasaka K, Hirabayashi T, Uyama S, Sato H, Kageyama T (1995) Efficacy of traditional herbal medicines in combination with acyclovir against herpes simplex virus type 1 infection *in vitro* and *in vivo.* Antiviral Res 27(1-2): 19-37

Li HY, Lee BK, Kim JS, Jung SJ, Oh SB (2008) Eugenol inhibits ATP induced P2X currents in trigeminal ganglion neurons. Korean J Physiol Pharmacol 12(6): 315-321

Liu BB (2015) Essential Oil of Syzygium aromaticum Reverses the Deficits of Stress-Induced Behaviours and Hippocampal p-ERK/p-CREB/ Brain-Derived Neurotrophic Factor Expression. Planta Medica 81(3): 185-192

Machado M (2011) Anti-Giardia activity of Syzygium aromaticum essential oils and eugenol: Effects on growth, viability, adherence and ultrastructure. Experimental Parasitology 127(4): 732-739

Mandal GP, Roy A, Patra AK (2014) Effects of feeding plant additives rich in saponins and essential oils on the performance, carcass traits and conjugated linoleic acid concentrations in muscle and adipose tissues of Black Bengal goats. Anim Feed Sci Technol 197: 76-84

Marcin A, Sustriková A, Mati R (2006) The effects of aromatic oils on growth performance and physiological parameters in the intestine of weaned pigs. Slovak J Anim Sci 39(1-2): 103-107

Mehr MA, Hassanabadi A, Moghadam NA, Kermanshahi H (2014) Supplementation of clove essential oils and probiotic on blood components, lymphoid organs, and immune response in broiler chickens. Res Opin Anim Vet Sci 4(4): 218-223

Moon SE, Kim HY, Cha JD (2011) Synergistic effect between clove oil and its major compounds and antibiotics against oral bacteria. Archives Oral Biol 56(9): 907-916

Morsy TA, Kholif SM, Matloup OH, Abdo MM, El-Shafie MH (2012) Impact of Anise, Clove and Juniper oils as Feed additives on the Productive Performance of Lactating Goats. International J Dairy Sci: 1811-9743.

Mukhtar AM (2011) The Effect of Dietary Clove Oil on Broiler Performance. Australian J Basic Appl Sci 5(7): 49-51

Neveu V, Perez-Jiménez J, Vos F, Crespy V, du Chaffaut L, Mennen L (1993) Phenol Explorer: an online comprehensive database on polyphenol contents in foods. doi: 10.1993/database/bap024.

Ordonez G, Llopis N, Penalver P (2008) Efficacy of eugenol against a Salmonella enterica serovar enteritisdis experimental infection in commercial layers in production. J Appl Poult Res 17: 376-382

Ouwehand AC, Tiihonen K, Kettunen H, Peuranen S, Schulze H, Rautonen N (2010) In vitro effects of es-sential oils on potential pathogens and beneficial members of the normal microbiota. Veterinarni Medicina 55: 71–78

Patra AK (2010) Meta-analyses of effects of phytochemicals on digestibility and rumen fermentation characteristics associated with methanogenesis. J Sci Food Agric 90(15): 2700-08.

Patra A, Yu Z (2012) Effects of essential oils on methane production, fermentation, abundance and diversity of rumen microbial populations. Appl Environ Microbiol 78(12): 4271-80

Patra AK, Kamra DN, Agarwal N (2009) Effects of extracts of spices on rumen methanogenesis, enzyme activities and fermentation of feeds in vitro. J Sci Food Agric 90: 511–520

Pérez-Conesa D, McLandsborough L, Weiss J (2006) Inhibition and inactivation of Listeria monocytogenes and Escherichia coli O157:H7 colony biofilms by micellar-encapsulated eugenol and carvacrol. J Food Prot 69(12): 2947-2954

Pina-Vaz C, Goncalves Rodrigues A,. Pinto E, S Costa-de-Oliveira C, Tavares L, Salgueiro, C Cavaleiro, Goncalves MJ,. Martinez-de-Oliveira J (2004) Antifungal activity of Thymus oils and their major compounds. J Eur Acad Dermatol Venereol 18: 73-78

Pinto E (2009) Antifungal activity of the clove essential oil from Syzygium aromaticumon Candida, Aspergillus and dermatophyte species. J Medical Microbiol 58 (11): 1454-1462

Pruthi JS (1980). Spices and condiments: Chemistry, microbiology technology. Advances in food research. Academic Press Inc., London.

Reiter M, Brandt W (1985) Relaxant effects on tracheal and ileal smooth muscles of the guinea pig. Arzneimittel-Forschung 35 (1): 408-414

Rofiq MN (2014). Combination Effect of Clove and Orange Peel Oils on in Vitro Digestion of Dairy Total Mixed Ration Using Ankom daisy. In Incubator. J Adv Agric Technol 1(1): 14-18

Rofiq MN, Gorgulu M (2012) The Effects of Clove and Cinnamon Oils on Milk Yield and Milk Composition of Dairy Goats. Animal Science Department, Cukurova University, Balcali, Adana, 01330, Turkey

Santos MB, Robinson PH, Williams P, Losa R (2010) Effect of addition of an essential oil complex to the diet of lactating dairy cows on whole tract digestion of nutrients and productive performance. Anim Feed Sci Technol 157: 64-71

Shan B, Cai YZ, Sun M, Corke H (2005) Antioxidant capacity of 26 spice extracts and characterization of their phenolic constituents. J Agric Food Chem 53(20): 7749-7759

Shabestari AH, Salamatdoustnobar R, Maheri-Sis N, Gorbani A, Ahari KM, Noshadi A, Samadi H, Nezhad JS (2011) Evaluation effects of clove methanol extract on methane production in the *in vitro* condition. Pakistan J Nutr 10(12): 1154-1157

Si W, Gong J, C Chanas S, Cui hyu, C Caballero, Friendship RM (2006) In vitro assessment of antimicrobial activity of carvacrol, thymol and cinnamaldehyde towards Salmonellaserotype Typhimurium DT104: Effects of pig diets and emulsification in hydrocolloids. J Appl Microbiol 101: 1282–1291

Singh G, Kapoor IP, Pandey SK, Singh UK. Singh RK (2002). Studies on essential oils: part 10; antibacterial activity of volatile oils of some spices. Phytother Res 16: 680-682

Sritabutra D, Soonwera M, Waltanachanobon S, Poungjai S (2011) Evaluation of herbal essential oil as repellents against Aedes aegypti (L.) and Anopheles dirus Peyton & Harrion. Asian Pac J Trop Biomed 1(Suppl 1): S124-S128

Tager LR, Krause KM, (2011) Effects of essential oils on rumen fermentation, milk production and feeding behavior in lactating dairy cows. J Dairy Sci 94: 2455-2464

Tariq H, Rao Raman, Raghuvanshi PV, Mondal RS, BC, Singh SK (2015) Effect of Aloe vera and clove powder supplementation on carcass characteristics, composition and serum enzymes of Japanese quails. Vety World 8(5): 664-668

Tartrakoon W, Sukkasem K, Meulen U, Vearasilp T (2003) Use of Essential Oil Extracted from Citronella, Cloves and Peppermint as Supplement in Weaner Pig Diets. "Technological and Institutional Innovations for Sustainable Rural Development". Deutscher Tropentag, G¨ottingen

Tassoul MD, Shaver RD (2009) Effect of a mixture of supplemental dietary plant essential oils on performance of periparturient and early lactation of dairy cows. J Dairy Sci 92: 1734-1740

Tedesco D (2001) The potentiality of herbs and plant extracts as feed additives in livestock production. Zootec Nutr Anim. 27: 111–133

Tedeshchi LO, Fox DG, Tyluki TP (2003) Potential environmental benefits of ionophores in ruminant diet. J Environ Qual 32: 1591-1602

Tiihonen K, Kettunen H, Bento MHL, Saarinen M, La-htinen S, Ouwehand AC, Schulze H, Rautonen N (2010) The effect of essential oils on broiler performance and gut microbiota. British Poult Sci 51: 381–392

Valero M, Salmeron MC (2003) Antibacterial activity of 11 essential oils against Bacillus cereus in tyndallized carrot broth. Int J Food Microbial 85: 73-81

❑❑❑

Chapter 12

Neem (*Azadirachta indica*)

Pramod Prabhakar

Department of Animal Husbandry, Mandan Bharati Agriculture College, Bihar Agricultural University, Saharsa-852201, India, E-mail: ppmbac@gmail.com

ABSTRACT

Azadirachta indica, commonly known as neem, has attracted worldwide prominence in recent years. Neem has been extensively used in Ayrveda, Unani and Homeopathic medicine and has become a cynosure of modern medicine. Neem contains numbers of phytochemicals *viz.* azadirachtin, nimbin, nimbidin, nimbidol, gedunin, salannin, quercetin, etc. These phytochemicals possess antibacterial, antifungal, anti-malaria, anti-inflammatory, antioxidant, antihistamine, anti-arthritic antifungal properties. All the parts of the neem tree-leaves, flowers, seeds, fruits, roots and bark have been traditionally for the treatment of inflammation, infections, fever, skin diseases and dental disorder. Parts of neem have been used as animal feed as they contain amounts of nutrients, protein and minerals required for animal health. Neem plant acts as a medicinal plant have been found effective in the treatment of bacterial, fungal, viral and other diseases and revealed the antibacterial, antifungal, antiviral, antimalarial, antiulcer and other biological activities. The lean, high protein meat can be produced by neem supplementation in birds. Neem is safe to mammals with low toxicity on predators and parsitoids used for biocontrol of pest. Neem plants are now growing popularity in the treatment of many infections.

Keywords: Neem, Antibacterial, Animal Health, Animal Feed.

12.1 Introduction

The neem plant is fast growing and long living tree. For Indians, the neem tree had many fascinating aspects. Neem (*Azadirachta indica*) is a native to the arid regions of the Indian subcontinent. It requires 130 mm of sufficient rainfall per annum for its normal growth. The seeds bark and leaves contain compounds with proven antiseptic, antiviral, antipyretic, anti-inflammatory, anti-ulcer and antifungal uses. Arista is the Sanskrit name for neem and it means 'perfect', complete and imperishable. Neem is recognized as a natural product which has much to offer in solving global, agricultural, and environmental and health problems. Natural properties of neem do not have any toxic reactions and so, they are well used in plant management of pests and diseases. All parts of neem like seed, flowers, bark and leaf can be used for plant protection and management. Neem products reduce insects' growth in crops and plants. Neem derivatives are used as neem insecticide, neem pesticide, neem pest fumigant, neem fertilizer, neem manure, neem urea coating agent and neem soil conditioner. Neem derivatives help in controlling several nematodes and fungi.

Indigenous Drugs Useful in the Treatment of Animals' 'published in 1929, lists the Veterinary applications of Neem. It notes that "leaves, bark and oil expressed from the seeds are generally used. Internally the preparations of the Neem tree are a good bitter tonic, antiperiodic and astringent and are used in combination with other drugs having similar properties. They are best administered in the form of a decoction. They are most useful in fever and debility. Externally, the leaves are used in varied forms, such as raw crushed mass, poultice and wash. The bruised leaves, mixed with charcoal or lime, form a good application to wounds, ulcers, pustular eruptions, such as epizootic aphtha, etc. The decoction of the leaves forms a valuable antiseptic and healing lotion to foul sores and ulcers. The leaves boiled with tamarind leaves are applied as a poultice to inflammatory swellings. The oil is applied to wounds as an antiseptic dressing. It is highly efficacious in parasitic diseases, cutaneous affections of all kinds and erysipelas, etc., as it contains sulphur in organic combination. It is also useful in removing maggots from the wounds. The oil is obtained from most of the bazaars". In the past few years, researchers have been studying ancient prescriptions like Neem with tools of modern bio-chemistry. In a recent trial at a University in Banguluru, it has been observed that alcohol based Neem leaf extract showed promising results *in vitro* trials as compared to other herbs.

Neem leaves and its extracts are being used as immuno stimulants in poultry flocks. In the poultry industry, use of Neem leaves is also made to prevent aflatoxicosis caused by *Aspergillus flavus*, which originates from oil cakes or maize, which are not dried properly and used as an ingredient of the feed. Use of Neem cake as a protein substitute has an economical advantage in those countries where it is abundant.

12.2. Taxonomy

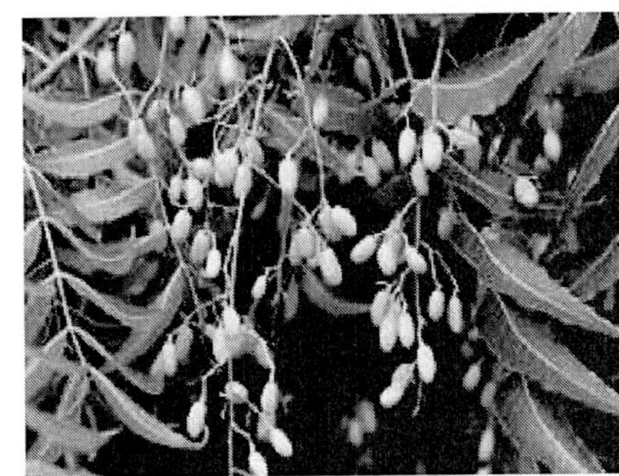

Order	:	Rutales
Suborder	:	Rutinal
Family	:	Maliaceae
Subfamily	:	Melioideae
Tribe	:	Melieae
Genus	:	*Azadirachta*
Species	:	*indica*

12.3. Chemistry

The chemical investigations of neem were undertaken by Indian pharmaceutical chemists in 1919, whereby they isolated acidic principle in neem oil, which they named as margosic acid. However, real chemical research originated in 1942 with isolation of three active constituents, viz, nimbin, nimbidin and nimbinene. Following the discovery of neem kernel as a locust feeding deterrent, its chemistry has grown considerably. Several compounds have been isolated and characterized. The main feature is that most of them are chemically similar and bio-genetically derivable from a tetracyclicterpenes. These are also called liminoids (azadirachtin, meliantrol, salanin, etc.) bitter principles and occur in other botanical species as well (Rutaceae and Simaroubaceae). The unraveling of high complex structural features and biogenetic inter-relationship represent classic piece of work on natural product chemistry. From the practical side these compounds also exhibit a wide variety of biological activity, for example, pesticides, antifeedants, and cytotoxic properties.

Leaves mainly yield quercetin (flavonoid) and nimbosterol (β-sitosterol) as well as number of liminoids (nimbin and its derivatives). Quercetin (a polyphenolic flavonoid) is known to have antibacterial and antifungal properties. This may perhaps account for the curative properties of leaves for sores and scabies. Limonoids like nimocinolide and isonimocinolide affect fecundity in house flies (*Musca domestica*) at a dose ranging between 100 and 500 ppm. They also show mutagenic properties in mosquitoes (*Aedes aegypti*) producing intermediates. Fresh matured leaves yield an odorous viscous essential oil, which exhibits antifungal activity against fungi (*Trichophyton mentagrophytes*) *in vitro*. White crystalline flakes obtained from petroleum ether extract of leaves consisting of a mixture of C 14, C 24, C 31 alkanes were found to exceed or equal the lavicidal activity of pyrethrum extract. The principal constituents of Neem leave include protein (7.1%), carbohydrates (22.9%), minerals, calcium, phosphorus, vitamin C, carotene, etc. But they also contain glutamic acid, tyrosine, aspartic acid, alanine, praline, glutamine and cystine like amino acids, and several fatty acids (dodecanoic, tetradecanoic, elcosanic, etc.). Besides, the essential oil consisting of sesquiterpene derivatives, the flowers contain nimbosterol and flavonoids like kaempferol, melicitrin, etc. Flowers also yield a waxy material consisting of several fatty acids, viz., behenic (0.7%), arachidic (0.7%), stearic (8.2%), palmitic (13.6%), oleic (6.5%) and linoleic (8.0%). The pollen of Neem contains several amino acids like glumatic acid, tyrosine, arginine, methionion, phenylalanine, histidine, arminocaprylic acid and isoleucine.

The trunk bark contains nimbin (0.04%), nimbinin (0.001%), nimbidin (0.4%), nimbosterol (0.03%), essential oil (0.02%), tannins (6.0%), a bitter principle margosine and 6-desacetyl nimbinene. The stem bark contains tannins (12-16%) and non-tannin (8-11%).The bark contains anti-inflammatory polysaccharide consisting of glucose, arabinose and fructose at a molar ratio 1:1:1 with molecular weight of 8,400. The bark also yields an antitumour polysaccharide. Besides polysaccharides, several diterpenoids, viz., nimbinone, nimbolicin, margocin, nimbidiol, nimbione, etc. have been isolated from stem bark and root bark.Besides β-sitosterol, 24-methylenelophenol and nimatone, the heartwood contains, calcium, potassium and iron salts (Ara *et al.*, 1989). The heartwood on destructive distillation gives charcoal (30%) and pyroligeneous acid (38.4%). Neem wood contains cellulose, hemicellulose (14.00%) and lignin (14.63%), while wood oil contains β-sitosterol, cycloeucalenol and 24-methyl encycloartenol.

The tree exudes a gum, which on hydrolysis yields, L-arabinose, L-fructose, D-galactose and D-glucoronic acid. The older tree exudes a sap containing free sugars (glucose, fructose, mannose and xylose), amino acids (alanine, aminobutyric acid, arginine, asparagines, aspartic acid, glycine, norvaline, praline, etc) and organic acids (citric, malonic, succinic and fumaric). The sap is reported to be useful in the treatment of general weakness and skin diseases. Seed is very important both because of its high lipid content as well as the occurrence of a large number of bitter principles (azadirachtin, azadiradione, fraxinellone, nimbin, salannin, salannol, vepinin, vilasinin, etc.) in considerable quantities. Azadirachtin has proven effectiveness as a pesticide against about 300 insect species and is reported as non-toxic to humans. Neem kernel lipids are similar to the normal glycerides from other oilseeds and contain oleic acid (50-60%), palmitic acid (13-15%), stearic acid (14-19%), linoleic acid (8-16%) and arachidic acid (1-3%). It is brownish yellow, non-drying oil with an acrid taste and unpleasant odour. The quality of the oil differs with the method of processing.

The composition of neem cake after the extraction of oil varies widely depending on the raw materials used for expelling, for example, whole dried fruits, seeds or kernels. The range of the proximate composition in percentage are: crude protein 13-35, carbohydrates 26-50, crude fibre 8-26, fat 2-13, ash 5-18, acid insoluble ash 1-7. The bitter cake has no value as animal or poultry feed. Extraction of cake with 70% alcohol followed by hexane yields a meal free from bitterness and odour, which will be satisfactory as feed. The neem cake is rich in most of the amino acids. It is a potential source of organic manure and contains many plant nutrients, viz., nitrogen 2-3%, phosphorus 1% and potassium 1.4%. It also contains 1.0-1.5% tannic acid and has the highest sulphur content of 1.07-1.36% among the oil cakes. The neem cake contains a large number of triterpenoids, more of which are being discovered.

12.4. Active Constitutent of Neem

There are many active compounds found in the neem tree which have diverse pharmaceutical properties (Sudhir *et al.*, 2010) as follows:

12.5. Biological Activities of Some Acctive Constitutent of Neem

Compounds Name	Source	Biological activity
Nimbidin	Seed oil	Anti-inflammatory Anti-arthritic, Diuretic, Hypoglycemic , Antifungal, Spermicidal, Antipyretic, Antibacterial, Anti-gastric ulcer
Azadirachtin	Seed oil	Anti-malarial
Nimbin	Seed oil	Spermicidal
Nimbolide	Seed oil	Anti-malarial, Antibacterial
Genuine	Seed oil	Anti-malarial, Antifungal
Mahmoodin	Seed oil	Antibacterial
Gallic acid and Catechin	Bark	Anti-inflammatory Immuno-modulatory
Margolone, mergolonone and Isomargolonone	Bark	Antibacterial
Cyclic trisulphide and cyclic tetrasulphide	Leaf	Antifungal
Polysaccharides G1A, G1B	Bark	Antitumour
Polysaccharides G2A, G3A	Bark	Anti-inflammatory
NB-2 Peptidoglucan	Bark	Immuno-modulatory
Quercetin	Bark	Anti-protozoal, antioxidant, anti-inflammatory, antibacterial

12.6. Biological Activities of Neem plant

12.6.1 *Antibacterial Activity*

Methanolic extract of Neem leaves was tested for its antibacterial, antisecretory and antihaemarrhagic activity against vibrio cholera (Thakurta *et al.*, 2007) .The hexane chloroform and methanol extracts of *Azadirachta indica* were screened for antibacterial activity against *Escherichia coli, Klebsiella pneumoniae, Proteus vulgaris, Micrococcus luteus, Bacillus subtilis.*

12.6.2 *Antifungal Activity*

The aqueous and ethanolic extracts of *Azadirachta indica* leaves have been shown to have antidermatophytic activity against dermatophytes (Ranganathan *et al.*, 1996) from the 88 clinical isolates with the help of agar dilution technique. The ethanolic extract showed more conspicuous activity as compared to aqueous extract. Antifungal characteristics was tested using methanolic and acetone extracts of

Azadirachta indica against two different fungal strains i.e. Aspergillus niger and Aspergillus fumigatus and it was reported that methanolic plant extract gives maximum antifungal activity as compared to acetonic extracts (Rao *et al.*, 1977). The seed and leaf extracts of *Azadirachta indica* (Neem were screened for antifungal activity against dermatophytes and the Minimum Inhibitory Concentration (MIC) of (*Azadirachta indica*) Neem seed extracts was found to be lower than that of Neem leaf, when screened against different species of Trichophyton and Epidermatophyton floccosum .Antifungal activity of aqueous ethanolic and ethyl acetone extracts of (*Azadirachta indica*) Neem leaves on growth of few human pathogens. *Aspergillus flavus, Candida albicans Aspergillus terreus, Aspergillus fumigates, Aspergillus niger, and Microsporum, gypseum* in vitro using different concentration and it was reported that these extracts prevented the growth of the test pathogenic organism and the effect gradually increased with increase in concentration. Gedunin isolated from Neem seed oil has been reported to have antifungal activity (Kher and Chaurasia, 1997). The compounds of Sulphur such as cyclic tetrasulphide and trisulphide isolated from the stem distillate.

12.6.3 *Antimalarial Activity*

Ball-shaped wood scrapings which is soaked in 5% Neem oil (*Azadirachta indica*) which is diluted in acetone and in 45 days the breeding of anopheles stephensi and aedes aegypti were controlled, when it is placed in water storage overhead tanks. Nimbolide isolated from Neem extracts shows the antimalarial activity by preventing the growth of plasmodium falciparum (Khalid *et al.*, 1989). Gedunin isolated from Neem seed oil has been reported to show antimalarial activities. Both aqueous and alcohol extracts of bark and leaves of Neem are effective antimalarial agents, particularly on chloroquine resistant strains.

12.6.4 *Antitumor and Antiviral Activity*

Scientist in India, Europe and Japan have now found that limonoids and polysaccharides found in neem seed oil, bark and leaves reduced tumours and cancers and revealed effectiveness against lymphocytic leukemia (Hassan *et al.*, 2010). Mitotic inhibition activity by the leaf extract was bserved. Several conclusions have also highlighted the pronounced antiviral effect of aqueous extract of neem leaves against Small Pox, Fowl Pox, Polio and HSV as assessed by virus prevention assay (98-100). Aqueous extracts of neem leaf and also the sum of fraction from neem oil (Nim-76) showed antiviral activity against HIV and Polio Viruses.

12.6.5 *Anti-inflammatory, Antipyretic and Analgesic Activities*

The chloroform extract of stem bark shows effectiveness against carrageen in induced paw oedema in rat and mouse ear Inflammation. Inflammatory stomatitis in children is treated by the bark extract (Bhargava *et al.*, 1970). Antipyretic activity has been reported in neem oil. A methanol extract of the leaves showed antipyretic effect, when it is administrated into male rabbits (David, 1969). Antipyretic and Anti-inflammatory activities in various extracts have been reviewed.

12.6.6 *Male Antifertility Activity*

The Neem seed oil (NSO) and leaf extracts used as powerful spermicide and significantly prevented spermatogenesis, decreased sperm mobility, count and cessation of fertility. No indicative or important effect on loss of libido or potency. Furthermore, NSO possess abortifacient and anti-implantation properties. The neem oil extract shows the spermicidal activity against human and rhesus monkey were found by Sinha *et al.* (1984). Vaginal biopsy reveals no side effect, while the studies of radio-isotope which indicate non-antiovulatory and non-absorption in the vagina. These research enabled Neem oil formulation "sensal" which is used as a powerful contraceptive in India.

12.6.7 *Antiulcer Activity*

The antiulcer effect was obtained with nimbidin in preventing acetylsalicyclic acid, indomethacin, serotonin-induced gastric lesions or streets as well as cysteamine induced duodenal ulcers or histamine (Dharmani and Palit, 2006). Leaf extract of *Azadirachta indica* (Neem) shows antiulcer effect were reported by Garg et al and the inhibition of mucus depletion and most cell defragmentation as possible mechanism.

12.6.8 *Medicinal Uses of Neem*

Neem plant shows the large number of medicinal uses. The non-wood products of Neem like flowers, leaves, bark, fruits, seeds (oil, cake), and gum also find various uses. The Neem plant shows various biological activities like antibacterial, antifungal, insecticidal and other activities (Tipu *et al.*, 2006).

12.7. Neem and its Applications

Neem leaves are used in storage of grains. It is also used as green leaf manure and in litter composite. The twigs/stem in the earlier stages are used as green manure after decomposing and widely incorporated in rice cultivation fields. Neem seed extracts are found to have insecticidal and fungicidal properties (Koul *et al.*, 1990). It is used in foliar spraying and treating seeds in rice cultivation. Neem bark and roots have medicinal properties. These are also used to control insects, fleas and sucking pests of rice crop. Neem seed cake, a residue of neem seeds after oil extraction is used for soil amendment and it enriches the soil with organic matter and reduced nitrogen losses by inhibiting the nitrification process. It also acts as a nematicide. Neem has anti-bacterial, anti-fungal and anti-nematicidal properties and positive effect in combating several diseases in rice cultivation and some more constituents of Neem which are further to be exploited.

12.7.1 *Neem as Manure*

Manure may be of animal or plant origin used to fertilise the land for improving the soil fertility and crop productivity. Neem manure is commanding popularity, as it is environmental friendly and also the compounds found in it help to increase the nitrogen and phosphorous content in the soil. It is rich in sulphur, potassium, calcium, nitrogen, etc. Neem cake is used to manufacture organic manure through high technology extraction methods like solvent extractions. It can be used directly by mixing with the soil or can be blended with urea and other organic manure like farmyard manure for best results.

12.7.2 *Neem as Urea Coating Agent*

Neem and its parts are being used to manufacture urea coating agent to improve and maintain the fertility of soil. The Neem urea helps to retard the activity and growth of the bacteria responsible for denitrification as a coating agent. It prevents the loss of urea in the soil. It can also be used to control a large number of pests such as beetles, caterpillars, leaf hoppers, borer, mites, etc. Urea coating is now available both in liquid form and powdered form (Musalia *et al.*, 2000). The properties of neem urea coating act as antifeedant, antifertility and pest growth regulator. These are excellent soil conditioners, natural or biopesticides, environmental friendly, non toxic, reduces urea consumption, convenient and easy to apply, high soil fertility and increases the yield of crops.

12.7.3 *Neem as a Fertilizer*

Neem is used as a fertilizer both for food crops and cash crops, particularly for rice, banana and sugarcane. The material left after oil is squeezed out from seeds and is known as seed cake. It acts as a bio fertiliser and helps in providing the required nutrients to plants. It is used widely to obtain a high yield of crops. Neem seed cake performs the dual function of both fertilizer and pesticide, acts as enriched of the soil reduces the growth of soil pests and bacteria, provides macro-nutrients essential for the plant growth, and increases the yield of plants in the long run. Government of India has recently allowed fertilizer firms to produce 100% Neem Coated Urea – a move aimed at helping farmers boost income & reducing subsidy bill by upto Rs. 6,500 crore. Government of India has done away with the cap on neem-coated urea & now it can be produced 100%. It is a win situation for all the players in the field- the industry, farmers & neem seed collection agencies. The countries like India having large number of neem trees are the major source of neem fruits and neem products. If commercial plantation and agro-forestry involving neem is popularized, the potential goes up significantly, with positive and large externalities for pesticides, fertilizers, livestock, dairying and other value-added products.

12.7.4 *Neem as Soil Conditioner*

Neem seed granules or powdered seeds are used to manufacture the soil conditioners. It can be applied during plant sowing, or sprinkled or raked into the soil. The process of sprinkling should be followed by proper irrigation, so that the product reaches the roots. It is a natural soil conditioner that helps to improve the quality of soil and enhances the growth of fruits. As a soil conditioner, it improves the soil quality .It helps the plants to grow and prevents them from being destroyed by certain pests and insects. Organic soil conditioner is gaining popularity in agricultural industry. Neem soil conditioner application in plantation crops is known to be a soil enhancer that helps to increase the fertility.

12.7.5. *Neem Leaves as Animal Feed*

Neem leaves contain appreciable amount of protein, minerals and carotene and adequate amount of trace minerals except zinc. These may be helpful in alleviating the copper deficiency, when feeding straw and dry fodder (Tipu *et al.*, 2006). Deoiled neem (Musali *et al.*, 2000) seed cake can considerably reduce the shortage of protein supplements in high producing animals. Seeds from neem yield sufficient oil and the residual cake is the major by-product. Neem cake consists of all essential and non-essential amino acids including sulphur containing amino acids but with negligible quantities of valine and tryptophan. The cake contains sulphur 1.07-1.36% which is more than other cakes (Christopher *et al.*, 1976). The nitrogen content varies from 2-3%. The cake has high crude protein, ether extract and fibre contents. Neem seed cake is a very good source of animal protein (upto 40%). The keeping quallity is good and it is not easily spoiled on storage nor is it attacked by fungi. The processed cake can be employed as a good poultry feed. Since the cake is bitter, it acts as a good appetizer. It is also a wormicide.

Goat and Camel relish lopped neem leaves and quite often these are fed as sole feed to them in winter season, when tree is not needed for shed. However, systematic studies are not available on neem feeding by these animals. Keeping in view these animals have the capability to thrive in hot and dry areas, there is considerable scope of rearing them on the neem leaves. The Neem leaves have appreciable quantity of digestible crude protein and total digestible nutrients. Cattle can be fed twigs and leaves in small quantities when mixed with other feeds.

Neem oil can be used in poultry rations. The fatty acid composition of oil indicates that it is a rich source of long chain fatty acids (Deepak *et al.*, 2002). It contains azadirachtin, meliantriol and salannin. Neem oil can be used in poultry rations. Fats and cholesterol have been associated with cardiovascular diseases in animals and birds. There is market pressure on the broiler industry to reduce the fat and cholesterol contents of its products due to greater consumer awareness about dietary fat/cholesterol and their perceived adverse effects on human health. The extent to which cholesterol intake influences total cholesterol levels is highly variable as part of it is synthesized in the body. Excessive level of LDL leads to the accumulation of cholesterol in tissues particularly the smooth muscle cells of the vascular system. It is, thus, involved in the arteriosclerotic process. In contrast, HDL functions in the removal of cholesterol from cells. This mechanism underlines its protective effects in Chronic Heart Diseases (CHD). The carcasses from broilers have excessive fat in abdominal/visceral regions and legs. Nutritional planes are known to influence fat, protein and ash deposition in broiler chickens.

12.7.6 *Neem in Animal Health*

For centuries Neem has been used in India provide health cover to livestock in various forms. It has also vary widely been used as animal feed. Ancient Sanskrit literature indicates that neem applications were used by Nakul and Sahadeva in the epic of Mahabharata as well as afterwards in a large number of indigenous prescriptions and formulations. The use of neem in veterinary medicine in India dates back to the times of the epic Mahabharata (300 B.C). According to scholars, two of the five Pandava brothers Nakul and Sahadeva, who practised veterinary medicine, used neem to treat ailing and wounded horses and elephants by applying poultices prepared from neem leaves and neem oil for healing the wounds, etc., during the battle of Mahabharata. Ancient Sanskrit literature indicates neem applications as feed and in a large number of prescriptions and formulations to provide health cover to livestock in various forms. Various neem preparations were standardized in the form of oils, liniments, powders and liquids. Ayurvedic scholars recommend the use of neem oil as antipyretic, sedative, anti-inflammatory, analgestic, anti-histaminic, antihelminthic and as an acaricide. Neem has been traditionally used against various livestock insects such as maggots, hornflies, blow-flies and biting flies (Dua *et al.*, 1995). Neem is also useful for controlling some bacteria of veterinary importance and against intestinal worms in animals. Patnaik, (1993) highlights the livestock friendly medicinal role of neem in the following: "the tree (Neem) is revered by Indian herdsmen as a gentle but effective veterinary poultice, a virtue confirmed by the 16th century Portuguese botanist and traveller, Garciada Orta in his "Coloquios".

Almost every part of the tree is bitter and finds application in indigenous medicine. Records exist that Neem has been used in a large number of ailments in animals ranging from systemic disorders to infections and injuries. In modern veterinary medicine, neem extracts are known to possess anti-diabetic, anti-bacterial and anti-viral properties and they have been used successfully in cases of stomach worms and ulcers. The stem and root bark and young fruits are reported to possess astringent, tonic and anti-periodic properties. The root bark is reported to be more active than the stem bark and young fruits. The bark is reported to be beneficial in cutaneous diseases.

12.8 Toxic Effect of Neem

The effects of Neem oil on mortality, survival and malformations of the non-target stink bug predator, *Podisus nigrispinus*. Neurotoxic and growth inhibitor insecticides were used to compare the lethal and sublethal effects from neem oil on this predator. Six concentrations of Neem oil were topically applied onto nymphs and adults of this predator. The mortality rates of third, fourth, and fifth instar nymphs increased with increasing neem oil concentrations, suggesting low toxicity to *P. nigrispinus* nymphs. Mortality of adults was low, but with sublethal effects of neem products on this predator. The developmental rate of *P. nigrispinus* decreased with increasing neem oil concentrations. Longevity of fourth instar nymphs varied from 3.74 to 3.05 d, fifth instar from 5.94 to 4.07 d and adult from 16.5 and 15.7 d with 0.5 and 50% neem doses. *Podisus nigrispinus* presented malformations and increase with Neem oil concentrations. The main malformations occur in wings, scutellum and legs of this predator. The neem oil at high and sublethal doses cause mortality inhibits growth and survival and results in anomalies on wings and legs of the non-target predator *P. nigrispinus* indicating that its use associated with biological control should be carefully evaluated.

12.8 Economic Potential of Neem

The Neem tree is now gaining the importance due to its wide scope of commercialization in the areas of agriculture, veterinary, cosmetics, medicine, toiletries and various industries. Neem is now becoming a popular in cosmetics and beauty aid. Some companies are now using neem products (Neem oil and leaves) for production of cosmetics like facial creams, nail polishes, nail oils, shampoos, conditioners, etc. The demand of neem products are increasing day by day. Agriculture sector is now becoming a major consumer of the neem products viz. neem oil, neem cake and neem based pesticides. Being eco-friendly and natural source of phytochemicals and nutrients it is preferred to apply neem manure and pesticide in agriculture especially in organic farming all over the world.

References

Ara I, Siddiqui BS, Faizi S, Sidddiqui S (1989) Structurally novel diterpenoid constituents from the stem bark of *Azadirachta indica* (melieceae). J Chem Soc Perkin Trans 343-345

Baswa M, Rath CC, Dash K (2001) Antibacterial activity of Karanj (Pongamiapinnata) and Neem (*Azadirachta indica*) seed oil; a preliminary report. Microbes 105: 183-189

Bhargava KP, Gupta MB, Gupta GP, Mitra CR (1970) Anti-inflammatory activity of saponins and other natural products. Indian J Med Res 58(6): 724-730

Bhide NK, Mehta DJ, Lewis RA (1958) Diuretic action of sodium nimbidinate. Indian J Medical Sci. 12: 141-145

Bhowmik D, Yadav CJ, Tripathi KK, Sampath KP (2010) Herbal remedies of *Azadirachta indica* and its Medicinal application. J Chem Pharm Res 2(1): 62-72

Biswas K, Chattopadhyay I, Banerjee KR, Bandyopadhyay U (2002) Biological Activities and medicinal properties of Neem (*Azadirachta Indica*). Current Sci 82: 1336-1345

Christopher, K.J., Ahmed, M.N. and Sastry, G.A. 1976. Effects of feeding deoiled *Neem* seed cake to chickens. Indian J Vet Path 1(1): 27-30

David SN (1969) Antipyretic activity of neem oil and its constituents. Mediscope 12: 25-27

Deepak G, Jogi S, Kumar A, Bais R, Vikas KS (2002) Effect of herbal liver stimulants on efficacy of feed utilization in commercial broiler chicken. Ind J Anim Res 36(1): 43-45

Dharmani P, Palit G (2006) Exploring Indian medicinal plant for anti-ulcer activity, Indian J Pharmacol. 38(2): 95-99

Dua VK, Nagpal BN, SharmaVR (1995) Repellant action of Neem cream against mosquitoes. Indian J Malaria 32: 47-53

Faiza A., Khalil, U. R., Mohammad, A and Muhammed, S. 2009. Antibacterial activity of various phyto-constituents of Neem. Pak J Agri Sci 46(3): 456-463

Fujiwara T, Takeda T, Ogihara Y, Shimizu M, Nomura T, Tomita Y (1982) Studies on the structure of polysaccharides from the bark of *Melia azadirachta*. Chem Pharm Bull 30: 4025-4030

Fujiwara T, Takeda T, Ogihara Y, Sugishita E, Shimizu M, Nomura T, Tomita Y (1984) Further studies on the structure of polysaccharides from bark of *Melia azadirachta*. Chem Pharm Bull 32: 1385-1391

Hassan A, Wafaa A, Helmy H, Taie A (2010) *In vitro* antitumor and antiviral activities of seeds and leaves from Neem (*Azadirachta indica*) extracts. International J Acad Res 2(2): 22-28

Jones I., Ley, S.V., Denholm, A.A., Lovell H., Wood A. and Sinden R. E. 1994. Sexual development of malaria parasites is inhibited *in vitro* by the neem extract azadirachtin and its semi-synthetic analogues. FEMS Microbiol Lett. 120(3): 267-273

Kakai T, Koho JP (1984) Anti-inflammatory Polysaccharides from *Melia azadirachta*. Chem Abstr 100: 913-50

Khalid SA, Duddeck H, Gonzalez-Sierra M (1989) Isolation and characterization of anti-malarial agent of the neem tree, *Azadirachta indica*. J Natural Product 52: 922-927

Kher A, Chaurasia SC (1997) Anti-fungal activity of essential oils of three medicinal plants. Ind Drug 15: 41-42

Koul O, Isman MB, Ketkar CM (1990) Properties and uses of Neem (*Azadirachta indica*). Can J Bot 68: 1-11

Mahmood DA, Hassanein NM, Youssef KA, Abou Zeid MA (2011) Antifungal activity of different Neem leaf extracts and the nimonal against some important human pathogens. Braz J Microbial 42(3): 113-117

Murthy SP, Sirsi M (1958) Pharmacological studies on Melia *Azadirachta indica*. Indian J Physiol Pharmacol 2: 387-396

Musalia LM, Anandan S, Sastry VRB, Agrawal DK (2000) Urea-treated neem *(Azadirachta indica)* Seed kernel cake as a protein supplement for lambs. Small Rum Res 35: 107-116

Pant N, Garg HS, Madhusudanan KP, Bhakuni D (1986) Fitoterapia, sulphurous compounds from *Azadirachta indica* leaves. Planta Medica 57: 302-304

Pillai NR, Santhakumari G (1981) Anti-arthritic and anti- inflammatory actions of nimbidin. Planta Medica 43: 59-63

Pillai NR, Suganthan D, Seshadri C, Santhakumari G (1978) Anti-gastric ulcer activity of nimbidin. Indian J Medical Res 68: 169-175

Pillai, N.R and Santhakumari, G. 1984. Effects of nimbidin on acute and chronic Gastro - duodenal ulcer models in experimental animals. *Planta Medica.* 50: 143-146.

Rachanakij S, ThebtarananthY, Yenjal CH, Yuthavong Y (1985) Nimbolide A constitute of *Azadirachta indica* inhibits Plasmodium falciparum in culture Southeast Asian J Med Public Health 16: 66-72

Ranajit R, Raut A, Sawant R, Jamge BB (2014) Anti-microbial activity of *Azadirachta indica* (Neem) against Pathogenic Microorganisms. J Acad Industrl Res 3(7): 327-329

Ranganathan S, Menon T, Balajee AM, Raja SM (1996) Anti-dermatophytic activities of *Azadirachta indica*: an in vitro and in vivo studies. Indian J Dermatolog 41(4): 113-117

Rao BS, Nazma, Rao MJ (1977) Anti-fungal activity of gedunin. Curr Sci 46: 714-716

Rojanapo W, Suwanno S, Somaree R, Glinsukon T, Thebtaranonth Y (1985) Screening of Antioxidants from some vegetables and herbs. J Sci Thailand 11: 177-188

Sharma P, Tomar L, Mukesh B, Bansal V (2011) Review on Neem *Azadirachta indica*): Thousand problems one solution. Inter Res J Pharm 12: 97-102

Sharma VN, Saksena KP (1959) Sodium nimbidinate *in vitro* study of its spermicidal action. *Indian J Medical Res* 1038-1042

Sharma VN, Saxena KP (1959) Spermicidal action of Sodium Nimbinate. Indian J Medical Res 47: 322-324

Srinivasan D, Nathan S, Suresh, P (2001) antibacterial activity of Neem (*Azadirachta indica*) and Tamarind (*Tamarindus indica*) leaves. Asian J Microbiol Biotech Environl Sci 3: 67-73

Sudhir KP, Mishra D, Ghosh G, Chandra, Panda S (2010). Biological action and medicinal properties of various constituent of *Azadirachta indica* (Meliaceae) an Overview. Annuals of Biological Res 1(3): 24-34

Thakurta P, Bhowmik P, Mukharjee S, Hajra TK, Patra A, Bag PK (2007) Antibacterial, antisecretary and antihaemorrhagic activity of *Azadirachta indica* used to treat cholera and diarrhoea in India. J Ethnopharmacol 111(3): 607-612

Tipu MA, Akhtar MS, Anjum MI, Raja ML (2006) New dimension of medicinal plants as animal feed. Pakistan Vet J 26(3): 144-148

Venugopal PV, Venugopal TV (1994) Anti-dermatophytic activity of Neem (*Azadirachta indica*) leaves *in vitro*. Indian J Pharmacol 26: 141-143

Vidyarthi VK, Nring K, Sharma VB (2008) Effect of herbal growth promoters on the performance and economics of rearing broiler chicken. Indian J Poult Sci 10: 297-300

Yogesh W, More RR, Raut AS, Taware A (2015) Review on biological activities of *Azadirachta indica* (neem) and its medicinal Uses. Intern J Infor Futuristic Res. 1327-1334.

□□□

Chapter 13

Thyme (*Thymus vulgaris*)

Kaushal Kumar[1] and Pankaj Kumar Singh[2]

[1] Department of Veterinary Pathology, Bihar Animal Sciences University, Patna- 800014, India, E-mail:drkaushal15@rediffmail.com

[2] Department of Animal Nutrition, Bihar Animal Sciences University, Patna- 800014, India, E-mail: vetpank@gmail.com

ABSTRACT

Thyme (*Thymus vulgaris*) is a medicinal plant which may be used as an effective alternative to antibiotics growth promoter for broiler as well as layer poultry flocks, because this herbal feed additive meets the needs of producers for increased broiler performance and the consumer's demands. Oil of thyme is the important commercial product obtained by distillation of the fresh leaves and flowering tops of thyme. Because of containing volatile oils such as thymol, carvacrole, and linaloel, as well as important digestive effect, *thymus vulgaris* has been known as a strong growth stimulant and as a good alternative for antibiotics in poultry industry across the world. In this chapter, effects of thyme on immune responses, serum biochemical parameters, haematology parameters, histomorphometry of small intestine, growth performance and carcass traits of poultry has been widely described.

Keywords: Poultry, Carvacrol, Phenols, Thymol, *Thymus vulgaris*.

13.1 Introduction

There is an increasing trend in the prevalence level of disease, by industrialization of poultry science and breeding chickens in a large scale. To cope with this problem and improve the biological and nutritional characters of chickens, chemical compounds like antibiotic have been used highly in poultry industry (Lee *et al.*, 2003). Unfortunately, over use of these products ended up with a lot of problems both for animals and consumers, for example, bacterial resistance to antimicrobial agents. Because of this problem, there have been made some restricted rules about the usage of these antibiotics, like ban and low use of antibiotics as feed additives (Kamel, 2001).

Organic poultry is a relatively new expression in western countries which is going to expand in other countries. In organic poultry farming, farmers do not use chemical compounds at all or in a very low level for the sake of consumers, instead they use alternatives like organic acids, probiotics, and medicinal plants, and despite of higher production cost of this method, these products have more fans in the costumers. There are a lot of reports indicating the positive effects of herbs like anti-coccidal, anti-oxidant, anti-fungi and anti-bacterial as well. Some of medicinal effects of herbs are related to their secondary metabolites such as phenols, necessary oils, saponins, etc. Herbs have been used for many diseases since long time ago because of availability, easy usage and no side effects. Many herbs have a long history of use even prehistoric, in preventing or treating human and animal diseases. Aromatic plants have been used traditionally in therapy of some diseases worldwide for a long time. Research on the use of herbal mixtures in broiler diets state significant positive effects on broiler performance (Peric *et al.*, 2008).

Due to the potentially undesirable effects of antibiotics as growth promoters in poultry production, researchers are looking for viable alternative to limit or replace their use. One such class of comparable alternative is natural source of herbs and medicinal plants. In the last decade, these alternatives have been increasingly used in broiler, layer and Japanese quail diets. Reports have variously claimed that medicinal plants, used as whole plant, their leaves or flowers, can enhance poultry performance. From the available literature, it can be concluded that thyme (*Thymus vulgaris*) belongs to such class of medicinal plant and may be an effective alternative to antibiotics growth promoter in poultry production. In this review, its effects on different parameters of growth performance in poultry are briefly discussed.

13.2 Description of Thyme

Garden thyme a member of *Lamiaceae* family and commonly known as Common Thyme, Du Thym, Echte Tijm, English Thyme, French Thyme, Garden Thyme, Kekik, Pile, Summer Thyme, Tati-Zyako-So, Thym Grandes Feuilles, Thyme, Tomillo, Winter Thyme, Zombi Nan Bois. It is a perennial type of herb which germinates easily in average soil type and grows well under full sun to partly shady areas. The content of essential oil varies drastically with climate, time of harvest and storage conditions. It can be used for culinary, antiseptic, anti bacterial, anti-spasmodic, tonic and carminative purposes (Mikaili *et al.*, 2010).

13.3 Taxonomic Hierarchy (USDA, NRCS. 2017)

Kingdom	:	Plantae
Sub-kingdom	:	Tracheobionta
Infrakingdom	:	Streptophyta
Superdivision	:	Spermatophyta
Division	:	Magnoliophyta
Class	:	Magnoliopsida
Sub-class	:	Asteridae
Order	:	Lamiales
Family	:	Lamiaceae
Genus	:	*Thymus*
Species	:	*Thymus vulgaris*

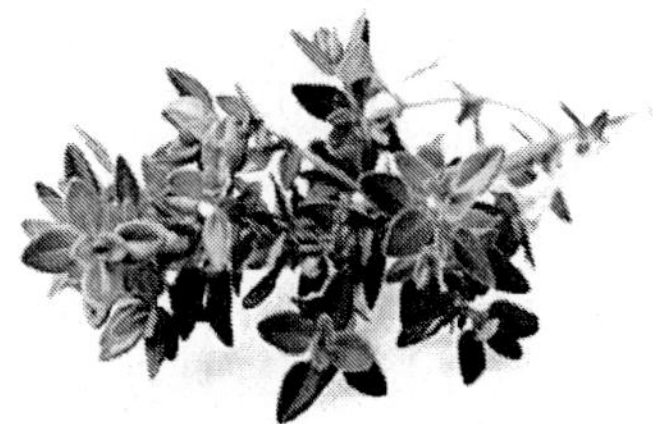
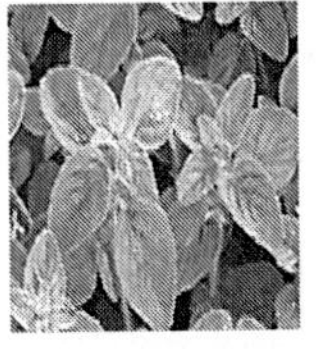
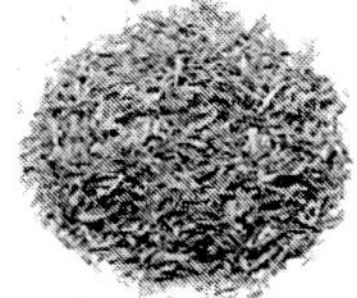

Figure : Garden thyme

The name Thyme, in its Greek form, was first given to the plant by the Greeks as a derivative of a word which meant 'to fumigate,' either because they used it as incense, for its balsamic odour, or because it was taken as a type of all sweet-smelling herbs. Others derive the name from the Greek word *thumus*, signifying courage, the plant being held in ancient and medieval days to be a great source of invigoration, its cordial qualities inspiring courage. The antiseptic properties of Thyme were fully recognized in classic times, there being a reference in Virgil's *Georgics* to its use as a fumigator, and Pliny tells us that, when burnt, it puts to flight all venomous creatures. This little plant, so familiar also in its wild form, has never been known in England by any familiar name, though occasionally 'Thyme' is qualified in some way, such as 'Running Thyme,' or 'Mother-of-Thyme'. 'Mother Thyme' was probably derived from the use of the plant in uterine disorders, in the same way that 'Motherwort' (*Leonurus Cardiaca*) has received its popular name for use in domestic medicine.

T. vulgaris is a perennial with a woody, fibrous root. The stems are numerous, round, hard, branched, and mostly from 5 to 10 inches high. The leaves are small, narrow and elliptical, greenish-grey in colour, reflexed at the margins, and set in pairs upon very small foot-stalks. The flowers terminate the branches in whorls. The calyx is tubular, striated, closed at the mouth with small hairs. The seeds are roundish and very small and they retain their germinating power for three years. The plant has an agreeable aromatic smell and a warm pungent taste. The fragrance of its leaves is due to an essential oil, which gives it its flavouring value for culinary purposes, and is also the source of its medicinal properties. There are three varieties usually grown for use, the broad-leaved, narrow-leaved and variegated: the narrow-leaved, with small, greyish-green leaves, is more aromatic than the broad-leaved, and is also known as Winter or German Thyme. The Garden Thyme is an 'improved' cultivated form of the Wild Thyme of the mountains of Spain and other European countries bordering on the Mediterranean, flourishing also in Asia Minor, Algeria and Tunis, and is a near relation to Wild Thyme (*Thymus serpyllum*), which has broader leaves (the margins not reflexed as in the Garden Thyme) and a weaker odour.

13.4 Cultivation of Thyme

Although Thyme grows easily, especially in calcareous light, dry, stony soils, it can be cultivated in heavy soils, but it becomes less aromatic. It dislikes excess of moisture. To form Thyme beds, choose uncultivated ground, with soil too poor to nourish cereals. If the soil does not suit it very well and is close and heavy, some material for lightening it, such as a little road-sand or sweepings, ensuring reasonable porosity, will be welcomed, and should be thoroughly incorporated - in a gritty soil it will root quickly, but it does not like a close, cold soil around its roots.

Sow in the middle of March or early April, in dry, mild weather, moderately thin, in shallow drills about 1/2 inch deep, and 8 or 9 inches apart, in good, light soil, in a warm position. Cover in evenly with the soil. Thyme thrives best with lots of room to spread in. It is well to make new beds annually. At the close of the summer, as soon as the herbs have been cut sufficiently, the beds should be attended to, all weeds cleared away and the soil well-forked on the surface. In winter, protect the plants from frost by banking up with earth. Thyme roots soon extract the goodness from the soil, hence whatever is sown or planted afterwards will seldom thrive unless the ground is first trenched deeper than the thyme was rooted, and is well-manured. According to Gattefosse, the Thyme is a faithful companion of the

Lavender. Generally speaking, the conditions most suitable to the growth of Thyme are identical with those favoured by Lavender. The plant is often overrun by Dodder (*Cuscuta epithymum*). If this happens, cut off the affected plants and burn them, or use a solution of sulphate of iron.

13.5 Nutritional Characterization of Garden Thyme

Thyme could be used as a whole, fresh and or dried. Flowering herb is used especially for production of oil of thyme. Leaves (Dry weight) of garden thyme per 100g contains energy : 276 Calories per 100g;Water : 7.8%; Protein: 9.1g; Fat: 7.4g; Carbohydrate: 63.9g; Fibre: 18.6g; Ash: 11.7g; Minerals-Calcium: 1890mg; Phosphorus: 201mg; Iron: 123.6mg; Magnesium: 220mg; Sodium: 55mg; Potassium: 814mg; Zinc: 6.2mg; Vitamins-A: 3800mg; Thiamine (B1): 0.51mg; Riboflavin (B2): 0.4mg; Niacin: 4.94mg; B6: 0mg; C: 0mg (Duke and Ayensu, 1985).

13.6 Chemical Constituents of Thyme

Oil of Thyme is the important commercial product obtained by distillation of the fresh leaves and flowering tops of *T. vulgaris*. Its chief constituents are from 20 to 25 per cent of the phenols Thymol and Carvacrol, rising in rare cases to 42 per cent. The phenols are the principal constituents of Thyme oil, being the most valuable for medicinal purposes, but carvacrol, an isomeric phenol, preponderate in some oils. The production of Thymol or Carvacrol seems to depend on some variation in the soil or climatic conditions which favours the formation of one or the other. Borneol and Linalol also have been detected in the high boiling fractions of the oil (Riebau *et al.*, 1997 and Boruga *et al.*, 2014).

The chemical composition of essential oils of the Albanian thyme (*Thymus vulgaris L.*) obtained by steam distillation of air-dried plant material and examined by GC and GC/MS detected over 86 compounds in the oils, from which more than 40 could be identified. The main components identified were: p-cymene: (7.76-43.75%), G-terpinene (4.20-27.62%), thymol (21.38-60.15%), carvacrol (1.15-3.04%) and Beta-caryophyllene (1.30-3.07%). Among the active compounds of the essential oil the major constituent is thymol, with lesser amounts of carvacrol, with 1,8-cineole, borneol, geraniol, linalool, bornyl and linalyl acetate, thymol methyl ether and a-pinene (Boruga *et al,* 2014). It also contains flavonoids; apigenin, luteolin, thymonin, naringenin and others and miscellaneous compounds like labiatic acid, caffeic acid and tannins, etc. Two commercial varieties of Thyme oil are recognized, the 'red,' the crude distillate, and the 'white' or colourless, which is the 'red' rectified by re-distilling. The yield of oil is very variable, from 2 per cent to 1 per cent in the fresh herb (100 lb. of the fresh flowering tops yielding from 1/2 to 1 lb. of essential oil) and 2.5 per cent in the dried herb. The phenols present in French and German oils consist mainly of Thymol, but under certain conditions the latter may be replaced by Carvacrol. The value of Thyme oil depends so much upon the phenols it contains.

13.7 Medicinal Properties and Uses

In herbal medicine, Thyme is generally used in combination with extracts of other herbs. Oil of Thyme is employed as a rubefacient and counter-irritant in rheumatism, etc. Thymol is a powerful antiseptic for both internal and external use; it is also employed as a deodorant and local anesthetic. It is extensively used to medicate gauze and wool for surgical dressings. Therefore, during recent years it has become one of the most extensively used antiseptics.

In respect of its physiological action, Thymol appears to stand between carbolic acid and oil of turpentine. Its action as a disinfectant is more permanent and at the same time more powerful than that of carbolic acid. It is less irritating to the skin, does not act as a caustic like carbolic acid, and is a less powerful poison to mammals. Veterinarians use it as a local irritant and anaesthetic to the skin and mucous membrane. It is used as an antiseptic lotion and mouth wash; as paint in ringworm, in eczema, psoriasis, broken chilblains, parasitic skin affections and burns; as an ointment, half strength, perfumed with lavender, to keep off gnats and mosquitoes. Thymol in oily solution is applied to the respiratory passages by means of a spray in nasal catarrh, and a spirituous solution may be inhaled for laryngitis, bronchial affections and whooping cough. It is most useful against septic sore throat, especially during scarlet-fever. Internally, it is given in large doses, to robust adults, in capsules, as a vermifuge, to expel parasites, especially the miner's worm, and it has also been used in diabetes and vesicular catarrh.

13.8 Role of Thyme in Poultry Production

13.8.1 Growth Performance

Sub-therapeutic dosages of antibiotics have been used extensively as growth promoters in livestock feeds for many years. They have been reported to increase growth rate and feed efficiency of poultry and other livestock as a result of improved gut health, nutrient utilization and improved feed conversion efficiency (Visek, 1978). However, there is the fear that the continuous and sub-therapeutic use of in-feed antibiotics could lead to the development of antibiotic resistant bacteria which are harmful to humans.

The pounded herb, if given to poultry broiler at the dose rate of 5g/kg body weight, the improvement in the body weight of broiler chicken could be attributed to thyme's positive effect on nutrient digestibility, as reported by Langhout (2000) and Toghyani *et al.* (2010). Other factors which could have contributed to the beneficial effects of the herbal products on the growth performance of birds are their probable antioxidant and antibacterial effects in the intestine (Nascimento *et al.,* 2000). Mechanism of action of herbal products is not very clearly defined yet, but there are suggestions that they alter the permeability of the cell membranes and cause a destruction of the pathogenic bacteria (Skandamis and Nychas, 2001). Helander *et al.* (1998) demonstrated that two isomeric phenols, i.e., carvacrol and thymol plays pivotal role in disintegrating the membrane of *E. coli* O157 and S. typhimurium, leading to the release of membrane-associated materials from the them to the external medium posing their antibacterial effects. A number of reports have provided evidence of the enhancement of feed conversion ratio (FCR) through the dietary addition of carvacrol (Lee *et al.,* 2003a) and a mixture of essential oils including oregano, cinnamon, thyme and capsicum (Zhang *et al.,* 2005). However, a higher dosage of thyme in the diet may have had an adverse effect on some beneficial microbial populations such as lactobacillus, preventing the herb from exhibiting its positive influence on performance and resulting in a poorer FCR. A significant improvement in body weight gain of broilers fed on diets containing thyme essential oil at 60 mg/kg had been recorded (Denli *et al.,* 2004) however, thyme oil at 400 mg/kg in the diet of broilers pose depressed feed intake (Ciftci *et al.,* 2009).

13.8.2 Carcass Traits

It has been found that the supplementation of the diet with thyme or thyme essential oil significantly decreased abdominal fat weight and abdominal fat percentage and hence a better carcass yield percentage (Toghyani *et al.*, 2010). Al-Kassie (2009) and Mansoob *et al.* (2011) found positive effect of thyme on the broilers live weight gain and the improvement of the poultry health, in addition to other performance traits, feed conversion ratio and feed intake.

The presence of harmful bacterial populations in the gastrointestinal tract may cause breakdown of amino acids and thereby reduce their absorption. Anti-microbial substances present in thyme reduce the harmful bacterial populations in the gastrointestinal tract and improve the levels of absorbed amino acids. Growth of organ like breast and thigh is more with increased amounts of absorbed amino acids (Khan, 2002). The carvacrol in thyme has stimulatory effects on pancreatic secretions by increasing the secretions of digestive enzymes thereby improve carcass traits. Increasing the percents of gizzard and liver by use of thyme can have positive effects via physically grinding and increasing bile secretion on nutrient digestion. The presence of antioxidants and phenolic substance in thyme may be the main cause of improvement in breast per cent of broilers carcass. Thus, broilers receiving thyme as feed additive may control and limit the growth and colonization of a variety of pathogenic and non-pathogenic species of bacteria in chicks gut. A more balanced biota population in gut could lead to a greater efficiency in digestibility and utilization of food, resulting in an enhanced growth and improved FCR.

13.8.3 Immune Responses

Thyme has been reported to have antibacterial and antifungal activities (Vincent, 2002; Basilico and Basilico, 1999). An increase in immune responses of chicks has been anticipated due to potent antioxidant properties of thymol and carvacrol containing thyme essential oil (Ragaa *et al.*, 2016). Although the dietary treatments did not induce any significant effect on immune related parameters yet no deleterious impact was detected as a result of thyme addition to the diet.

13.8.4 Serum Biochemical Parameters

Serum biochemistry is a labile biochemical system which can reflect the condition of the organism and the changes happening to it under influence of internal and external factors. Toghyani *et al.* (2010) found that triglyceride concentration tended to decrease in a dose dependent manner by addition of thyme, although the changes did not reaches statistical significance. Similarly, Radwan *et al.* (2008) reported that the addition of 1% thyme to broiler diet resulted in a marked decrease in plasma total lipids.

On contrary to these reports, Ali *et al.* (2007) found that adding thyme to hen's rations significantly decreased plasma HDL, total cholesterol, triglycerides and total lipids. The reduction of triglycerides and cholesterol noticed with thyme in animal studies was attributed to the lowering effect of thymol or carvacrol on HMG-Co A reductase the rate-limiting enzyme of cholesterol synthesis (Case *et al.*, 1995; Lee *et al.*, 2003b). But Lee *et al.* (2003b) indicated that dietary carvacrol, and not thymol, reduces plasma triglycerides and phospholipids and suggested that carvacrol may have more impact on lipogenesis than on cholesterol biosynthesis. However, Bolukbas *et al.* (2006) reported that dietary thyme oil increases plasma level of triglycerides, LDL-cholesterol and HDL-cholesterol in broilers. Thus, further study is needed to clarify the mechanism of hypolipidemic actions.

13.8.5 Haematology Parameters

Blood parameters are good indicators of physiological, pathological and nutritional status and changes in haematological parameters have the potential of being used to elucidate the impact of nutritional factors and additives supplied in diet on an individual. For example leucocytes are known to increase sharply, when infection occurs, as they are one of the first lines of defense of the body (Ganong, 1999).

Reports on the effect of thyme supplementation on blood haematological parameters are very scarce. Studies have indicated no detrimental impact of thyme on erytherocyte and leukocyte counts, haemoglobin content and hematocrit percentage (Toghyani *et. al.*, 2010). However, Al-Kassie (2009) showed that feeding diet supplemented with thyme extract and cinnamon to broilers, significantly increased haematocrit, hemoglobin values, erytherocyte and leukocyte count compared with the control group. It could be suggested that supplementing broilers diet with thyme could indicate favourable influences of antibiotic growth promoter effect on performance of broilers without any detrimental impact on blood parameters.

13.8.9 Histomorphometry of Small Intestine of Poultry

Demir *et al.* (2005) also found that the depth of crypts in ileum was significantly reduced by inclusion of garlic and thyme in diets in comparison to diets supplemented with antibiotic growth promoter. The crypt can be regarded as the villi factory and a large crypt indicates fast tissue turnover and a high demand for new tissue (Ragaa *et al.*, 2016). Any additional tissue turnover increases the nutrient requirement for maintaince. It has been postulated that a reduction in crypt depth in the ileum of broilers given dietary natural growth promoters such as garlic and thyme might leave the energy conserved by the reduced turnover rate of the epithelial cells for the lean tissue mass synthesis, which imply improvements in body weight gain and feed efficiency.

13.9 Conclusions

The use of antibiotics as growth promoters in poultry feed has led to some unwanted advances in antibiotic resistance. Therefore, it has been envisaged to find alternatives for antibiotics. Because of containing volatile oils such as thymol, carvacrole, and linaloel, as well as important digestive effect, thymus vulgaris has been known as a strong growth stimulant and as a good alternative for chemical materials in poultry industry across the world. Thyme may be used as alternatives to an antibiotic growth promoter for broiler as well as layer poultry floks, because these herbal feed additives meet the needs of producers for increased broiler performance and the consumer's demands that broiler production should be conducted under environmentally friendly conditions. In conclusion, future research efforts should continue to evaluate the effectiveness of the dietary herbal growth promoters and their specific effects on performance, blood parameters, the histologic parameters and the concentrations of micro-organisms in the intestine of broiler chickens that are kept under litter conditions.

References

Ali MN, Hassan MS, Abdel-Ghany FA (2007) Effect of strain, type of natural antioxidant and sulphate on productive, physiological and hatching performance of native laying hens. Int J Poult Sci 6: 539-554

Al-Kassie GAM (2009) Influence of two plant extracts derived from thyme and cinnamon on broiler performance. Pak Vet J 29(4): 169-173

Basilico MZ, Basilico JC (1999) Inhibitory effects of some spice essential oils on Aspergillus ochraceus NRRL 3174 growth and ochratoxin-A production. Lett Appl Microbiol. 29: 238-241

Bolukbas SC, Erhan MK, Özkan A (2006) Effect of dietary thyme oil and vitamin E on growth, lipid oxidation, meat fatty acid composition and serum lipoproteins of broilers. South Africa J Anim Sci 36(3): 189-196

Boruga O, Jianu C, Misca C, Golet, I, Gruia, AT, Horhat, FG (2014) Thymus vulgaris essential oil: chemical composition and antimicrobial activity. Journal of Medicine and Life 7(3): 57-60

Case GL, He L, Mo H, Elson CE (1995) Induction of geranyl Pyrophosphate pyrophosphatase activity by cholesterol suppressive isoprenoids. Lipids. 30: 357-359

Ciftci M, Guler T, Gulcihani Simsek U, Nihat Ertas O, Dalkilic B, Bicer Z (2009) The effect of *thymus vulgaris l.* oil as growth promoter in broilers. Indian Vet J 86(9): 930-932

Demir E, Sarica S, Özcan MA, Suiçmez M (2005) The use of natural feed additives as alternative to an antibiotic growth promoter in broiler diets. Arch fur Geflugelkunde. 69(3): 110-116

Denli M., Okan F, Uluocak A.N. 2004. Effect of dietary supplementation of herb essential oils on the growth performance, carcass and intestinal characteristics of quail. South Africa. J. Anim. Sci. 34(3): 174-179

Duke JA, Ayensu, ES (1985) *Medicinal Plants of China*. 2 Vols. 705 S, 1300 Strichzeichnungen Publ, Inc. Algonac. Michigan

Ganong WF (1999) Review of Medical Physiology. 19th ed. Stanford, Connecticut, Appleton and Lange: 353

Helander IM, Alakomi HL, Latva-Kala K, Mattila-Sandholm T, Pol I, Smid EJ, Gorris LGM, Von-Wright A (1998) Characterization of the action of selected essential oil components on Gram-negative bacteria. J Agric Food Chem. 46: 3590-3595

Kamel CT (2001) Modes of action and roles of plant extracts in non-ruminants. Recent advances in animal nutrition: P. C. Garnssworthy and J. Wiseman, Nottingham Univ. press, Nottingham, UK. Nutraceuticals: 19-21

Khan RU, Naz S, Nikousefat Z, Tufarelli V, Laudadio V (2012) Study: Thyme as antibiotic alternative in poultry feed.World's Poultry Science Journal. 68(03): 401-408

Langhout P (2000) New additives for broiler chickens. World Poult Elsevier, 16(3): 22-27

Lee KW, Everts H, Kappert HJ, Frehner M, Losa R, Beynen AC (2003a) Effects of dietary essential oil components on growth performance, digestive enzymes and lipid metabolism in female broiler chickens. Br Poult Sci. 44: 450-457

Lee KW, Everts H, Kappert HJ, Frehner M, Losa R, Beynen AC (2003b) Dietary Carvacrol lowers body weight gain but improves feed conversion in female broiler chickens. J Appl Poult Res. 12:394-399

Lee KW, Everts H, Beyen AC (2003) Dietary carvacrol lowers body gain but improves feed conversion in female broiler chickens. Journal of Applied Poultry Research. 12(4): 394-399

Mansoub, NH, Myandoab, MP (2011) The effects of different levels of Thyme on performance, carcass traits, blood parameters of broilers. Annals of Biological Research. 2(4):379-385

Mikaili P, Mohammad Nezhady MA, Shayegh J, Asghari MH (2010) Study of antinociceptive effect of *thymus vulgaris* and *Foeniculum vulgare* essential oil in mouse. *International* Journal of Academic Research, 2: 374-376

Nascimento GGF, Locatelli J, Freitas PC, Silva GL (2000) Antibacterial activity of plant extracts and phytochemicals on antibiotic-resistant bacteria. Brazil J Microbial. 31(4): 247-256

Peric L, Milosvic N, dukic-Stojcic M, Bledov S (2008) Effect of phytogenic products on performance of broiler chicken. World Nutrition Forum, Mayrhofen, Austria: Nottingham University Press, 18-20: 325

Ragaa NM, R M.SKorany, FF Mohamed (2016) Effect of Thyme and/or Formic Acid Dietary Supplementation on Broiler Performance and Immunity. Agriculture and Agricultural Science Procedia 10: 270-279

Radwan NL, Hassan RA, Qota EM, Fayek HM (2008) Effect of natural antioxidant on oxidative stability of eggs and productive and reproductive performance of laying hens. Int J Poult Sc. 7: 134-150.

Riebau, FJM, Berger MB, Yegen O, Cakr C (1997) Seasonal variations in the chemical compositions of essential oils of selected aromatic plants growing wild in Turkey. J Agri Food Chem. 45: 4821-4825

Skandamis PN, Nychas GJE (2001) Effect of oregano essential oil on microbiological and physico-chemical attributes of minced meat stored in air and modified atmospheres. J Appl Microbiol 91: 1011-1022

Toghyani M, Tohidi M, Gheisari AA, Tabeidian SA (2010) Performance, immunity, serum bio-chemical and haematological parameters in broiler chicks fed dietary thyme as alternative for an antibiotic growth promoter. African Journal of Bio-technology 9(40): 6819-6825

USDA, NRCS (2017) The Plants Database http://plants.usda.gov, National Plant Data Team, Greensboro, NC 27401-4901 USA

Vincent HV (2002) Carvacrol and thymol reduce swine waste odour and pathogens stability of oils. Current Microbiol. 44: 38-43

Visek WJ (1978) The mode of growth promotion by antibiotics. J. Anim.Sci. 46: 1447-1469.

Zhang KY, Yan F, Keen CA, Waldroup PW (2005) Evaluation of microencapsulated essential oils and organic acids in diets for broiler chickens. Int J Poult Sci 4(9): 612-619.

□□□

Chapter 14

Essential Oils in Poultry Feeding

Deben Sapcota

Debarment of Poultry Science, Assam Agricultural University, Khanapara Campus, Guwahati-781022, Assam, India, E-mail: debensapcota@yahoo.com

ABSTRACT

Antimicrobial feed additives have been used for decades in poultry production as growth promoter to improve zootechnical parameters and decrease morbidity. However, long use of such products tantamount to the development of antibiotic-resistant bacteria in the bio- system and residual effects in their products. Such a situation has resulted in the development of non-antibiotic feed additives that may improve poultry performance as alternative to antibiotic growth promoters. In recent years, aromatic plants/herbs and their extracts have received increasing attention as growth and health promoters. It has been established that most of their properties are due to the essential oils and other secondary plant metabolites. Essential oils improve production of digestive secretions, stimulate blood circulation, exert antioxidant properties, decrease levels of pathogenic bacteria and act as immuno-stimulant. Looking into the banning of antibiotic growth promoters in poultry husbandry, the prospects of essential oils as non-antibiotic growth promoters appears to be bright.

Keywords: Essential oils, Antimicrobials, Immunity, Production, Poultry.

14.1 Introduction

In-feed antibiotics have been used in sub therapeutic dosages for growth promotion and prophylaxis against enteric pathogens in large-scale livestock and poultry production for the last almost 60 years. Since the 1990s, it has become obvious that their continuing use as performance enhancers in animals contributed to a growing resistance among human pathogens and commensal micro-organisms (EC 2007).

Of late, animal production in many countries has faced restrictions in the use of antibiotic growth promoters. This additive has been banned in the European Union since 2006 and the USA is banning it from 2017. Based on the strong European regulations and the increasing movements in the USA, a worldwide ban of antibiotic growth promoters seems likely on the horizon (Bastiaanse, 2005). The second reason behind the regulations concerning feed additives, especially the ban of antibiotics and hormones, is a response to consumer pressures to eliminate all xenobiotic agents from food-producing animals and their respective food chains.

Such a situation necessitates a search for safe and natural alternatives. In recent years, aromatic plants and their extracts have been receiving growing attention as performance and health promoters. It is known that most of their properties are due to the essential oils (EOs) and other secondary plant metabolites, consisting of low-boiling-phenylpropenes and terpenes. They are particularly associated with characteristic plant essences and fragrances. The EOs -also called volatile or ethereal oils- are aromatic oily liquids obtained from plant material (flowers, buds, seeds,leaves, twigs, bark, herbs, wood, fruits, and roots). The term 'essential' was proposed by Paracelsus in his theory of '*quintaessentia*', and described that this quintessence could be an effective element for medical use (Oyen and Dung, 1999).

They are typically extracted by distillation methods, in particular steam distillation (Greathead, 2003). An estimated 3000 EOs are known, of which about 300 are commercially important and are used mainly in the flavours and fragrances market (Van de Braak and Leijten, 1999). Apart from their traditional use, a host of beneficial effects have been reported by experimental studies during the past three decades. Among these are their beneficial influence on lipid metabolism, ability to stimulate digestion, antioxidant propertiesand anti-inflammatory potential (Acamovic and Brooker, 2005).Yet some researchers have found that many herbs and botanicals are able to improve growth rate through increased feed intake (Wenk, 2006).

EOs enhance production of digestive secretions, stimulate blood circulation, exert antioxidant properties, reduce levels of pathogenic bacteria, impact positively on gut microbiota and welfare, and may enhance immune status. Some of their biological activities include antibacterial, antiviral, anti-fungal, antiparasitic, anti-oxidant, anti-toxigenic, insecticidal and anti-inflammatory effects amongst others. The EOs also have the odour and ammonia control properties (Varel, 2002).

14.2 Composition and Activities of Essential Oils

The composition of EOs, from the chemical point of view, are quite complex, constituted by several dozens of components, and this complexity makes it often difficult to explain their activities (Senatore 1996; Russo *et al.*, 1998). They are variable mixtures of mainly terpenoids (linalool, geraniol, thujanol, borneol, menthol, citronnillol, á-terpineol), and a variety of low molecular weight aliphatic hydrocarbons (e.g. phenols as thymol, carvacrol, eugenol, gaiacol, and aromatic aldehydes as cinnamaldehyde, cuminal and phellandral) (Dorman and Deans, 2000). Baring minor components present in trace amounts the overwhelming components (upto 85%) are comprised of two or three components at fairly high concentrations (Senatore, 1996; Bauer *et al.*, 2001). Generally, the main constituents reflect the biophysical and biological features of the EOs from which they were isolated.The phenolic components are primarily responsible for the antibacterial properties of EOs (Cosentino *et al.*, 1999). The EOs possess characteristic odour, and are soluble in organic solvents. Most of the oils are lighter than water with a specific gravity between 0.8-1.17. These oils are sensitive to heat and light, therefore should be stored in dark bottles and cool places (Krishnan and Narang, 2014).

The major components of a number of EOs, according to Chao *et al.* (2000), are presented in Table 1. These components shown to have antibacterial activity.There is some evidence that the activity of the main components is modulated by other minor molecules. Some studies have concluded that whole EOs have a greater antibacterial activity than the major components mixed (Gill *et al.*, 2002; Mourey and Canillac, 2002), which suggests that the minor components are critical to the activity and may have a synergistic effect or potentiating influence. This has been found to be the case for sage (Marino *et al.*, 2001), certain species of Thymus (Lattaoui and Tantaoui-Elaraki, 1994; Paster *et al.*, 1995; Marino *et al.*, 1999) and oregano (Paster *et al.*, 1995).

14.3 Factors Affecting Chemical Composition of EOs

There are many factors affecting chemical composition of the plant containing EOs. Some of them are: soil type, climate, use of chemical (fertilizers), genetics, harvesting time, season and methods, species, subspecies and age of the plant, part used, chemotype, geographical location and method of extraction. In many cases, the antimicrobial activity results through a complex interaction between different classes of compounds such as aldehydes, ketones, phenols, esters, alcohols, hydrocarbons or ethers found in the EOs. It was reported that EOs having phenols or aldehydes, for example, cinnamaldehyde, carvacrol, citral, thymol or eugenol as major components could show considerable antibacterial activity (Dormans and Deans, 2000). The efficacy of EO mixture also depends upon the compatibility with the other ingredient(s) of the mixture in the feed (Wang *et al.*, 1998).

14.4 Effects of using EOs in Poultry Ration

Various reports on the use of EOs in poultry ration indicate variable results. A summary of recent publications on the effect of EOs on productive performance parameters have been reported by Windisch *et al.* (2008). The majority of experimental results indicate reduced feed intake at largely unchanged body weight gain or final body weight, leading to an improved feed conversion ratio, when feeding EOs. No influence on performance parameters has been

Table 1: Some essential oils and their major components (Chao *et al.*, 2000)

Essential oils	Main components	Total (%)	Essential oil	Main components	Total (%)
Angelica root	[illegible]	24.7	Mandarine	Limonene	79.5
	β-3-carene	10.5		γ -Terpinene	9.7
	α-Phellandrene +myrcene	10.8	-	-	-
	Limonene	12.9	-	-	-
	β -Phellandrene	10.4	-	-	-
	ρ-Cymene	7.7	-	-	-
Bergamot	β -Pinene	7.7	Nutmeg	α-pinene	26.0
	Limonene + phellandrene	39.4		[illegible]	15.0
	γ-Terpinene	8.6		Sabinene	27.1
	Linalool	11.1		Myristicin	5.9
	Lynalil acetate	28.0	-	-	-
Cinnamon bark	(E)-Cinnamaldehide	77.1	Orange	Limonene	91.5
	Eugenol	7.2	-	-	-
Coriander	ρ -Cymene	6.1	Pepper	α-Pinene	9.0
	Linalool	72.0		β –Pinene	10.4
-	-	-		Sabinene	19.4
-	-	-		δ-3-Carene	5.4
-	-	-		Limonene	17.5

-	-	-		β-Caryophyllene	14.7
Dill (Indian)	Limonene	50.9	Pine (Scotch)	α -Pinene	9.0
	Trans-Dihydrocarvone	10.4		β -Pinene	10.4
	Carvone	20.3		δ-3-3-carene	21.6
	Dillapiole	36.3		Myrcene + α-terpin	5.8
Eucalyptus	Citronellal	72.8	Rosemary	α -Pinene	7.4
	Citronellol	14.5		β -Pinene	10.4
-	-	-		1,8-Cineole	21.6
-	-	-		Camphor	5.8
Geranium	Isomenthone	6.4	Rosewood	Linalool	80.0
	Citronellol	42.0	-	-	-
	Geraniol	5.5	-	-	-
	Cytronellylfor-mate	14.2	-	-	-
Ginger	Camphene	14.1	Sage	Cineole	8.4
	Neral	4.9		α -Thujone	31.8
	Geranial + bornyl acetate	8.1		β -Thujone	33.2
	Bisabolene	22.1	-	-	-
	Ar-Curcumene	14.5	-	-	-
	β -Eudesmol	5.4	-	-	-
Juniper berry	α – Pinene	33.7	Savory	ρ -Terpinene	7.4
	Sabinene	27.6		Cymene	25.9
	Myrcene	5.5		Carvacrol	37.7
Lime	Geranial	6.0	Tarragon	(Z)- β -Ocimene	7.3
	Limonene	55.5		(E)-β -Ocimene	6.9
	β -Pinene	11.0		Methyl chavicol	77.6
	Terpinene	14.5	-	-	-

reported by different authors (Botsoglou *et al.*, 2002a; Lee *et al.*, 2003; Hernández *et al.*, 2004; Shanmugavelu *et al.*, 2004; Jang *et al.*, 2007) using oregano essential oil, thymol, cinnamaldehyde, pepper, garlic powder and a commercial blend of EO containing thymol.

The positive effect of plant extracts (capsaicin and polyphenols) on broiler performance has been published by Kamel (2000, 2001). Similarly, the inclusion of a plant extract containing capsaicin, cinnamaldehyde, and carvacrol (Jamroz *et al.*, 2003), garlic powder (Lewis *et al.*, 2003; Cross *et al.*, 2004, Borgohain *et al.*, 2016), garlic and thymol powder (Demir *et al.*, 2003), and a combination of EOs (Alcicek *et al.*, 2003, 2004) as well as numerous field studies (Bassett, 2000; Langhout, 2000; Kamel, 2001) observed improvements in the performance of broilers and carcass yield and a reduction in the intestinal weight. Demir *et al.* (2003) attributed this improvement to the significant reduction in the depth of the crypts in the ileum with the inclusion of thyme andgarlic.

In early maturing turkeys, Bampidis *et al.* (2005) also showed that dietary oregano leaves improved feed conversion ratio. Sarma *et al.* (2003) observed health promoting effect by feeding a mixture of herbs on zootechnical broiler chickens. In certain series of trials Sapcota *et al.* (2005a, 2005b, 2006a and 2006b) used *Andrographis paniculata, Ocimum sanctum, Emblica officinalis* or *Piper nigrum,* respectively in counteracting experimental aflatoxicosis in broiler chickens and obtained encouraging results. Whereas, Islam *et al.* (2006), Ahmed *et al.* (2007) and Gogoi *et al.* (2010) recorded counteractive properties of *Emblicaofficinalis, Allium sativum* and *Curcuma longa,* respectively against aflatoxin B1 in broiler chickens.

14.5 Antimicrobial Activities and Modulation of Gut Microbiota by using EOs

EOs are marginally more effective against Gram-positive as compared to Gram-negative food pathogens (Burt, 2004) because they have an outer membrane surrounding the cell wall which limits the intrusion of hydrophobic compounds through its lipopolysaccha-ride structures (Vaara, 1992). Many EOs stimulate growth of beneficial microbes and limit number of pathogenic bacteria in poultry (Wenk, 2006). Cerisuelo *et al.* (2014) showed a clear effectiveness of low doses of EOs and sodium butyrate in *Salmonella* control in broilers. Table 2 shows the *in vitro* studies of EOs for its antimicrobial activity and minimum inhibitory concentration (MIC).

Table 2: Antibacterial activity and minimum inhibitory concentration (MIC, ppm) of essential oils

Micro-organisms	MIC values (ppm)			References
	Carvacrol	Thymol	Cinnamadehyde	
Escherichia coli	450	450	396	Helander *et al.* (1998)
Escherichia coli	225	225	NT	Cosentino *et al.* (1999)
Staphylococcus aureus	450	225	NT	Cosentino *et al.* (1999)
Candida albicans	150	150	NT	Ali-shtayeh *et al.* (1997)
Candida albicans	113	113	NT	Cosentino *et al.* (1999)
Candida albicans	200	NT	200	Ferhout *et al.* (1999)
Pseudomonas aeruginosa	500	500	NT	Ali-shtayeh *et al.* (1997)
Pseudomonas aeruginosa	>900	>900	NT	Cosentino *et al.* (1999)
Salmonella typhimurium	150	150	396	Helander *et al.* (1998)
Salmonella typhimurium	225	56	NT	Cosentino *et al.* (1999)
Streptococcus mutans	125	250	250	Didry *et al.* (1994)
Streptococcus mitis	125	125	125	Didry *et al.* (1994)

NT = Not tested. (Krishnan and Narang, 2014)

An important characteristic of EOs and their components is their hydrophobicity, which enables them to partition lipids in the bacterial cell wall and mitochondria, disturbing the structures and rendering them more permeable. Generally, the EOs possessing the strongest antibacterial properties against food borne pathogens containing a high percentage of phenolic compounds such as carvacrol, eugenol (2-methoxy-4-(2-propenyl)phenol) and thymol (Farag *et al.*, 1989a, 1989b; Thoroski *et al.*, 1989; Cosentino *et al.*, 1999; Dorman and Deans, 2000; Juliano *et al.*, 2000; Lambert *et al.*, 2001).

References

Acamovic T, Brooker JD (2005) Bio-chemistry of plant metabolites and their effects in animals. Proc Nutr Soc 64: 403–412

Ahmed SU, Sapcota D, Phukan B (2007) Effect of feeding garlic (*Allium sativum*) on carcass characteristics and nutrient utilization in broilers in induced aflatoxicosis. Indian J Anim Nutr 24: 99-103

Alcicek A, Bozkurt M, Cabuk M (2003) The effect of herbal essential oils, an organic acid or a probiotic on broiler performance. S Afr J Anim Sci 34: 217–222

Alcicek A, Bozkurt M, Cabuk M(2004)The effect of an essential oil combination derived from selected herbs growing wild in turkey and broiler. S Afr J Anim Sci 33: 89–94

Ali-shtayeh MS, Yaghmour, R M R, Faidi Y R, Salem K,Al-Nuri MA (1997) Antimicrobial activity of 20 plants used in folkloric medicine in the Palestinian area. JEthnopharmacology 60: 265-271

Bampidis VA, Christodoulou V, Florou-Paneri P, Christaki E, Chatzopoulou PS, Tsiliglianni T, Spais AB (2005) Effect of dietary dried oregano leaves on growth performance, carcass characteristics and serum cholesterol of female early maturing turkeys. Br Poult Sci 46: 591–601

Basílico MZ, Basílico JC (1999) Inhibitory effects of some spice essential oils on *Aspergillus ochraceus* NRRL 3174 growth and ochratoxinA production. Lett ApplMicrobiol 29: 238–241

Bassett R (2000) Oregano's positive impact on poultry production. World Poult 16: 31–34

Bastiaanse HB (2005) In: International Conference for the Feed and Food Chain, Noordwijk, The Netherlands

Bauer K, Garbe, D, Surburg H (2001) Common Fragrance and Flavour Materials: Preparation, Properties and Uses, Fourth ed. Wiley-VCH, Weinheim.

Borgohain B, Mahanta JD, Sapcota D, Sharma M, Borah MC (2016) Effect of feeding garlic (*Allium sativum*) as prebiotic on the performance of commercial broiler chickens. Souvenir cum Compendium of National Symposium, XXXIII Annual conference of IPSA, Nov. 3- 5, Khanapara: abstract No. OP-II-17, Page No 89 (Abstr.)

Botsoglou NA, Florou-Paneri P, Christaki E, Fletouris, DJ, Spais AB (2002) Effect of dietary oregano essential oil on performance of chickens and on iron-induced lipid oxidation of breast, thigh and abdominal fat tissues. Br Poult Sci 43: 223–230

Burt S (2004) Essential oils: their antibacterial properties and potential applications in foods - a review. International J Food Microbial 94: 223-253

Cerisuelo A, Marín C, Sánchez-Vizcaíno F, Gómez E A, de la Fuente J M, Durán R, and Fernández C (2014) The impact of a specific blend of essential oil components and sodium butyrate in feed on growth performance and Salmonella counts in experimentally challenged broilers. Poult Sci 93: 599-606

Chao SC, Young D G, and Oberg C J (2000) Screening for inhibitory activity of essential oils on selected bacteria, fungi and viruses. J Essential Oil Res 12: 639–649

Cosentino S, Tuberoso CIG, Pisano B, Satta M, Mascia V, Arzedi E, Palmas F(1999) *In vitro* antimicrobial activity and chemical composition of Sardinian Thymus essential oils. Lett Appl Microbiol 29: 130–135

Cowan MM(1999) Plant products as antimicrobial agents. Clinic Microbiol Rev 12: 564–582

Cross DE, Hillman K, Fenlon D, Deans SG, McDevitt RM, Acamovic T(2004). Antibacterial properties of phytochemical in aromatic plants in poultry diets. In: Acamovic T, Stewart C S, Pennycott T W (Eds.) Poisonous Plants and Related Toxins, Wallingford. CAB International, Oxon, pp. 175–180

Demir E, Sarica S, Ozcan MA,Suicmez M, (2003) The use of natural feed additives as alternatives for antibiotic growth promoter in broiler diets. Br Poult Sci 44: S44–S45

Didry N, Dubreuil L, Pinkas M (1994) Activity of thymol, carvacrol, cinnamaldehyde and eugenol on oral bacteria. Pharmaceutica Acta Helvetiae 69: 25-28

Dorman HJ, Dand Deans SG (2000) Antimicrobial agents from plants: antibacterial activity of plant volatile oils. J Appl Microbial 88: 308–316

European Community (EC) European Regulations Nos. 834 (2007), 889 (2008) and 1831 (2003). Community Register of Feed Additives (2008).

Farag RS, Badei AZM, Hewedi FM, El-Baroty GSA (1989a). Antioxidant activity of some spice essential oils on linoleic acid oxidation in aqueous media. J Am Oil Chem Soc 66: 792–799

Farag RS, Daw ZY, Hewedi F M,and El-Baroty, GSA (1989b). Antimicrobial activity of some Egyptian spice essential oils. J Food Protect 52: 665–667

Ferhout H, Bohatier J, Guillot J, and Chalchat J C (1999) Antifungal activity of selected essential oils, cinnamaldehyde and carvacrol against Malassezia furfur and Candida albicans. J Essential Oil Res 11: 119-129

Gill A O, Delaquis P, Russo P and Holley R A (2002) Evaluation of antilisterial action of cilantro oil on vacuum packed ham. Int J Food Microbial 73: 83–92

Gogoi R, Sapcota D and Gohain A K (2010) Efficacy of dietary *Curcuma longa* in aflatoxicosis in broilers. Indian Vet J87: 681-83

Greathead H (2003) Plants and plant extracts for improving animal productivity. Proc Nutr Soc 62: 279–290

Helander I M, Alakomi H L, Latva-Kala K, Mattila-Sandholm T, Pol I, Smid E J, Gorris L G M, Vonand Wright A (1998) Characterization of the action of selected essential oil components on Gram-negative bacteria. J Agric Food Chem 46: 3590–3595

Hernández F Madrid J, Garcia V, Orengo J, and Megias M D, (2004) Influence of two plant extracts on broiler performance, digestibility, and digestive organ size. Poult Sci 83: 169–174

Islam R, SapcotaD, Upadhyay TN (2006) Induced aflatoxicosis& its amelioration by *Pipernigrum* & methomin in broiler chickens: Haemato-biochemical, organ weight& leg/feather score studies. Indian J Anim Sci 76: 408-412

Jamroz D, Orda J, Kamel C, Wiliczkiewicz A, Wertelecki T, and Skorupinsk J (2003) The influence of phytogenic extracts on performance, nutrient digestibility, carcass characteristics, and gut microbial status in broiler chickens. J Anim Food Sci 12: 583–596

Jang I S, Ko YH, Kang SY,Lee CY (2007) Effect of commercial essential oils on growth performance, digestive enzyme activity and intestinal microflora population in broiler chickens. Anim Food Sci Technol 134: 304–315

Juliano C, Mattana A, Usai M (2000) Composition and *in vitro* antimicrobial activity of the essential oil of Thymus herba-baronaLoisel growing wild in Sardinia. J Essential Oil Res 12: 516–522

Kamel C (2000) Extractos de plantasnaturales: Remediosclásicos que aportansolucionesmodernas a la producción animal. In: III Conferencia-Salón de Fabricantes de Piensosdel Mediterráneo, Reus (Tarragona).

Kamel C (2001) Tracing modes of action and the roles of plant extracts in non-ruminants. Recent Advances in Animal Nutrition. Nottingham University Press, pp. 135–150.

Krishan G, Narang A (2014) Use of essential oils in poultry nutrition: A new approach. J Adv Vet Anim Res 1(4): 156-162

Lambert R J W, Skandamis PN, Coote P, Nychas GJE (2001) A study of the minimum inhibitory concentration and mode of action of oregano essential oil, thymol and carvacrol. J Appl Microbial 91: 453–462

Langhout P (2000) New additives for broiler chickens. World Poult 16: 22–27

Larrondo JV, Agut MandCalvo-Torras M A (1995) Antimicrobial activity of essences from labiates. Microbiol 82: 171–172

Lattaoui N, Tantaoui-Elaraki A (1994) Individual and combined antibacterial activity of the main components of three thyme essential oils. RivistaItaliana EPPOS 13: 13–19

Lee KW, Everts H, Kappert HJ, Frehner M, Losa R, Beynen AC (2003) Effects of dietary essential oil components on growth performance, digestive enzymes and lipid metabolism in female broiler chickens. Br Poult Sci 44: 450–457

Lewis MR, Rose SP, MaCkenzie AM, Tucker LA (2003) Effects of dietary inclusion of plant extracts on the growth performance of male broiler chickens. Br Poult Sci 44: S42–S43

Marino M, Bersani C, Comi G (1999) Antimicrobial activity of the essential oils of *Thymus vulgaris* L. measured using a bio-impedometric method. J Food Protect 62: 1017–1023

Marino M, Bersani C, Comi G(2001) Impedance measurements to study the antimicrobial activity of essential oils from Lamiacea and Compositae. Int J Food Microbiol 67: 187–195

Mourey A, Canillac N (2002) Anti-Listeria monocytogenes activity of essential oils components of conifers. Food Control 13: 289–292

Nenoff P, Haustein UF, Brandt (1996) Antifungal activity of the essential oil of *Melaleuca alternifolia* (tea tree oil) against pathogenic fungi in vitro. Skin Pharmacol 9: 388–394

Oyen L P A, and Dung N X (1999) Plant resources of South East Asia No. 19. Essential oil plants. Backhuys Publishers

Paster N, Menasherov M, Ravid U andJuven B (1995) Antifungal activity of oregano and thyme essential oils applied as fumigants against fungi attacking stored grain. J Food Protect 58: 81–85

Rota C, Carraminana J J, Burillo J, Herrera A (2004). *In vitro* antimicrobial activity of essential oils from aromatic plants against selected food borne pathogens. J Food Protect 67: 1252–1256

Russo M, Galletti GC, Bocchini P,Carnacini A (1998) Essential oil chemical composition of wild populations of Italian oregano spice (*Origanum vulgare* ssp. hirtum (Link) letswaart): A preliminary evaluation of their use in chemotaxonomy by cluster analysis: 1. Inûorescences. J Agric Food Chem 46: 3741–3746

Sapcota, D, Islam R, Medhi A K (2005a) Efficacy of *Andrographis paniculata* in ameliorating aflatoxicosis in broilers. Indian Vet J 82: 529-32

Sapcota, D, Islam R, Baruah KK, Upadhyay TN (2005b) Effect of dietary *Ocimum sanctum* against aflatoxin B1 contaminated feed in broilers. Indian J Poult Sci 40: 282-284

Sapcota, D, Islam R, Upadhyay T N (2006a) Dietary supplementation of *Emblica officinali* sfor amelioration of experimental aflatoxicosis in commercial broilers. Anim Nutr Feed Technol 6: 65-71

Sapcota, D, Islam R and Upadhyay T N, Bora M (2006b) Induced aflatoxicosis and its amelioration by dietary Piper nigrum and methomin in broiler chickens: Haemato-biochemical, organ weight and leg/feather score studies. Indian J Anim Sci 76: 408-412

Sarma M, Sapcota D, Sarma S, Dutta KK, Gohain AK (2003) Herbal growth promoters on haemato-biochemical constituents in broilers.Indian Vet J 82: 946-948

Senatore F (1996) Inûuence of harvesting time on yield and composition of the essential oil of a thyme (*Thymus pulegioides* L.) growing wild in Campania (Southern Italy). J Agric Food Chem 44: 1327–1332

Shanmugavelu S, Acamovic, Cowieso AJ (2004). Effect of thyme oil and garlic powder on the nutritive value of soybean meal. Br Poult Sci 45: S54–S55

Tabak M, Armon R, Neeman I (1999) Cinnamon extracts' inhibitory effect on *Helicobacter pylori*. JEthnopharmacol 67: 269–277

Thoroski J, Blank, G, Biliaderi C (1989) Eugenol induced inhibition of extracellular enzyme production by *Bacillus cereus*. J Food Protect 52: 399–403

Vaara M (1992) Agents that increase the permeability of the outer membrane. Microbiol Rev 56: 395-411

Van de BraakS AAJ, Leijten GC(1999) Essential Oils and Oleoresins: A Survey in the Netherlands and other Major Markets in the European Union.CBI, Centre for the Promotion of Imports from Developing Countries, Rotterdam.

Varel VH (2002) Livestock manure oder abatement with plant-derived oils and nitrogen conservation with urease inhibitors: a review. J Anim Sci 80: E1-E7

Wang R, Li D, Bourne S (1998) Can 2000 years of herbal medicine history help us solve problems in the year 2000? Biotechnology in the feed industry. Proceedings of Alltech's 14th Annual Symposium. Kentucky, USA; pp. 273-291

Wenk C (2006) Are herbs, botanicals and other related substances adequate replacements for antimicrobial growth promoters? In: Barug D, de Jong, J Kies, A K, Verstegen MWA (Eds.) Antimicrobial Growth Promoters. Wageningen Academic Publishers, The Netherlands, pp. 329–340

Windisch W, Schedle K, Plitzner C, Kroismayr A (2008) Use of phytogenic products as feed additives for swine and poultry. J Anim Sci 86 (E. Suppl.): E140–E148.

❑❑❑

Chapter 15

Indian Goose Berry (*Emblica officinalis*)

Dinesh Kumar[1] and Brishketu Kumar[2]

[1] Department of Veterinary Science & Animal Husbandry, Jawaharlal Nehru Agricultural University,Tikamgarh, Madhya Pradesh, India, E-mail: kr.dinesh7@gmail.com

[2] Department of Animal Sciences, College of Agriculture, Nevsari Agricultural University, Bharuch-392011, Gujarat, India

ABSTRACT

Indian gooseberry (*Phyllanthus emblica*) is a valuably most important medicinal plant in Indian Ayurveda. Various parts of the plant are used to treat a range of diseases or used as feed additives in animals but the most important part is fruit. The fruit is rich in quercetin, phyllaemblic compounds, gallic acid, tannins, flavonoids, pectin and vitamin C and also contains various polyphenolic compounds. A wide range of phytochemical components including terpenoids, alkaloids, flavonoids and tannins have been shown to possess useful biological activities. The fruit is used either alone or in combination with other plants and have wide range of action such as antipyretic, analgesic, antitussive, antiatherogenic, adaptogenic, cardioprotective, gastroprotective, antianemia, antihy percholesterolemia, wound healing, antidiarrheal, antiatherosclerotic, hepatoprotective, nephroprotective and neuroprotective properties. Amla is also reported to possess radiomodulatory, chemomodulatory, chemopreventive effects, free radical scavenging, antioxidant, anti-inflammatory, antimutagenic and immuno-modulatory activities. In this review, we have focused our interest on use of amla as phytogenic feed additive for efficient livestock production.

Keywords: Amla, Querecetin, Livestock, Antioxidant, Anti-inflammatory.

15.1 Introduction

Amla has been regarded as the sacred tree in India. The tree was worshipped as Mother Earth and is believed to nurture mankind because the fruits are very nourishing. The leaves and fruits are used in worship in India. According to Indian mythology, it is believed to be the first tree created in the universe. The medicinal properties of amla have been mentioned in the old Ayurvedic text such as Charaksanhita and Sushrutsanhita. Amla is a monoecious glabrous or pubescent deciduous tree belongs to the family Euphorbiaceae. The name of the family Euphorbiaceae comes from Euphorbus, physician to Juba, King of Mauritania. The plant is commonly known as Amla and found throughout plains of India, Pakistan, Nepal, Uzbekistan, Sri Lanka, SE Asia, China and Malaysia at an elevation of 610-1390 m above the sea level (Stainton, 1997; Sahni, 1998). The Persian name of Emblica is amlah (from Sanskrit amla) but, as the Arabic amlaj suggests, probably in older Persian amlag, and hence, Emblica. Garcia de Orta says it was called embelgi by the Arab physicians. In Sanskrit amla has many synonym: Dhatriphala (dhatri means female supporter, a nurse; phala means fruit); Vayahstha (means strong, vigorous, 'being in the bloom of age'); Amritaphala (amrita means immortal); Amala (means pure or clean); Amla (sour) all these synonymous words show how important this plant is in traditional Indian medicine, in fact it is the most common Ayurvedic plant (Monier-Williams, 1997).

The Amla fruits are sour, astringent, bitter, acrid, sweet, cooling and anodyne in nature and used as ophthalmic, carminative, digestive, stomachic, laxative, alterant, aphrodisiac, rejuvenative, diuretic and antipyretic purposes. They are useful in vitiated conditions of tridosha, diabetes, cough, asthama, bronchitis, cephalalgia, ophthalmopathy, dyspepsia, colic, flatulence, hyperacidity, peptic ulcer, erysipelas, skin diseases, leprosy, haematogenesis, inflammations, anaemia, emaciation, hepatopathy, jaundice, strangury, diarrhoea, dysentery, haemorrhages, leucorrhoea, menorrhagia, cardiac disorders, intermittent fevers and greyness of hair.

15.2 Taxonomy

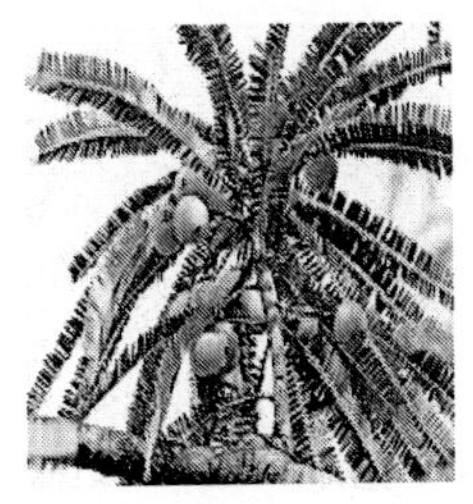
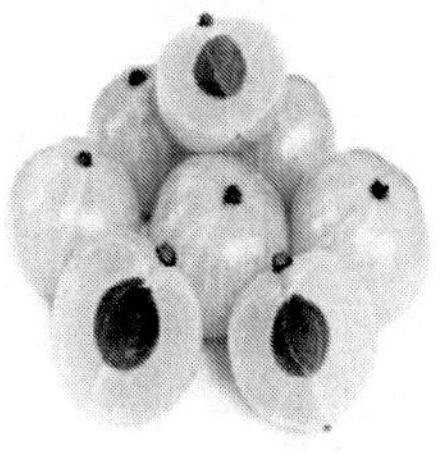

Kingdom : Plantae
Division : Angiosperm
Class : Magnoliopsida
Order : Euphorbiales
Family : Euphorbiaceae
Genus : *Phyllanthus*
Species : *emblica L*

Because of all these properties amla is explored as herbal feed additive to enhance the livestock and poultry production. Very less work is reported in case of ruminant animals as compared to monogastric animals. The herbal feed supplement (feed additive) is a substance or mixture used in minor quantity other than basic feed in order to complement certain nutrients for improving performance of the animals and birds (Narhari, 1992). The efficiency of poor quality roughages utilization can be maximized by the supply of deficient nutrients like nitrogen, micronutrients, feed additives, *etc.* in the ration of animals. Recently, growth promoters have been banned in animal nutrition. With the ban on use of antibiotics as growth promoter by European Union from March 2006, it has become need of the hour to produce drug/chemical free products. There are two principal reasons behind the changes in legislation on the use of in-feed antibiotic growth promoters. The first is to try to combat the development of microbial resistance to antibiotic drugs and its consequences on human health. The second is a response to consumer pressures to eliminate the use of all non-plant xenobiotic agents from the animal diets but at the same time, we can't afford to compromise with the production level because of increasing demand of animal products due to increasing human population and awareness of consumer regarding the importance of animal protein. Reviews on the usage pattern of phytochemicals reveals that tannins, saponins, essential oils, anthraquinones, flavonoids are the major plant secondary metabolites studied in ruminants (Calsamiglia *et al.*, 2007; Patra and Saxena, 2010). These phytochemicals could act alone or a combination of the following potential mechanisms on animal system: (i) increased feed intake (ii) improved feed efficiency (iii) improved gut function leading to reduced incidence of digestive disturbances (iv) stimulation of digestion (v) methane inhibition (vi) immune modulation (vii) antioxidant and (viii) antimicrobial effect. Usually mixture of several herbs rather than single one is more effective for better and sustainable performance of animals.

15.3 Nutritional Composition of Amla

Amla is well known for its nutritional qualities. It is rich in polyphenols, minerals and is regarded as one of the richest source of vitamin C (200 900mg/100g of edible portion), therapeutic potential of the fruits was attributed to their high content of ascorbic acid (Jain *et al.*, 2000). Amla is often incorporated in the herbal formulation called "Triphala", which contain the equal proportion of the fruits of *E. officinalis, Terminalia chebula & Terminalia belerica*. Amla fruits contain moisture 81.2%, protein 0.5%, fat 0.1%, mineral matter 0.7%, fiber 3.4%, carbohydrates 14.1%, Ca (0.05%), K (0.02%), Fe (1.2 mg/100g), nicotinic acid (0.2 mg/100g), vitamin C (600mg/100g) (Khan 2009). Amla fruit powder contains 4.23% protein, 0.5% fat, 2.38% ash, 0.32% AIA, 27.94% NDF, 19.32% ADF, 8.62% HC, 92.87% T-CHO, 0.07% Ca and 0.008% P (Kumar *et al.*, 2016). Its ascorbic acid level ranges from 3.0 to 5.43 g/100 g of dried powder (Mishra *et al.*, 2009).

15.4 Chemistry of Amla

The active ingredient that has significant pharmacological action in amla is designated by Indian scientist as "Phyllemblin". The fruit is rich in quercetin, phyllaemblic compounds, gallic acid, tannins, flavonoids, pectin and vitamin C and also contains various polyphenolic compounds. A wide range of phytochemical components including terpenoids, alkaloids, flavonoids and tannins have been shown to possess useful biological action (Kim *et al.*, 2005). The fruits, leaves and bark are rich in tannins. The root contains ellagic acid and lupeol and bark contains leucodelphinidin. The seeds yield a fixed oil (16%) which is brownish-yellow in colour. It contains linolenic acid (8.8%), linoleic acid (44.0%), oleic acid (28.4%), stearic acid (2.15%), palmitic acid (3.0%) and myristic acid (1.0%) (Thakur *et al.*, 1989). The phytochemicals of this plant include hydrolysable tannins (Emblicanin A, Emblicanin B, punigluconin, pedunculagin) (Ghosal *et al.*, 1996), flavonoids (Rahman, 2007), alkaloids (Phyllantidine and phyllantine) (Khanna *et al.*, 1975). Gallic acid, ellagic acid, chebulinic acid, quercetin, chebulagic acid, corilagin together with isostrictinnin, were isolated from the fruit of Phyllanthus emblica (Zany, 2003). It contains two new hydrolysable tannins with low molecular weight

(<1000), called emblicanin A (37%), emblicanin B (33%), punigluconin (12%) and pedunculagin (14%) (Ghosal *et al.*, 1996). These two new tannins (emblicanins A and B) have a very strong antioxidant action (Bhattacharya *et al.*, 1999; Santos *et al.*, 1999) and found to preserve erythrocytes against oxidative stress induced by asbestos, generator of superoxide radical.

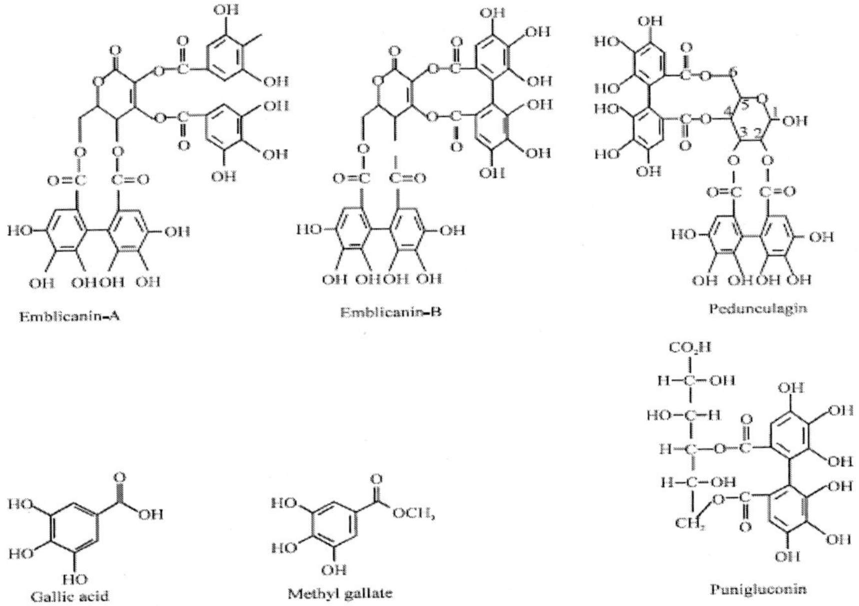

Emblicanin-A Emblicanin-B Pedunculagin

Gallic acid Methyl gallate Punigluconin

Fig. Important phytochemicals of amla

Tannins traditionally been considered as anti-nutritional factors but now a days they are more known in ruminant nutrition for their beneficial effects on ruminal modification (Animut *et al.*, 2008). They are classified into hydrolysable and condensed tannins and are considered to have both adverse and beneficial effects depending on their concentration and nature besides other factors such as animal species, physiological state of the animal and composition of the diet (Makkar, 2003). Feeding of tannin rich diet also induced a shift in rumen microbial profile with increased population of tannin tolerant bacteria (Singh *et al.*, 2011). The whole concept of farming during the last two decades or so has undergone a sea of changes. The poultry industry has now emerged as a highly structured and market-oriented enterprise. The major objective of livestock and poultry farming is to increase the profit margin in business by improving feed efficiency and growth rate keeping the health status of animals.

15.5 Preparation of the Amla Powder

Sorting and grading is essential to get suitable quality of fruit which was done by hand. The fruits were first washed to remove the dirt. Grading of fruit was done based on soundness, firmness, cleanliness, size, maturity, weight, colour, shape and freedom from foreign matters, insect damage and mechanical injury. From the graded amla the pulp was extracted manually. It was homogenized in a mixer to obtain fine pulp or dry in oven at 60°C, then grind to obtained amla powder.

15.6 Effects on Digestion

The Amla fruits have well known action as carminative, digestive, stomachic, laxative and tonic in nature. The regular use of Amla can strengthen digestion, absorption and assimilation of food. But it works more slowly and gently than ginger or other digestion-enhancing herbs. In addition, it improves assimilation of iron for healthy blood. Amla purify the Rasa Dhatu (nutrient fluid) and Rakta Dhatu (blood), thus supporting the functions of the liver. It also strengthens the liver and helps in detoxification and removal of toxins from the body (Pramyothin *et al.,* 2006).

Amla as feed additives have no side effects on the health of birds. The dietary use of herbal growth promoter increases the performance of broiler by improving digestion, metabolism and absorption of certain nutrients which ultimately improve live weight gain and FCR (Samarth *et al.,* 2002). Herbs have a complex mode of action on various organs or systems due to active ingredients present in them. They are supposed to have greater impact on different factors which promote growth and health, by improving physiological and immunological functions of body. Kumar and Singh, (2005) conducted an experiment on day old broiler chicken of Hubbard strain to evaluate the efficacy of amla fruit on the productive performance of broiler chicken. The production was comparatively higher in amla fed group as evidence by higher body weight gain and FCR. The mortality percentage was zero in treatment groups, whereas 5% mortality was recorded in control group. Likewise, Daisy *et al.* (2007) supplemented amla fruit powder in water and observed growth performance of broiler. The result showed better growth and feed utilization in treated groups as compared to control.

Wadhwa *et al.* (2007) observed the effect of amla fruit powder in feed of broiler at level of 250 (AM_1), 500 (AM_2) and 750 (AM_3) gm/ton and compared it with zinc bacitracin supplemented and non-supplemented groups. The body weight was significantly high in amla treated group, then zinc bacitracin treated birds but there was no significant difference from weight of broiler reared without antibiotic. Feed consumption was high in birds supplemented with amla powder. During the last two weeks of age, however, the broilers in AM_3 gain significantly highest weight than rest of treatments. Singh *et al.* (2008) conducted an experiment under hot and humid climate to study the effect of density, protein and amla levels on performance of broilers. Body weight was significantly influenced by density at earlier (2 to 3 wk) and later ages (5 and 6 wk) during hot humid climate. At earlier age D_2 medium density was optimum, whereas in later of age sixth week body weight was significantly high in D_3 low density than D_1 high and D_2 medium density groups. Effect of protein was significant on weight gain. Amla additive improved body weight by 14 gms at 6 weeks of age. D_3 low density has significantly better feed efficiency than D_1 high density. Tiwari *et al.* (2008) studied the effect of probiotic and herbal supplement on growth and immuno competence traits of commercial broilers. The bird of the first group were fed on a basal diet supplemented with probiotic (Biovet YC @ 50 g/quintal of the basal diet) while the second group birds were fed on a basal diet supplemented with herbal mixture (1% amla pulp powder, 0.5 % turmeric powder, 0.5 % neem leaf powder). The herbal supplemented group had apparently higher body weight gain compared to the control group throughout the experiment and at 6th week of age, the average weekly body weight gain was significantly higher in the herbal supplemented group compared to the probiotic and control groups. No significant differences in the weekly FCR of commercial broilers among different treatment groups were observed during the experimental period except at 6th week, where herbal supplemented group had significantly better FCR compared to the probiotic and control group. HA titre was significantly higher in the herbal supplemented group compared to the probiotic and control group at 6 weeks of age.

Ghavate *et al.* (2009) conducted an experiment to study the effect of feeding different levels of amla on performance of broilers during 0-6 weeks of age. There was significant effect of supplementation on gain in body weight of broilers in T_2 group as compared to those in

T_1 and T_0 (control) groups. Feed intake was also significantly higher in T_2 group than in T_1 and control T_0 groups. The supplementation of amla powder @ 15 kg/t of feed T_2 group significantly improved FCR compared to T_1 group (2.66). It was concluded that the effect of addition of amla powder on live weight gain, feed intake and feed conversion ratio was significant due to supplementation of amla powder @ 10 kg/t and 15 kg/t of feed but costly as compared to control group. Similarly, Ghule *et al.* (2010) conducted a comparative study of amla and vitamin C on performance of broilers under nutritional stress for a period of 42 days, and found that birds fed low energy (5% than control) rations with supplements amla and Vitamin C showed apparently higher body weight gain in fourth and sixth week than control and low energy group without supplementation. Patel *et al.* (2016) also reported similar result and concluded that, dietary addition of amla fruit powder (@ 0.4 and 0.8%) had a positive effect on growth performance and net profit per bird in commercial broiler chickens as compared to control group. Similarly, Tangade (2007) studied the effect of supplementation of herbal amla and synthetic vitamin C on performance of broilers during intense summer conditions. Control group T_0 received corn soya based standard ration. Group T_1, T_2 and T_3 received corn soya based standard ration supplemented with 150, 200 and 250 mg/kg synthetic vitamin C respectively. Group T_4, T_5 and T_6 received corn soya based standard ration supplemented with 150, 200 and 250 mg/kg vitamin C equivalent to synthetic vitamin C through amla. He finds that the group T_5 (200 mg/kg herbal (amla) vitamin C) showed significant improvement over all groups in body weight, weekly gain in body weight, feed consumption and FCR.

Other than health promoting function of amla, some phytogenic feed additives have also shown the effect on the rumen ecosystem of ruminants, which resulted in reduced methanogenesis (Kamra *et al.*, 2008; Bodas *et al.*, 2009) and also increased the feed utilization efficiency (Lopez *et al.*, 2010). The overall literature review showed that the use of amla fruit powder as herbal supplement was beneficial in livestock and poultry for its encouraging results in relation to growth performance. The overall performance and economical benefits were better due to addition of this herb to poultry rations.

15.7 Gastroprotective Effects

An ethanol extract of amla was examined for its antisecretory and antiulcer activities employing different experimental models in rats, including pylorus ligation Shay rats, indomethacin, hypothermic restraint stress induced gastric ulcer and necrotizing agents (80% ethanol, 0.2 M NaOH and 25% NaCl). Oral administration of amla extract @ 250 mg/kg and 500 mg/kg significantly inhibited the development of gastric lesions in all test models used. It also caused significant decrease of the pyloric-ligation induced basal gastric secretion, titratable acidity and gastric mucosal injury. Histopathological analyses are in good agreement with pharmacological and biochemical findings. The results indicate that amla extract possesses antisecretory, antiulcer and cytoprotective properties.

15.8 Hypolipidaemic Effect

The lipid lowering and antiatherosclerotic effects of amla fresh juice were evaluated in cholesterol fed rabbits (rendered hyperlipidaemic by atherogenic diet and cholesterol feeding). Fresh juice of amla was administered @ 5 ml/kgBW/day for 60 days. Serum cholesterol, TG, phospholipid and LDL levels were lowered by 82, 66, 77 and 90%, respectively (Mathur *et al.,* 1995). Similarly, the tissue lipid levels showed a significant reduction following amla juice administration. Aortic plaques were regressed. Amla juice treated rabbits excreted more cholesterol and phospholipids, suggesting that the mode of absorption was affected. Similarly, beneficial effects of amla fruit extract on serum and tissue lipid parameters have also been reported by others (Bhandari, 1989). Amla fruits are a rich source of ascorbic acid (600 mg %) and acts as an antioxidant to prevent the oxidation of LDL cholesterol and thus slows atherogenesis. A substantial reduction in the risk of atherosclerosis in subjects with high plasma concentrations of vitamin C has been well established (Riemersma *et al.,* 1991).

15.9 Antioxidant Effect

As a result of metabolic reactions and diseases, there is generation of free radicals in the form of reactive oxygen species and reactive nitrogen species within the animal's body. Free radicals are chemical entities, which contains one or more unpaired electrons due to which they are highly unstable and cause damage to other molecules by extracting electrons from them in order to attain their stability. Reactive oxygen species (ROS) are highly reactive oxidizing agents belonging to the class of free-radicals. The free-radical initiate chain reactions by removal of an electron from another molecule to complete its own orbital. The most common ROS that have potential implications in reproductive health includes superoxide anion (O^{-}_{2}), hydrogen peroxide (H_2O_2), hydroxyl radical (OH^{-}) and nitric oxide (NO^{+}). An increased production of ROS by any cell beyond the capacity of the cellular antioxidant defense leads to oxidative stress (OS), which ultimately cause significant cell damage through irreversible modification of vital cellular structures such as lipids, proteins and nucleic acids. This higher shift of oxidative stress may lead to several disorders and could be pre-disposing factor for them (Irshad and Chaudhuri, 2002). The natural mechanism to counteract the effect of reactive oxygen species is via antioxidant compounds (vitamin C, vitamin E, carotene, uric acid) and enzymes (catalase, superoxide dismutase, glutathione peroxidase/reductase). Herbs are known to contain large amounts of different families of antioxidants of which flavanoids and tannins are most recurring followed by phenolics, ascorbic acid and alkaloids (Ali *et al.*, 2008).

Because of two new tannins, amla have a very strong antioxidant action. The two emblicanins A and B have been found to preserve erythrocytes against oxidative stress induced by asbestos, generator of superoxide radical. Emblicanin A oxidates, when put in contact with asbestos becoming emblicanin B and together they have a stronger protective action to erythrocytes than vitamin C. Moreover, they improve the efficacy of vitamin C in reducing dihydroascorbic acid to ascorbic acid. The same recycling process has been observed in the rutin- vitamin C combination. Antioxidant compounds can help to protect DNA from the damage associated with free radicals which are highly reactive compounds.

Amla and other rasayanas are effective broad spectrum antioxidants and free radical scavengers, helping to reduce disease and slow the aging process. The use of amla as an antioxidant has been examined by a number of authors (Kumaran *et al.*, 2006). Adaptogenic herbs like Amla, Ashwagandha, Tulsi and Ginseng etc. are being used as anti-stress factors for long years in human and animal medicines with proven results (Ranade and Desai, 2005). These compounds in herbs have the capacities to quench lipid peroxidation, prevent oxidative DNA damage, and scavenge ROS, such as superoxide, hydrogen peroxide and hydroxyl radicals (Yoo *et al.*, 2008). The oral administration of flavonoids from amla at a dose of 10 mg/kg showed significant antioxidant action in cholesterol fed experimental rats. The activities of free radical scavenging enzymes were significantly elevated and lipid peroxide content was significantly decreased in flavonoid treated hypercholesterolemic rats (Anila and Vijayalakshmi, 2003). This antioxidant activity of the amla extract has been found to be both dose and concentration dependent. Administration of amla (@ 500 mg/kg BW for 30 days) prevents the restrain stress induced oxidative stress and elevation of corticosterone levels (Thangraj *et al.*, 2007). Maini *et al.* (2007) conducted a trail on commercial broiler chicks. Control group was given basal diet and treatment groups were supplemented with either vitamin E (200mg/kg feed), dried mint leaves (10g/kg and 30g/kg feed) or amla-electrolyte mix (1g/kg feed) from day 1 to seven weeks of age. Antioxidant supplemented groups showed significantly reduced level of lipid peroxidation in erythrocytes both at 3rd and 5th week, whereas in control group at 3rd and 5th week showed high concentration of lipid peroxidation and low activity of glutathione (GSH) and superoxide dismutase (SOD) in erythrocytes, heart, liver and brain cortex.

15.10 Effect on Immune Modulation and Immune Response

Immunity is a homeostatic process, a series of delicately balanced complex, multicellular and physiologic mechanisms that allow an individual to distinguish foreign material from "self" and neutralize and/or eliminate the foreign matter (Kaminski *et al.*, 2008). The immune system is primarily concerned with resistance against foreign invaders and protection against neoplastic cells. Whereas, immuno-modulator is an agent that intensifies or diminishes the immune responses and such effect is called as immuno-modulatory effect. Immunomodulation using medicinal plants could provide an alternative to conventional chemotherapy for a variety of diseases, especially when host defence mechanism has to be activated under the conditions of impaired immune response or when a selective immunosuppression is desired in situations like autoimmune disorders (Alamgir and Uddin, 2010). Amla acts as strong immunity booster, antibacterial, antifungal, antiviral medical studies conducted on amla fruit suggest that it has antiviral properties (Udupa, 1993) and also functions as an anti-bacterial and anti-fungal agent (Treadway, 1994).

Amla fruit powder as feed additive has been reported to possess antistress, adaptogenic, immunogenic and growth-stimulating properties resulting in better performance of broiler (Sapcota *et al.*, 2005 and Wadhwa *et al.*, 2007).

15.11 Anticancer and Antiulcer Effects

It was tested *in vivo* in wistar rats treated with carcinogen Diethylnitrosamine (DEN) (200mg/kg b.wt i.p) to induce liver cancer. The results showed that pretreatment of methanolic fruit extract (100 and 200 mg/kg b.wt) exhibited significant pathological manifestations at both the doses. Amla has the potential to be useful in ameliorating the carcinogen induced response in rat (Sarwat *et al.*, 2008). Similarly, potential anticancer effects of aqueous fruit extract of amla was tested in several different human cancer cell lines such as A549 (lung), HepG2 (liver), HeLa (cervical), MDA MB 231 (breast), SKOV3 (ovarian) and SW620 (Colorectal). Amla extract significantly inhibited the growth of several human cancer cell lines at doses of 50 100 μg/ml (Ngamkitidechakul *et al.*, 2010). Research found that amla is benecifical to treat different types of cancers. Garima *et al.* (2005) also reported chemopreventive potential of amla against skin carcinogenesis. Similarly, Banu *et al.* (2004) also experimentally evaluated ethanolic extract of amla against genotoxicity induced by DMBA. Amla fruit administered orally at different concentrations (100, 250, 500 mg/kg b.wt) for seven consecutive days in Swiss albino mice prior to a single intraperitoneal injection of DMBA decreased the frequency of bone marrow micronuclei. The protection provided by amla may be due to its antioxidant capacity and through its modulatory effect on hepatic activation and detoxifying enzymes.

15.12 Antimicrobial Effects

Herbal growth promoters due to their multi-directional actions are also useful in controlling pathogenic bacteria without possibility of development of resistance and are also safe for animals and humans. In such manner they can work as herbal anti-microbial agents with other advantages like more economical, free from possibility of resistance, maintaining normal functions, improving production performance in broilers, improving egg size, lymphocyte percentage and egg weight in layers (Reddy *et al.*, 2002 and Shon *et al.*, 2002). Saeed *et al.* (2007) also reported that, aqueous infusion and decoction of amla exhibited potent antimicrobial activity against different strains of *Staphylococcus aureus, S. haemolyticus, S. saprophyticus, Micrococccus varians, M. lylae, M. roseus, M. halobius, M. sedenterius, Bacillus subtilis, B. megaterium* and *Candida albicans.*

15.13 Conclusions

Research on herbal plants has gained a renewed focus recently. The prime reason is that other system of feed additives although effective with a number of side effects along with residue in final products that often lead to serious complications in human being as well as welfare of animals. Plant based phytogenic feed additive being natural does not pose this serious problems. Though amla has various medicinal applications, but it is the need of hour to explore its additive values at nutritional as well as molecular level with help of various bio-technological tools and techniques. Amla has variety of phytochemical such as tannins, flavonoids, terpenoids and alkaloids are reported to indicate several pharmacological properties such as carminative, digestive, stomachic, laxative, antioxidant, antitumor, antigenotoxic and anticarcinogenic effects. It is considered to be safe herbal feed additives without any adverse effects. Further studies should be needed to standardize the inclusion levels in livestock's especially in large ruminants.

References

Al Rehaily AJ, Al Howiriny TS, Al Sohaibani MO, Rafatullah S (2002) Gastroprotective effects of 'Amla' *Emblica officinalis* on *in vivo* test models in rats. Phytomedicine 9(6): 515-522

Alamgir MA, Uddin SJ (2010) Recent advances on the ethnomedicinal plants as immuno-modulatory agents. Ethnomedicine: A Source of Complementary Therapeutics 37: 227-244

Ali SS, Kasoju N, Luthra A, Singh A, Sharanabasava H, Sahu A, Bora U (2008) Indian medicinal herbs as sources of antioxidants. Food Res Int 41: 1-15

Anila L, Vijayalakshmi NR (2003) Antioxidant action of flavonoids from *Manifera indica* and *Emblica officinalis* in hypercholesterolemic rats. Food Chemistry 83: 569-574

Animut G, Puchala R, Goetsch AL, Patra AK, Sahlu T, Varel VH, Wells J (2008) Methane emission by goats consuming diets with different levels of condensed tannins from lespedeza. Anim Feed Sci Tech 144: 212-227

Banu SM, Selvendiran K, Singh JP, Sakthisekaran D (2004) Protective effect of *Emblica officinalis* ethanolic extract against 7, 12- dimethylbenz (a) anthracene (DMBA) induced genotoxicity in Swiss albino mice. Hum Exp Toxicol 23(11): 527-31

Bhattacharya A, Chatterjee A, Ghoshal S, Bhattacharya SK (1999) Indian J Exp Biol 37: 676-680

Bodas R, Frutos P, Giraldez FJ, Hervas G, Lopez S (2009) Effect of sodium bicarbonate supplementation on feed intake, digestibility, digesta kinetics, nitrogen balance and ruminal fermentation in young fattening lambs. Spanish J Agricultural Res 7(2): 330-341

Calsamiglia S, Busquet M, Cardozo PW, Castillejos L, Ferret A (2007) Essential oils as modifiers of rumen microbial fermentation. J Dairy Sci 9: 2580-2595

Daisy K, Patel M, Ashok K, Bhardwaj RK, Hore SK (2007) Effect of amla (*Emblica officinalis*) on performance of broiler. XXIV Annu. Conf. of IPSA and National symposium 25-27 April 2007 Ludhiana, pp. 99-100

Ghavate AM, Wankhede SM, Deshmukh SV (2009) Effect of feeding different levels of *Emblica officinalis* (Amla) on performance of broilers.13th biennial Conference of ANSI, Dec. 17-19, 2009 NIANP, Bangalore. Vol. II, pp. 207

Ghosal S, Rao G, Sarvana V, Nira Mishra M, Dipak R (1996) A possible chemical mechanism of the bioactivities of mangiferin. Indian J Chem 35(6): 561

Ghule (2010) Comparative study of *Emblica officinalis* (amla) and vitamin C on Performance of Broilers under Nutritional Stress. Unpublished M.V.Sc. Thesis submitted to Maharashtra Animal and Fishery Sciences University, Nagpur

Irshad M, Chaudhuri PS (2002) Oxidant-antioxidant system: role and significance in human body. Indian J Expt Biology 40: 1233-1239

Kaminski NE, Faubert Kaplan BL, Holsapple MP (2008) Toxic responses of the immune system. In: Casarett and Doull's Toxicology The Basic Science of Poisons. Edited by Klassen C.D. Seventh Edition, McGraw- Hill Medical Publishing Division, USA. pp. 485-556

Kamra DN, Patra AK, Chatterjee PN, Kumar R, Agarwal N, Chaudhary LC (2008) Effects of plant extract on methanogenesis and microbial profile of the rumen of buffalo: a brief overview. Australian J Expt Agriculture 48: 175-178

Khan KH (2009) Role of *Emblica officinalis* in Medicine-A Review. Botany Res Int 2(4): 218-228

Kumar D, Singh P, Chaturvedi VB, Verma AK (2016) *In Vitro* Digestibility and Rumen Fermentation Parameters of Feeds as Affected by Supplementary Amla Powder and Fenugreek Seeds. Indian J Anim Nutr 33(1): 64-69

Maini S, Rastogi SK, Korde JP, Madan AK, Shukla SK (2007) Evaluation of oxidative stress and its amelioration through certain antioxidants in broilers during summer. J Poult Sci 44: 339-347

Makkar HPS (2003) Effects and fate of tannins in ruminant animals, adaptation to tannins, and strategies to overcome detrimental effects of feeding tannin-rich feeds. Small Ruminant Res 49: 241-256

Manoj Kumar, Singh KCP (2005) Effect of supplementation of herbal product on the production potential of chickens. Indian Poult. Sci. Asso., XXIII Annual Conf. and National Symposium, held at Hyderabad from 2-4 Feb., 2005. pp. 67

Mishra P, Srivastava V, Verma D, Chauhan OP, Rai GK (2009) Physicochemical properties of Chakiya variety of Amla (*Emblica officinalis*) and effect of different dehydration methods on quality of powder. African J Food Sci 3: 303-306

Monier-Williams M (1997) A Sanskrit-English Dictionary. Motilal Banarsidass Publishers Pvt., New Delhi

Ngamkitidechakul C, Jaijoy K, Hansakul P, Soonthornchareonnon N, Sireeratawong S (2010) Antitumour effects of *Phyllanthus emblica* L: induction of cancer cell apoptosis and inhibition of *in vivo* tumour promotion and *in vitro* invasion of human cancer cells. Phytother Res 24: 1405–1413

Patra AK, Saxena J (2010) A new perspective on the use of plant secondary metabolites to inhibit methanogenesis in the rumen. Phytochem 71: 1198-1222

Ranade AS, Desai DN (2005) Natural products for enhanced poultry productivity. IPSACON – 2005 available from poultvet.com

Reddy R, V Reddy, Reddy KS (2002) Unpublished data, Nagarjuna Poultry Farm, Shahanshabad, Hyderabad

Saeed S, Tariq P (2007) Antimicrobial activities of *Emblica officinalis* and *Coriandrum sativum* against gram positive bacteria and candida albicans. Pak J Bot 39(3): 913-917

Sahni KC (1998) The Book of Indian Trees. Bombay Natural History Society, Oxford University Press, Mumbai

Samarth VR, Jagtap DG, Dakshinkar NP, Nimbalka MV, Kothekar MD (2002) Effect of Ashwagandha root powder (*Wtihania somnifera)* on performance of broiler. Indian Vet J 79: 733-734

Santos AR, De-Campos RO, Miguel OG, Cechinel FV, Yunes RA, Calixto JB (1999) Eur J Pharmacol 379: 7-17

Sapcota D, Upadhyaya TN, Islam R, Dev KB (2005) Effect of dietary *Emblica officinalis* in ameliorating aflatoxicosis in broiler chicken: gross and histopathological studies. Indian Poult. Sci. Asso., XXIII Annual Conf. and National Symposium, held at Hyderabad from 2-4 Feb. 2005. pp. 97-98

Shon KS, Knon OS, Min BJ, Cho JH, Chen YJ, Kim IH, Kim HS (2002) Unpublished data, Department of Animal Resources and Sciences, Dankook University, Cheonan, Korea

Singh S, Atkare SS, Bhardwaj JK, Parmar SNS (2008) Effect of density protein and amla additive on growth and feed efficiency of broiler during hot humid climate. Indian Poult. Sci. Asso., Silver Jubilee Annual Conf. and National Symposium held at Anand from 10-12 Dec 2008, pp. 409

Singh VK, Patanaik AK, Sharma K, Saini M (2011) Effect of dietary energy intake on erythrocytic antioxidant defence in growing lambs fed a wheat strawbased diet. Anim Prod Sci 51: 642-649

Stainton A (1997) Flowers of the Himalaya: A Supplement. Oxford India, New Delhi

Tangade SU (2007) Effect of herbal and synthetic vitamin C supplementation on the performance of broilers under intense summer condition. Unpublished M.V.Sc. Thesis submitted to Maharashtra Animal and Fishery Sciences University, Nagpur

Thangraj R, Ayyapan SR, Manikandan P, Bhaskaran J (2007) Antioxidant property of *Emblica officinalis* during experimentally induced restain stress in rats. J Health Sci 53: 496-499

Tiwari M, Singh HN, Bhattacharyya A, Goswami M (2008) Effect of probiotic and herbal supplement on growth and immuno-competence traits of commercial broilers. Indian Poult Sci. Asso., Silver Jubilee Annual Conf. and National Symposium held at Anand from 10-12 Dec., 2008, pp. 419

Wadhwa D, Sood S, Meena K, Sharma VK, Chounan J S (2007) Effect of supplementation of gooseberry (*Emblica officinalis*) powder supplementation on biological performance of commercial broilers. XXIV Annu. Conf of IPSA and National Symposium 25-27 April, 2007. Ludhiana. pp. 95

Yoo KM, Lee CH, Lee HJ, Moon BK, Lee CY (2008) Relative antioxidant and cytoprotective activities of common herbs. Food Chem 106: 929-936.

❑❑❑

Chapter 16

Ginger (*Zingiber officinale*)

Lipismita Samal and N.C. Behura

Post-Graduate Department of Poultry Science, College of Veterinary Science & Animal Husbandry, Orissa University of Agriculture and Technology, Bhubaneswar-751003, India, E-mail: lipismitasamal@gmail.com

ABSTRACT

Ginger (*Zingiber officinale*) is widely used as a cooking spice, condiment, culinary herb and medical treatment for certain diseases. Ginger is native to southern China but is also cultivated in many tropical and subtropical regions of the world. Fresh ginger contains 80.9% moisture, 2.3% protein, 0.9% fat, 1.2% minerals, 2.4% fibre and 12.3% carbohydrates. In the crude plant material of ginger, several other sulfonated compounds, diarylheptanoids and shogasulfonic acids are found. The powdered rhizome contains 3-6% fatty oil, 9% protein, 60-70% carbohydrates, 3-8% crude fibre, 8% ash, 9-12% water and 2-3% volatile oil. In Ayurveda, ginger has been recommended for use as carminative, diaphoretic, anti-splasmodic, expectorant, peripheral circulatory stimulant, astringent, appetite stimulant, anti-inflammatory agent, diuretic and digestive aid. It has been suggested as an effective treatment for cataracts, amenorrhea, heart disease, migraines, stroke, angina, Athlete's foot, colds, bursitis, chronic fatigue, tendinitis, flu, coughs, depression, dizziness, fever, erectile difficulties, infertility, kidney stones, hypertension, obesity, diabetes, osteoarthritis, Raynaud's disease, sciatica, Alzheimer's disease, and bacterial and viral infections. Ginger has a lot of useful effects on animals' health such as anti-dyspepsia, anti-bloating, anti-vomiting, anti-diarrhoea and anti-spasm. It shows various pharmacological effects including immune-modulatory, anti-tumorigenic, anti-inflammatory, anti-apoptotic, anti-hyperglycemic, anti-lipidemic and antiemetic effects.

Keywords: *Zingiber officinale,* Rhizome, Gingerols, Shagoal, Volatile oils, Hypercholesterolaemia.

16.1 Introduction

Ginger (*Zingiber officinale*) is widely used as a cooking spice, condiment and culinary herb (Larsen *et al.*, 1999) and medical treatment for certain diseases (Mohdyusof *et al.*, 2002; Masuda *et al.*, 2004; Tapsell *et al.*, 2006) in South Asia. The medical form of ginger historically was called *'Jamaica ginger'*. It is a tropical plant with green and purple flowers and an aromatic underground stem, called rhizome (ginger root). Ginger is native to southern China but is also cultivated in many tropical and subtropical regions of the world. China and India lead the world in fresh ginger production with a global share of over 50%, followed by Indonesia, Nepal and Nigeria. Other major producers of ginger include Bangladesh, Japan, Thailand, Philippines, Cameroon, Sri Lanka, Korea and Fiji. In India, it is mainly cultivated in Kerala, Karnataka, Tamil Nadu and North Eastern states. Kerala is the largest ginger producing state, accounting for about 33 per cent of the total production in India. In Sanskrit, ginger is known as *Sringavera*, referring to the horned appearance of the knobby, irregular rhizome. Over time the name changed to *Zingiberi* in Greek and to the Latin *Zingiber*, a name more reflective of the area in southern India where ginger was believed to have originated. Ginger has been used as medicine since the 4th century BC and is called 'maha aushadhi', means the great medicine. In Ayurveda, ginger has been recommended for use as carminative, diaphoretic, antispasmodic, expectorant, peripheral circulatory stimulant, astringent, appetite stimulant, anti-inflammatory agent, diuretic and digestive aid. It has been suggested as an effective treatment for cataracts, amenorrhea, heart disease, migraines, stroke, angina, Athlete's foot, colds, bursitis, chronic fatigue, tendinitis, flu, coughs, depression, dizziness, fever, erectile difficulties, infertility, kidney stones, Raynaud's disease, sciatica, Alzheimer's disease, cancer and viral infections. The Greek physician Galen used ginger as a purificant of body. He used ginger to treat conditions caused by imbalances in body (Langner *et al.*, 1998). Ginger has a lot of useful effects on animals' health such as anti-dyspepsia, anti-bloating, anti-vomiting, anti-diarrhoea and anti-spasm. Ginger can increase digestion and can cure gastric problems. It shows various pharmacological effects including immune-modulatory, anti-tumorigenic, anti-inflammatory, anti-apoptotic, anti-hyperglycemic, anti-lipidemic and antiemetic effects (Ali *et al.*, 2008). The ginger has been listed as 'Generally Recognised as Safe' (GRAS) by the Food and Drug Administration (FDA) of United States.

16.2 Taxonomy

Domain : *Eukarya*
Kingdom : *Plantae*
Phylum : *Magnoliophyta*
Class : *Lilopsida*
Order : *Zingiberales*
Family : *Zingiberaceae*
Genus : *Zingibe*
Species : *Officinale*

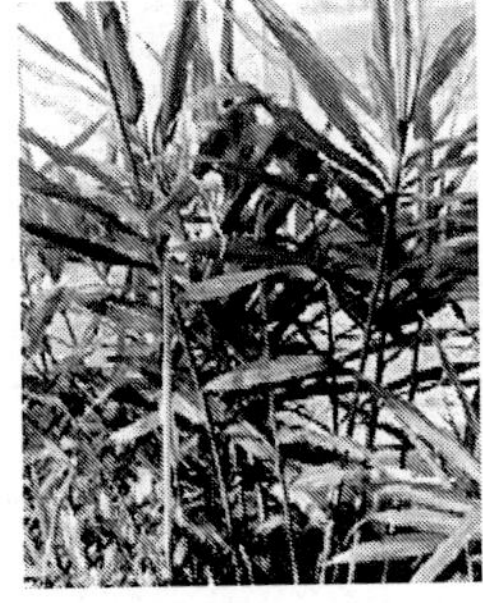

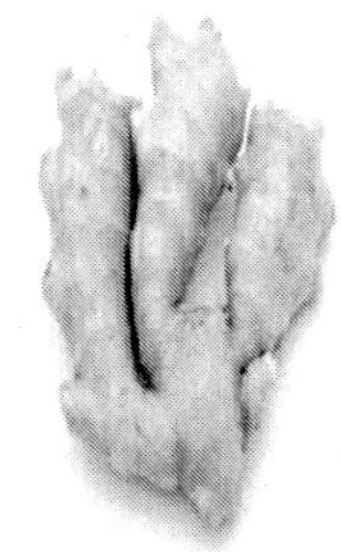

16.3 Different Ginger Preparations

Ginger is available in a variety of forms including fresh root, root extract, oil, oleoresins, dried, pickled, preserved, crystallised or candied, steamed, roasted, powdered or ground, processed, coated or unscraped, unbleached (natural) and bleached ginger. Processed ginger including dried ginger, confectionary ginger and ginger extracts such as oils and resins are traded, largely for their flavouring and medicinal properties. Different improved cultivars of ginger from the Indian Institute for Spice Research (IISR) are Rejathaa, Mahimab, IISR-Varada, Suprabha, Suruchi, Suravi, Himagiri and Rio-de-Janeiro. Cochin ginger and Calicut ginger are the popular Indian ginger varieties in the world market. Other promising varieties are Nadia, Maran, China, Wynad Kuruppampadi, Ernad and Varad.

16.4 Chemistry of Ginger

The composition varies with the type, variety, agronomic conditions, curing methods, drying and storage conditions. The quality and quantity of biologically active constituents of ginger depend on its cultivation practices and post-harvest treatment. Fresh ginger contains 80.9% moisture, 2.3% protein, 0.9% fat, 1.2% minerals, 2.4% fibre and 12.3% carbohydrates. In the crude plant material of ginger, several other sulfonated compounds, diarylheptanoids and shogasulfonic acids are found. The powdered rhizome contains 3-6% fatty oil, 9% protein, 60-70% carbohydrates, 3-8% crude fibre, 8% ash, 9-12% water and 2-3% volatile oil. Ginger is comprised of key components including amino acids, fibre, volatile oils (monoterpenes, sesquiterpenes, paradols, zingiberol, gingerol, shagoals) and minerals (chromium, magnesium, zinc). Gingerols, in particular 6-gingerol, is the active ingredient of ginger and is also responsible for its characteristic taste. Gingerols have cardio-tonic, analgesic, anti-inflammatory and anti-pyretic activity (Young *et al.,* 2005). Shagoal has antioxidant and anti-hepatotoxic activities (Ahmad *et al.,* 2006; Yemitan *et al.,* 2006). The volatile oil consists of mainly camphene, β-phellandrene, curcumene, cineole, geranyl acetate, terphineol, terpenes, borneol, geraniol, zingiberol, eucalyptol, citral, limonene, linalool, monoterpenoids (α-pinene, cineole, borneol, geraniol, geranial and neral), sesquiterpenoids, gingerol, oleoresin (gingerin), zingiberol, zingerone, shagaol, α-zingiberene, β-sesquiphellandrene, β-bisabolene, α-farmesene, ar-curcumene and -farnesene,-bisabolene and -esquiphellandrene. Monoterpenes are compounds that contain 10-carbon skeleton often arranged in a ring. Sesquiterpenoids have a 15-carbon skeleton. In the fresh ginger rhizome, the gingerols are the major active components and 6-gingerol [5-hydroxy-1-(4-hydroxy-3-methoxy phenyl)-decan-3-one] is the most abundant constituent in the gingerol series and this is more pungent than 8-or 10-gingerol. There are many other gingerols, including methylgingerol, gingerdiol, dehydrogingerdione, gingerdiones, diarlyheptanoids, diterpenlactones, zingiberone, bisabolene, camphene, geranial, linalool, borneol and galanolactone (Chrubasik *et al.,* 2005). Fresh ginger may also contain a 5-deoxy derivative of ginger called paradol. In dried ginger powder and semi-dried ginger plant, shogaol (a dehydrated or degraded product of gingerol) is the predominant constituent (Kiuchi *et al.,* 1993; Mustafa *et al.,* 1993). These shogaols are much more pungent than gingerols. Gingerols are thermally labile. Heating converts gingerol to the less pungent zingerone; drying converts it to shogaol, which is about twice as strong-tasting. Zingerone is also a degradation product and it causes the ginger product to smell bad as it ages. Oleoresin, which is isolated by acetone and ethanol extraction, contains 6-Gingerol, 8-gingerol, 10-gingerol, 6-shogaol, zingerone, zingiberol, paradol, zingiberene, gingediol, diarylheptanoids, vitamins, resins and phytosterols. The acetone extract of ginger contains zingerberone and ether extract contain zingerone. The fresh rhizome is less hot and contains more of the flavour components such as triterpenoids and volatile oils which act on the peripheries of the body. The dried rhizome is quite hot from its concentration of pungent gingerols and acts centrally. The minerals present in ginger are iron, calcium, chromium, magnesium, sodium, potassium, zinc and phosphorous. It also contains vitamins such as vitamin A, thiamine, riboflavin, niacin and vitamin C.

16.5 Biological Activities of Ginger in Livestock and Poultry

16.5.1 Anti-inflammatory Effect

It contains some of the most potent anti-inflammatory fighting substances and is a natural powerful painkiller. In Ayurveda, ginger is reported to be useful in treating inflammation and rheumatism. *In vitro* experiments (Aktan *et al.*, 2006; Frondoza *et al.*, 2004) and several animal studies (Mustafa *et al.*, 1993; Ojewole *et al.*, 2006; Funk *et al.*, 2009) provide suggestive evidence that ginger and its active ingredients i.e. gingerols, shagoals, zingerone and diarylheptanoids have the capacity to decrease symptoms of inflammation-associated conditions such as osteoarthritis, muscle soreness, osteoporosis, rheumatoid arthritis, sore throat, toothache, joint and muscle pain. Ginger can also benefit those experiencing other diseases caused by or fuelled by inflammation such as obesity, diabetes, cancer and cardiovascular disease. Two *in vitro* studies point to potential benefits of ginger in alleviating neurological disorders such as Alzheimer disease (Kim *et al.*, 2007; Ghayur *et al.*, 2008). Another cell culture study demonstrated anti-inflammatory actions of ginger extract in mouse microglial cells (Jung *et al.*, 2009). This anti-inflammatory effect may be due in part to its inhibition of cyclooxygenase, inducible nitric oxide synthase and 5-lipoxygenase (5-LO) activities, as well as suppression of inflammatory prostaglandin and leukotriene biosynthesis (Kiuchi *et al.*, 1992) and interference in cytokine signalling (Jung *et al.*, 2009). The 5-lipoxygenase and cyclooxygenase enzymes are needed to convert arachidonic acid into prostaglandins and leukotrienes. Ginger is more effective than non-steroidal anti-inflammatory drugs (NSAID) without the adverse events reported such as gastric mucosal irritation and ulceration. Research has shown that ginger may provide migraine relief due to its ability to stop prostaglandins from causing pain and inflammation in blood vessels.

16.5.2 *Anti-diabetic Effect*

Abnormal metabolic products of aldose reductase enzyme are believed to be responsible for many diabetic complications. Ginger has been found to have 5 components which work as aldose reductase inhibitors (Kato *et al.*, 2006). It has been shown to possess anti-diabetic activity in a variety of animal studies. A study found that when rats were given ginger juice for 6 weeks, the risk for developing diabetes was reduced. The researchers found that treatment with ginger significantly increased insulin levels and decreased fasting glucose levels (Srinivasan, 2005). It is insulinotropic rather than hypoglycemic (Islam and Choi, 2008). Treatment with ginger also produced other favourable effects in diabetic rats, including decreases in serum cholesterol, triglycerides and blood pressure.

In streptozotocin (STZ)-induced diabetic rats, specific extracts of ginger lowered blood glucose, cholesterol and triglyceride levels and increased high-density lipoprotein cholesterol concentrations (Akhani *et al.*, 2004; Al-Amin *et al.*, 2006). Furthermore, dietary intakes of dried ginger (0.5-2.0% wt/wt) by STZ-treated diabetic rats was superior to the anti-diabetic actions of garlic (Islam and Choi, 2008). Similar results have been observed in other rodent models of hyperglycemia, hyperlipidemia and hyperinsulinemia, effects that in part may be due to 6-gingerol (Kadnur *et al.*, 2005; Ojewole *et al.*, 2006). *In vitro* studies using adipocytes point to gingerol as having insulin-sensitizing and glucose uptake-enhancing actions (Sekiya *et al.*, 2004). The zingiberone also produced lower blood glucose levels, body weight and parametrial adipose tissue weight in ovariectomized rats (Han *et al.*, 2008).

16.5.2 *Alleviation of Constipation and Diarrhoea*

The active components of ginger are reported to stimulate digestion, absorption, relieve constipation and flatulence by increasing muscular activity in the digestive tract (Stewart *et al.*, 1991). Ginger can enhance gastro-intestinal transport of a meal and can significantly inhibit serotonin-induced diarrhoea. Zingerone is likely to be the active constituent against enterotoxigenic *Escherichia coli* heat-labile enterotoxin-induced diarrhoea.

16.5.3 *Anti-emetic*

Ginger extracts and its constituents (gingerols, â-carotene, capsaicin and shogaols) demonstrate strong anti-emetic effects. Ginger is thought to act directly on the digestive tract and has been used for centuries for the treatment of nausea caused by motion sickness, morning sickness, seasickness, chemotherapy and surgery. It can increase gastric contractility, speeding up gastric emptying and therefore, increasing the gastro-intestinal transit time of meals, which can decrease the nausea (Chrubasik *et al.*, 2005). Animal experiments, suggest that ginger has anti-emetic activity, when nausea is induced by cisplatin or cyclophosphamide. There are several mechanisms which could explain the possible anti-emetic effects of ginger. In an animal model, it was demonstrated that 6-gingerol enhanced gastrointestinal transport (Yamahara *et al.*, 1990). This and other compounds of ginger have also been shown to have anti-hydroxy-tryptamine (HT) activity in isolated guineapig ileum. Galanolactone, another constituent of ginger, is a competitive antagonist at ileal 5-HT3 receptors. Thus, anti-emesis could be brought about by effects on the gastric system through 5-HT3 antagonism (Yamahara *et al.*, 1989; Huang *et al.*, 1991; Ghayur and Gilani, 2006). There may also be effects on the central nervous system. Two studies performed on rats have yielded contradictory results. The study done by Weidner and Sigwart (2001) concluded that ginger extract in doses of upto 1000mg/kg body weight administered to pregnant rats, during the early weeks of pregnancy and organogenesis, caused neither maternal nor foetal toxicity nor complications and was thus, safe during pregnancy. In contradiction, the study conducted by Wilkinson (2000) also performed on rats, concluded that ginger tea of upto 50g per litre posed no risk for maternal toxicity, but the embryonic loss in the treatment group was double that of the control group. Strangely, the surviving foetuses exposed to ginger were heavier and had more advanced skeletal development. In rodents, ginger extracts have been demonstrated to possess cholinergic agonist actions, muscarinic antagonist-like effects and anti-serotonin actions.

16.5.4 *Improvement of Asthama*

Ginger is approved by FDA as drug for asthama (Chang *et al.*, 1995). It is placed in FDA list of herbal drugs. The gingerol analogs through increasing heart output are beneficial for asthamatic patients.

16.5.5 *Anti-allergy Effect*

Ginger acts as anti-histamine and aids in the treatment of allergies. The ginger juice effectively suppresses hypersensitivity response produced in response to exogenic or endogenic allergens.

16.5.6 *Hypotensive Effects*

Findings from several animal studies suggest that ginger may have beneficial effects on blood pressure (Ali *et al.*, 2008). The mechanism for ginger's effect in lowering blood pressure may be mediated by inhibition of voltage-dependent calcium channels as well as by stimulating muscarinic receptors.

16.5.7 *Maintenance of Normal Blood Circulation*

Ginger contains chromium, magnesium and zinc which can help to improve blood flow, as well as help prevent chills, fever, and excessive sweat. It stimulates blood circulation throughout the body by powerful stimulatory effect on the heart muscle and by diluting blood. The improved circulation is believed to increase the cellular metabolic activity, thus contributing to the relief of cramps and tension.

16.5.8 *Anti-platelet Agent*

There are few investigations into ginger's capacity to alter blood clotting. Ginger reduced the formation of prostaglandins and thromboxane, thus lowering the clotting ability of the blood (Bordia *et al.,* 1997). Based upon *in vitro* inhibitory effects on thromboxane synthesis, the interactions between ginger and anti-thrombotic drugs including warfarin and aspirin have also been suggested.

16.5.9 *Treatment of Acid Reflux*

Rather than interfering with or removing stomach acid barrier (and thereby deactivating proteolytic enzymes and increasing risk of infection), ginger inhibits acid reflux and contains potent proteolytic enzymes.

16.5.10 *Anti-oxidative Property*

Ginger contains a number of antioxidants such as gingerols, gingerdiol, zingerone, gingerdione, shogaols, â-carotene, ascorbic acid, terpenoids, alkaloids and polyphenols such as flavonoids, flavones glycosides, rutin and several phenolic ketone derivatives. In case of water extracts of raw ginger, boiling results into reduction while roasting has no significant effect on the antioxidant levels. In case of acetone extracts, the antioxidant level of raw ginger is reduced on boiling and increased on roasting. Ginger extract can scavenge superoxide anion and hydroxyl radicals. It was found to inhibit the activity of lipoxygenase and peroxidation (Topic *et al.,* 2002). Ginger and some specific constituents have demonstrated antioxidant effects in several cell culture systems (Aeschbach *et al.,* 1994; Kim *et al.,* 2007). Furthermore, there are animal studies showing that ginger extracts and individual ginger constituents such as 6-gingerol can protect several tissues and organs against damage due to a variety of oxidation-inducing stressors (Ahmed *et al.,* 2000; Kim *et al.,* 2007). In rats, ginger extract also ameliorated acetic acid-induced ulcerative colitis, likely due to its anti-oxidant and anti-inflammatory actions (El-Abhar *et al.*, 2008). Quinone reductase is another important phase II detoxification enzyme which participates in the anti-oxidative process. Stimulation of the quinone reductase activity suggests that 5% ginger feeding can effectively counteract the oxidative damage in tissues of liver and lungs. Dietary oxidation stability and egg mass of laying hens responded to ginger powder supplementation in a dose-dependent manner. Optimum concentrations of ginger powder in the diet of laying hens were found to be 10 to 15 g/kg of diet for enhancing serum and egg yolk oxidative stability and 10 g/kg of diet for increasing egg mass (Zhao *et al.*, 2011).

The aqueous ginger extract showed an ameliorative effect against cadmium bromide induced hepatotoxicity and nephrotoxicity in adult female albino rats. Ginger also has been reported to decrease chemically induced liver toxicities in rodents (Yemitan and Izegbu, 2006; Verma and Asnani, 2007). This protective effect could be attributed to the fact that ginger contains high content of anti-oxidants that makes it a free radical scavenger. The anti-oxidant activity of ginger might be due to not only radical scavenging activity of anti-oxidants but also their affinity to the substrates. Barakat and Mohammed (2011) showed ability of ginger to protect the liver against the oxidative stress and hepato-cellular injury.

16.5.11 *Nephro-protective Activity*

Ginger extracts contain flavonoids which enhances the renal mitochondrial antioxidant system (Stoilova *et al.*, 2007). Dried fresh ginger juice extract along with gentamicin normalized the gentamicin-induced increase in serum creatinine, serum uric acid and blood urea nitrogen and serum urea levels. Ethyl acetate extract and dried fresh ginger extracts possess a significant nephro-protective activity and significantly protect rat kidneys from gentamicin-induced histo-pathological changes (Lakshmi and Sudhakar, 2010). Ethanol extract of ginger alone and in combination with vitamin E partially ameliorated cisplatin-induced nephrotoxicity as the activities of SOD, CAT, GPx and level of GSH were elevated and level of MDA declined significantly. This protection is mediated either by preventing the cisplatin-induced decline of renal antioxidant defense system (Ajith *et al.*, 2007). A study done on diabetic rats found that those rats given ginger had a reduced incidence of diabetic nephropathy.

16.5.12 *Cardio-protective Activity*

Based on evidence primarily from animal and *in vitro* studies, ginger may have beneficial effects towards cardiovascular disease through its multiple actions counteracting inflammation, hyperlipidemia, platelet aggregation and hypertension. It may have blood thinning and cholesterol lowering properties that may make it useful for treating heart disease. Animal studies suggest that ginger may also help alleviate problematic blood lipid levels associated with heart disease. Ginger reduces the level of cholesterol and lipid peroxidation following intake of cholesterol-rich diet. Animal studies suggest that ginger extract may provide some protection against statin-associated liver function abnormalities in hypercholesterolaemic patients.

16.5.13 *Effect on Microbes*

Ginger contains anti-bacterial, anti-viral, anti-fungal, anti-parasitic and anti-toxic properties. It inhibits gut pathogens while it encourages beneficial flora. Two natural antibiotics are found in ginger. In animal studies, ginger extracts exhibited the capacity to protect mice against infections caused by several microbes (Jageta *et al.,* 2003; Chen *et al.,* 2007). With regard to anti-fungal activity, ginger has been reported to be effective in some but not all studies (Ficker *et al.,* 2003; Pozzatti *et al.,* 2008). Likewise, reports on the capacity of ginger to suppress virus growth are inconsistent (Imanishi *et al.,* 2006; Schnitzler *et al.,* 2007). A study showed that ginger possessed *in vivo* anti-parasitic activity in sheep given at a dose of 1 to 3 g of ginger powder/kg body weight (Iqbal *et al.,* 2006).

Ginger can kill bacteria including *Salmonella* internally and topically as an antiseptic. It contains zingibain that dissolves parasites and their eggs. It was observed that the antimicrobial effect of plant extract varies from one plant to another in different researches carried out in different regions of the world. This may be due to many factors such as, the effect of climate, soil composition, age and vegetation cycle stage, on the quality, quantity and composition of extracted product, different bacterial strains. Moreover, different studies found that the type of solvent has an important role in the process of extracting.

Ginger showed stimulation activity on *Bacillus subtilis* (gram-positive bacteria) and *Candida albicans* (yeast). Ginger ethanolic extracts had no activity against *Bacillus spp., S. aureus* and *E. coli,* whereas

Sebiomo *et al.* (2011) found ginger ethanolic extracts inhibit the growth of *S. aureus* and *E. coli*. *Pseudomonas aeruginosa* was resistant to ethanolic extract of ginger. *In vitro* studies have shown that active constituents of ginger inhibit multiplication of colon bacteria. These bacteria ferment undigested carbohydrates causing flatulence. Ginger inhibits the growth of *Escherichia coli, Proteus* sp., Staphylococci, Streptococci and *Salmonella*. Ginger inhibits *Aspergillus* which produces aflatoxin, a carcinogen. Fresh ginger juice showed inhibitory action against *A. niger, S. cerevisiae, Mycoderma* sp. and *Lactobacillus acidophilus* at 4, 10, 12 and 14%, respectively at ambient temperatures. Ginger extracts and individual constituents have been reported in *in vitro* studies to suppress the growth of a variety of common infectious bacteria including *Staphylococcus aureus* and *Listeria monocytogenes* (Norajit *et al.*, 2007). 10-Gingerol was also able to enhance the antimicrobial efficacy of drugs in the treatment of drug-resistant enterococci (Nagoshi *et al.*, 2006). Gingerols and phenolic metabolites can inhibit growth of *Helicobacter pylori* and enhance the effectiveness of drugs targeting this bacterium, suggesting a new potential use of ginger in combating *H. pylori* and related gastrointestinal diseases. The combined treatment of antibiotics and ginger were tested for the control and treatment of *H. pylori* infections. The treatment was effective and was shown to inhibit *H. pylori* with synergistic or additive activity.

16.5.14 *Immuno-modulatory Effects*

Ginger promotes normal production of thromboxanes and leukotrienes which explains its action on the immune system as well as its ability to promote healthy circulation and inflammatory responses. Using ginger rhizome powder increased humoral immunity at 35th day in Ross 308 broilers. Adding 10 g/kg ginger rhizome powder improved the immune response to Newcastle disease vaccines (NDVB1). Nidaullah *et al.* (2010) observed that aqueous extract of ginger rhizome mixed in water plays better performance as immune stimulant against ND, infectious bronchitis (IB), infectious bursal disease (IBD) and coccidiosis. Ademola *et al.* (2009) observed that ginger at 1% caused significant decrease in white blood cells of chickens. Essential oil of ginger has a positive impact on the gut microflora. Tekeli *et al.* (2010) observed that supplemental ginger increased the number of lactic acid bacteria in the jejenum. Thayalini *et al.* (2011) found that, higher lactic acid content was observed with the supplementation of ginger.

16.5.15 *Prevents Cold and Flu*

Ginger has long been used as a natural treatment for colds, flu and stomach flu or food poisoning. The intake of ginger helps stimulate the secretion of mucus. Ginger is a natural decongestant. It seems to provide a measure of relief from cold symptoms by dilating constricted bronchial tubes. It's often included in herbal decongestant blends that are designed for sinusitis and other respiratory complaints.

16.5.16 *Anti-tumour Property*

The occurrence of induced gastric ulcer can be prevented by the ingestion of ginger extract. Roasted ginger used in the extract has a stronger anti-ulcer tendency than dry ginger. Ginger may be powerful weapon in the treatment of ovarian cancer. It inhibits cell growth and modulates angiogenic factor in ovarian cancer cells. The component 6-shogaol may also slow the growth of colorectal carcinoma cells. Animal studies show that gingerol inhibits carcinogenesis in the gastrointestinal tract, skin and mammary gland. The molecular targets involved in chemoprevention like the inhibition of NF-êB activation via impairing nuclear translocation, suppresses cIAP1 expression, increases caspase-3/7 activation, arrests cell cycle in G2 + M phases, up-regulates Cytochrome-c, Apaf-1, activates PI3K/Akt/I kappaB kinases IKK, suppresses cell proliferation and induces apoptosis and chromatin condensation. Ginger extract has demonstrated the capacity in numerous cancer cell culture systems to suppress cell proliferation and induce cell death (Shukla and Singh, 2007). Ginger supplemented rats had a significantly smaller number of tumours and cancer incidence in rats. In addition, supplemented rats had significantly less lipid oxidation and higher level of enzymatic and non-enzymatic anti-oxidants. The component 6-gingerol was found to be effective for inhibiting angiogenesis and may be useful in the treatment of tumours and other angiogenesis-dependent diseases. When mice were injected with 6-gingerol, the growth of cancerous melanoma cells was reduced. Ginger inhibits 5-LO enzymes and so prevent prostate cancer cells. It is beneficial to prevent constipation-related cancer, lung cancer. It is an effective anti-tumour agent in leukemia cells. Gingerols inhibited pancreatic cell growth, inhibited the growth of *H. pylori* associated with dyspepsia, peptic ulcer disease and the development of gastric and colon cancer. Ginger extract raises significantly the thymus index, spleen index, percentage of phagocytosis and thus, improves the immunologic function relating to tumours. Gingerol inhibits cell adhesion, invasion, motility and activities of breast cancer cell lines. It induces viability reduction (killed) gastric cancer cells. Due to its promotion of mucus secretion, ginger protects against the development of ulcers, unwanted holes in the lining of stomach. A ginger extract causes apoptosis of breast carcinoma cells. Ginger suppresses metastasis in any type of cancer cell including leukemic, skin, kidney, lung and pancreatic cancer cells.

16.5.17 *Effect on Gastro-intestinal Tract*

Ginger's effect on the digestive system is complex. The aromatic, spasmolytic and absorbent properties of ginger suggest that it has direct effects on gastrointestinal tract (GIT). Ginger has been reported to improve animals' nutrient digestion and absorption because of the positive effects on the gastric and pancreatic enzyme secretions (pancreatic lipase, intestinal lipase, disaccharidases, sucrase and maltase), bile secretion, enterokinesia and digestive enzyme activities (Patel and Srinivasan, 2000). The active components of ginger are reported to stimulate digestion, absorption, relieve constipation and flatulence by increasing muscular activity in the digestive tract. Ginger contains potent digestive enzymes, most notably the proteolytic enzyme, zingibain, which aid in digestion and the prevention of cramps. It also reduces total gastric juice volume as H_2-receptor antagonists (e.g., Zantac, Pepcid, Tagamet) do, but without disturbing pepsin-pH interaction. Ginger is often used to treat severe stomach ailments such as dyspepsia or colic. The shogoals and gingerols are believed to stimulate the flow of saliva, bile and gastric secretions, to neutralize stomach acids and tone the muscles of the digestive tract. Ginger also has been found to suppress gastric contractions and improve intestinal muscle tone and peristalsis. Ginger is taken generally to combat digestive problems and stomach related issues.

16.5.18 *Effect on Gastro-intestinal Tract*

Dietary supplementation of ginger powder improved laying performance. The optimum supplementation rate of ginger powder in the diet of laying hens appeared to be between 10 and 15 g/kg of diet (Zhao *et al.*, 2011). The supplementation of ginger powder increased (P<0.05) the serum and egg yolk anti-oxidant enzymatic activities of laying hens on d 35 and 70 and enhanced dietary oxidation stability in a dose-dependent manner.

16.5.19 *Protection against the Toxic Effect of Xenobiotics*

The stimulation of protective enzyme glutathione S-transferase (GST) due to ginger feeding in liver and lungs and to some extent in intestine and kidney indicates that ginger feeding can confer protection against the toxic effect of xenobiotics. The GST group of enzymes play a major role in the detoxification pathway and help in the conversion of reactive chemicals to non-reactive polar compounds which can be excreted from the body. Since liver is the major site of xenobiotic metabolism and transformation, stimulatory effect of ginger feeding on liver and intestine enzyme levels are significant.

16.6 *Potential Adverse Effects*

The ingestion of whole, fresh ginger has relatively few adverse effects, since it is not usually ingested in large enough amounts to cause any effects. Reported adverse effects may include stomach upsets or intestinal blockage. High doses of concentrated ginger in the form of powder or herbal tinctures can increase bleeding risk by decreasing platelet-aggregation and also increase stomach acid production, especially if taken with other herbs or medicines with the same effect. Very high doses of ginger powder can increase exfoliation of gastric epithelial cells which cause gastric irritation and can lead to gastric bleeding. Inhalation of ginger-dust may produce IgE-mediated allergy. Studies done on rats showed a higher risk for spontaneous abortions in pregnant rats being supplemented with ginger, possibly because of its blood-thinning properties. Doses of ginger tea up to 50g/L posed no risk for maternal health but the embryonic loss was more than double that of the control group. Contrastingly, the foetuses who survived the exposure to the ginger tea were significantly heavier than the controls and their skeletal development was more advanced (Chrubasik *et al.*, 2005). For ginger oil the acute oral LD50 (lethal dose 50%) in rats and the acute dermal LD_{50} in rabbits exceeded 5g/kg body weight (Chrubasik *et al.*, 2005). Heartburn, drowsiness, dizziness, headache, belching, gastrointestinal distress and diarrhoea, allergic reaction, dehydration and oral irritation were reported as side effects. Intake of large amounts of ginger may affect blood sugar levels.

16.8 Conclusions

Consumption of ginger has beneficial effects in heart disease, cancer, hypertension, obesity, diabetes, osteoarthritis and bacterial infections. The potential of ginger as a cancer protective agent is of growing interest. Other recent research relates to possible applica-tions of ginger in ulcerative colitis, liver disease, hypercholesterolaemia, as a radioprotective and as an antimicrobial. Now scientific evidences in favour of some of these beneficial properties are emerging which would support their consumption and use to ameliorate certain disorders.

References

Ademola SG, Farinu GO, Babatunde GM (2009) Serum lipid, growth and haematological parameters of broilers fed garlic, ginger and their mixtures. World J Agri Sci 5: 99-104

Aeschbach R, Loliger J, Scott B, et al (1994) Anti-oxidant actions of thymol, carvacrol, 6-gingerol, zingerone and hydroxytyrosol. Food Chem Toxicol 32: 31–36

Ahmad N, Sulaiman S, Mukti N, Murad N, Hamid N, Yusof Y (2006) Effects of ginger extract (*Zingiber officinale* roscoe) on anti-oxidant status of hepatocarcinoma. Indu Malaysian J Biochem Mol Biol 14: 7–12

Ahmed R, Seth V, Pasha S, Banarjee B (2000) Influence of dietary ginger (*Zingiber officinale* Rosc.) on oxidative stress induced by malathion in rats. Food Chem Toxicol 38: 443–450

Ajith TA, Nivitha V, Usha S (2007) *Zingiber officinale* Roscoe alone and in combination with alpha-tocopherol protect the kidney against cisplatin-induced acute renal failure. Food Chem Toxicol 45(6): 921–927

Akhani S, Vishwakarma S, Goyal R (2004) Anti-diabetic activity of *Zingiber officinale* in streptozotocin-induced type 1 diabetic rats. J Pharm Pharmacol 56: 101–105

Aktan F, Henness S, Tran V, Duke C, Roufogalis B, Ammit A (2006) Gingerol metabolite and a synthetic analogue capsarol inhibit macrophage NF-kappaB-mediated iNOS gene expression and enzymatic activity. Plant Med 72: 727–734

Al-Amin Z, Thomson M, Al-Qattan K, Peltonen-Shalaby R, Ali M (2006) Anti-diabetic and hypolipidaemic properties of ginger (*Zingiber officinale*) in streptozotocin-induced diabetic rats. Br J Nutr 96: 660–666

Ali BH, Blunden G, Tanira MO, Nemmar A (2008) Some phytochemical, pharmacological and toxicological properties of ginger (*Zingiber officinale* roscoe): A review of recent research. Food Chem Toxicol 46: 409–420

Barakat LAA, Maha MM (2011) Ginger, cumin and mustard seeds modulate Acetaminophen-induced acute hepatic injury in rats. J Appl Sci Res 7(9): 1368–1374

Bordia A, Verma SK, Srivastava KC (1997) Effect of ginger (*Zingiber officinale* Roscoe) and fenugreek on blood lipids, blood sugar and platelet aggregation in patients with coronary artery disease. Prostaglandins Leukot Essent Fatty Acids 56: 379

Chang DP, Chang JY, Wang FY, Chang JG (1995) The effect of chinese medicinal herb Zingiber rhizome extract on cytokine Secretion by human peripheral blood mononuclear cells. J Ethnopharmacol 48: 13–19

Chen J, Huang L, Wu S, Kuo S, Ho T, Hsiang C (2007) Ginger and its bioactive components inhibit enterotoxigenic *Escherichia coli* heat-labile enterotoxin-induced diarrhoea in mice. J Agric Food Chem 55: 8390–8397

Chrubasik S, Pittler MH, Roufogalis BD (2005) Zingiberis rhizome: A comprehensive review on the ginger effect and efficacy profiles. Phytomedicine 12: 684–701

El-Abhar H, Hammad L, Gawad H (2008) Modulating effect of ginger extract on rats with ulcerative colitis. J Ethnopharmacol 118: 367–372

Ficker C, Smith M, Akpagana K, *et al.* (2003) Bioassay-guided isolation and identification of anti-fungal compounds from ginger. Phytother Res 17: 897–902

Frondoza C, Sohrabi A, Polotsky A, Phan P, Hungerford D, Lindmark L (2004) An *in vitro* screening assay for inhibitors of pro-inflammatory mediators in herbal extracts using human synoviocyte cultures. *In vitro* Cell Dev Biol Anim 40: 95–101

Funk J, Frye J, Oyarzo J, Timmermann B (2009) Comparative effects of two gingerol-containing *Zingiber officinale* extracts on experimental rheumatoid arthritis (perpendicular). J Nat Prod 72: 403–407

Ghayur M, Gilani M (2006) Species differences in the prokinetic effects of ginger. Int J Food Sci Nutr 57: 65–73

Ghayur M, Gilani A, Ahmed T, *et al.* (2008) Muscarinic Ca(++) antagonist and specific butyrlcholinesterase inhibitory activity of dried ginger extract might explain its use in dementia. J Pharm Pharmacol 60: 1375–1383

Han L, Morimoto C, Zheng Y, Li W, Asami E, Okuda H, Saito M (2008) Effects of zingiberone on fat storage in ovariectomized rats. Yakugaku Zasshi 128: 1195–1201

Huang Q, Iwamoto M, Aoki S, Tanaka N (1991) Anti-5-hydroxytriptamine effect of galanolactone diterpenoid isolated from ginger. Chem Pharm Bull 39: 397–399

Imanishi N, Andoh T, Mantani N, *et al.* (2006) Macrophage-mediated inhibitory effect of *Zingiber officinale* Rosc., a traditional oriental herbal medicine, on the growth of influenza A/Aichi/2/68 virus. Am J Clin Med 34: 157–169

Iqbal Z, Lateef M, Akhtar M, Ghayur M, Gilani A (2006) *In vivo* anti-helminthic activity of ginger against gastro-intestinal nematodes of sheep. J Ethnopharmacol 106: 285–287

Islam MS, Choi H (2008) Comparative effects of dietary ginger (*Zingiber officinale*) and garlic (*Allium sativum*) investigated in a type 2 diabetes model of rats. J Med Food 11(1): 152–159

Jageta G, Baliga M, Venkatesh P, Ulloor J (2003) Influence of ginger rhizome (*Zingiber officinale* Rosc.) on survival, glutathione and lipid peroxidation in mice after whole body irradiation. Radiat Res 160: 584–592

Jung H, Yoon C, Park K, Han H, Park Y (2009). Hexane fraction of Zingiberis rhizoma crudus extract inhibits the production of nitric oxide and pro-inflammatory cytokines in LPS-stimulated BV2 microglial cells via the NFkappaB pathway. Food Chem Toxicol 47: 1190–1197

Kadnur S, Goyal R (2005) Beneficial effects of *Zingiber officinale* Roscoe on fructose-induced hyperlipidemia and hyperinsulinemia in rats. Indian J Exp Biol 43: 1161–1164

Kato A, Higuchi Y, Goto H, et al (2006) Inhibitory effects of *Zingiber officinale* Roscoe derived components on aldose reductase activity *in vitro* and *in vivo.* J Agric Food Chem 54: 6640–6644

Kim D, Kim J, Han Y (2007) Alzheimer's disease drug discovery from herbs: neuroprotectivity from beta-amyloid (1-42) insult. J Altern Complement Med 13: 333–340

Kim J, Kim Y, Na K, Surh Y, Kim T (2007) [6]-Gingerol prevents UVB-induced ROS production and COX-2 expression *in vitro* and *in vivo.* Free Radic Res 41: 603–614

Kiuchi F, Iwakami S, Shibuya M, Hanaoka F, Sankawa U (1992) Inhibition of prostaglandin and leukotriene biosynthesis by gingerols and diaryl heptanoids. Chem Pharm Bull 40: 387

Kiuchi F, Shibuya M, Sankawa V (1993) Inhibitors of prostaglandin biosynthesis from ginger. Chem Pharm Bull 30: 754

Lakshmi B, Sudhakar M (2010) Protective effect of *Zingiber officinale* on gentamicin-induced nephrotoxicity in rats. Int J Pharmacol 6: 58–62

Langner E, Greifenberg S, Gruenwald J (1998) Ginger: History and use. Adv Ther 15: 25

Larsen K, Ibrahim H, Khaw SH, Saw LG (1999) Gingers of Peninsular Malaysia and Singapore. Kota Kinabalu: Natural History Publication, pp. 135

Masuda Y, Kikuzaki H, Hisamoto M, Nakatani N (2004) Antioxidant properties of gingerol related compounds from ginger. Biofactors 21: 293–296

Mohdyusof YA, Sieh S, Murad NA, Wan Ngah WZ (2002) Anticancer effect of ginger extract (Zingiber officinale) on liver cancer cell lines. Malays J Biochem Mol Biol 7: 38-42

Mustafa T, Srivastava KC, Jensen KB (1993) Drug Development Report (9): Pharmacology of ginger, *Zingiber officinale*. J Drug Dev 6: 24

Mustafa T, Srivastava K, Jensen K (1993) Drug development report: pharmacology of ginger, *Zingiber officinale*. J Drug Devel 6: 25–89

Nagoshi C, Shiota S, Kuroda T, et al (2006) Synergistic effect of [10]-gingerol and aminoglycosides against vancomycin-resistant enterococci (VRE). Biol Pharm Bull 29: 443–447

Nidaullah H, Durrani FR, Ahmad S, Jan IU, Gul S (2010) APRN J Agri Biol Sci 5: 53

Norajit K, Laohakunjit N, Kerdchoenchuen O (2007) Anti-bacterial effect of five Zingiberaceae essential oils. Molecules 12: 2047–2060

Ojewole J (2006) Analgesic, anti-inflammatory and hypoglycemic effects of ethanolic extract of *Zingiber officinale* (Roscoe) rhizomes (Zingiberaceae) in mice and rats. Phytother Res 20: 764–772

Patel K, Srinivasan K (2000) Influence of dietary spices and their active principles on pancreatic digestive enzymes in albino rats. Nahrung 44: 42–46

Pozzatti P, Scheid L, Spader T, Atayde M, Santurio J, Alves S (2008) *In vitro* activity of essential oils extracted from plants used as spices against fluconazole-resistant and fluconazole-susceptible *Candida* spp. Can J Microbiol 54: 950–956

Schnitzler P, Koch C, Reichling J (2007) Susceptibility of drug-resistant clinical herpes simplex virus type 1 strains to essential oils of ginger, thyme, hyssop, and sandalwood. Anti-microbe. Agents Chemother 51: 1859–1862

Sebiomo A, Awofodu AD, Awosanya AO, Awotona FE, Ajayi AJ (2011) Comparative studies of antibacterial effect of some antibiotics and ginger (*Zingiber officinale*) on two pathogenic bacteria. J Microbiol Antimicrobials 3(1): 18–22

Sekiya K, Ohtani A, Kusano S (2004) Enhancement of insulin sensitivity in adipocytes by ginger. Biofactors 22: 153–156

Shukla Y, Singh M (2007) Cancer preventive properties of ginger: a brief review. Food Chem Toxicol 45: 683–690

Srinivasan K (2005) Plant foods in the management of diabetes mellitus: spices as beneficial anti-diabetic food adjuncts. Int J Food Sci Nutr 56(6): 399–414

Stewart J, Wood MJ, Wood CD, Mims ME (1991) Effects of ginger on motion sickness susceptibility and gastric function. Pharmacol 42: 111–120

Stoilova I, Krastanov A, Stoyanova A, Denev P, Gargova S (2007) Antioxidant activity of a ginger extract (*Zingiber officinale*). Food Chem 102: 764–770

Tapsell LC, Hemphill I, Cobiac L, Patch CS, Sullivan DR, Fenech M, Roodenrys S, Keogh JB, Clifton PM, Williams PG, Fazio VA, Inge KE (2006) Health benefits of herbs and spices: The past, the present, the future. Med J Aust 185: 4–24

Tekeli A, Kutlu HR, Celik L, Doran F (2010) Determination of the Effects of Z. officinale and Propolis Extracts on Intestinal Microbiology and Histological Characteristics in Broilers. Int J Poult Sci 9: 898

Thayalini K, Shanmugavelu S, Saminathan PM, Masidayu MS, Idayusni Y, Zianuddin H, Akmal CA, Wong HK (2011) Effect of ginger powder rhizome on homural immunity of broiler chickens. Mal J Anim Sci 14: 43

Topic B, Tani E, Tsiakitzis K, Kourounakis PN, Dere E, Hasenohrl RU, Hacker R, Mattern CM, Huston JP (2002) Enhanced maze performance and reduced oxidative stress by combined extracts of *Zingiber officinale* and gingko biloba in the aged rat. Neurobiol Aging 23: 135–143

Verma R, Asnani V (2007) Ginger extract ameliorates paraben induced bio-chemical changes in liver and kidney of mice. Acta Pol Pharm 64: 217–220

Weidner MS, Sigwart K (2001) Investigation of the teratogenic potential of a *Zingiber officinale* extract in the rat. Reproductive Toxicol 15: 75–80

Wilkinson JM (2000) Effect of ginger tea on the foetal development of Sprague-Dawley rats. Reproductive Toxicol 14(6): 507–512

Yamahara J, Huang QR, Li Y, Xu L, Fujimura H (1990) Gastro-intestinal motility enhancing effect of ginger and its active constituents. Chem Pharm Bull 38: 430–431

Yamahara J, Rong H, Iwamoto M, Kobayashi G, Matsuda H, Fujimura H (1989) Active components of ginger exhibiting anti-seratoninergic action. Phytother Res 3: 70–71

Yemitan OK, Izegbu MC (2006) Protective effects of *Zingiber officinale* (Zingiberaceae) against carbon tetrachloride and acetaminophen-induced hepatotoxicity in rats. Phytother Res 20: 997–1002

Young HY, Luo YL, Cheng HY, Hsieh WC, Liao JC, Peng WH (2005) Analgesic and anti-inflammatory activities of [6]-gingerol. J Ethnopharmacol 96: 207–210

Zhao X, Yang ZB, Yang WR, Wang Y, Jiang SZ, Zhang GG (2011) Effects of ginger root (*Zingiber officinale*) on laying performance and anti-oxidant status of laying hens and on dietary oxidation stability. Poult Sci 90: 1720–1727.

❑❑❑

Chapter 17

Peppermint (*Mentha piperita*)

K.Merina Devi[1] and Jyoti Palod[2]

[1] Department of Poultry Science, College of Veterinary Sciences, Assam Agricultural University, Guwahati, Assam, India, E-mail: merinadevi.90@gmail.com

[2] Department of Livestock Production Management, G B Pant University of Agriculture & Technology, Pantnagar, India

ABSTRACT

Pepper mint (*Mentha piperita*) is one of the oldest plants in the history that dates back to traditional medicine thousands years ago. Peppermint leaves contains menthol, p-menthone, menthofuran, terpene oxides, caffeic acid, flavonoids, polymeried polyphenols, carotenes, tocopherols, betaine, choline and tannins and other phytochemicals. In addition, it also contains major quantity of carvone, limonene, 1,8-cineole, linalool, etc. having a strong antibacterial and antioxidant activities. Compounds in peppermint like cineole, nerol, anethole, eugenol, caffeic acid, carvacrol, menthol, sabinene, etc. have antiseptic property. The essential oil of peppermint enhances digestive system by alleviating the disorders like anti-spasmodic, anti-bloat, ulcer, etc. and have profound effect such as anticancer, anaesthetic properties, etc., improves ascites and stimulated growth and immune system. The essential oil of peppermint also reduces the serum content of glucose, cholesterol and triglycerides in livestock and poultry.

Keywords: *Mentha piperita,* Menthol, Anti-oxidant, Anti-bacterial, Livestock, Poultry.

17.1 Introduction

The use of medicinal herbs in healing is as old as mankind itself. The utility of medicinal plants is a consequence of struggle against illnesses since many centuries owing to which man ultimately learned to obtain drugs from barks, seeds, fruit bodies, other parts of the plants, etc. Since time immemorial, people have wrangle to find medications to alleviate pain and cure different diseases. Scientific experiments were first documented on the antimicrobial properties of plant components in late 19th century (Zaika, 1975). In every successive century from the development of mankind and advanced civilizations, the healing properties of certain medicinal plants were identified, recorded, and imparted to the successive generations and more recent discoveries were made about the beneficial effects of such herbal plants which upgraded the old properties year after year. This interest primarily stems from the belief that medicines derived from plant are safe and dependable, compared with costly synthetic drugs that have adverse effects (Gordon and David, 2001). Since ancient times, herbs and their essential oils have been known for their varying degrees of antimicrobial activity (Juven *et al.*, 1994; Change, 1995). Structure of plants contains certain bio-active compounds *viz* alkaloids, bitters, bioflavonoids, flavonoids, glycosides, mucilage, saponins, tannins (Vandergrift, 1998), guinones, phenols, phenlic acids, coumarins, terpenoids, lectins, essential oil, polypeptides (Cowan, 1999), etc. Which are believed to act against microbes, insects, fungi and herbivores (Cowan, 1999). They also have the property to stimulate appetite and enhance feed intake (Abdel-Wareth and Lohakare, 2014), improve the endogenous digestive enzyme secretion, activate the immune responses of the body with less to strong antioxidant properties. Peppermint (*Mentha piperita*), known as one of the oldest plants in the history that dates back to traditional medicine thousands years ago. This medicinal plant has an aromatic fragrance, grows almost exclusively perennial, rarely annual and are widely distributed in many environments (Brickell and Cole, 2002). The peppermint plant is sterile in nature due to the reason that they are a hybrid of two other *Mentha* species *viz.* water mint (*M. aquatica*) and spearmint (*M. spicata*) and easily distinguished from spearmint by its menthol fragrance.

17.2 History of Peppermint

Peppermint was first described by Carl Linnaeous in 1753 and classified as a separate species (Linnaeous, 1753).The word 'Mint' comes from the Latin word *Mentha*, which is rooted in the Greek word *minthe*, exemplified in Greek mythology as Minthe, a river nymph in the Cocytus river who was transformed into a mint plant by Persephone who was jealous that her husband Pluto was showing affection to Minthe. While Pluto could not reverse the curse that his wifefling, he imparted Minthe with a sweet smell plant. The herb is popularly known as *Pudina* in many Indo-Aryan_ languages. In Spain and Central and South America, mint is generally familiar, as *Menta.* Mint is also known as Hierbabuena which means good herb in Central and South America. In Portugal, the herb is named as Hortela.

The remains of the peppermint were found in a bouquet in ancient Egyptian tomb as early as 1035-332 B.C. (Brown, 2015). Peppermint is thought to have originated in Northern Africa and the Mediterranean regions. The medicinal benefits were recorded since time immortal and there was a long history of cultivation of mint and has been used in cooking and herbal medicine since about 1500 B.C. In England, *Mentha pipperita.* L. was first recognized and published as a distinct species in 1696 and was admitted to the London Pharmacopoeia in I791 as *Mentha piperitissupore*. Peppermint was eventually introduced to Europe where it also became a popular culinary and medicinal herb. In India, the primary medical system of treatment called Ayurveda which has been known for nearly 5000 years ago, includes the used of diets and herbs while emphasizing the body, mind and spirit in disease prevention and treatment (Morgan, 2002).The Roman philosopher Pliny wrote that peppermint had property to stimulate appetite stirring and quoted "the mind and appetite to a greedy desire of food". And also added that mint binds around the head as a crown stimulates the mind and the soul. Greeks believes that mint have an aphrodisiac property and prohibits its consumption by soldiers in order to manage control. In European history, it was recorded that tea made from peppermint is used to treat indigestion, nausea, diarrhoea, colds, cramps and was traditionally offered to guests upon their arrival. Tea made from the mint leaves was believed to cure digestive upset. Cultivation of peppermint in the United States began shortly after 1816 in New York, gradually extended to Ohio, North India then to Michigan which eventually became the biggest producer, and finally to the Pacific North-west (Landing, 1969). Other countries which have produced peppermint include Japan, Germany, France, Italy. Russia, China and southern India. As early as 1938, Bulgaria stood the third rank in the world in terms of peppermint oil production. Today, India occupies the top place in exporting and producing highest quantity of peppermint oil in world (Srivastava, 2009). Gently, the medicinal usages of peppermint were diffused to every nook and corner of the world and hence, attain its popularity.

17.3 Taxonomy

The taxonomic classification of peppermint is listed below:

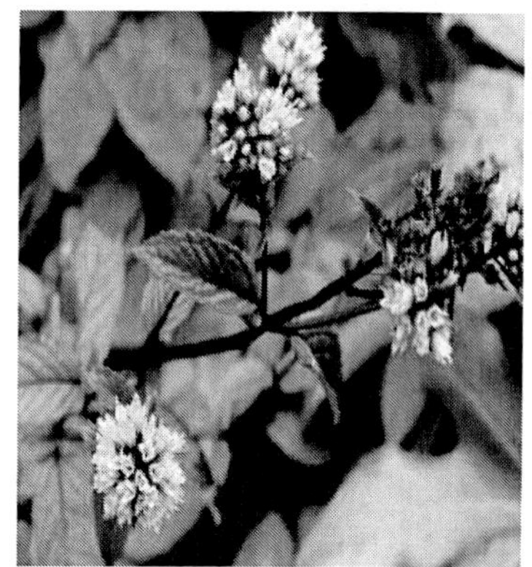

Kingdom	:	Plantae
Subkingdom	:	Tracheobionta
Superdivision	:	Spermatohyta
Phylum	:	Angiospermophyta
Class	:	Magnoliopsida
Order	:	Lamiales
Family	:	Lamiaceae
Genus	:	Mentha
Species	:	*Piperita*

17.4 Chemical Composition

Peppermint contains a large number of active ingredients which contributes to its medicinal properties. The active virtues of the mint depend on the abundant volatile oil that contains a wide variety of terpenes and terpenoids, which are usually found in concentration ranges from 0.5% to 4.6%. The volatile oil was demonstrated to contain a hydrocarbon thymol and higher oxygenated compound (Galib, 2010). The active component found in the leaves and flowering tops of peppermint plant is the menthol (molecular formula of menthol is $C_{10}H_{20}O$) which is the alcoholic constituents responsible for the characteristic quality producing cooling effect besides its medicinal properties. Peppermint leaves contains about 0.5–4% mint essential oil, that is composed of 25–78% menthol, 14–36% menthone, 1.5-10% isomenthone. Peppermint leaves contains 2.8–10% menthyl acetate, 3.5–14% cineol (Grigoleit and Grigoleit, 2005).

Menthol is oxidised to menthone in presence of oxidising agents such as chromic acid or dichromate, however, in certain conditions the oxidation can go further and break open the structural ring. Secondly, menthol is readily dehydrated and yield the principal compound namely, 3-menthene in presence of 2% sulphuric acid. Pulegone is a central intermediate in the bio-synthesis of menthol which is regarded as the most significant component of peppermint essential oil. Depending upon environmental conditions, this branch point metabolite may be reduced to menthone route to menthol, by pulegone reductase, or oxidized to menthofuran, by menthofuran synthase (Scavroni *et al.*, 2005) concluded that peppermint plant cultivated in presence of biosolid favoured menthofuran formation.

Besides being a highly potent antimicrobial substance mainly due to menthol (63 %) and p-menthone (19.5%), other pharmacologically active compounds includes ketones, monoterpenes (and the class of such chemicals are collectively called as sesquiterpenes), menthofuran, and terpene oxides (Inouye *et al.*, 2001; Kêdzia, 2007) and bitter substances, caffeic acid, flavonoids (12%), polymeried polyphenols (19 %), carotenes, tocopherols, betaine, choline and tannins (Shimade *et al.*, 1992; Karuza *et al.*, 1996; Sokovic *et al.*, 2009), etc. In addition, it also contains major quantity of carvone (67.3 %), limonene (13.5 %), 1,8-cineole (5.4 %), linalool (2.8 %), etc. indicating a strong antibacterial and antioxidant activities (Durrani *et al.*, 2008). According to the book, "Healing Herbal Tea", it was published that besides volatile oils of peppermint, it contains the following constituents viz. beta-carotene, vitamin B complex, falcanoid (lutein, rutin), resin, luteolin and romaine acid various methyl esters, particularly methyl acetate which imparts familiar minty aroma. Concentration of methyl acetate is greater when the plant is grown in areas with long, warm and bright summer days and adds characteristic flavour to mint. The composition of menthol and peppermint essential oil is significantly differ depending upon its availability, climatic conditions, latitude and maturity of the plant.

17.5 Nutritive Value of Dried Peppermint (as-fed basis)

Nutrient	Percentage	Nutrient	Percentage
Dry matter	92.12	Total ash	11.0
Crude protein	25.0	Calcium	1.97
Crude fibre	14.60	Phosphorus	0.31
Ether extract	2.40		

(Khempaka *et al.*, 2015)

17.6 Pharmacological Effects

In 1704, Ray, in his famous publication *Historia Plantarum* explained that peppermint designated as *M. Palustris* considered as an exceptionally superior mint for treating "stomach weakness" and diarrhoea. By 1721, peppermint leaves had gained popularity and accepted officially in the *London Pharmacopoeia*, although spearmint was still the medicinal mint of choice. In the year 1789, *The Edinburgh New Dispensatory* recommended that leaves of "Aqua *Menthe sativa*" (spearmint water) heated over low flame with water 3 times its weight, considered as a remedy for strengthening a weak stomach and curing vomiting proceeding from cold viscous phlegm. The actual commercial cultivation of the plant was reported to start about 1750 at Mitcham. Surrey in London (Holly, 2010). In 1848, the *U.S. Dispensatory* called peppermint as "a very grateful aromatic stimulant" and recommended it for alleviating nausea, allaying spasmodic pains, evacuating gas, and also significantly use for covering the taste of medicines. The fresh mint plant as a whole was believed as a remedy for curing cholera in children. Certain pharmacological effects of peppermint are listed below:

17.6.1 *Carminative Effect*

Carminative activity of peppermint refers to the ability of peppermint to relax the lower esophageal sphincter which leads to release gas pressure in the stomach (Pizzorno, 1999). The mechanism of action of peppermint is not well studied but it is believed that the components such as carvacrol, thymol and menthol content of peppermint have combine effects to release intestinal gaseous by relaxing the esophageal sphincter, alleviate symptoms of bloat and by facilating gas eructation. The mechanism of peppermint as carminative is related to a local stimulatory effect of essential oil on the GIT. As studied by Harries *et al.* (1978), Smerville *et al.* (1984), the carminative effect of peppermint is related to its anti- foaming properties and antispasmodic effects. The carminative effect of peppermint essential oil has been linked to the relief of flatulence (Martindale, 1989). Now-a-days, peppermint capsule are available that have been designed to dissolve in intestine insteadof in stomach, thus directly acting to the local site and improve digestion avoiding typical phenomena of flatulence or bloating related to malabsorption of fats.In other words, mint oil causes relaxation of the lower esophageal sphincter and equalization of intragastric and intraesophageal pressures inside the body (Mills and Bone, 2000).

17.6.2 *Anti-spasmodic Effect*

In the *Ebers Papyrus*, an ancient Egyptian medical text dating to 1550 BC, mint is listed as calming to stomach pains. Peppermint exhibits anti-spasmodic byactivation of sensory neurons of transient receptor potential (TRP) channels in particular melstatin8 (TRPM8) (Fareo and Grundmann, 2013). In a study conducted by Papathanasopoulos *et al.* (2013) further explained the mechanism behind this effect and added that the influx of Ca2+ ion influx through the TRPM8 channels expressed in dorsal root ganglia, sensory neurons, vagal afferent neurons, gastric fundus, small intestine, colon, etc. was induced by menthol. At specific dose of peppermint oil, 0.1-0.24ml, when administered topically (intraluminal) or orally is enough to provoke antispasmodic effect (Grigoleit and Grigoleit, 2005). The spasmolytic property of peppermint has been established against many convulsant drugs, including acetylcholine, histamine, serotonin etc. Essential oils of peppermint, ethanol extracts and the flavonoids content of peppermint leaf have shown antispasmodic property *in vitro* study (ESCOP, 1997). Peppermint is widely used in curing various intestinal diseases like irritable bowel syndrome by inhibiting hypercontractibility of intestinal smooth muscle, therefore, maintaining muscles tonacity. Recently, enteric coated peppermint oil capsule is available for curing IBS in juvenile.The enteric coated peppermint capsules were found to dissolve in colon and gelatin coated peppermint capsules in human stomach. To be effective in the treatment of spastic colon syndromes, the oil must reach colon in unmetabolized state (Somerville *et al.,* 1984). In 1996, in German double-blind placebo controlled trial, 45 subjects suffered from IBS were treated with enteric coated peppermint capsules and concluded that there was a significant improvement of the pain symptoms with 89.5%.The administration of peppermint oil decreased the number of deudenal contractions and contraction amplitudes (Micklefield *et al.,* 2000) reduces painful muscle spasm in patients undergoing endoscopy. The antispasmodic effects are the most desirable in lower small intestine and colon as essential oil acts by local mechanism. Another source claimed that intracolonic administration of peppermint oil has shown a significant reduction of spasmolytic effect (Asao *et al.,* 2003).

17.6.3 *Antioxidant Effect*

Peppermint oil and its constituent such as menthone and isomenthone present antioxidant property. Mint composes numerous chemical compounds which are antioxidant, disease preventing and health promoting properties. The antioxidant activity of the essential oil and extracts of peppermint was analysed by its ability to scavenging 2,2-diphenyl-1-picrylhydrazyl stable radicals (DPPH) by using method described previously (Shimada *et al.*, 1992). In addition of the above, peppermint is a rich source of antioxidant vitamins viz. vitamin A, beta carotene, vitamin C and vitamin E. Total antioxidant strength (ORAC) of fresh peppermint herb is recorded to be 13,978 μmol TE/ 100g. The manganese and copper contents of the peppermint works as co-factors for the anti-oxidant enzyme superoxide dismutase. Various research works have been conducted on the antioxidant properties of peppermint on poultry and the results come out with an appreciating results (Khempaka *et al.*, 2013).

17.6.4 *Choleretic Effect*

The choleretic property of peppermint was contributed by the active ingredients like flavanoids (Lucida and Wallace, 1998), menthol and other related terpenes. A drug, Rowachol (a mixture of six cyclic monoterpenes menthol, pinene, menthone, borneol, cineol and camphene)were reported to treat cholesterol bile in gallbladders and bile ducts (Ellis and Bell, 1981).The components have the ability to stimulate liver by enhancing the release of bile duct,thereby facilitates digestion. The production of bile in liver is enhanced by peppermint oil and leaf based falconoid to a very significant degree. Some mono-terpenes like mentholand limoneneinhibit hepatic 3-hydroxy-3-methylglutaryl (HMG) CoA- reductase activity (Clegg *et al.*, 1980) which in return reduces cholesterol level in serum.

17.6.5 *Intestinal Relaxation Effect*

Relaxing property of tannin, antispasmodic ability of menthol has soothing effect upon the lining and muscles of intestine and colon and alleviates cases like diarrhoea, spastic colon, etc.

17.6.6 *ExternalAnalgesic Effect*

The analgesic properties of menthol are mediated through a selective activation of ê-opioid receptors (Galeottia *et al.*, 2002). Menthol has been found to participate in the synergistic excitation of GABA receptors and sodium ion channels resulting to analgesia (Farco and Grundmann, 2013). In 1879, it was first published in the British Medical Journal lancet, the use of peppermint oil as an anodyne or analgesic to cease headache.The external analgesic and counterirritant property of peppermint oil is contributed by its menthol content. When peppermint oil or menthol is applied externally, it stimulates nerves that receive cold, dilates blood vessels (Eccles, 1994; Wasner *et al.*, 2004) causing sensation of coolness and simultaneously alleviates pain sensation. This effect has been used to aid penetration of topical drugs; higher diffusion of tetracaine has been demonstrated with menthol-enhanced gel (Liu *et al.*, 2005). Now-a-days, in certain commercially available topical musculo-skeletal products the sensory effects of menthol are incorporated (Kraemer *et al.*, 2005).Thus, it is used in treatment of rheumatic and muscular pain, headache, neck and back pain, sore throat, etc. On hairless mice, menthol (1-5% w/v) enhances the absorption of cortisone, mannitol, indomethacin, morphine hydrochloride, & propranolol (Katayama *et al.*, 1992; Morimoto, 1993; Kunta *et al.*, 1997). In human data, menthol moderates oral sensations of warmth and coldness. In further explanation, at low concentrations, topical application of menthol causes a cooling sensation, while in high concentrations it has the ability to cause irritation and local anaesthetic effects (Eccles, 1994). Adam *et al.* (2006) demonstrates the combined effect of peppermint and caraway which regulate post-inflammatory visceral hyperalgesia in rat. Menthol has been found to participation of synergistic excitation of GABA receptors and sodium ion channels resulting to analgesia (Farco and Grundmann, 2013).

17.6.7 *Emmenagogue Effect*

Emmenogogues are the substances which provokes a normal menstrual function in female. Peppermint is categorized as one of such substances which greatly relieves cramping and pain that accompany the process (Sara, 2013).

17.6.8 *Cholelithiasis, Hypocholesterolemic and Hypoglycaemic Effects*

Researchers have demonstrated cholelithiaisis effect of peppermint is due to the formula containing menthol and terpenes (menthone, pipene, borneol, cineol and camphene) which have the efficacy of preventing and dissolving gallstones (Ellis and Bell, 1981). These mentioned above compounds reduce bile cholesterol levels and simultaneously increases bile acid and lecithin concentrations in the gallbladder and thereby dissolves gallstones and ureteric stones (Srivastava, 2009). The hypocholesterolemic effect of mint plants were also demonstrated by different researchers in laying hens (Abdel and Lohakare, 2014; Devi *et al.*, 2017). The herb contains no cholesterol; however, it is rich in essential oils, vitamins and dietary fiber which helps to control blood cholesterol and blood pressure. Also, as the herb is an excellent source of minerals like potassium, it maintains normalheart rate and blood pressure. Barbalho *et al.* (2011) reported the hypoglycaemic property of peppermint supplemented in livestock animal. According to them, the offspring from diabetic dam treated with peppermint showed significant decrease in glucose level. Also, the same effect of peppermint was also reported by Khamisabadi *et al.* (2015) by feeding an extract of peppermint in broiler chicken.

17.6.9 *LocalAnesthetic Effect*

The local anaesthetic effect of menthol using a conjunctival reflex test in rabbit was demonstrated by Galeotti *et al.* (2001). According to the study, there was an increased number of stimuli necessary to induce conjunctival reflex in swiss albino mice.The administration of ethanolic extract of peppermint inhibited acetic acid induced analgesic activity. Menthol has been found to participation of synergistic excitation of GABA receptors and sodium ion channels resulting to analgesia (Farco and Grundmann, 2013).

17.6.10. *Antiviral Effect*

Peppermint is also found to have antiviral and fungicidal activity (Chaumont and Senet, 1978). Menthol is virucidal against influenza, herpes and other viruses. Aqueous extracts of peppermint leaves demonstrated significant antiviral activity against Influenza A, Newcastle disease, *Herpes simplex, Vaccinia,* Semliki Forest and West Nile viruses in egg and cell culture system (Herrmann and Kucera, 1967). The tannin content of the herb has an affinity for Newcastle virus and mumps virus; and a non-tannin fraction called polyphenolshave an antiviral effects against herpes simplex. Another source suggests that the monoterpenes and phenols present in peppermint essential oils possess noticeable anti-microbial, anti-fungal and antiviral activity.

17.6.11. *Antifungal Effect*

Separate groups of researchers (Pattnaik *et al.*, 1996) demonstrated that peppermint is found to contain both fungistatic and fungicidal effects. *M. piperita* has been shown to possess strong anti-fungal activity, even when compared to commercial fungicide bifonazole (Mimica-Dukie *et al.,* 2003). The fungicidal activity of peppermint oil when used in combination with salt and heat (Inouye *et al.*, 2007) acts against *Trichophytonmentagrophytes*, this activity is similar to lavender and clove oil. The fungicidal actions of menthol and peppermint oil are against *Candida albicans, Aspergillus albus* and *Dermatophyticfungi* (Janssen, 1986), *A. niger, Alternariaalternata* and *Fusarium sp.*, etc. (Aqil *et al.*, 2001). Moderate antifungal property of peppermint was also observed against *Aspergillus niger, Aspergillus candidus, Rhizopus-stolonifer, Botrytis cinerea, Penicillin species, Fusariumculmorum* (Braun and Cohen, 2015) but the herb was reported to have high antifungal activity against *Candida albicans* (Braun and Cohen, 2015). The chemical responsible for this action was mainly contributed by the active ingredient, menthone (Sokovic *et al.*, 2009). At different concentrations of peppermint oil, about 85-90% Aflatoxin B production can be inhibited when evaluated activities against *Aspergillus parasiticus* and *Aspergillus flavus* (peppermint oil, about 85-90% Aflatoxin B production can be inhibited when evaluated activities against *Aspergillus parasiticus* and *Aspergillus flavus* (Bluma *et al.*, 2008).

17.6.12. *Antibacterial Effect*

Peppermint oils are regarded as natural oils available with highest antibiotic property so far tested. Peppermint oil contains not only the significant antibacterial activity (Mimica-Dukie *et al.*, 2003) but also the juice provokes the same effect (Braun and Cohen, 2015). Antibacterial activity of peppermint may likely to be associated with a high concentration of menthol (ether and chloroform extracts), phenols or flavanoids (chloroform and ethyl acetate extracts) but a synergistic effect of the other constituents of peppermint oil cannot be ruled out.Peppermint oil and menthol have moderate antibacterial effects against both Gram-positive and Gram-negative bacteria (Pattnaik, 1996; Moleyar and Narasimham, 1992). Peppermint extracts are bacteriostatic against *Streptococcus thermophilus* and *Lactobacillus bulgaricus* (Bayoumi, 1992), *Streptococcus pyrogens, Streptococcus aureus, Streptococcus pyrogens, Serratiamarcescens, E.coli* and *Mycobacterium avium* (Gotshall, 1949), also inhibit *Salmonella enteritidis, Listeria monocytogens* and also many other strains of *Micrococcus flavus*and *Shigellasonnei* (Minica-Dukie *et al.*, 2003), *Helicobacter pylori, E.coli* (Mohsenzadeh, 2007) and other gram positive and gram negative bacteria. Peppermint was also recorded to inhibit the intestinal bacterial induced production of methanethiol (MeSH), hydrogen sulphide in pig large intestine.The candy prepared from peppermint and other such substances have found to contain less micro-organisms, due to the germicidal properties of its flavour.

17.6.13. *Diaphroretic Effect*

Diaphroretic property of peppermint is associated with the ingredients called menthol. It is used in the treatment of common cold, flu like symptoms, etc. reducing body temperature by means of sweat evaporation. The ability of menthol the well-known cooling sensation it provokes when inhaled, eaten, or applied to the skin (Eccles, 1994). Another source claims that peppermint has antipyretic and antiulcer properties due to the presence of Azulene, residue of peppermint oil (Lucida and Wallace, 1998). Azulene upon distillation has a marked antipyretic action. At dose rate 0.1 gm/kg, Azulene injected intramuscularly, was effective against hot water burns on the ear of a rabbit.

17.6.14. *Antitussive Effect*

Menthol is available in a variety of non-prescription products (e.g. chest rubs, inhalations, lozenges, syrups) for the treatment of colds and related congestion and cough. A decrease in cough was demonstrated in children, when inhalation of menthol was compared with placebo (Houghton and Beardsmore, 1998). The combine properties of antitussive effect of peppermint is contributed thymol, luteolin, cineole, carvacrol and also soothing and antispasmodic properties of menthol, etc. are useful to relief cough, respiratory distress symptoms such as asthma, pharyngitis, bronchitis, etc. by clearing and opening the respiratory passage. Menthol inhalation can cause a subjective nasal decongestant effect without any objective decongestant action (Eccles, 1994). In lozenges, the main action of menthol appears to be a subjective sensation of improved nasal airflow (Eccles, 1994). In vitro data, menthol vapour lowered the surface tension on synthetic surfactant films and menthol may affect lungs surface tension and lungs function (Zanker, *et al.*, 1980).

In guinea-pigs who received a cough-inducing citric acid challenge, menthol vapour significantly decreased cough in a dose-dependent fashion (Laude *et al.*, 1994). It was shown that the mixture of aromatic oils including menthol applied as a chest rub significantly reduced citric acid-induced cough for 30 and 60 minutes after administration (Zanker *et al.*, 1980).

17.6.15. *Fly Repellent*

Peppermint oil has a high concentration of natural pesticides, mainly polygone and menthone (Krieger, 2001) which acts as fly repellents. Head lice (*Pediculus humanusvarcapitis*) were successfully treated with peppermint oil (Canyon and Speare, 2007). A combined lotion incorporating 5% peppermint oil and 5% eucalyptus oil in 50% ethanol also act against head lice (Gonzalez Audino *et al.*, 2007). *Giardia trophozoites* were inhibited by peppermint extracts (Vidal *et al.*, 2007). Peppermint oil was recorded to show moderate effect against *Culexpipiens* (Erler *et al.*, 2006) and the menthol and its derivatives also have act as moisquitocidal against *Culex quinquefasciatus, Aedesaegypti, Anopheles tessellates* (Samarasekera *et al.*, 2008) etc. In pigs and goats, the aqueous extracts of peppermint is used against GI nematodes (Lans *et al.*, 2007). Besides anti-nematodal property, peppermint exerts antigiardial effect. The antigiardial property of dichlormethane extracts of peppermint *in-vitro* condition is mediated by causing alterations on the plasma membrane surface of parasite and inhibiting its adhesion (Vidal *et al.*, 2007). In comparison with other essential oils of plant having high levels of phenolic compounds, peppermint has weaker anti-giardial effect. The anthelmentic activity of peppermint when used *in vivo* has no significant result.

17. 6.16. *Antiseptic Effect*

Compounds in peppermint like cineole, nerol, anethole, eugenol, caffeic acid, carvacrol, menthol, sabinene, etc., have antiseptic property. It produces a sense of relief and freshness and thus, decreases itching sensation.

17.6.17. *Skin Disease Treatment*

Mint essential oils are generally used externally for treating antipruritic, rubefacient, astringent, antiseptic and anti-microbial purposes for the treatment related to neuralgia, myalgia headches and migraines (Hendriks, 1998). Menthol enhances the efficacy of ibuprofen in topical applications via vasodilation, which reduces skin barrier function (Brain *et al.*, 2006). Peppermint has capacity to balance the pH levels of the skin. This property balances the production of excessive oils in the skin, thereby reducing overall acne and breakouts. Peppermint water has been studied for prevention of nipple cracks in breast-feeding women (Melli *et al.*, 2007). In addition, peppermint is a rich source of Vitamin A and vitamin C and contains folates and omega 3 fatty acids which help in fighting sun related problems like sun tan and sun burn.

17.6.18. *Anti-tumour Effect*

Peppermint is a potential anti-cancer agent. It contains perillyl alcohol, a phytonutrient, which is known to stop tumours growth in pancreas, mammary, skin, colon, lungs and liver. Vitamin C content in peppermint is the main water soluble anti-oxidant which significantly decreases the level of free radicals causingcell damage and also performs a moderate role in decreasing colon cancer. Beta carotene and other cartenoids have also shown to reduce the risk of developing colon and rectal cancer. Cartenoids are also known to increase cell differentiation and protect the cells against carcinogenic chemicals that could damage DNA. It was also found to reduce the incidence and multiplicity of benzo[α]pyrene-induced lung carcinogenicity and mutagenicity (Samarth *et al.*, 2006). Menthol was found to synergize with vitamin D in blocking the growth of prostate cancer cells by cooperatively modulating expression of bcl-2 and p21 proteins (Park *et al.*, 2009).

17.6.19. *Anti-inflammatory Effect*

Peppermint contains menthol which has vasodilatory effects that stimulates capillary dilation and dilates the constricted blood vessels. This action causes skin redness by drawing blood from deeper tissues and organs, thereby helps to relieves skin congestion and inflammation, also it was used to prevent headache and migraine. Mint oil (oil obtained from *Menthaspicata*) also inhibits the inflammatory consequences of lipopolysaccharide (LPS), including inhibition of interleukin-1 (IL-1), prostaglandin E2 (PGE2), leukotriene B4 (LTB4) production by LPS-stimulated human monocytes.

17.6.20. *Astringent and Anti-enemetic Effect*

Peppermint was reported to contain strong astringent and decongestive actions which alleviate stuffiness and catarrh. In September 1997, according to the Journal of Advanced Nursing, inhalation of peppermint oil vapour significantly reduced post-operative nausea and the requirement for pharmacologic antiemetics following gynaecologic surgery (Tate, 1997). An allosteric effect of menthol and peppermint oil on the 5-HT $_3$ receptor may explain its antiemetic action; however, the effect was weak and may not be clinically relevant (Heimes *et al.*, 2011).

17.6.21. *Dyspepsia Treatment*

Peppermint oil alone and in combination with other herbs was more effective than placebo in reducing symptoms of dyspepsia in adults and children (Madisch *et al.*, 2004; Campo, 2005). Gastric emptying was accelerated by peppermint oil added to a test meal (Inamori *et al.*, 2007). Also, the leaves of peppermint or its oil were recorded to alleviate abdominal pain and dyspepsia. The suspension of barium sulphate and peppermint oil eliminated the residual spasm in the patients undergoing double contrast barium enema examination (Asao *et al.*, 2003).

17.6.22. *Neuro-psychiatic Effects*

Peppermint oil blocks smooth muscle contraction induced by serotonin and substance. In frogs, menthol non-competitively blocked neuromuscular transmission (Futami, 1984). The combination of peppermint oil, eucalyptus oil and ethanol have cognitive performance and had a muscle relaxing and mentally relaxing effect, but had little influence on pain sensitivity. Peppermint oil and ethanol exerted a significant analgesic effect and reduction in sensitivity to headache (Goebel, 1994). According to researchers, the vasodilatory effect of peppermint helps in dilation of constricted blood vessels and thus it is used as a common trigger of headches and migraines.

17.6.23. *Endocrine Effects*

Certain researches reported that there was a statistically significant increase in the secretion of endocrine hormonesby peppermint (Robbers *et al.*, 1999). Akdogan *et al.* (2004) also explained in his theory that the tea prepared from peppermint have a significant effect in enhancing the hormonal levels of Follicle Stimulating Hormone and Luteinising Hormone; also noticeably minimizes the total testosterone levels in rats.

17.6.24. *Effect on Production Performances*

Laying birds fed with peppermint in various form (dried powder, leaves, extract, etc.)either alone or in combination with some other plants was recorded to enhance the performance *et al.* percentage, eggshell thickness and Haugh unit of hens (Abdel and Lohakare, 2014). Similarly, when the same herb when added to the broiler birds resulted better performance in terms of body weight gain, feed conversion ratio, dressing per cent (Galib, 2010) and certain bio-chemical parameters (Abdel and Lohakare, 2014).

17.6.25. *Effect on Blood Parameters*

There is limited literature showing the effect of peppermint on haematological parameters. In animal, peppermint essential oil in combination with chromium picolinate or peppermint alone reduced the serum concentration of glucose and triglycerides in broiler birds. The mechanism may be associated with the antioxidant properties of peppermint and chromium picolinate (Akbari and Torki, 2014).

17.6.26. *Other Effects*

Experiments conducted in mice explained and conclusion of those experiments says that spray-dried peppermint infusion has been recorded to be a weak diuretic and also shown a weak sedative property (Della *et al.*, 1990). Another well known action of peppermint extracts is that it alleviates the side effects of arsenic induced hepatopathy (Sharma *et al.*, 2007). According to new research, peppermint oil exhibits more inhibitory actions against acetyl-cholinesterase and butyrycholinesterase than activity employed by individual components of oil (Orhan *et al.*, 2008).

The use of peppermint on a daily basis results improper absorbed of the drugs like oral anticholinergics, tetracycline derivatives, phenothiazines, digoxin, phenytoin, isoniazid and warfarin. The urinary excretion of alkaline drugs like quinidine or amphetamines, may be inhibited by the antacid nature of the herb (peppermint). The analgesic property of this herb may be reduced or even eliminated with the administration of phenobarbital, p-chlorophenylalanine and cyproheptadine HCl. Conversely, the CNS-depressant tendency of this analgesic may be potentiated by chlorprothixene hydrochloride, haloperidol, and tranquilizers. Peppermint oil is also reported to use in construction and plumbing to test for the tightness of pipe lines and disclose leaks by its odour (Kains, 1912). Peppermint is also widely used in the treatment of toothache, mastitis in animal (Archuleta, 2012) and ascites or anti-bloat (Akbari *et al.*, 2015). Peppermint itself being anti-inflammatory, astringent and vulnerary, it is used in curing of external haemorrhoids. Peppermint possesses various aromatic substances that offers a strong and exceptional flavour. Menthol can ensconce halitosis by stimulating secretion of saliva and check odour causing bacteria. Also, treats xerostomia, dry mouth, teeth decay and gingivitis.Peppermint oil extract is effective in preventing the development of biofilm that contributes to cavities.

17.7 Peppermint Interactions

Peppermint interacts with many compounds. Antacids may compromise the enteric coating of some commercially available peppermint oil capsules. H2-receptor antagonists and proton pump inhibitors may interact in the same manner.The manufacturers of certain enteric-coated peppermint oil preparations suggest that enteric coated peppermint oil should not be taken at the same time with the indigestion remedies (antacids) because there may be rise in pH caused by antacids. This may cause premature dissolution of the enteric coating and release of the peppermint oil in the stomach which in turn increases the risk of heartburn.

Menthol content of peppermint slightly delays the absorption of caffeine (Gelal *et al.*, 2003). Peppermint oil may influence metabolism of felodipine via inhibition of CYP3A4, elevating felodipine plasma concentrations and increasing the pharmacologic effects and adverse reactions such as light-headedness, headache, and flushing. Peppermint oil 600 mg in water increased the area under the curve (AUC) of felodipine 40% (Dresser *et al.*, 2002). However, a study claims that menthol have no effect on felodipine pharmacokinetics in healthy adults (Gelal *et al.*, 2005). *In vitro* experiments suggest that peppermint oil is a moderate inhibitor of nifedipine metabolism (Herb-drug interaction, 2011).

Cyclosporin is an immuno-suppresent drug. The concentration of cyclosporine was reported to be reduced in a patient consuming herbal tea containing peppermint and 8 other herbs (Nowack and Nowak, 2005). Peppermint oil elevates the plasma concentration of simva195 statin via inhibition of CYP3A4 mechanism and thereby increases the pharmacologic & adverse reactions (Dresser *et al.*, 2002).

Many herbal medicines including peppermint contain cardiac glycosides, which could have additive effects with digitoxin or digoxin, or interfere with their assays. However, few such interactions have been reported so far.

The manufacturers of certain enteric-coated peppermint oil preparations suggest that such peppermint oil should not be taken immediately after meal. This is assumed that the presence of food in the stomach may delay gastric emptying and cause premature dissolution of the enteric coating resulting to release of the peppermint oil before it reaches the intestine for absorption. This may lead to indigestion.Tea prepared from Peppermint appears to reduce the absorption of iron similarly to conventional tea.

17.8 Toxicity

Peppermint is included on the FDA's list of herbs generally recognized as safe (GRAS) only times when it is used as a beverage or food. Pulegone (potentially toxic compound in pennyroyal) is also found in peppermint in much lesser proportions. In rats, pulegone at the dose rate of 80 and 160 mg for 28 days can resulted to weight lost, atonia, reduced blood creatinine level and histopathological changes in hepatic cells and white matter of cerebellum. In rats, menthol was found to cause hepatocellular changes (Thorup *et al.*, 1983). Allergic reactions associated with peppermint have been reported in certain group of human.

Adverse reactions to enteric coated peppermint oil capsules are quite uncommon, however, can include contact dermatitis, heartburn, hypersensitivity reaction, abdominal pain, perianal burning, bradycardia, muscle tremor heartburn, etc. (Murray, 1995). Menthol upon inhalation can cause apnea and larygoconstriction. In certain case, patients were reported to have contact sensitivity to menthol and peppermint with oral symptoms likerecurrent oral ulceration, burning mouth syndrome, or a lichenoid reaction. The excessive inhalation of mentholated preparation of peppermint has caused anorexia, reversible nausea,ataxia,cardiac problems and other CNS related disorders. Peppermint oil is contraindicated in gallbladder inflammation, obstruction of the bile ducts and severe liver damage (Lucida and Wallace, 1998).

17.9 Summary and Conclusions

Peppermint is regarded as one of the most essential herbs due to its varying degrees of medicinal properties and extensive uses. The essential oil of peppermint enhances digestive system by alleviating the disorders like anti-spasmodic, anti-bloat, ulcer, IBS, etc., have profound effect such as anticancer, anaesthetic properties, etc., improves ascites and stimulated growth and immune system. Peppermint has antioxidant and anti-microbial properties that can effectively be used as natural anti-microbial and anti-oxidant in food and beverages. The essential oil of peppermint also reduces the serum content of glucose, cholesterol and triglycerides in animals and in poultry.

References

Abdel-Wareth AAA and Lohakare JD (2014) Effect of dietary supplementation of peppermint on performance, egg quality, and serum metabolic profile of Hy-Line Brown hens during the late laying period. Anim Feed Sci Tech 197: 114-120

Adam B, Liebregts T, Best J, Bechmann L, Lackner C, Neumann J, Koehler S, Holtmann G (2006) A combination of peppermint oil and caraway oil attenuates the post-inflammatory visceral hyperalgesia in a rat model. Scandinavian JGastroenterol 41: 155-160.

Akbari M, Ezati P, Nazari M, Moradikor, N(2015) Physiological and pharmaceutical properties of peppermint as a multi-purpose and valuable medicinal plant.Scientific J MedSci 4: 413-420

Akbari M, Torki M(2014) Effects of dietary chromium picolinate and peppermint essential oil on growth performance and blood biochemical parameters of broiler chicks reared under heat stress condition. Int JBiometeor 58: 1383–1391

Akdogan M, Ozquner M, Kicak A, Oncu M, Cicek E (2004) Effects of peppermint teas on plasma testosterone, follicle-stimulating hormone, and luteinizing hormone levels and testicular tissue in rats.Urol 64: 394-398

Aqil F, Beg AZ, Ahmad I(2001) In vitro toxicity of plant essential oils against soil fungi. J Med Arom Plant Sci 22/23: 177–181

Archuleta D (2012) The benefits of the use of peppermint in herbal preparations, pp. s1-20

Asao T, Mochiki E, Suzuki H, Nakamura J, Hirayama I, Morinaga N, Shoji H, Shitara Y, Kuwano H (2001) An easy method for the intraluminal administration of peppermint oil before colonoscopy and its effectiveness in reducing colonic spasm.Gastroint Endo 53: 172–177

Asao T, Kuwano H, Ide M, Hirayama I, Nakamura JI, Fujita KI,_HoriutiR (2003) Spasmolytic effect of peppermint oil in barium during double-contrast barium enema compared with BuscopanClin Rad 58: 301-305

Barbalho SM, Damasceno DC, Spada APM, Martuchi VS, Oshiiwa KA, Machao M, Mendes CG (2011) Metabolic profile of offspring from diabetic wistar rats treated with *Menthapiperita* (peppermint). Evid Based Complement. Alternat. Med. 5: 1-6

Bayoumi S (1992) Bacteriostatic effect of some spices and their utilization in the manufacture of yoghurt.ChemieMikrobiologieTechnologie der Lebensmittel 14: 21-26

Bluma R, Amaiden MR, Daghero J, Etcheverry M (2008) Control of Aspergillus section Flavi growth and aflatoxin accumulation by plant essential oils. J Appl Microbiol 105: 203–214

Brain K, Green DM, Dykes PJ, Bola TS (2006) The Role of Menthol in Skin Penetration from Topical Formulations of Ibuprofen 5% in vivo. Skin Pharmacolphysiol 19: 17-21

Braun L, CohenM (2015) Herbs and natural supplements: An evidence-based guide. 2: 739

Brickell C, Cole, T (2002) *The American Horticultural Society: Encyclopedia of Plants & Flowers*. New York, DK Publishing, ISBN 0789489937

Brown D (2015) Herbal: The Essential Guide to Herbs for Living. Pavilion Books, June 11

Campo JV (2005) Coping with ignorance: exploring pharmacologic management for pediatric functional abdominal pain. *Pediatric Gastroenterol Nutr* 41: 569-574

Canyon DV, Speare R (2007) A comparison of botanical and synthetic substances commonly used to prevent head lice (*Pediculushumanus var. capitis*) infestation. Int J Dermatol 46: 422-426

Chang HW (1995) Anti-bacterial effect of spices and vegetables.Food Indus 27: 53-61

Chaumont JP, Senet JM (1978) Antagonistic properties of higher plants against fungal parasites of man from food contaminants: screening of 200 fungi. Plant Med Phytother 12: 186-196

Clegg RJ, Middleton B, Bell D, White DA (1980) Inhibition of hepatic cholesterol synthesis and S-3-hydroxy-3-methylglutaryl-CoA reductase by mono and bicyclic monoterpenes administered *in vivo.* Biochem Pharmacol 29: 2125-2127

Clegg RJ, Middleton B, Bell D,White DA (1982) The mechanism of cyclic monoterpene inhibition of hepatic 3-hydroxy-3-methylglutaryl coenzyme A reductase *in vivo* in the rat. J Biol Chem 257: 2294-2299

Cowan M (1999) Plant Products as Antimicrobial Agents.Clin Microbiol Rev 12: 564-582

Della LR, Tubaro A, Lunder TL (1990) Evaluation of some pharmacological activities of a peppermint extract. Fitoterapia 61: 215-221

Devi KM, Palod J, Singh, DV, Singh CB, Dar AH, Singh PK, Singh VS (2017) Effect of pudina (*Mentha arvensis*) on bio-chemical parameters in White Leghorn.Int J Livest Res 7: 2016-216

Dresser GK, Wacher V, Wong S, Wong HT, Bailey DG (2002) Evaluation of peppermint oil and ascorbyl palmitate as inhibitors of cytochrome P4503A4 activity *in vitro* and *in vivo.* Clin Pharmacol Therapeu 72: 247-255

Durrani FR, Abidullah Chand, N., Durrani Z. and Akhtar, S (2008) Haematological, bio-chemical, immuno-modulatory and growth promoting effect of feed added wild mint (*Mentha longifolia*) in broiler chicks.Sarhad J Agricult 24: 661-664

Eccles R (1994) Menthol and related cooling compounds. J Pharm Pharmacol 46: 618-630

Ellis WR, Bell GD (1981) Treatment of biliary duct stones with a terpene preparation. Bri Med J 282: 611

Erler F, Ulug I, Yalcinkaya B (2006) Repellent activity of five essential oils against *Culexpipiens*.Fitoterapia 77: 491-494

ESCOP (1997) Monograph: *Mentha epiperita eaetheroleum* (Peppermint Oil), Exeter (UK)

Fareo JA, Grundmann O (2013) Menthol—pharmacology of an important naturally medicinal "cool". Mini Rev Med Chem 13: 124–131

Futami T (1984) Actions of counterirritants on the muscle contractile mechanism and nervous system. Nippon Yakurigaku Zasshi 83: 207-218

Galeotti N, Ghelardini C, Cesare D, Mannalli L, Mazzanti G, Baghiroli L, Bartolini A (2001) Local anaesthetic activity of (+) and (-) menthol. Planta Med 67: 174-176

Galeottia N, Mannellia LDC, Mazzantib G, Bartolinia A, Ghelardini C(2002) Menthol: a natural analgesic compound. Neurosci Let 322: 145-148

Galib AM, Al-Kassie 2010. The role of peppermint (*Menthapiperita*) on performance in broiler diets. AgriculBiol North Amer 1: 1009-1013

Gelal A, Balkan D, Ozzeybek D,BenowitzNL(2005) Effect of menthol on the pharmacokinetics and pharmacodynamics of felodipine in healthy subjects. Euro J ClinPharmacol 60: 785-790

Gelal A, Guven H, Balkan D, Artok L, Benowitz NL(2003) Influence of menthol on caffeine disposition and pharmacodynamics in healthy female volunteers. EuroJ ClinPharmacol 59: 417-422

Gonzalez AP, Vassana C, Zerba E, Picollo M (2007) Effectiveness of lotions based on essential oils from aromatic plants against permethrin resistant *Pediculus humanuscapitis*.Arch Dermatolo Res 299: 389-392

Gordon MC, David JN (2001) Natural product drug discovery in the next millennium. PharmaceuBiol 139: 8-17

Gotshall RY, Lucas EH, LickfeldtA, Roberts JM (1949) The occurrence of anti-bacterial substances active against *Mycobacterium tuberculosis* in seed plants.J Clin Invest 28: 920-923

Grigoleit HG, Grigoleit P (2005) Gastrointestinal clinical pharmacology of peppermint oil.Phytomed 12: 607-611

Harborne JB (1998) Phytochemcial methods: a guide to modern techniques on plant analysis. Kluwer Academic Publishers, 3rd Edn, United Kingdom, p. 299–312

Harries N, James KC, Pugh WK (1978) Antifoaming and carminative actions of volatile oils.Brit J Sur 2: 171-177

Heimes K, Hauk F, Verspohl EJ (2011) Mode of action of peppermint oil and menthol with respect to 5-HT3 receptor subtypes: binding studies, cation uptake by receptor channels and contraction of isolated rat ileum. Phytother Res 25: 702-708

Hendriks H (1998) Pharmaceutical aspects of some *Mentha* herbs and their essential Oils.PerfumFlav 23: 15-23

Herrmann EC, Kucera LS(1967) Antiviral substances in plants of the mint family (Labiatae). III. Peppermint (*Menthapiperita*) and other mint plants. Proceedings of The Society for Experimental Biology and Medicine 124: 874-878

Holly SL (2010) Grow herbs, feel better. Gardening, pp. 25-26

Houghton TM, Beardsmore CS(1998) The effect of menthol on nasal airflow, perception of nasal patency, and cough receptor sensitivity in children aged 10 and 11 years. *Thorax* 53(suppl 4): 9A

Inamori M, Akiyama T, Akimoto K, Fujita K, Takahashi H, Yoneda M, Abe Y, Kubota K, Saito S, Ueno N, Nakajima A (2007) Early effects of peppermint oil on gastric emptying: a crossover study using a continuous real-time 13C breath test (Breath ID system). J Gastroenterol 42: 539-542

Inouye S, Takizawa T, Yamaguchi H (2001) Antibacterial activity of essential oils and their major constituents against respiratory tract pathogens by gaseous contact. J Antimicro*Chemother* 47: 565–573

Inouye S, Uchida K, Nishiyama Y, Hasumi Y, Yamaguchi H Abe, S (2007) Combined effect of heat, essential oils and salt on the fungicidal activity against *Trichophyton mentagrophytes* in foot bath. *Japanese J Med Myco* 18: 27-36

Janssen AM, Chin NL, Scheffer JJ, Svendsen A (1986) Screening for anti-microbial activity of some essential oils by the agar overlay technique.Pharmaceu *Week blad Sci* 8: 289-292

Juven BJ, Kanner J, Schved F, Weisslowicz H(1994) Factors that interact with the anti-bacterial action of thyme essential oil and its active constituents. J Applied Bacteriol 76: 626–631

Kains MG (1912) American Agriculturist, ed. Culinary Herbs: Their Cultivation Harvesting Curing and Uses. Orange Judd Company

Karuza N, Blazevic Z, Soljic (1996) Isolation and structure of flavonoids from peppermint (*Mentha piperita*) leaves. Acta Pharmaceu 46: 315–320

Katayama K,Takah AO, Matsui R, Moriqaki S, Aiba T, Kakemi M, Koizumi T (1992) Effect of l-menthol on the permeation of indomethacin, mannitol and cortisone through excised hairless mouse skin.Chem Pharmaceu Bulletin 40: 3097-3099

Kêdzia A (2007) The activity of peppermint oil (*Oleum Menthaepiperitae*) to anaerobic bacteria. Post Fitoterapia 4: 182–186

Khamisabadi H, Kafilzadeh F, Charaien B (2015) Effect of thyme (*Thymus vulgaris*) or peppermint (*Menthapiperita*) on performance, digestibility and blood metabolites of fattening Sanjabi lambs. Biharean Biologist (online first): art. 151408

Khempaka S,Pudpila U, Molee W (2013) Effect of dried peppermint (*Menthacordifolia*) on growth performance, nutrient digestibility, carcass traits, anti-oxidant properties, and ammonia production in broilers. J Appl Poult Res 22: 904-912

Kraemer WJ, Ratamess NA, Maresh CM (2005). A cetylated fatty acid topical cream with menthol reduces pain and improves functional performance in individuals with arthritis. J Strength Cond Res 19: 475-480

Krieger RI (2001) Handbook of Pesticide Toxicology: Principles. Academic Press, p. 823

Kunta JR, Goskonda VR, Brotherton HO, Khan MA, Reddy IK (1997) Effect of menthol and related terpenes on the percutaneous absorption of propranolol across excised hairless mouse skin.JPharmaceuSci 86: 1369-1373

Landing JE (1969) American Essence; A History of the peppermint and spearmint industry in the United States, Kalamazoo, Michigan: Kalamazoo Museum

Lans C, Turner N, Khan T, Brauer G (2007) Ethnoveterinary medicines used to treat endoparasites and stomach problems in pigs and pets in British Columbia, Canada.Vet Parasitol 148: 325–340

Laude EA, Morice AH, Grattan TJ (1994) The antitussive effects of menthol, camphor and cineole in conscious guinea-pigs.PulmPharmacol 7: 179-184

Linnaeous C (1753) Species Plantarum, 2: 576-577

Liu Y, Ye X, Feng X, Zhou G, Rong Z, Fang C, Chen H (2005) Menthol facilitates the skin analgesic effect of tetracaine gel. Int J Pharmaceu 305: 31-36

Lucida GM, Wallace JM (1998) In: Herbal medicines, a clinician guide, pharmaceutical products. Press, New York, London, p. 85-86

Madisch A, Holtmann G, Mayr G, Vinson B, Hotz J (2004) Treatment of functional dyspepsia with a herbal preparation. A double-blind, randomized, placebo-controlled, multicenter trial.Digest 69: 45-52

Martindale(1989) The Extra Pharmacopoeia. London: The Pharmaceutical press. 29th Ed. p. 1060

Melli S, Rashidi M, Delazar MR, Madarek A, Maher KE, Ghasemzadeh MH, Tahmasebi Z (2007) Effect of peppermint water on prevention of nipple cracks in lactating primiparous women: A randomized controlled trial. Int Breastfeed J 2: 2-7

Micklefield GH, Greving I, May B (2000) Effect of peppermint oil and caraway oil on gastroduedenal motility. Phytother Res 14: 20-23

Mills S, Bone K(2000) Principles and practice of phytotherapy.Churchill livingstone 2: 507-514

Mimica-Dukic N, Bozin B, Sokovic M, Mihailovic B, Matavulj M (2003) Antimicrobial and antioxidant activities of three *Mentha* species essential oils. Planta Medica 69: 413-419

Mohsenzadeh M (2007) Evaluation of antibacterial activity of selected Iranian essential oils against Staphylococcus aureus and Escherichia coli in nutrient broth medium. Pakistan J BiolSci 10: 3693-3697

Moleyar V, Narasimham P(1992) Antibacterial activity of essential oil components.Int J Food Microbial 16: 337-342

Morgan K (2002) Medicine of the Gods: Basic Principles of Ayurvedic Medicine. Available from: http://www.compulink.co.uk/mandrake/ayurveda.htm

Morimoto Y (1993) A new enhacer-coenhancer system to increase skin permeation of morphine hydrochloride *in vitro*. Int JPharmacol 91: 9-14

Murray MT (1995) The healing power of herbs: the enlightened person's guide to the wonders of medicinal plants. Rocklin, CA: Prima Publication:xiv, 410.

Nowack R, Nowak B (2005) Herbal teas interfere with cyclosporin levels in renal transplant patients. Nephrol Dial Transplant 20: 2554-2556

Orhan I, Kartal M, Kan Y,Sener B (2008) Activity of essential oils and individual components against acetyl and butyylcholinesterase. Zeitschriftfür Naturforschung 63: 547-553

Papathanasopoulos A, Rotondo A, Janssen P, Tack J (2013) Effect of acute peppermint oil administration on gastric sensorimotor function and nutrient tolerance in health.Neurogastroenterol Mot 25: 263-271

Park EJ, Kim SH, Kim BJ, Kim SY, So I, Jeon JH(2009) Menthol enhances an antiproliferative activity of 1alpha, 25-dihydroxyvitamin D (3) in LNCaP cells. J ClinBiochemNutri 44: 125-130

Patnaik S, SubramanyamVR, Kole C (1996) Antibacterial and antifungal activity of ten essential oils in vitro.Microbios 86: 237-246

Pizzorno JJE (1999) Textbook of natural medicine. Churchill Livingstone 1: 827-830

Robbers JE, Tyler VE (1999) Tyler's Herbs of choice: the therapeutic use of phytomedicinals. New York: Haworth Herbal Press, p. 287

Samarasekera R, Weerasinghe IS, Hemalal P (2008) Insecticidal activity of menthol derivatives against mosquitoes. Pest Management Sci 64: 290-295

Sara I (2013) Can peppermint cause a miscarriage?/www.livestrong.com

Scavroni J, Boaro CSF, Ferreira LC (2005) Yield and composition of the essential oil of *Menthapiperita* L. (Lamiaceae) grown with biosolid. Brazilian J Plant Physiol 17: 345-352

Sharma A, Sharma MK, Kumar M (2007) Protective Effect of *Menthapiperita* against Arsenic-Induced Toxicity in Liver of Swiss Albino Mice. Basic Clin Pharmacol Toxicol 100: 249–257

Shimada K, Fujikawa K, Yahara K, Nakamura T (1992) Antioxidative properties of xanthan on the antioxidation of soybean oil in cyclodextrin. J Agri Food Chem 40: 945–948

Shrivastava A (2009) A review on peppermint oil.Asian J PharmaceuClin Res 187: 27-33

Sokovic MD, Vukojevic J, Marin PD, Brkic DD,Vajs V, Van Griensven LJLD (2009) Chemical composition of essential oils of Thymus and *Mentha* species and their anti-fungal activities. Molecules 14: 238–249

Somerville KW, Richmond CR, Bell GD (1984) Delayed release peppermint oil capsule (Colpermin) for the spastic colon syndrome: a pharmakinetic study. Bri JPhamacol 18: 638-640

Tate S (1997) Peppermint oil: a treatment for post-operative nausea. J AdvNurs 26: 543-549

Thorup I, Wurtzen G, Cartensen J, Olsen P (1983) A short term toxicity study in rats doed with pulegone and menthol.ToxicolLet 19: 207-210

Vandergrift B (1998) Bio-technology in the feed industry.Proceedings of Altech's 14th Annual Symposium, Altech Technical Publications Nottingham University Press, Nicholasville, p. 293-300

Vidal F, VidalJC, Gadelha AP, Lopes CS, Coelho MG, Monteiro-Leal LH(2007) *Giardia lamblia*: the effects of extracts and fractions from Mentha x piperita Lin. (Lamiaceae) on trophozoites. ExperiParasitol 115: 25-31

Wasner G, Schattschneider J, Binder A, Baron R (2004) Topical menthol—a human model for cold pain by activation and sensitization of C nociceptors.Brain 127: 1159-1171

Zaika LL (1975) Spices and herbs: their antimicrobial activity and its determination. JFood Safety 9: 97-118

Zanker KS, Tolle W, Blumel G, Probst J (1980) Evaluation of surfactant-like effects colds. Respiration 39: 150–157.

❑❑❑

Chapter 18

Wheat Grass (*Triticum aestivum*)

K. Merina Devi[1] and Jyoti Palod[2]

[1] Department of Poultry Science, College of Veterinary Sciences and Animal Husbandry, Assam Agricultural University, Guwahati-781022, Assam, India, E-mail: merinadevi.90@gmail.com

[2] Department of Livestock Production Management, College of Veterinary Sciences and Animal Husbandry, GB Pant University of Agricultural University, Pantnagar-263145, India

ABSTRACT

Wheat grass (*Triticum aestivum*) is an annual grass and is considered as one of the so-called green foods that are widely used as health foods due to its great source of nutrients. Wheat grass contains high proportion of amino acids such as aspartic acid, glutamic acid, arginine, alanine and serine. The grass has double the measure of vitamin A as in carrots and is richer in vitamin C than in oranges. Wheat grass has antioxidant action due to its bio-flavonoids like apigenin, quercitin and luteolin. Other notable ingredients which make this grass therapeutically effective, is the presence of indole compounds, apigenin and laetrile, alkaloids, carbohydrates, saponins, gum and mucilages. Wheat grass has anti-oxidant, anti-inflammatory, hepatoprotective role and haempoietic role and hypoglycaemic role. As wheat grass contains over 80 enzymes used for digestion, all the B group of vitamins and rich in major and minor minerals. Therefore, supplementation of wheat grass to birds result in superior performance due to better utilization of nutrients.

Keywords: *Triticum aestivum*, Antioxidant, Bioflavonoids, Haempoietic.

18.1 Introduction

Plant medicines have been widely used in the treatment of various ailments since time immemorial. In the present world, many drugs obtained from plant origin, either in the form of plant extracts, powder or juice form, others are synthesized to mimic a natural plant compound or the plant itself are widely included not only in the feed of human but also incorporated in the animals. Wheatgrass (*Triticum aestivum*), a subspecies of the family Poaceae (Shanker and Singh, 2000), is considered to be one of the so-called green foods that are widely used as health foods due to its great source of nutrients. This grass has been an integral part of Indian culture for thousands of years, and has been known to have remarkable healing properties as well. The history of wheat grass is over 5000 years, to ancient Egypt and possibly even early Mesopotamian civilizations (Jurgen, 2016). It is believed that ancient Egyptians found sacred the young leafy blades of wheat and prized them for their positive effect on their health and vitality. The consumption of wheatgrass in the Western world began in the 1930s as a result of experiments conducted by Charles F. Schnabel. He demonstrated an experiment by using wheat grass on a dying hen. The result was an encouraging where he found that when supplemented wheat grass in sicked hen not only improved the health condition of the bird but also doubled the egg production. Later, by 1940, he started promoting his discovery by selling cans of Schnabel's powdered grass in major drug stores throughout the United States and Canada (Meyerowitz and Steve, 1999). Simultaneously, a woman named Ann also advocated the consumption of wheat grass as a part of a raw food diet. Wigmore, the founder of the Hippocrates Health Institute, proposed that wheat grass not only help to clean toxins in the body but also maintains a proper balance of nutrients as a whole food.

Wheat grass contains high chlorophyll content which accounts for 70% of its total chemical constituents (Swati *et al.*, 2010; Kothari *et al.*, 2008). The molecular structure of chlorophyll in wheat grass and haemoglobin in the human body is identical, due to which wheat grass is called 'Green Blood' (Ferruzzia and Blakesleeb, 2007). The only difference is that the central element in chlorophyll is magnesium while in haemoglobin it is iron. Chlorophyll, not only being soluble in fat particles, but also has the same pH value that of blood (7), therefore, it is quickly absorbed into blood stream via the lymphatic system and replenishes the body with electrolytes which benefits the body.

18.2 Taxonomy of Wheat Grass

Triticum is a genus of annual and biennial grasses. In early growth stages, the wheat grass consists of a much-compressed stem or crown and numerous narrowly linear or linear lanceolate leaves. Leaves are about 1.2 m tall, flat, narrow, 20-38 cm long and 1.3 cm broad. Each mature leaf comprises the sheath, wrapping around the subtending leaf, and a lamina (blade). Wheat grass culms are simple, hollow or pithy, glabrous. At the junction of the sheath and lamina, there is a membranous structure, the ligule, and a pair of small, hairy projections, the auricles. The base of the leaves on the culm is thickened to form a hard knot or pulvinus. The spikes are long, slender, dorsally compressed and somewhat flattened.

Kingdom	:	Plantae
Subkingdom	:	Tracheobionta
Superdivision	:	Spermatophyta
Division	:	Magnoliophyta
Class	:	Liliopsida
Subclass	:	Commelinidae
Order	:	Cyperales
Family	:	Poaceae
Genus	:	Triticum L.
Species	:	*Aestivum*

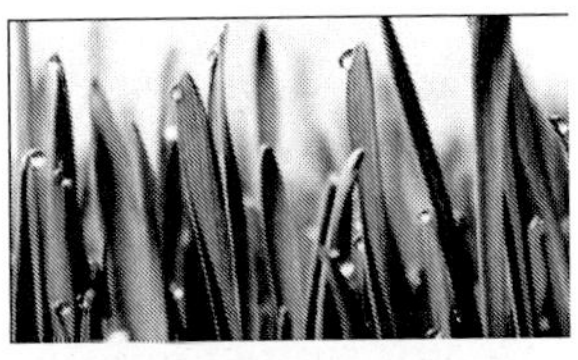

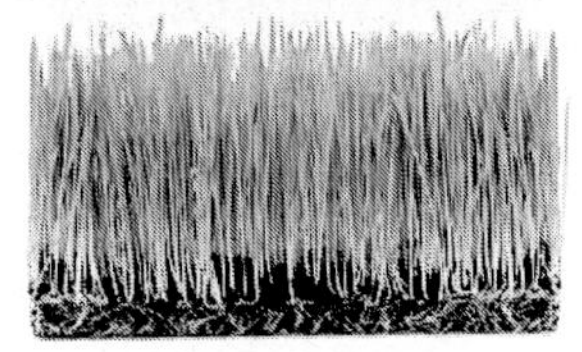

Wheat grass is a young green grass of the common wheat plant, *Triticum aestivum,* whereas wheat is a grain. Wheat grass contains no wheat gluten (Mogra, 2013) but wheat contains the gluten (protein). During germination, vitamins, minerals, and phenolic compounds including flavonoids are synthesized in wheat sprouts and attains the maximum antioxidant potential (Aate *et al.*, 2017). Although grass germinated from grain, it undergoes a complete transformation into a vegetable (Wigmore, 1985). Wheatgrass is a nutrient-rich type of young grass in the wheat family, is many times richer in levels of vitamins, minerals and proteins as compared to seed kernel, or grain products of the mature cereal plant (Tirgar *et al.*, 2011).

18.3 Cultivation and Harvest of Wheat Grass

Wheat grass is normally grown in open fields or indoors using few inches of soil with less effort. A common method for sprout production indoors is often on trays in a growth medium such as a potting mix. With the development of various agricultural techniques, the grass is also well-adopted in hydroponics methods. It was successfully grown in growth chambers and in field conditions at temperature of 18 to 26R" C and a relative humidity of 40 to 50%. The genus *Triticum* yields various types of wheat, which are native to Southwest Asia and the Mediterranean region and also grown throughout temperate regions of North America and Europe (Durairaj *et al.*, 2014). In India, it is the most commonly found herb. Generally, 15-20 species are recognized, of which about 8 have been reported to occur in India. Wheat grass (common or Bread wheat), is known by different names across India. In Hindi, Manipuri and Urdu, it is called as Gehun, in Kannada as Godhi; Sanskrit as Arupaand, Godhuma; Tamil- Godumai; and in Telugu-Godumalu (Aate *et al.*, 2017).

Harvesting of the grass can be done when the leaves develop a "split" as another leaf emerges; in an around 6-10 days or when the grass is about 15-25cm tall, by cutting at 2-3 cm above the soil and leaving the roots. Peak nutrition is reached by harvesting just prior to the 'jointing stage' which is the period when the plant switches from vegetative growth to reproductive growth, as the blade develops a second stem. Sometimes, third cutting may be possible but may be tougher and have lesser sugars than the first. Harvested wheat grass can be stored for about a week but the maximum nutritional benefits are obtained only from freshly cut grass.

18.4 Nutrients Composition of Wheat Grass

Wheat grass has higher nutritive value than broccoli and spinach. It is reported that "15 pounds of wheat grass is equal in overall nutritional value to 350 pounds of ordinary garden vegetables" as it contains various essential and nonessential amino acids, vitamins, minerals, chlorophyll and enzymes (Meyerowitz, 1992). For instance, the wheat grass has double the measure of vitamin A as in carrots and is richer in vitamin C than in oranges (Thammana *et al.*, 2016). It has 20 per cent of aggregate calories originating from protein (poly peptides, simple and short chains of amino acid) which are utilized all more productivity as a part of the circulation system and tissue. About 3.5 g of the wheat grass provides 860 mg protein, 18.5 mg chlorophyll, 15 mg calcium, 38 mg lysine, 7.5 mg vitamin C along with B complex vitamins and amino acids. Wheat grass is considered to have higher levels of vitamins, minerals and proteins as compared to the seed kernel, or grain products of the mature cereal plant (Tirgar *et al.*,

2011).The various enzymes responsible for its pharmacological properties are protease, amylase, lipase, cytochrome oxidase, transhydrogenase, superoxide dismutase. Wheat grass contains high proportion of amino acids such as aspartic acid, glutamic acid, arginine, alanine and serine (Bar-Sella, 1998). The major clinical utility of wheat grass juice is due to its antioxidant action which is derived from its high content of bioflavonoids like apigenin, quercitin and luteolin. Other notable ingredients which make this grass therapeutically effective, is the presence of indole compounds, apigenin and laetrile, alkaloids, carbohydrates, saponins, gum and mucilages. Scientific reports on nutritional analysis of wheat grass have been published frequently in various journals (Hamilton *et al.*, 1988; Kohler, 1994).

In a study conducted to determine the elemental concentration profile of wheatgrass using instrumental neutron activation analysis, it was observed that the concentration of elements such as K, Na, Mg and Ca increased linearly in the shoots with the growth period whereas the concentrations of the elements, namely Zn, Mn and Fe remained constant in shoots after 8th day of plantation. However, it was observed that the shoot to root concentration ratio in all the conditions increased linearly for K, Na, Ca, Mg and Cl and decreased for Zn, Fe, Mn, and Al with growth period (Kulkarni *et al.*, 2006).

18.5 Different forms of Wheat Grass

Wheat grass can be consumed on its own or used in combination with other juices, vegetable drinks or supplements. Considering it to be a "superfood," several forms of wheat grass are becoming more widely available which comprise- juice, capsules, powder, pills, tablets, etc. However, the best way to consume all foods is as close to their natural state as possible. Consumption of fresh obtained wheatgrass juice would be preferred over consuming it in either tablet or powder forms. In absence of fresh juice, wheat grass powder makes a good second option.

18.5.1 Wheat Grass Juice

Wheat grass juice is an extract squeezed from the mature sprouts of wheat seed (Chauhan, 2014). Juice is considered to be the finest medicine available in the nature. The wheat grass supplements and freeze dried powders are only 2 per cent as effective as fresh juiced when consumed shortly within 15 minutes of preparation. Henceforth, it is advisable to consume the juice proximately because the nutrients present in it get quickly oxidise. The powerful nutrients present in the grass can prevent destruction of DNA and protects from the ongoing effects of pre-mature aging and cellular breakdown.

In order to develop a holistic approach for the treatment of chronic diseases, extensive studies have been conducting to evaluate the efficacy of wheat grass (either in the form of powder or juice) and also for the better understanding of therapeutic potential of this medicinal grass (Rajesh and Ramesh, 2011).

Table 1: Physical Characteristics of wheat grass juice (Ashok, 2011)

Physical constants	***Triticum aestivum***
Nature	Grass
Colour	Bright/ Dark green
Odour	Characteristic odour
Taste	Acrid
Loss on drying (%w/w)	21.1%

18.5.2 Wheat Grass Powder

The dry powder form of wheat grass is a method for preservation of nutrients. The powder form has achieved protein assays greater than 40 per cent and optimal high levels of live enzymes, readily absorbable minerals as well as trace minerals which are used in maintaining good health and enhanced resistance to various ailments (Kulkarni *et al.*, 2006). 100g wheat grass powder obtained from 1 kg of fresh wheat grass, can provide nourishment equal to that obtained from 23 kg of selected vegetables. Wheat grass powder is rich in dietary fiber and thus, functions to maintain blood sugar level, cholesterol level and also prevents constipation. However, owing to its high fibrous nature which is indigestible by human, wheat grass must be liquefied before it is consumed.

Table 2: Nutrients present in *Triticum aestivum* powder

Nutrients composition (g)	Per 100 g
Moisture	6.30
Protein	25.00
Fat	0.90
Carbohydrate	33.00
Mineral ash	4.80
Fiber	30.00
Moisture	6.30

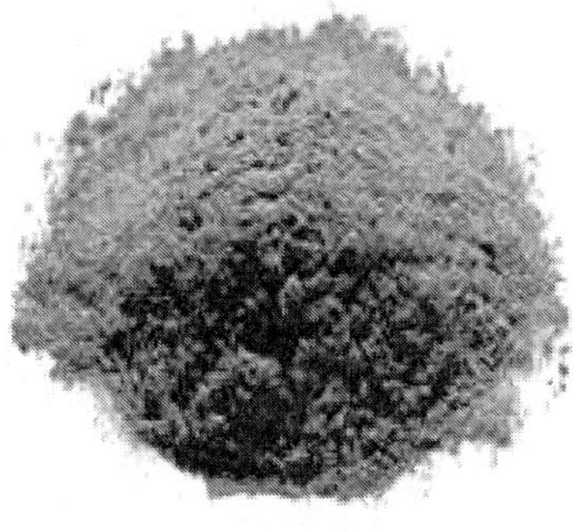

(Jain and Jain, 2014)

18.6 Pharmaceutical Properties of Wheat Grass

Epidemiological studies reported that wheatgrass has been shown to have number of medicinal properties (Millen *et al.*, 2007) which are discussed below.

18.6.1 *Hepatoprotective Role*

Triticum aestivum either in the form of leaf extract (Arya and Kumar, 2011), fresh juice (Jain *et al.*, 2007) or tablets (Rana *et al.*, 2011) have been reported to have hepatoprotective potential. The leaf extract of wheat grass affects the activities of liver enzymes as well as lipid peroxidation (Arya *et al.*, 2011).The significant hepatoprotective role of the grass was shown with a dose of 100 mg/kg/day in terms of SGOT, SGPT, ALP and bilirubin in serum (Jain *et al.*, 2007). Oral administration of wheat grass showed its protective nature on liver tissue by reducing the elevated levels of SGOT and SGPT. Treatment with wheat grass was reported to prevent the increase in liver enzymes activities depending upon the dose rate of the grass (Kamboj *et al.*, 2011). The presence of three compounds *viz.* choline, magnesium and potassium which are found abundantly in wheat grass, are responsible to keep the liver vital and healthy. As choline functions to prevent the deposition of fat and magnesium works to draw out excess fat in the same way. Magnesium sulphate (Epsom salts) is reported to draw pus from any infection while potassium acts as an invigorator and stimulant (Wingmore, 1985).

18.6.2 *Haematopoetic Role*

According to various researches conducted on the haemopoetic actions of the wheat grass showed that regular administration of chlorophyll derivatives of wheat grass increased 70-83% in red blood cells count within 10-16 days of the experiment (Kelentei *et al.*, 1958). Kelentei *et al.* (1998) demonstrated that chlorophyll injection could improve the red blood cell count with normal haemoglobin counts in animals. Results of experiment conducted by Singh (2006) on broilers confirm the findings of results. The chlorophyll molecule obtained from wheat grass not only has similar structure with that of haemoblobin of the blood (Ferruzzia and Blakesleeb, 2007), but also the same pH factor of human blood (7.4) (Singh *et al.*, 2010). Hence, feeding of wheat grass for long time might promote absorption of mineral elements which are building stones for heme pigment resulting in formation of haemoglobin and ultimately improved haemoglobin values.

Juice obtained from the fresh wheatgrass have been proved to increase haemoglobin, WBC and differential WBC counts in thrombocytopenic rats as study conducted by Tirgar (2011) and also in guinea fowl (Sindhe, 2014), Sethi *et al.* (2010) reported that same results. Higher TLC in wheat grass supplemented group may be attributed to Co-chlorophyll content of wheat grass which was believe to increase the leukocyte count and directly or indirectly stimulated haematopoiesis.

18.6.3 *Anti- inflammatory Role*

Wheat grass has been shown to have potential anti-inflammatory and anti-aging properties (Smith, 2000). Wheat grass extract which is a topical anti-inflammatory immuno-modulator, substance P inhibitor, topical hemostatic agent, and a stimulant of fibroblastic action, has abroad range of healing properties (Rana *et al.*, 2011). The cream extract from the grass have been claimed to reduce skin toxicity from radiotherapy. Chlorophyll in (water-soluble salts which are semi-synthetic derivatives of chlorophyll) has bacteriostatic properties that aids in wound healing. It has been used to treat various kinds of skin lesions, burns, and ulcers, where it acts as a wound-healing agent, stimulating granulation tissue and epithelialization (Wingmor, 1985). Its anti-inflammatory properties exert a positive effect on bone and joint problems, reducing pain and swelling (Nenonen *et al.*, 1998).The same findings was also reported by Balint *et al.* (2006).

18.6.4 *Hypocholesterolemic Role*

The hypocholesterolemic properties of wheat grass have been reported in total blood in rats fed with wheat grass (Sethi *et al.*, 2010). Same results was also reported by Kothari (2008) and Shirude (2011) in serum of rats fed with wheat grass juice, and in wheat grass powder by Shinde (2014). The hypocholesterolemic properties may be attributed to the role of wheat grass in ameliorating hyperlipidemia. It is believed that the fibre content of wheat grass may be one of the main roles to play in the reduction of cholesterol levels (Tasi *et al.*, 1976). Addition of wheat grass juice was found to decrease triglycerides level in broilers (Singh, 2006), in rats (Jain *et al.*, 2007; Kothari, 2008) and in guinea fowl (Shinde, 2014).

18.6.5 *Hypoglycemic Role*

Persistent hyperglycemia is a key contributor to metabolic alterations that directs to the development of diabetic complications. One of the key enzymes in the catabolism of glucose is hexokinase, which phosphorylates glucose and converts it into glucose-6-phosphatase (Laakso *et al.*, 1995). Administration of wheat grass to diabetic rats resulted in an increased activity of liver hexokinase. The increased activity of hexokinase helps in accelerating glycolysis and increasing utilization of glucose for energy production. Another source reported that the possible mechanism of action of the grass could be potentiating the pancreatic secretion of insulin from â-cells of islets, resulting to significantly lowering the level of glucose (Mohan *et al.*, 2013). Wheat grass has been observed to reduce the levels of glucose in the blood (Chude *et al.*, 2001) in rats treated with wheat grass juice (Jain *et al.*, 2007), in alloxan induced diabetic rats treated with wheat grass juice (Mukhopadhyay *et al.*, 2009) and in guinea fowl (Sindhe, 2014). The decrease in the concentration of blood glucose in wheat grass-treated rats also can be due to increased glycolysis (increased liver hexokinase activity). The antidiabetic ability to regenerate the pancreatic β-cell has already been proved (Chika and Bello, 2010). Reduction in serum glucose level might be attributed to abundance of natural fiber in wheat grass which optimizes blood sugar levels. Wheat grass also influences insulin growth factor and thereby balances glucose level in blood. The presence of chlorophyll, a pharmacologically active component in wheat grass, acts as an anti-diabetic agent (Shaikh *et al.*, 2012; Ashok, 2011).

18.6.5 *Anti-oxidant Role*

Wheat grass has the potential to reduce the oxidative stress and thereby improves antioxidant concentrations in the body (Kamboj *et al.*, 2011). The juice extract from wheat grass has a potent antioxidant activity due to its high content of bioflavonoids and polyphenols (Zendehbad *et al.*, 2014) which makes it one of the best functional foods that can be used as an excellent adjuvant in therapeutic regimens. In a study published in "Phytotherapy Research" in 2006, researchers evaluated the antioxidant activity of flavonoid-containing extracts made from wheat grass grown under several conditions for various lengths of time. They found that the grass has highest antioxidant activity after fifteen days of growth in soil with added nutrients compared to grass cultivated in other conditions and added that the extract has higher antioxidant activity than other natural extracts prepared from a variety of plants and vegetables. The ethanolic extract of *Triticum aestivum* exhibited significant antioxidant activities in streptozotocin-induced diabetic rats as reported by Mohan *et al.* (2013). The grass is loaded with vitamins A, C, and E which may acts as natural antioxidants and retards ageing of cells. The major clinical utility of wheat grass juice is due to its antioxidant action which is derived from its high content of bio-flavonoids like apigenin, quercitin and luteolin.

18.6.6 *Anticarcinogenic Role*

The extract of wheat grass contains chlorophyll which is an antioxidant that may affect in the prevention of development of cancer. Inclusion of wheat grass in the dietary programme claims that it can regress cancer and prolong lives of people (Millen *et al.*, 2007). The active component in wheat grass extract, chlorophyll, inhibits the metabolic activity of carcinogens (Manju *et al.*, 2005). Moreover, selenium and lactrile present in wheatgrass have anticarcinogenic potentials. Selenium builds the immune system and thereby decreases the risk of cancer. The cancerous degeneration of cells has been revealed to be from the destruction of a specific respiratory enzyme, cytochrome oxidase (Kane *et al.*, 1997). Another study reported that superoxide dismutase in the wheat grass converts two superoxide anions into a hydrogen peroxide molecule, which has an extra oxygen molecule to kill cancer cells. P4D1, a glycoprotein present in wheat grass, also acts similarly to antioxidants, which stimulates the renewal of RNA and DNA. In animal experiments, anticarcinogenic effect of the wheat grass was also studied (Bar-Sela *et al.*, 2015).

18.6.7 *Miscellaneous Roles*

Chlorophyllin, a semi-synthetic derivatives of chlorophyll, has bacteriostatic properties that aids in wound healing (Young *et al.*, 2006). It has been used to treat various kinds of skin lesions, burns, and ulcers, where it acts as a wound-healing agent, stimulating granulation tissue and epithelialization (Chernomorsky and Segelman, 1988). Epidemio-logical studies have shown regular consumption of wheat grass juice potentiates the digestion and promotes general well-being (Ben *et al.*, 2002). Wheat grass is used to treat a number of problems like the common cold, cough, bronchitis, fever, infections, inflammed mouth, throat, skin disorders like haemorrhoids, psoriasis, ivy, eczema, burns and thalassemia (Meyerowitz, 1999). As studied by Ben *et al.* (2002) confirmed that administration of the extract of wheat grass in the patient showed significant improvement in rectal bleeding and abdominal pain associated with ulcerative colitis, Flavenoids, anti-inflammatory agents-apigenin and agropyrene contained in wheat grass, played role in alleviation of symptoms. Wheat grass also contains another flavonoid indole, which helps in synthesis of enzymes and deactivates carcinogens in the liver. Wheat grass contains all the essential amino acids, particularly alanine, aspartic acid, glutamic acid, arginine and serine which help to provide a sufficient protein in the body. Other benefits of wheat grass include toxin removal from the body, blood sugar level balance, prevention of tooth decay, maintainence of healthy hair, improvement in digestion and reduction of high blood pressure (Kelentei *et al.*, 1998). It is also a boon in the treatment of thalassemia patients (Singh *et al.*, 2010). It was also documented that young grasses and other chlorophyll-rich plants are safe and effective treatment for ailments such as high blood pressure, certain cancers, obesity, diabetes, gastritis, ulcers, pancreas and liver problems, fatigue, anemia, asthama, eczema, hemorrhoids, skin problems, halitosis, body odour and constipation (Wigmore, 1985). Chlorophyll present in the wheat grass protects the body from carcinogens also; it strengthens the cells, detoxifies the liver and blood stream and neutralize the polluting elements (Borisenko and Sofonova, 1995). It has the ability to neutralize toxins in the body, cleanses the lymphatic system and oxygenates the blood.

18.7 Wheat Grass and Performance of Animals

As wheat grass contains over 80 enzymes used for digestion, all the B group of vitamins and rich in major and minor minerals, it helps to improve performance index, FCR of broilers (Singh, 2006), also seen in guinea fowl (Shinde, 2014). Therefore, supplementation of wheat grass to birds resulted in superior performance due to better utilization/availability of nutrients and also believes to restore good health.

18.7.1 *Improved Feed Intake*

Incorporation of wheat grass in the diet of guinea pigs (Morgan 1992) and guinea fowl (Shinde, 2014) claimed that there was reduction in the amount of feed intake. However, in another study initiated by Singh (2006) reported that there was increase in feed intake in wheat grass juice supplemented broiler chicks as compared to control groups.

18.7.2 *Growth Performance*

Researchers conducted several experiments by feeding of form of wheat grass supplemented on broilers (Singh, 2006) and in guinea fowl (Shinde, 2014) reported that there was gain in body weight in target animals. Increase in body weight may be contributed to the high concentrations of chlorophyll, active enzymes, vitamins as well as other nutrients in wheat grass by which it improves digestion power and in return increases body growth rate. Better weight gain in wheat grass supplemented groups may be attributed to general tonic properties of wheat grass as well.

18.7.3 *Carcass Quality*

The evaluation of carcass quality in animals fed with wheat grass is prime important evaluation from economic point of view. Singh (2006) and Shinde (2014) in their experiments concluded that feeding of wheat grass resulted in higher dressed yield, higher thigh, breast, drumstick and back carcass yield. The better dressed yield in wheat grass supplemented groups may be due to better feed utilization and growth in wheat grass. Lee *et al.* (2003) reported that there was better protein utilization, mobilization and retention due to green supplementation resulting in better yield of cut up parts. Another researcher, Choct and Naylor (2004) studied that better protein metabolism in vitamin E and selenium supplemented broilers resulting in better yield of cut up parts. Wheat grass is also rich in vitamin E and selenium. Therefore, higher cut up part values in present investigation may be attributed to vitamin E and selenium content of wheat grass.

18.8 Toxicity of Wheat Grass

There is no much information available about the toxicity of wheatgrass. However, it can cause nausea, inappetance, constipation in certain cases. Wheat grass juice generally contains no harmful substances with the exception of a possible allergic reaction. The consumption of wheat grass in pregnant woman and breast feeding mothers is restricted unless advised by the practitioner (Aste *et al.*, 2017). Wheat allergies are generally a response to the gluten (a protein) found in the wheat berry.

18.9 Summary and Conclusions

Herbal based foods or their products are extensively used in order to treat various diseases. Wheat grass is not only considered to be as one of the herbs that are esteemed by well-being of people as an incredible source of nutrients, proteins, essential amino acids, minerals, vitamins, chlorophyll and active enzymes but also have been used in the therapeutic treatments of various ailments. Widespread data from a number of studies suggest that as the wheat grass is loaded with various essential nutrient supplements, awareness should be done among the people about the availability, nutritional and therapeutic values to promote the inclusion of it on daily dietary intake in order to explore its maximum benefits. Since there is limited works done in animals and birds, extensive research works is needed to discover its potential in normal physiological conditions and as therapeutic application in various diseases.

References

Aate J, Urade P, Potey L, Kosalge S (2017) *A review: Wheat Grass and its Health Benefits.* Int J Pharm Pharma Res 9: 288-298

Arya P, Kumar M (2011) Chemoprevention by *Triticum aestivum* of mouse skin carcinogenesis induced by DMBA and croton oil- Association with oxidative status. Asian Pac J Cancer Prev12: 143-148

Ashok SA (2011) Phytochemical and pharmacological screening of wheatgrass juice (*Triticum aestivum* L.) Int J Pharma Sci Rev Res 9: 159-164

Bálint G, Apáthy A, Gaál, Telekes A, Resetár A, Blazsó G, Falkay G, Szende B, Paksy A, Ehrenfeld M, Shoenfeld Y, Hidvégi, M (2006) Effect of Avemar—a fermented wheat germ extract—on rheumatoid arthritis. Preliminary data. Clin Exp Rheumatol 24: 325-8

Bar-Sella P (1998) Rejuvenation—Health According to Dr. Ann Wigmore's Teachings. Kiryat Ono, Israel: Shachar Ltd.Int J ChemStudies, p. 142–152

Bar-Sella G, Cohen M, Ben-Arye E, Epelbaum R (2015) The medical use of wheat grass: Review of the gap between basic and clinical applications. Mini Rev Med Chem 15: 1002-1010

Ben AE, Goldin E, Wengrower D, Stamper A, Kohn R, Berry E (2002) Wheat grass juice in the treatment of active distal ulcerative colitis, a randomized double-blind placebo-controlled trial. Scand J Gastroenterol 37: 444-449

Durairaj V, Muddasarul H, Garima S, Sankar P, Preedia B, Rukkumani R (2014) Phytochemical screening and analysis of antioxidant properties of aqueous extract of wheatgrass. Asian Pac J Trop Med 7: 398-404

Ferruzzia, MG, Blakesleeb J (2007) Digestion, absorption and cancer preventive activity of dietary chlorophyll derivatives. Nutr Res 27: 1-12

Hamilton E, Whitney E, Sizer, F(1988) Nutrition: Concepts and Controversies. 4th edn, West Publishing Co., St. Paul, Minn

Jain B, Jain N (2014) Nutritional composition, phytochemical analysis and product. Indian J Ancient Med Yoga 7(1): 23-27

Jain G, Argal A, Pathak AK, Singh VK, Kannojia P (2007) Hepatoprotective activity of wheatgrass juice. The harmacist 2: 29-30

Jurgen (2016) Wheat grass Powder. Remedies health store

Kamboj JK, Rana SV, Dhawan DK, Vahiphei K (2011) Role of wheat grass in prevention of carbon tetrachloride induced hepatotoxicity in rats. J Clin Exp Hepatol 1: 51

Kane DJ, Sarafian TA, Anton R (1997) Bcl-2 inhibition of neural death: decreased generation of reactive oxygen species. Sci 262: 1274–1277

Kelentei B, Fekete I, Kun S (1998) Influence of copper chlorophyll in on experimental anaemia. Acta Pharm Hung 28: 176-180

Kelentei B, Fekete I, Kun (1958) Influence of copper chlorophyll in on experimental anemia. Acta Pharm Hung 28: 176-180

Kent S (2013) "Wheat grass (*Triticum aestivum*)". *Illinois State University*

Kohler G (1944) The effect of stages of growth on the chemistry of the grasses. J Biol Chem 152: 215-223

Kothari S, Anand KJ, Mehta SC, Tonpay SD (2008) Effect of fresh *Triticumaestivum* grass juice on lipid profile of normal rats. Indian JPharmacol 40: 235-236

Kulkarni SD, Acharya R, Nair AGC, Rajurkar N, Reddy AVR (2006) Determination of elemental concentration profiles in tender wheat grass (*Triticum aestivum*) using instrumental neutron activation analysis. Food Chem 95: 699-707

Laakso M, Malkki M, Deeb SS (1995) Amino acid substitutions in hexokinase II among patients with NIDDM. *Diabetes* 44: 330–334

Lee KW, Everts H, Kappert HJ, Frehner M, Losa R, Beynen AC (2003) Effects of dietary essential oil components on growth performance, digestive enzymes and lipid metabolism in female broiler chickens. Br Poult Sci 44: 450-457

Manju V, Balasubramaniyan V, Nalini N (2005) Rat colonic lipid peroxidation and antioxidant status the effects of dietary luteolin on 1, 2-dimethylhydrazine challenge. Cell Mol Biol Lett 10: 535-551

Meyerowitz, S (1999) Nutrition in Grass-Wheat grass Nature's Finest Medicine: The Complete Guide to Using Grass Foods & Juices to Revitalize Your Health. Healthy Living Publications, pp. 186-187

Meyerowitz S(1999) "Nutrition in grass". Wheatgrass nature's finest medicine. The Complete Guide to Using Grass Foods & Juices to Revitalize Your Health, 6th ed. Book Publishing Company. ISBN 1-878736-97-3

Meyerowitz S (1992) Nutrition in grass" Wheat grass Nature's Finest Medicine: The complete Guide to using Grass Foods & Juices to Revitalize Your Health.6th ed. Great Barrington (Massachusetts): Sproutman Publications

Millen AE, Subar AF, Graubard BI, Peters U, Hayes RB, Weissfeld JL, Yokochi LA, Ziegler RG (2007) PLCO Cancer Screening Trial Project Team: Fruit and vegetable intake and prevalence of colorectal adenoma in a cancer screening trial. Am J Clin Nutr 86: 1754-64

Mogra R (2003) Health benefits of wheat grass - a wonder food. Int J Food NutriSci 2: 10-13

Mohan Y, Jesuthankaraj GN, Narendhirakanna RT (2013) Antidiabetic and Antioxidant Properties of *Triticum aestivum*in Streptozotocin-Induced Diabetic Rats. AdvPharmacolSci 26: 703-716

Mohan Y, Jesuthankaraj GN, Narendhirakannan RT (2013) Antidiabetic and antioxidant properties of *Triticum aestivum* in Streptozotocin-Induced Diabetic Rats. Adv. PharmacoSci10.1155/2013/716073PMCID: PMC3876669

Morgan CA (1992) Manipulation of fatty acid composition of pig meat lipids by dietary means. J Sci Food Agri 58: 357-368

Mukhopadhya YS, Basak J, Kar M, Mandal S, Mukhopadhyay A(2009) The role of iron chelation activity of wheat grass juice in patients with myelodysplastic syndrome. J Clin Oncol 7012-7014

Nenonen T, Helve T, Rauma T, Nninen H(1998) Uncooked, Lactobacilli-Rich, Vegan Food and Rheumatoid arthritis. Brit J Rheum 37: 274–281

Rajesh M, Ramesh BB (2011) A study on wheat grass and its Nutritional value. Food Science and Quality Management. Food Sci Qual Manag

Rana S, Kamboj JK, Gandhi V(2011) Living life the natural way-Wheat grass and health. Funct Foods Health Dis. 1: 444-456

Ravi (2010) "Wheat grass therapy", Phama Tutor pp. 1-5

SethiJ, Yadav M, Dahiya K, Sood S, Singh V, Bhattacharya SB(2010) Antioxidant effect of *Triticumaestivium* (wheat grass) in high-fat diet-induced oxidative stress in rabbits. ExpClinPharmacol 32: 233-235

Sethi J, Yadav M, Dahiya K, Sood S, Singh V, Bhattacharya SB (2010) Antioxidant effect of *Triticumaestivium* (wheat grass) in high-fat diet-induced oxidative stress in rabbits. Exp ClinPharmacol 32: 233-235

Shaikh MRN, Quazi M (2012) Hypoglycemic effect of wheatgrass juice in alloxan induced diabetic rats. FS J Pharm Res 1: 39-40

Shanker G, Singh H (2000) Anxiolytic profile of standardized Brahmi extract. Indian J Pharmacol: 32: 152

Shinde, PR (2014) Study on wheat grass supplementation on the performance ofguinea fowl. Ph.D. Thesis. G.B.P.U.A. & T., Pantnagar, India

Singh K, Pannu MS, Singh P, Singh J (2010) Effect of wheat grass tablets on the frequency of blood transfusions in Thalassemia Major. Indian J Pediatr. 77: 90-101

Singh VS (2006) Dietary modulation for management of poultry cocciodiosis. Ph.D. Thesis submitted to G.B.Pant University of Agriculture and Technology, Pantnagar

Smith BH (2000) Generalization of spatially variant apodization to non-integral Nyquist sampling rats. IEEE Trans Image Process 9: 1088-1093

Swati P, Sushma D, Indira R, Alka G, Mamta, D (2010) Multitude potential of wheat grass juice (Green Blood): An overview. Chronicles of young scientists 1: 23-28

Tasi AC, Elias J, Kelly RC, Lin K, Robson RJ (1976) Influence of certain dietary fibers on serum and tissue cholesterol levels in rats. J Nutr 106: 118-123

Thammana M, Seshamma S, Nambaaru, S (2016) A mini review on wheatgrass. J Pharmacog Phytochem 12: 2347-2332

Tirgar PR, Thumber BL, Desai TR (2011) Isolation, characterization and biological evaluation of Iron chelator from *Triticum aestivum* (Wheat Grass). Intern J Pharma Biol Sci 2: 288-296

Wigmore A (1985) The Wheatgrass Book. Avery publishing group Inc. Wayne, New Jersey

Young MA, Cook JL, Webster KE (2006) The effect of topical wheatgrass cream on chronic plantar fasciitis: a randomized, double-blind, placebo-controlled trial.Complement Ther Med 14: 3-9

Zendehbad SH, Mehran MJ, Malla S (2014) Flavonoids and phenolic content in wheat grass plant (*Triticum aestivum*). Asian J Pharm Clin 7: 184-187.

❑❑❑

Chapter 19

Holy Basil (*Ocimum sanctum L.*)

Amitav Bhattacharyya and Garima Shukla

Department of Poultry Science, College of Veterinary Science and Animal Husbandry, U P Pt. Deen Dayal Pashu Chikitsa VigyanVishwavidyalya, Mathura- 281001, India, E-mail: amitav16@rediffmail.com

ABSTRACT

Holy Basil (*Ocimum sanctum* L.), the queen of herbs is one of the holiest and most cherished of the many healing and healthy giving herbs of the orient. The leaf of holy basil contains eugenol, euginal, urosolic acid, carvacrol, linalool, limatrol, caryophyllene, methyl carvicol while the seed volatile oil have fatty acids and sitosterol. In addition, the seed mucilage contains some levels of sugars and the anthocyans are present in green leaves. The sugars are composed of xylose and polysaccharides. The plant extract has antioxidant, antibacterial, immuno-modulatory, antidiabetic, anti-inflammatory and anticancerous effects. Holy basil extracts are used in Ayurvedic remedies for pain, fever, vomiting, bronchitis, ear ache, common colds, headaches, stomach disorders, inflammation, diseases of heart and blood, various forms of poisoning and malaria. It is also used in case of diabetes, arthritis and asthama. Extract of holy basil have been used as growth promoter and immunomodulatory agent in poultry.

Keywords: *Ocimum sanctum*, Eugenol, Carvacrol, Immuno-modulation, Poultry.

19.1 Introduction

Holy Basil (*Ocimum sanctum* L.), also known as or Tulsi leaves has been used for thousands of years in Ayurveda for its diverse healing properties. Tulsi, the queen of herbs is one of the holiest and most cherished of the many healing and healthy giving herbs of the orient. The sacred basil, Tulsi, is renowned for its religious and spiritual sanctity, as well as for its important role in the traditional Ayurvedic and Unani system of holistic health and herbal medicine of the East. Tulsi is an important symbol in many Hindu religious traditions, which link the plant with Goddess figure. The name 'Tulsi' in Sanskrit means 'the incomparable one'. The presence of a Tulsi plant symbolizes the religious bend of a Hindu family. It has been mentioned by Charaka in the Charaka Samhita, an Ayurvedic text. Tulsi is considered to be an adaptogen, balancing different processes in the body and helpful for adapting to stress. Marked by its strong aroma and astringent taste, it is regarded in Ayurveda as a kind of 'elixir of life' and believed to promote longevity. Tulsi extracts are used in Ayurvedic remedies for pain, fever, vomiting, bronchitis, ear ache, common colds, headaches, stomach disorders, inflammation, diseases of heart and blood, various forms of poisoning and malaria. It is also used in case of diabetes, arthritis and asthama. Fresh leaves taken with black pepper are used as a prophylactic against malaria and a decoction of the root are recommended for malarial fever. The leaf juice is used in chronic fever, haemorrhage, dysentery and dyspepsia. It is used also as an anthelmenthic and is topically used for ringworm and skin diseases. Its pounded leaves are mixed with sandalwood and applied topically for relief in headache. Tulsi seeds are used in anti leucoderma preparations. Traditionally, *tulsi* is taken in many forms *viz.* herbal tea, dried power or fresh leaf. For centuries, the dried leaves of Tulsi have been mixed with stored grains to repel insects.

19.2 Botanical Description

Tulsi is a member of the family *Lamiaceae* (*Labiatae*) and is closely related to the common basil (*Ocimum basilicum*). Tulsi is an erect, much branched sub-shrub 30-60 cm tall covered with soft hairs and have simple opposite green or purple leaves that are strongly scented. The stems are square in transaction. The leaves are opposite, elliptical-oblong with relatively long petioles and serrated leaf margins. Leaves have petiole, up to 5 cm long and are usually somewhat toothed. The flowers appear in racemes arising in whorls on the terminal part of the stem and are labiates, bilaterally symmetrical and purplish in colour.

Classification

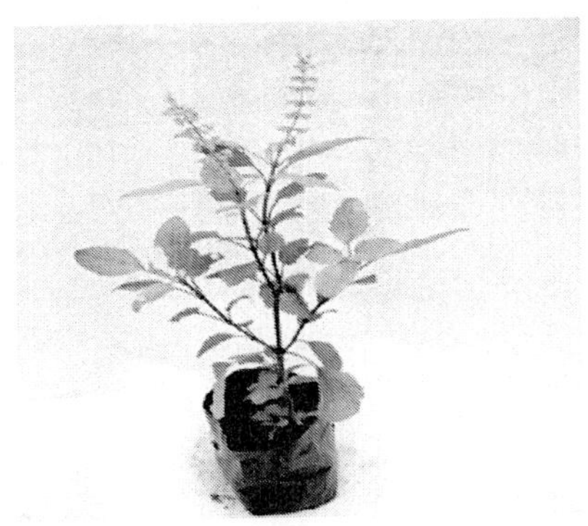

Kingdom	:	Plantae
Division	:	Magnoliophyta
Class	:	Magnoliopsida
Order	:	Lamiales
Family	:	Lamiaceae
Genus	:	*Ocimum*
Species	:	*Sanctum*

19.3 Geographical Distribution

Tulsi is widespread as a cultivated plant and an escaped weed throughout the world tropics. It is cultivated for religious and medicinal purposes and for its essential oil. Tulsi is found throughout India and it is said to have been grown profusely in Vrindavan, Uttar Pradesh, India. It is also grown in many part of old world tropics and also occur in the warmer part of Australia.

Vernacular names

English	:	Holy basil, Monk basil, Rough basil, sacred basil
Hindi	:	Tulsi or Tulasi, Vrinda
Sanskrit	:	Ajaka, Arjaka, Gauri, Gramya, Haripriya, Laxmi, Krishanamula, Madhvi, Vaishnavi
Tamil	:	Alungai, Karut, Tulasi, Kullai, Karut
Bengali	:	Kalatulsi, Kural, Tulshi, Tulsi
Malayalam	:	Krishnatulsi, Kunnakam, Punya, Shivatulsi, Trittavu
Gujrati	:	Tulsi, Tulasi
Arabic	:	Dohsh, Shadjant, Vasub
Kanada	:	Kalatulsi, Karitulsi, Sritulsi, Tulasi

19.4 Phytochemical Constituents

The chemical composition of tulsi is highly complex, containing many nutrients and other biologically active compounds, the proportions of which may vary considerably between strains and even among plants within the same field. Furthermore, the quantity of many of these constituents is significantly affected by differing growing, harvesting, processing and storage conditions that are not yet well understood. The nutritional and pharmacological properties of the whole herb in its natural form, as it has been traditionally used, result from synergistic interactions of many different active phytochemicals. Consequently, the overall effects of Tulsi cannot be fully duplicated with isolated compounds or extracts. Because of its inherent botanical and bio-chemical complexity, Tulsi standardization has, so far, eluded modern science.

Tulsi contains eugenol, carvacrol, methylchavicol. Tulsi contains a volatile oil consisting of about 70% eugenols as well as methyl eugenol and caryophyllene. Other constituents with likely pharmacological activity include the triterpenoidursonic acid, rosmarinic acid, alkalids, saponins, flavonoids (including apigenin and luteolin and glycosides thereof), phenylpropane glucosides and tannins. The seeds of tulsi contain affixed oil containing five fatty acids, including about 17% linolenic acid and just over 50% linoleic acid. The leaf volatile oil contains eugenol (1-hydroxy-2-methoxy-4-allylbenzene), euginal (also called eugenic acid), urosolic acid (2,3,4,5,6,6a,7,8,8a,,10,11,12,13,14b-tetradecahydro-1H-picene-4a-carboxylic acid), carvacrol (5-isopropyl-2-methylphenol), linalool (3,7-dimethylocta-1,6-dien-3-ol) limatrol, caryophyllene, methyl carvicol (also called Estragol) while the seed volatile oil have fatty acids and sitosterol. In addition, the seed mucilage contains some levels of sugars and the anthocyans are present in green leaves. The sugars are composed of xylose and polysaccharides.

Although tulsi is known as a general vitalizer and increases physical endurance, it contains no caffeine or other stimulants. The stem and leaves of holy basil contain a variety of constituents that may have biological activity, including saponins, flavonoids, triterpenoids, and tannins (Jaggi *et al.*, 2003). Two water-soluble flavonoids, Orientin (8-C-beta-glucopyranosyl-3′,4′,5,7-tetrahyd-roxyflav-2-en-3-one) and Vicenin (6-C-beta-D-xylopyranosyl-8-C-beta-D-glucopyranosyl apigenin), have been shown to provide protection against radiation-induced chromosomal damage in human blood lymphocytes (Uma *et al.*, 2000).

19.5 Therapeutic Applications

Tulsi has a long history of medicinal use and is mentioned in ancient Ayurvedic text such as Charak Samhita. Tulsi is used for treatment of variety of conditions including pain, fever, vomiting, bronchitis, earache and diseases of heart and blood. It is also used in case of diabetes, arthritis and asthma. Whole plant (leaves, stem, flower, root) has therapeutic use. The leaves are acrid and bitter. Fresh leaves taken with black pepper used as a prophylactic against malaria and a decoction of the root are recommended for malarial fever. The leaf juice is used in chronic fever, haemorrhage, dysentery and dyspepsia. Its pounded leaves are mixed with sandalwood and applied topically for relief in headache. Tulsi seeds are used in anti leucoderma preparations. Zheljazkov *et al.* (2008) reported that essential oil containing *O.bacilium* as component had *in vitro* activity against *Leishmania donovani*. Tulsi has different types of action. It has anti stress activity and it improves resistance to different types of stress. It is also regarded as herbal antibiotic. It has antipyretic activity and it is very effective in case of malarial fever. It also helps in relieving during respiratory problems as bronchitis and asthama. Many studies show that it has antioxidant activity. It also has the anti inflammatory and analgesic activity. It has anti-diabetic action because tulsi leaves have been reported to reduce blood glucose when administered to rat and human beings with diabetes. It helps in healing of wounds. Tulsi is a dipana, an herb that improves the digestive fire, and also acts as an appetizer and digestive. It also acts as an adaptogen. It significantly increases cell-mediated immunity, both in the number of immune defense cells and also in their activity.

The whole plant of *Ocimum Sanctum* has medicinal value (Gordon and Dravid, 2001), although mostly the leaves, and sometimes the seeds, are used. Earlier studies with tulsi have indicated that the plant has hypoglycaemic (Wink, 2000), hypolipidaemic (Cor *et al.*, 1970), adaptogenic (Warrier, 1995), anti-cancer (Biswas and Biswas, 2005), radioprotective (Sen, 1993), analgesic (Gupta *et al.*, 2002) and anti-inflammatory properties. Village women and Ayurvedic physicians have been reported to be using tulsi leaves for anti-fertility effect (Chopra *et al.*, 1956), but this type of traditional practice has been limited to rural areas of India (Anbarasu *et al.*, 2007). A rational approach to this traditional practice with modern scientific methods is not available in medical literature in spite of the easy availability of *Ocimum Sanctum* in India. Leaves of tulsi have antizygotic, anti-implantation and early abortifacient effect in women and in experimental animals.

19.5.1 *Antidiabetic Effect*

Ethanolic extract of *tulsi* significantly decreases the blood glucose, glycosylated haemoglobin and urea with a concomitant increase in glycogen, haemoglobin and protein in streptozotocin-induced diabetic rats. This extracts also resulted in an increase in insulin and peptide levels and glucose tolerance. The constituents of *O. sanctum* L. leaf extracts have stimulatory effect on physiological pathways of insulin secretion, which may underlie its reported antidiabetic action.

Grover *et al.* (2005) suggested that treatment with *O. sanctum* L. extract for 30 days to normal rats fed with fructose for 30 days significantly lowered serum glucose level in comparison with control group. However, *O. sanctum* L. extract has no significant effect on hyperinsulinemia. Gholap and Kar (2004) unraveled the possible mechanism of glucose-lowering activity of *O. sanctum* L. in male mice. The study suggested that *O. sanctum* L. decreases the serum concentration of both cortisol and glucose and also exhibited antiperoxidative effect. Therefore, *O. sanctum* L. may potentially regulate corticosteroid- induced diabetic mellitus. Vats *et al.* (2004) reported that administration of *O. sanctum* L. extracts in rats @ 200 mg/kg for 30 days lead to decrease in plasma glucose levels by approximately 9.06 and 24.4% on 15th and 30th day. Chattopadhyay (1993) also reported that oral administration of alcoholic extract of leaves of *O. sanctum* L. led to marked lowering of blood sugar level in normal, glucose-fed hyperglycemic and streptozotocin-induced diabetic rats. Furthermore, the extract potentiates the action of exogenous insulin in normal rats. The activity of the extract was 91.55 and 70.43% of that of Tolbutamide in normal and diabetic rats, respectively.

19.5.2 *Wound Healing Activity*

Ethanolic extract of leaves of *O. sanctum* L. was investigated for normal wound healing and dexamethasone-depressed healing. The extract significantly increased the wound breaking strength, wound epithelializes fast and wound contraction was significantly increased along with increase in wet and dry granulation tissue weight and granulation tissue breaking strength (Udupa *et al.*, 2006).

19.5.2 *Genotoxicity*

In vivo cytogenetic assay in *Allium cepa* root tip cells has been carried out to detect the modifying effect of *O. sanctum* L. aqueous leaf extract against chromium (Cr) and mercury (Hg)-induced genotoxicity (Babu and Uma, 2006). It was observed that the roots post-treated with the leaf extract showed highly significant recovery in mitotic index (MI) and chromosomal aberrations. When compared to pre-treated (Cr/Hg) samples, the lower doses of the leaf extract were found to be more effective than the higher doses.

Jena *et al.* (2003) reported that Immu-21, a poly-herbal formulation containing *O. sanctum* L. and other herbal extracts when given at 100 mg per kg daily over 7 days and 300 mg/kg daily over 14 days inhibited both cyclophosphamide (40 mg/kg i.p.)-induced classical and non-classical chromosomal aberration (40–60% of control). This also reduces the increase in micronuclei in the bone marrow erythrocytes of mice treated with cyclophosphamide.

19.5.3 *Antioxidant Activity*

Geetha and Vasudevan (2004) noted that aqueous extract of *O. sanctum* L. inhibits the hypercholesterolemia-induced erythrocyte lipid peroxidation activity in a dose-dependent manner in male albino rabbits. Oral feeding also provides significant leaver and aortic tissue protection from hypercholestrolemia-induced peroxidative damage. The effect of methanolic extract of *O. sanctum* L. leaves in cerebral reperfusion injury as well as long-term hypoperfusion was studied by Yanpallewar *et al.* (2004). *Osimum sanctum* L. pre-treatment (200 mg/kg/day for 7 days) prevented reperfusion-induced rise in lipid peroxidation and superoxide dismutase.

19.5.4 *Antimicrobial Activity*

Singh et al. (2005) in his study suggested that higher content of linoleic acid in *O. sanctum* L. fixed oil could contribute towards its antibacterial activity. The oil shows good antibacterial activity against *Staphylococcus aureus, Bacillus pumius* and *Pseudomonas aeruginosa,* where *S. aureus* was the most sensitive organism Geeta *et al.* (2001) reported that the aqueous extract of *O. sanctum* L. (60 mg/kg) show wide zones of inhibition compared to alcoholic extract against *Klebsiella, E. coli, Proteus, S. aureus* and *Candida albicans,* when studied by agar diffusion method. Alcoholic extract showed wider zone for *Vibrio cholerae.*

19.5.5 *Immunomodulatory Effect*

Godhwani *et al.* (1988) investigated the immunoregulatory profile of methanolic extract and an aqueous suspension of *O. sanctum* L. leaves to antigenic challenge of *Salmonella typhosa* and sheep erythrocytes by quantifying agglutinating antibodies employing the Widal agglutination and sheep erythrocyte agglutination tests and E-rosette formation in albino rats. The data of the study indicate an immuno-stimulation of humoral immuno-genic response as represented by an increase in antibody titer in both the Widal and sheep erythrocyte agglutination tests as well as by cellular immunologic response represented by E-rosette formation and lymphocytosis.

19. 5.6 *Anti-inflammatory Activity*

Singh (1998) in his study reported that linoleic acid present in different amount in the fixed oil of different species of *O. sanctum* L. has the capacity to block both the cyclooxygenase and lipoxygenase pathways of arachidonate metabolism and could be responsible for the anti-inflammatory activity. A methanolic extract (Godhwani *et al.*, 1987) and an aqueous suspension of *O. sanctum* L. (500 mg/kg) inhibited acute as well as chronic inflammation in rats as tested by carrageenin-induced pedal edema and cratonoil -induced granuloma and exudates, respectively, and the response was comparable to the response observed with 300 mg/kg of sodium salicylate.

19.5.7 *Anticancer Activity*

Prashar *et al.* (1998) in their study reported that *O. sanctum* L. leaf extract blocks or suppresses the events associated with chemical carcinogenesis by inhibiting metabolic activation of the carcinogen.

19.6 Role of Tulsi in Livestock and Poultry

Tulsi may reduce infections in cows (Kumar *et al.*, 2011), poultry (Sadekar *et al.*, 1998), goats (Deka, 2009). Immunotherapeutic potential of aqueous extract of O. sanctum L. leaf in bovine sub-clinical mastitis (SCM) was investigated after intramammary infusion of aqueous extract. The results revealed that the aqueous extract of *O. sanctum* L. treatment reduced the total bacterial count and increased neutrophil and lymphocyte counts with enhanced phagocytic activity and phagocytic index (Mukherjee *et al.*, 2005). Tulsi may also be used in combination with other herbs for the treatment of various ailments and elicit production in animals and birds.

One such example has been mentioned below:

Tephrosia purpurea	40%
Eclipta alba	20%
Andrographis paniculata	10%
Terminalia chebula	10%
Ocimum santum	10%
Excipients	Q.S.

Indications

- As a liver tonic.
- To improve liver functions in hepatic disorders.
- To improve feed conversion ratio (FCR).
- As a growth promoter in broiler and layer

Administration & dosages

To be given orally.

Cattle and Buffaloes : 5-10 g. once daily for 10 days.

Sheep and Goat : 3-5 g. once daily for 10 days.

Broilers / Layers : 100g. in kilogram feed concentrate regularly

(Anonymous, 2015).

Poultry

Gupta and Charan (2007) studied the non toxic doses of *Ocimum sanctum* in broiler chicken. Broiler chicken at two weeks of age were divided in to seven groups and supplemented with different doses *viz.* 0, 100, 200, 300, 400, 500, and 600 mg of Tulsi leaf powder per chicken for 15 days. It was found that maximum weight gain was observed in the group of chickens treated with 200 mg of dried leaves powder per birds daily for 15 days as compared to control group.

Rao *et al.* (1999) studied the effect of Zeetress, a polyherbal preparation containing *Withania somnifera, Ocimum sanctum, E. officinalis* on chicken and found that administration of zeetress minimized stress and had a positive effect on weight gain, feed conversion, general resistance and livability. Babu *et al.* (2002) studied the effect of zeetress, a poly herbal compound containing (*Ocimum sanctum, Withania somnifera* and *Emblica officinalis*) against cypermethrin induced immunosuppression and reported that cypermethrin significantly reduced the phagocytic, opsonic indices and body weight, where as zeetress significantly restored the affected phagocytic, opsonic indices and body weight.

Batra and Gupta (2004) studied the clinicopathological and immunological effect of *Ocimum sanctum* in chicken. Tulsi leaf powder supplemented @ 5 gm/kg feed did not cause any pathological lesion in the tissue. Delayed type hypersensitivity response against di nitro chloro benzene antigen was significantly increased in the *Ocimum sanctum* leaf powder group, indicating the immuno modulatory activity of tulsi leaf. Sapcota et al. (2005) noted that *Ocimum sanctum* fed in the diet as (0.1%, 0.15%, 0.2% and 0.25%) showed ameliorating effect on aflatoxicosis in broilers at a dose related fashion. Among the various doses, 0.20% was found to be the best. The herb also yielded beneficial effects on various zoo technical parameters in broilers when fed singly.

Hindustani and Singh (2006) reported that Zeetress, a herbal preparation containing extract of *Ocimum sanctum* and *Withania somnifera* as major ingredient added to the drinking water @ 5mg per bird from day 3 to 28 and 10mg/bird from day 29 to 42 had immuno-potentiating effect in vaccinated chicken with better immune response to Newcastle disease virus vaccine, lower lesion scores, improvement in live weight gain and feed conversion efficiency. Mamta and Mishra (2006) reported that administration of tulsi dry leaf powder @ 5 g/kg of feed enhanced cell mediated immune response as observed by DTH in terms of increased foot pad thickness to sonicated bacterial cell protein (sbcp) antigen. It also enhanced humoral immune response against *S. pullorum* plain antigen as detected by standard tube agglutination (SAT) test. The present findings indicate that tulsi dry leaf powder has an immunopotentiating effect.

Lanjewar *et al.* (2008) reported that supplementation of tulsi leaf powder @ 0.5% and 1.0% significantly increased the final body weight and weekly body weight gain in broiler chicken. Feed conversion ratio also improved in 1.0% tulsi leaf powder group. They also noted that serum HDL cholesterol level was significantly increased with supplementation of tulsi in diet. The net profit found was more in birds supplemented with 0.5% Tulsi leaf powder than 1.0% tulsi leaf powder. They concluded that supplementation of tulsi leaf powder @

1.0% in broiler diet for 42 days reduced the meat and serum cholesterol with increase in serum HDL–cholesterol. Kumar *et al.* (2012) concluded that 0.5% TLP may be supplemented to elicit growth performance and immune response of commercial broilers.

19.8 Conclusions

In recent years, there has been a resurgence of interest in investing the traditional health promoting uses of Tulsi. The nutritional and pharmacological properties of the whole herb in its natural form, as it has been traditionally used, may result from synergistic interactions of many different active phytochemicals. Consequently, the overall effects of Tulsi cannot be fully duplicated with isolated compounds or extracts. Because of its inherent botanical and bio-chemical complexity, Tulsi standardization has, so far, eluded modern science. Tulsi is also known as a general vitalizer and increase physical endurance, it contains no caffeine or other stimulant.

References

Anbarasu K, Vijayalakshmi G (2007) Improved shelf life of protein-rich Ocimum sanctum (tulsi) extracts to benefit Indian rural population. J Food Sci 72: M 300-305

Anonymous (2015) http://www.vetsfarma.com/ philippines_livestock4. html. 2015

Babu BJ, Kalakumar B, Reddy KS, Rao AS (2002) Effect of zeetress on cypermethrin induced suppression of growth and immunity in broiler birds. Indian J Toxicology 9(1): 35-38

Babu K, Maheshwari KC (2006) *In vivo* studies on the effect of Ocimum sanctum L. leaf extract in mordifying the genotoxicity induced by chromium and mercury in Allium root meristems. J Environ Biol 27: 93–95

Batra M, Gupta RP (2004) Effect of ocimum sanctum (TLP) on clinicopathological and immune response in chickens. Haryana Veterinarian 43: 48-50

Biswas NP, Biswas AK (2005) Evaluation of some leaf dusts as grain protectant against rice weevil Sitophilus oryzae (Linn.). Environ Ecol 23: 485–488

Chattopadhyay RR (1993) Hypoglycemic effect of Ocimum sanctum leaf extract in normal and streptozotocin diabetic rats. Indian J Exp Biol 31: 891–893

Chopra RN, Nayer SI, Chopra IC (1956) Glossary of Indian Medicinal plants CSIR,New Delhi

Cor JS, Beach JF, Blair A, Clark AJ, King J, Lee TB (1970) Disodium chromoglycate. Adv Drug Res 5: 190–196

Deka RS (2009) Influence of tulsi (*Ocimum sanctum*) and ashwagandha (*Withania somnifera*) supplementation on production of organic meat in goats. Vet Practitioner 10: 57–59

Geetha RK, Vasudevan DM (2004) Inhibition of lipid peroxidation by botanical extracts of Ocimum sanctum: In vivo and in vitro studies. Life Sci 76: 21–28

Gholap S, Kar A (2004) Hypoglycemic effects of some plant extracts are possibly mediated through inhibition in corticosteroid concentration. Pharmazie 59: 876–878

Godhwani S, Godhwani JL, Vyas DS (1987) Ocimum sanctum: An experimental study evaluating its anti-inflammatory, analgesic and antipyretic activity in animals. J Ethnopharmacol 21: 153–63

Godhwani S, Godhwani JL, Vyas DS (1998) Ocimum sanctum: A prelimnary study evaluating its immuno-regulatory profile in albino rats. J Ethnopharmacol. 24: 193–198

Gordon MC, David JN (2001) Naturan product drug discovery in the next millennium. Pharm Biol 39: 8–17

Grover JK, Vats V, Yadav SS (2005) Pterocarpus marsupium extract (Vijayasar) prevented the alteration in metabolic patterns induced in the normal rat by feeding an adequate diet containing fructose as sole carbohydrate. Diabetes Obes Metab 7: 414–420

Gupta G, Charan S (2007). Exploring the potential of ocimum sanctum (Shyama tulsi) as a feed supplememt for its growth promoter activity in broiler chickens. Indian J Poult Sci 42(2): 140-143

Gupta SK, Prakash J, Srivastava S (2002) Validation of traditional claim of Tulsi, Ocimum sanctum Linn. as a medicinal plant. Indian J Exp Biol 40: 765–773

Hindustani SC, Singh KC (2006) Immuno-modulatory effect of zeetress in IBD vaccinated broiler chicken. Indian Vet J 83(7): 711-715

Jaggi RK, Madaan R, Singh B (2003) Anticonvulsant potential of holy basil, Ocimum sanctum Linn. and its cultures. Indian J Exp Biol 41: 1329–1933

Jena GB, Nemmani KV, Kaul CL, Ramarao P (2003) Protective effect of a polyherbal formulation (Immu-21) against cyclophosphamide-induced mutagenicity in mice. Phytother. Res 17: 306–310

Kumar S, Gupta HP, Prasad S, Rajora VS, Prasad JK (2011) Antibacterial properties of garlic and tulsi in repeat breeding crossbred cows. Indian Vet J 88: 28–30

Kumar S, Singh HN, Bhattacharyya A (2012) Comparative efficacy of antibiotic and tulsi leaf powder supplement on the growth, immune response and carcass characteristics of commercial broilers. IPSACON Souvenir, Dec 5-7, Hyderabad pp. 32

Lanjewar RD, SZanzad AA, Ramteke BN, Ingewar SM, Patankar RB (2008) Effect of dietary supplementation of tulsi (*Ocimum sanctum*) leaf powder on meat cholesterol and serum lipid profile in broilers. Ildex India

Mamta and Mishra SK (2006) Effect of tulsi (O. sanctum) dry leaf powder on immune response to broiler chickens experimentally infected with Salmonella gallinarum. J Immunol Immunopathol 6: 13-14

Mukherjee R, Dash PK, Ram GC (2005) Immuno-therapeutic potential of Ocimum sanctum (L) in bovine subclinical mastitis. Res Vet Sci 79(1): 37-43

Prashar R, Kumar A, Hewer A, Cole KJ, Davis W, Phillips D (1998) Inhibition by an extract of *Ocimum sanctum* of DNA-binding activity of 7,12-dimethylbenz anthracene in rat hepatocytes in vitro. Cancer Lett 128: 155–60

Rao NR, Pande CB, Kiran (1999) Effect of zeetress on broiler performance. Pashudhan 14(2): 4-7

Sadekar RO, Pimprikar NM, Bhandarkar, AG, Barmase BS (1998) Immuno-modulating effect of Ocimum sanctum linn. Dry leaf powder on humoral immune response in poultry naturally infected with IBD virus. Indian Vet J 75: 73–74

Sapcota D, Islam R, Baruah KK, Upadhyaya TN (2005) A study on the efficacy of dietary Ocimum sanctum against aflatoxin B contaminated feed in broilers. Indian J Poult Sci 40(3): 282-284

Sen P (1993) Therapeutic potential of Tulsi: From experience to facts. Drug News Views 1: 15–21

Singh S (1998) Comparative evalution of anti-inflammatory potential of fixed oil of different species of Ocimum and its possible mechanism of action. Indian J Exp Biol 36: 1028–1031

Singh S, Malhotra M, Majumdar DK (2005) Antibacterial activity of Ocimum sanctum L.fixed oil. Indian J Exp Biol 43: 835–837

Udupa SL, Shetty S, Udupa AL, Somayaji SN (2006) Effect of Ocimum sanctum Linn.on normal and dexamethasone suppressed wound healing. Indian J Exp Biol 44: 49–54

Vasudevan DM, Kedlaya R, Deepa S, Ballal M (2001) Activity of Ocimum sanctum (the traditional Indian medicinal plant) against the enteric pathogens. Indian J Med Sci 55: 434–448

Vats V, Yadav SP, Grover JK (2004) Ethanolic extract of Ocimum sanctum leaves partially attenuates sterptozotocin-induced alterations in glycogen content and carbohydrate metabolism in rats. J Ethnopharmacol 90: 155–160

Warrier PK (1995) In: Indian Medicinal Plants. CBS publication, New Delhi. pp. 168.

Wink M (2000) Introduction Bio-chemistry, role and bio-technology of secondary products. In: Bio-chemistry of secondary product metabolism (Wink, M., eds.), Florida: CRC press, Boca Raton. pp. 1–16

Yanpallewar SU, Rai S, Kumar M, Acharya SB (2004) Evaluation of antioxidant and neuroprotective effect of Ocimum sanctum on transient cerebral ischemia and long-term cerebral hypoperfusion. Pharmacol Bio-chem Behav 2(79):155–164

Zheljazkov VD, Cantrell CL, Tekwani B, Khan SI (2008) Content, composition and bio-activity of the essential oils of three basil genotypes as a function of harvesting. J Agric Food Chem 56(2): 380-338.

□□□

Chapter 20

Giloy (*Tinospora cordifolia*)

Dinesh Jain[1] and Tara Bothra[2]

[1] Department of Animal Nutrition, College of Veterinary and Animal Sciences, Rajasthan University of Veterinary and Animal Sciences, Bikaner, Rajasthan, India, E-mail: ddineshvet@gmail.com

[2] Department of Livestock Production and Management, College of Veterinary and Animal Sciences, Rajasthan University of Veterinary and Animal Sciences, Bikaner, Rajasthan, India

ABSTRACT

Tinospora cordifolia is a large deciduous, extensively spreading climbing shrub with a number of coiling branches. The plant contains many phytoconstituents such as diterpene, tinosporone, tinosporic acid, cordifolisides, syringen, berberine, giloin, gilenin, etc. These phytoconstituents have different type of activity such as neuro-protective, immunomodulatory, antioxidant, anti-inflammatory, hepatoprotective and antimicrobial activity. This plant is used to improve the immune system and body resistance against infections. In ruminants the herb improves milk yield and milk quality by relegating heat stress, stimulating milk secretion, suppressing mammary infection, improving nutrient utilisation, and boosting immune function. *Tinospora cordifolia* alone and in combination with other herbs have been effectively used to improve immunity and growth performance in poultry.

Keywords: Tinosporone, Immunomodulation, Poultry, *Tinospora cordifolia.*

20.1 Introduction

Herbal plants have been in major demand due to their great efficiency of herbal remedies. Herbs play a significant role especially in modern times and primary healthcare needs of nearly 80% of the world's population relies mainly on plant-based-traditional-medicines (Anonymous, 2003). India is bestowed with enormous bio-diversity of medicinal plants. Plants and plant derived products being natural, non toxic or residue free have multiple effects on animal including appetite stimulator, enhanced secretary activity of GIT, immuno-stimulant, bactericidal, antiviral, antioxidants and are termed as phytogenics (Hashemi and Davoodi, 2011). Among them *Tinospora cordifolia* has a wide range of bioactive principles and occupies the top of the list of 'Ayurvedic Materia Medica' because of its extraordinary power of healing. *T. cordifolia* is described as a potential healer of many diseases in the ancient texts of Ayurveda. It is known as heart leaved Moonseed plant in English, Guduchi in Sanskrit, Giloy in Hindi and there is so many local names as depicted in Table 1 (Bhattacharya and Bhattacharya, 2013). *Tinospora cordifolia* belonging to the family Menispermaceae, is a climbing shrub widely distributed throughout India. *T. cordifolia* can be propagated by seeds and vegetative cuttings and it can be grown in almost all climates but mostly favours warm climate with medium black or red soil for its cultivation. Planting is usually done during rainy season (July to August). *Tinospora cordifolia* is also called as Neem Giloy because of its climber nature with Neem (*Azadirachta indica*) and it also incorporate the medicinal virtue of Neem (Anonymous, 1982). Due to its high demand, *T. cordifolia* has been listed in 178 medicinal plant species in high Volume Trade by NMPB, New Delhi, India. Every part of the plant has therapeutic value, but the stem is the most frequently used part of the medicinal preparations (Mittal *et al.*, 2014).

20.2 Botanical Description

The genus Tinospora Miers (Menispermaceae) is represented by four species in India *i.e. T. cordifolia, T. sinensis, T. crispa and T. glabra. T. cordifolia* and *T. sinensis* resemble each other in many microscopic characters but can be differentiated by some characters as depicted in Table 2.

Taxonomic Descriptions of *T. cordifolia*

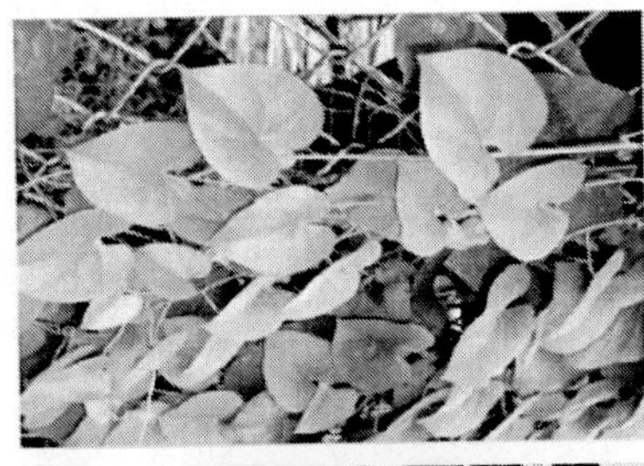

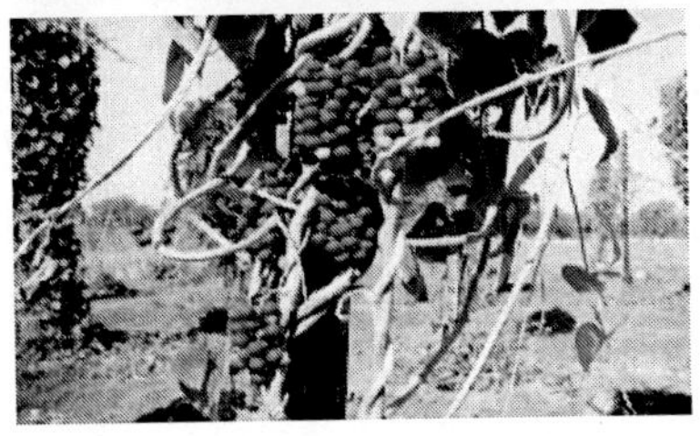

Kingdom	:	Plantae
Subkingdom	:	Tracheophyta
Superdivision	:	Spermatophyta
Division	:	Magnoliophyta
Class	:	Magnoliopsida
Subclass	:	Polypetalae
Series	:	Thalamiflorae
Order	:	Ranales
Family	:	Menispermaceae
Genus	:	*Tinospora*
Species	:	T. *cordifolia*

Tinospora cordifolia is a large deciduous, extensively spreading climbing shrub with a number of coiling branches. Different parts of *Tinospora cordifolia* is presented in Fig. 1. Stem of this plant is rather succulent with long, filiform, fleshy and climbing in nature. Aerial roots arise from the branches. The bark is creamy white to grey in colour. Aerial roots are characterized by tetra to penta-arch primary structure. Leaves simple, alternate, exstipulate, long petioles up to 15cm long, roundish, pulvinate, at both the base and apex with the basal one longer and twisted partially and half way around. Flowers are unisexual, recemes, greenish yellow in colour, appears when plant is leafless. Male flowers are clustered and female flowers exist in solitary inflorescence. Sepals are 6 in 2 series of 3 each, outer ones being smaller. Petals are also 6, smaller than sepals, free and membranous. Flowering occurs during March to June. Fruits aggregate of 1-3, ovoid smooth drupelets on thick stalk with subterminal style scars, scarlet or orange coloured.

Table 1: Local names of *Tinospora cordifolia*

Language		Name in local language
Assamese	:	Hoguni-Lot, Amarlot, Amarlata, Aor-Lota
Bengali	:	Gadancha, Gulancha, Giloe, (In Bangladesh: Pipolti, Gulunchi, Pipulti, Padma Gulancha, Pipul-Morich, Gulocho)
English	:	Heart-Leaf-Moonseed, Tinospora
Himachal Pradesh	:	Galoein, Guljya
Meghalaya	:	Poddho-Guloncho
Gujarati	:	Gado, Galo, Gadu Navel
Hindi	:	Giloe, Gulbel, Gulvel, Gurcha, Chinna, Chinnarhuha, Giloy, Giloya, Gudach, Gulancha, Guluncha, Gurch, Amara, Jivanti, Jivantika, Pittagni, Tiktaparvan, Vajra, Amritvalli, Chinnodebha, Vatsadani
Kashmiri	:	Gilo
Konkani	:	Amritvel
Malayalam	:	Amrytu, Sittamrytu
Manipuri	:	Ningthou Khongli
Marathi	:	Ambarvel, Giroli, Gulvel, Amrita, Amritavalli, Gudochi, Guduchi
Mijo	:	Theisawntlung
Oriya	:	Gulancha
Punjabi	:	Gilo
Sanskrit	:	Amrita, Guduchi, Chinna, Giloy, Jivanti, Jivantika, Jvara-Arihi, Vajra, Vatsahani
Tamil	:	Amridavalli, Niraidarudian, Akaca-K-Karutan, Akaca-Valli, Akaci, Acanamirta-Tailam, Akaya-Valli, Amarai, Amudom, Amirtai, Amirta-K-Koti, Amirtavalli, Shindil Kodi
Tamang	:	Gurju
Telugu	:	Tippa-Teega, Tippatheega, Gudapaala, Guduchi, Iruluchi
Urdu	:	Guruch, Gilo and 'Abb-E-Hyat'

Table 2: Distinguished microscopic characters of *Tinospora cordifolia* and *Tinospora sinensis*

Microscopic characters	*Tinospora cordifolia*	*Tinospora sinensis*
Sclerenchymatous sheath	Disintegrated into scattered irregular patches in the cortical Regions	Broken into areas capping the vascular bundle
Crysatal	Absent	Large crystal of calcium oxalate is present within the lumen of each cork cell
Mucilaginous cells	More	Less
Vascular Strands	Fewer	More
Xylem	Well developed	Poorly developed
Pith	Narrow	Wide
Starch content	More	Less

20.3 Nutritional Composition

The proximate and mineral composition of *Tinospora cordifoila* herb is pictured in Table 3. The variation in the proximate parameters might be due to the varietal differences, agro climatic conditions, maturity and the time of the harvesting (Nordeide *et al.*, 1996; Kutbay and Ok, 2001). The following data represents good nutritional value of *Tinospora cordifolia* for body building and boosting of immune response.

20.4 Ethno Botanical Uses of *T. cordifolia*

Ethnoveterinary alternatives are an option for livestock farmers to prevent minor health problems of livestock by the use of herbs. The use of plants as medicine is widespread throughout the world. Ethno-veterinary and herbal medicinal products ideally have multiple effects and are helpful in a variety of disease conditions as well as

Table 3: Chemical composition of Tinospora cordifoila

Particulars	**Stem** (Chauhan *et al.*, 2014)	**Stem** (Sood and Shilpa, 2015)	**Stem** (Nile & Khobragad, 2009)	**Stem** (Mahima *et al.*, 2014)	**Stem** (Hussain *et al.*, 2009)	**Leaves** (Pandey *et al.*, 2016)
Chemical composition (% dry matter basis)						
Moisture	69.40	10.63	18.34	34.39	-	9.64
EE	1.03	1.92	3.10	0.91	1.99	1.05
CP	1.85	2.13	4.50	7.74	13.32	5.23
NFE	9.05	-	-	-	-	7.53
Ash	3.60	6.35	12.40	7.96	-	5.88
CF	14.83	5.72	15.90	56.42	23.30	52.30
Cellulose	-	-	-	23.02	-	-
NDF	-	24.80	-	58.31	-	-
ADF	-	25.20	-	54.61	-	-
Minerals ((mg/100g)						
Ca	212	-	-	10.22	-	210
P	193	-	-	2.48	-	-
Na	205	-	-		-	-
K	0.97	-	-		-	-
Fe	0.089	-	-	2.61	-	22.55
Cu	32	-	-	0.37	-	-
Zn	143	-	-	0.73	-	-
Mn	0.29	-	-	1.22	-	-
Mg	6.34	-	-	-	-	-
Vitamin C	17.01	-	-	-	-	16
Beta carotene (µg)	-	-	-	-	-	428.5
Energy (kcal)	-	-	-	-	-	240

for beneficial effects on animal health. The paste of stem of the *T. cordifolia* and the roots of *Solanum surattense* was used in the treatment of fever (Singh and Maheshwari, 1983) by the tribals Baiga of Varanasi district. The tribals of Bombay and the fishermen along the sea coast use *T. cordifolia* as drug in the treatment of fever, jaundice, chronic diarrhoea and dysentry (Shah, 1984). The whole plant is beneficial in treatment of dysentery (Singh *et al.,* 2002; Jain *et al.,* 2009), urinary diseases (Rai and Gupta 1967), gout (Choudhary *et al.,* 2013), Skin diseases (Pandit 2010; Gupta *et al.,* 1967) and anamia (Nayampalli *et al.,* 1986).

20.5 Phytochemical Constituents of *T. cordifolia*

Knowledge of the chemical constituents of plants is desirable for the discovery of its therapeutic agents. Phytochemical composition of *Tinospora cordifolia* is depicted in Table 4. *T. cordifolia* contains a large number of different types of phytoconstituents which may vary according to geographical location of plant, includes alkaloids (Jadeja *et al.,* 2006; Pandey *et al.,* 2012), glycosides (Pandey *et al.,* 2012; Singh, 2005), diterpenoid lactones (Pandey *et al.,* 2012), aliphatic compounds (Sankhla *et al.,* 2012), carbohydrates polysaccharides (Singh, 2005; Subramanian *et al.,* 2002) and phenols (Ghate *et al.,* 2013). Important phytoconstituents are diterpene, tinosporone, tinosporic acid, cordifolisides A to E, syringen, berberine, giloin, gilenin, crude giloinin, arabinogalactan polysaccharide, picrotene, bergenin, gilosterol, tinosporol, tinosporidine, cordifol, heptacosanol, octacosonal, tinosporide, columbin, chasmanthin, palmarin, palmatosides C and F, amritosides, cordioside, tinosponone, berberine, ecdysterone, makisterone A, magnoflorine, tembetarine, syringine, sitosterol, glucan polysaccharide, syringine apiosylglycoside, isocolumbin, palmatine, tetrahydropalmaitine and jatrorrhizine. These phytoconstituents have different type of activity such as neuroprotective effect (berberine, choline, tembetarine, tinosporin, palmitine, jatrorrhizine), immunomodulatory activity (cordifolioside A, tinocordiside, syrigin), antioxidant activity (tinosporin, isocolumbin, palmatine), anti-inflammatory activity (furanolactone, tinosporin, tinosporide, jateorine, columbin, clerodane derivatives), hepatoprotective activity (tinosporin, isocolumbin, palmatine, tetrahydropalmatine) and antimicrobial activity (furanolactone, tinosporon, jateorine, columbin).

This plant is used to improve the immune system and body resistance against infections because of its various pharmacological activities including antimicrobial (Manjusha *et al.*, 2011), anti-diarrhoel (Kumar *et al.*, 2010), antiprotozoal (Sawangjaroen and Sawangjaroen, 2005), anti-stress (Sarma *et al.*, 1995), hepatoprotective (Dahanukar *et al.*, 2004), hypocholesterolemic (Nagaraja *et al.*, 2008) and immunomodulator (Desai *et al.*, 2002). Ethanolic extract of aerial part have neuroprotective effect (Kosaraju and Roy, 2014). Aqueous extract of whole plant have immuno-modulatory activity (Gupta and Sharma, 2011) and hepatoprotective activity (Stance *et al.*, 2011), while ethanolic extracts have antioxidant activity (Ramesh *et al.*, 2015). Studies reported aqueous extracts of stem have anti-infammatory activity (Patgiri *et al.*, 2014) antibacterial activity (Xavier and Anand, 2003) while its ethanolic extracts have radioprotective, cytoprotective and antibacterial activity (Xavier and Anand, 2003).

Table 4: Phytochemical composition of *Tinospora cordifolia*

Phytochemicals	***Tinospora cordifolia* leaves***	***Tinospora cordifolia* stem****
Polyphenols (mg/100g)	12.2	5700
Flavanoids(mg/100g)	18.28	-
Anti- Radical Activity (%)	19.75	21.72
Saponin (%)	-	1.92
Tanin (%)	-	0.56
Alkaloid (%)	-	0.25
Flavonoids (%)	-	0.81
Carotenoids (mg/100gm β-carotene)	-	0.98
(*Pandey *et al.*, 2016 ** Chauhan *et al.*, 2014)		

20.6 Role of *Tinospora cordifolia* in Animal Feeding

Nowadays, phytogenic feed additives are being used in animal feeding to improve the productivity of livestock through amelioration of feed properties, promotion of the animal's production performance and improving the quality of food derived from those animals (Windisch *et al.*, 2008).

20.6.1 Influence on Animal Performance

Herbs are used as feed additives for a better growth instead of antibiotics due to the wide variety of active components present in them which affect digestion processes in various ways. Most of them stimulate the secretion of saliva and enhances the synthesis of bile acids in the liver and their excretion in bile, which further beneficially effects the digestion and absorption of lipids. Supplementation of *Tinospora cordifolia* stem powder have significant effect on overall feed intake in broiler birds as reported by Kulkarni *et al.* (2011) and Bhushan *et al.* (2013) while Sarag *et al.* (2001), Vidyarthi *et al.* (2008) and Bhardwaj et al. (2011) reported no improvement in feed intake and feed conversion ratio in broiler birds. Supplementation of Superliv concentrate premix containing *Tinospora cordifolia* is beneficial for broiler production and optimum feed utilization (Singh *et al.*, 2009). Singh (2014) reported that *Tinospora cordifolia* alone and in combination with other herbs is an effective feed additive for better broiler production.

20.6.2 Antioxidant Activity

The antioxidant activity of *T. cordifolia* (Soni and Chauhan, 2015) stem is due to presence of phenolics, flavonoids, alkaloids, tannins and carbohydrate. It also possesses good DNA protective potential. *Tinospora cordifolia* has the ability to scavenge free radicals generated during aflatoxicosis and provide protection against aflatoxin-induced nephrotoxicity due to the presence of alkaloids (Gupta and Sharma, 2011). On administration of aqueous extract of roots of *T. cordifoila* in alloxan diabetic rats for six weeks, Stanley and co-workers (1999) found significant reduction of serum and tissue cholesterol, phospholoipids, and free fatty acids in alloxan diabetic rats.

20.6.3 Antimicrobial Activity

Antibacterial activity of *T. cordifolia* extract has been reported by many researchers against *Escherichia coli, Staphylococcus aureus, Klebsiella pneumonia, Proteus vulgaris, Salmonella typhi, Shigella flexneri, Salmonella paratyphi, Salmonella typhimurium, Pseudomonas aeruginosa, Enterobacter aeruginosa, Enterobacter aerogene* (Narayan *et al.*, 2011; Jayachandran *et al.*, 2003; Ambekar *et al.*, 2009). Sengupta *et al.* (2009) reported improved phagocytic and intracellular bacterial capacities of neutrophils against bacterial growth in mice. Shakya *et al.* (2014) studied *in vivo* antibacterial effect of *T. cordifolia* in broiler orally challenged by *E. coli* and found better protection and survival rate as compared to control. Soni and Chauhan (2015) obtained maximum diameter of zone of inhibition (24mm at 1g/ml) with organic extract of *Tinospora cordifolia*. Likewise Kaur *et al.* (2016) studied the antibacterial properties for *Tinospora cordifolia* stem extracts and showed marked dose dependent antimicrobial activity *in vitro* against both Gram +ve bacteria (*Staphylococcus aureus*) and Gram–ve bacteria (*Escherichia coli*).

20.6.4 Immuno-modulatory Activity

Tinospora cordifolia has been well-documented for its immuno-modulatory response by many researchers (Tripathi *et al.*, 1997; Bishayi *et al.*, 2002; Subramanian *et al.*, 2002). Rege *et al.* (1999) reported the significant adaptogenic activity of the whole and aqueous extracts of *T. cordifolia* on a variety of biological, physical and chemical stressors on different animal models. Aqueous *T. cordifolia* extracts have been reported to influence the cytokine production, mitogenicity, stimulation and activation of immune effector cells (Upadhyaya *et al.*, 2011). Arabinogalactan polysaccharide (Chintalwar *et al.*, 1999) isolated from the dried stem, appeared to induce tolerance against endotoxic shock by modulation of cytokines and nitric oxide. Subramanian *et al.* (2002) also observed good protective effect of arabinogalactan polysaccharide against iron mediated lipid peroxidation of rat brain homogenate. Significant immuno-modulatory effect of *Tinospora cordifolia* on the functions of macrophages obtained from mice treated with the carcinogen ochratoxin A have been investigated by Dhuley (1997). Sudhakaran *et al.* (2006) observed that the fish injected with ethanol and petroleum ether extract of leaves at a dose of 8 mg/kg were protected against experimental infection with virulent *A. hydrophila* and concluded that the *T. cordifolia* leaf extract is useful as an immunoprophylactic to prevent diseases in finfish aquaculture. Kolte *et al.* (2007) studied the effect of feeding *T. cordifolia* herb in broiler, which were immuno-suppressed with cyclophosphamide and found a significant increase in antibody titer level against ND virus with augmentation of inflammatory reaction to skin contact sensitivity test. Dietary supplementation of *T. cordifolia* in broiler diet enhances immunity as an alternative to antibiotics (Rajkumar *et al.*, 2009). *T. cordifolia* stem extract for its property of immuno-modulation like levamisole can also be used potentially before mass vaccination of the chicks (Bhardwaj *et al.*, 2011).

20.6.5 Anti-inflammatory Activity

Girish and Priyadarshini (2012) investigated the effect of *T. cordifolia* on wound healing in albino rats and concluded that *T. cordifolia* promotes healing of wounds and peri-operative use of *T. cordifolia* gives better results in healing of surgical wounds.

20.6.6 Hepato Protective Activity

A formulation having *T. cordifolia* has been reported to express hepatoprotective properties in adult goats of either sex (Nasare *et al.*, 2001). Rege *et al.* (1984) studied the use of *T. cordifolia* in the hepatic damage induced by carbon tetra chloride (CCl_4) and found effective results in preventing fibrous changes and promoting regeneration by parenchymal tissue. *T. Cordifolia* as drug is useful in relieving the symptoms as well as normalization of altered liver function test (Prakash and Rai, 1996).

20.6.7 Herbal Galactogogue

Recently, *T. cordifolia* has also been studied for its use as a galactogogue in dairy animals in India. Supplementation of ration with *T. cordifolia* significantly improves milk yield and milk quality by relegating heat stress, stimulating milk secretion, suppressing mammary infection, improving nutrient utilisation, and boosting immune function. *Tinospora cordifolia* with its lactogenic properties and other health benefits have been mentioned as indispensable herb in Indian system of medicine (Sehgal and Sood, 2013). Mir *et al.* (2014) reported average milk yield (kg/day) in *T. cordifolia* supplemented group (8.07) was significantly ($P<0.05$) higher than the control (7.16) in Murrah buffaloes. The dietary supplementation of *T. cordifolia* results in improved milk production and reduction in somatic cell count (Mallick and Prakash, 2011) in crossbred cattle. Sharma (2017) reported significantly higher milk phosphorus values in *T. cordifolia* supplemented Jersey crossbred animals as compared to control group on day 60 of experiment while no significant difference was observed in any other mineral during the course of herbal supplementation.

20.6.8 Effect on Blood Parameters

The supplementation of root extract of *T. cordifolia* resulted in hypoglycemic and hypolipidaemic effect in alloxan diabetic rats (Stanley *et al.*, 1999) with reduction in serum and tissue cholesterol, phospholipids and free fatty acids (Stanley *et al.*, 2000). The study of

Wadood *et al.* (1991) revealed no significant effect on total lipid levels in normal as well as in alloxan-treated diabetic rabbits by supplementation of extract of *T. cordfolia* leaves. They also reported that extracts of the leaves of *T. cordfolia* have insulin-like action and can significantly reduce the blood glucose in normal rabbits and in alloxan-induced diabetic rabbits. The alcoholic extract of *T. cordifolia* (500mg/kg body weight, orally) resulted in decreased levels of serum creatinine, blood urea nitrogen and alkaline phosphatase in cisplastin induced nephrotoxicity in rats (Khanam *et al.*, 2011). Dhingra *et al.* (2011) reported lower triacylglycerol levels in rats treated with *T. cordifolia* stem extract. The plasma lipid profile (TAG, Total Cholesterol, HDL and LDL) values of *T. cordifolia* fed animals remained lower in comparison to control group but the differences were non-significant (Sharma, 2017) likewise Vetrivadivelan *et al.* (2012) revealed that the aqueous extract of *T. cordifolia* was found to increase HDL concentrations in blood of streptozocin-induced diabetic rats. Sharma (2017) also reported the significantly lower plasma glucose levels and lower A:G ratio in the *T. cordifolia* fed group of Jersey crossbred than the control group animals. Sharma and Pandey (2010) reported that *T. cordifolia* stem extract significantly increased the value of Hb and PCV in mice. Similarly, Manjrekar *et al.* (1999) reported increased leukocyte count in mice by aqueous extract of *T. cordifolia.*

20.6.9 Carcass Traits and Organometry

Singh (2014) reported significant improvement in dressing weight percentage by supplementation of *T. cordifolia* in broiler. There was no adverse effect found on the internal organs i.e. liver, heart, gizzard and giblet per cent in broiler in the *T. cordifolia* herb supplementation group due to the antistress effect of *T. cordifolia* supplementation (Kulkarni *et al.*, 2011; Dhore *et al.*, 2014).

20.7 Summary and Conclusions

The livestock sector has an important role in the overall economy of the nation. Livestock serve as a key factor in the nation's overall development in the agriculture sector. Animal husbandry practices are generally done by rural farmers. Small land holdings, low income, poor veterinary facilities and a minimal exposure to new technology make it difficult for the farmers to have high economic gains. Objective of most of the research work, in India, is based on the use of by-products and the upgrading of ingredients. Apart from this, using supplements based on herbs is best suited for marginal farmers.

Ayurveda has listed various herbal plants and out of which *Tinospora cordifolia* is easily and abundantly available in every part of India and is used by many communities due to its proven medicinal property as mentioned in many ancient text of Ayurveda. A thorough study about *Tinospora cordifolia* as herbal feed additive shall pave a way towards a cheap, economic and easily accessible way of augmenting livestock production. Keeping in mind the different phytoconstituents and nutritional values present in it, furthermore research is needed to explore the potential of *T. cordifolia* in optimum livestock production.

References

Ambekar DH, Khante BS, Chandak BR, Titare AS, Baralkar SS, Aghadte SN (2009) Screening of antibacterial potential of some medicinal plants from Melghat forest in India. Afr J Trad Comp Altern Med 6: 228-232

Anonymous (1982) Pharmacognosy of Indigenous Drugs, Vol. 1, Edited by K Raghunathan and Roma Mitra, (Central Council for Research in Ayurveda & Siddha, New Delhi), 321

Anonymous (2003) World Health Organization. Traditional medicine-growing needs and potential. WHO policy perspectives on medicine, No. 2. WHO/EBM/2002. Geneva. (WHO, 2003, Revised Traditional Medicine Facts. Sheet No.134.http://www.who.int/mediacentre/factsheets/fs134/en

Bhardwaj U, Tiwary BK, Prasad A, Ganguly S (2011) Use of Tinospora cordifolia as poultry feed supplement. Intern J Bio-Med Life Sci Res 1(1): 18–22

Bhattacharyya C, Bhattacharyya G (2013) Therapeutic potential of Giloe, *Tinospora cordifolia* (willd.) Hook. F. & Thomson (Menispermaceae): The magical herb of ayurveda. International J Pharmac Bioll Arch 4(4): 558-584

Bhushan SS, Ramnivas, Sigh DP, Bisen B (2013) Impact of herbal based diets on production efficiency of broiler. The Bioscan 8(1): 119–22

Bishayi B, Roychowdhury S, Ghosh S, Sengupta M (2002) Hepatoprotective and immuno-modulatory properties of *Tinospora cordifolia* in CCl_4 intoxicated mature albino rats. J Tox Sci 27(3): 139-146

Chauhan DK, Puranik V, Mishra, V (2014) Analysis of stem of *Tinospora cordifolia,* leaves of *Andrographis paniculata* and root and leaves of *Boerhaavia diffusa* for nutritional and phytochemical composition. Intern J Food Nutr Sci 3(4): 104-111

Chintalwar G, Jain A, Sipahimalani A, Banerji A, Sumariwalla P, Ramakrishnan R, Sainis, K (1999) An immunologically active arabinogalactan from *Tinospora cordifolia*. Phytochem 52(6): 1089-1093

Dahanukar SA, Rege NN, Oak, MA (2004) *In-vitro* effect of *Tinospora cordifolia* on leukemia cell proliferation. Indian J Pharmacol 95: 130-135

Desai VR, Kamat JP, Sinis KB (2002) An immuno-modulator from *Tinospora cordifolia* with antioxidant activity in cell free system. Indian J Exper Biol 114: 713-720

Dhingra D, Vaneeta J, Sharma S, Kumar HR (2011) Evaluation of antiobesity activity of *Tinospora cordifolia* stems in rats. Int J Res Ayurv Pharma 2(1): 306-311

Dhingra D, Goyal PK (2008) Evidences for the involvement of monoa-minergic and GABAergic system in antidepressant like activity of *Tinospora cordifolia* in mice. Indian J Pharm Sci 70(6): 761-767

Dhore RN, Tangade SU, Dhok AP (2014) Effect of herbal and synthetic vitamin C supplementation on performance of broilers under intense summer conditions. Indian J Poult Sci 49(1): 48-51

Dhuley JN (1997) Effect of some Indian herbs on macrophage functions in ochratoxin A treated mice. J Ethnopharmacol 58(1): 15-20

Ghate NB, Chaudhuri D, Mandal N (2013) *In vitro* assessment of *Tinospora cordifolia* stem for its antioxidant, free radical scavenging and DNA protective potentials. Int J Pharm Bio Sci 4(1): 373-388

Girish M, Priyadarshini K (2012) The influence of *Tinospora cordifolia* on wound healing in albino rats. Int J Pharma Biosci 3(2): 379-384

Gupta R, Sharma V (2011) Ameliorative effects of *Tinospora cordifolia* root extract on histopathological and bio-chemical changes induced by aflatoxin-b (1) in mice kidney. Toxicol Int 18: 94-98

Gupta SS, Verma, SC, Garg VP, Rai M (1967) Anti-diabetic effects of *Tinospora cordifolia*. Effect on fasting blood sugar level, glucose tolerance and adrenaline induced hyperglycemia. Indian J Med Res 55: 733-745

Hashemi SR, Davoodi H (2011) Herbal plants and their derivatives as growth and health promoters in animal nutrition. Vet Res Commun 35: 169-180

Hussain J, Khan AL, Rehman N, Hamayun M, Shinwari ZK, Ullah W, Lee IJ (2009) Assessment of herbal products and their composite medicinal plants through proximate and micronutrients analysis. J Med Plants Res 3(12): 1072-1077

Jadeja BA, Odedra NK, Odedra KR (2006) Herbal remedies used for haemorrhoids by tribals of Saurashtra, Gujarat. Indian J Traditional Knowledge 5(3): 348-352

Jain SC, Jain R, Singh R (2009) Ethnobotanical survey of sariska and siliserh regions from Alwar district of Rajasthan. India Ethnobotanical Leaflets 1(21)

Jayachandran R, Xavier TF, Anand, SP (2003) Antibacterial activity of stem extracts of *Tinospora cordifolia* (willd.) Hook. F. and Thoms. Ani Sci Life 22: 40-43

Kaur H, Amini MH, Suttee A (2016) Evaluation of antioxidant and anthelmintic properties of *Caesalpinia sappan* L. Leaves. Int J Pharm Phytocheml Res 8(2): 362-368

Khanam S, Mohan NP, Devi K, Sultana R (2011) Protective role of *Tinospora cordifolia* against cisplastin induced nephrotoxicity. Int J Pharm Pharmaceut Sci 3(4): 98-70

Kolte AY, Siddiqui MF, Mode SG (2007) Immuno-modulating effect of *Withania somnifera* and *Tinospora cordifolia* in broiler birds. Indian J Vet Medi 27(1): 33-37

Kosaraju J, Roy PD (2014) Neuroprotective effect of *Tinospora cordifolia* ethanol extract on 6-hydroxydopamine induced parkinson disease. Int J Pharmacol 46: 176-80

Kulkarni RC, Mandal AB, Munj CP, Dan A, Saxena A, Tyagi PK (2011) Response of coloured broilers to dietary addition of Geloi (*Tinospora cordifolia*) during extreme summer. Indian J Poult Sci 46(1): 70-74

Kumar R, Sharma RJ, Bairwa K, Roy RK, Kumar A (2010) Pharmacological review on natural antidiarrhoel agents. Der Pharma Chemica 2(2): 66-93

Kutbay HG, Tolga OK (2001) Foliar N and P resorption and nutrient levels along an elevational gradient in Zelkova carpinifolia (Pall.) C. Koch subsp. yomraensis Ansin and Gercek. Annals of Agri Bio Research 6(1): 1-8

Mahima, Rahul A, Prakash A, Verma AK, Kumar V, Roy D (2014) Proximate and elemental analysis of *Tinospora cordifolia* stem. Pakistan Journal of Biological Sciences 17(5): 744-747

Mallick S, Prakash BS (2011) Influence of feeding *Tinospora cordifolia* peripartum on lactation parameters in crossbred cows. Journal of Animal Physiology Animal Nutrition 96(6): 1112-1120

Manjrekar PN, Jolly CI, Narayan S (1999) Comparative studies of the immuno-modulatory acivities of *Tinospora cordifolia* and *Tinospora sinensis*. Fitoterapia 71(3): 254-257

Manjusha GV, Rajathi K, Alphonse JKM, Meera KS (2011) Antioxidant potential and antimicrobial activity of *Andrographis paniculata* and *Tinospora cordifolia* against pathogenic organisms. J Pharm Res 4(2): 452-55

Mir AN, Kumar P, Rather SA, Sheikh FA, Wani SA (2015) Effect of supplementation of *Tinospora cordifolia* on lactation parameters in early lactating Murrah buffaloes. Buffalo Bulletin 34(1): 17-20

Mir AN, Parveen K, Wani SA, Shergojry SA, Ashutosh, Aarif O (2014) Milk production status of lactating murrah buffaloes on *Tinospora cordifolia* supplemented diet with special reference to immunological, metabolic and hormonal profile. Anim Sci Rep 8(1): 18-25

Mittal J, Sharma MM, Batra A (2014) *Tinospora cordifolia*: a multipurpose medicinal plant- A review. J Med Plants Studies 2(2): 32-47

Nagaraja PK, Kammar KF, Sheela DR (2008) Efficacy of *Tinospora cordifolia* (Wild.) extracts on blood lipid profile in streptozotocin diabetic rats. Is it beneficial to the heart? Biomed Res 19(2): 92-96

Narayanan AS, Raja SS, Ponmurugan K, Kandekar SC, Maripandi A (2011) Antibacterial activity of selected medicinal plant against multiple antibiotic resistant uropathogens: A study from Kolli Hills, Tamil Nadu, India. Benef. Microbes 2: 235-243

Nasare P, Lal SB, Sharma MC (2001) Therapeutic efficacy of an indigenous drug formulation in experimental hepatopathy and nephropathy in goats. Indian J Anim Sci 71: 819-822

Nayampalli SS, Desai SS, Ainapure (1986) Dry barks of *T. cordifolia* has anti-spasmodic, anti-pyretic, anti-allergic and anti-leprotic properties. Indian J Pharm 18: 250-252

Nile H, Shivraj, Khobragade NC (2009) Determination of nutritious value and mineral elements of some important medicinal plant from western part of India. J Med Plants 8: 1-6

Nordeide MB, Hatloy A, Folling E, Lied E, Oshaug A (1996) Nutrient composition nutritional importance of green leaves and wild food resources in an agriculture district, Koutiala, in southern Mali. Int J Food Sci Nutr 47: 455-469

Pandey M, Surendra K, Chikar MKV, Rohit S, Gulab ST, Bisen PS (2012) *Tinospora cordifolia*: A climbing shrub in health care management. Int J Pharm Bio Sci 3(4): 612-628

Pandey M, Paul V, Singh P, Ali Z (2016) Evaluation of nutritional composition and antioxidant activity of herbal leaves. World J Pharm Pharmaceut Sci 5(8): 1396-1402

Pandit PK (2010) Inventry of ethno veterinary medicinal plants of Jhargram division, West Bengal, India

Patgiri B, Umretia BL, Prajapati PK, Shukla VJ (2014) Anti-inflammatory activity of aqueous extract of *Tinospora cordifolia*. Ayurveda 35: 108-110

Prakash S, Rai NP (1996) Role of *Tinospora cordifolia* (Willd.) Miers (Guduchi) in the treatment of infective hepatitis. J Res Ayurv Siddha 17(1-2): 58

Rai M, Gupta SS (1967) Experimental evaluation of *Tinospora cordifolia* (guduchi) for dissolution of urinary calculi. J Res Ind Med 2(1): 115-116

Rajkumar RS, Yadav AS, Kirupasankar M, Saxena VK, Singh S (2009) Effect of *Tinospora cordifolia* supplementation on immunity of broiler chicks. Indian Vet J 86(12): 1244-1245.

Ramesh V, Jayaprakash R, Sridhar MP (2015) Antioxidant activity of ethanol extract of *Tinospora cordifolia* on N-nitrosodiethylamine induced lier cancer in male wistar albino rats. J Pharmac Bioallied Sci 1: 45-50

Rege N, Dahanukar S, Karandikar SM (1984) Hepatotoxic effects of *Tinospora cordifolia* against carbon tetrachloride induced liver damage. Indian Drugs 21(12): 544

Rege NN, Thatte UM, Dahanukar SA (1999) Adaptogenic properties of six rasayana herbs used in Ayurvedic medicine. Phytother Res 13(4): 275-291

Sankhala LN, Saini, RK, Saini BS (2012) A review on chemical and biological properties of *Tinospora cordifolia*. I.J.M.A.P. 2(2): 340-344

Sarag AN, Khobragade RS, Rekhate DH, Dhok AP (2001) Supplementation of *T. cordifolia* (0.5%) and *L. reticulata* (0.5%) has positive effects on live weight gain and feed efficiency of broilers. Punjabrao Krishi Vidyapeeth Res J 25(2): 114-115

Sarma DNK, Khosa RL, Chansauria JPN, Sahai M (1995) Antiulcer activity of *Tinospora cordifolia Miers* and *Centella asiatica Linn* extracts. Phyto Res 9(8): 589-590

Sawangjaroen N, Sawangjaroen, K (2005) The effects of extracts from anti-diarrheic Thai medicinal plants on the *in vitro* growth of the intestinal protozoa parasite: *Blastocystis hominis*. J Ethnopharm 98: 67-72

Sehgal AB, Sood SK (2013) Ethnoveterinary practices for herbal cure of livestock used by rural populace of Hamirpur, (H.P.) India. J Agric Vet Sci 3(1): 7-14

Sengupta S, Mukherjee A, Goswami R, Basu S (2009) Hypoglycemic activity of the antioxidant saponarin, characterized as alpha-glucosidase inhibitor present in *Tinospora cordifolia*. J Enzyme Inhib Med Chem 24: 684-690

Shah GL (1984) Some economically important plants of salsette island near Bombay. J Econ Tax Bot 5: 753

Shakya P, Sharma V, Sharma RK, Sharda R, Misraulia KS, Bamnele R (2014) *In vivo* antibacterial activity of cow urine with medicinal herbs. Environ Eco 32(1): 146-149

Sharma A, Kumar N, Dogra PK, Saklani S (2017) Effect of feeding Giloy (*Tinospora Cordifolia*) and Fenugreek (*Trigonella Foenum-Graecum*) on lipid profile in jersey crossbred cows. Explor Anim Med Res 7(2): 142-147

Sharma V, Pandey D (2010) Beneficial effects of *Tinospora cordifolia* on blood profiles in malemice exposed to lead. Toxico Intern 17(1): 8–11

Singh KK, Maheshwari JK (1983) Traditional phytotherapy amongst the tribals of varanasi distric, U.P. Journal of Economic & Taxonomic Botany 4: 829

Singh RK (2005) *Tinospora cordifolia* as an adjuvant drug in the treatment of hyper-reactive malarious splenomegaly: Case reports. J. Vector Borne Dis. 42: 36-38

Singh A (2014) Effect of Bael (*Aegle Marmelos*) and Giloy (*Tinospora Cordifolia*) alone and in combination on growth and feed conversion of Broiler Chicks. Global J Res Analysis 3(11): 96-99

Singh, AK, Raghubanshi AS, Singh, JS (2002) Medical ethnobotany of the tribals of sonaghati of sonbhadra district, Uttar Pradesh, India. J Ethnopharmacol 81(1): 31-41

Singh VK, Chauhan SS, Ravikanth K, Maini S and Rekhe DS (2009) Effect of dietary supplementation of polyherbal liver stimulant on growth performance and nutrient utilization in broiler chicken. Vet World 2(9): 350-352

Soni AP, Chauhan GN (2015) Study of antioxidant and antimicrobial activity of medicinal plants utilized in cancer treatment. Res J Recent Sci 4: 15-21

Sood S, Shilpa (2015) Studies on preparation and evaluation of value added products from Giloy (*Tinospora cordifolia*). Himachal J Agric Res 41(1): 30-35

Stance MH, Nagy AA, Tosa M, Vlad L (2011) Hepatoprotective effect of orally administered melatonin and *Tinospora cordifolia* in experimental jaundice. Chirurgia (bucur) 106(2): 205-210

Stanely M, Prince P, Menon VP, Gunasekaran G (1999) Hypolipidaemic action of *Tinospora cordifolia* roots in alloxan diabetic rats. J Ethnopharmacol 64(1): 53-57

Stanely P, Prince M, Menon VP (2000) Hypoglycaemic and other related actions of *Tinospora cordifolia* roots in alloxan-induced diabetic rats. Journal of Ethnopharmacol 70: 9-15

Subramanian M, Chintawar GJ, Chattopadhyay S (2002) Antioxidant properties of *Tinospora cordifolia* polysaccharide against iron-mediated lipid damage and gamma-ray induced protein damage. Redox Rep 7: 137-143

Sudhakaran DS, Srirekha P, Devasree LD, Prem Singh S, Michael RD (2006) Immuno-stimulatory effect of *Tinospora cordifolia* Miers leaf extract in *Oreochromis mossambicus*. Indian J Exp Bio 44 (9): 726-732

Tambekar DH, Khante BS, Chandak BR, Titare, AS, Boralkar SS, Aghadte SN (2009) Screening of antibacterial potentials of some medicinal plants from Melghat forest in India. African J Trad Complem Altern Med 6(3): 228-232

Tripathi YB, Sharma M, Manickam (1997) Rubia 5 din, a new antioxidant from rubiacordifolia. Ind J Biochem Biophy 34: 302-30.

Upadhyaya R, Sharma PRV, Anita KV (2011) Assessment of the multifaceted immuno-modulatory potential of the aqueous extract of *Tinospora cordifolia*. Res J Chem Sci 1:71–79

Vetrivadivelan K, Venkateswaran KV, Selvasubramanian S, Sesh PSL (2012) Antihyperlipidemic effect of *Tinospora cordifolia* extract in streptozotocin induced diabetic rats. Indian J Pharmaceut Sci Res 3(5): 1423-1429

Vidyarthi VK, Nring K, Sharma VB (2008) Effect of herbal growth promoters on the performance and economics of rearing broiler chicken. Indian J Poult Sci 43(3): 297–300

Windisch, WK, Schedle, C Plitzner and Kroismayr, A (2008) Use of phytogenic products as feed additives for swine and poultry. J Anim Sci 86(14): 140–148

Wadood N, Wadood A, Shah SAW (1991) Effect of *Tinospora cordifolia* on blood glucose and total lipid levels of normal and alloxan-diabetic rabbits. Planta Medica 58: 131-136

Xavier TF, Anand SP (2003) Antibacterial activity of stem extracts of *Tinospora cordifolia.* Ancient science Life 23: 40-43.

❑❑❑

Chapter 21

Medicinal Aloe (*Aloe vera*)

Ashok Kumar Patil, R.P.S. Baghel and Sunil Nayak

Department of Animal Nutrition College of Veterinary Science and Animal Husbandry, Nanaji Deshmukh Pashu Veterinary Science University, Jabalpur-482001, India, E-mail: ashokdrpatil@gmail.com

ABSTRACT

Aloe vera is a tropical or subtropical plant which has been used for its medicinal value for several thousand years. Aloe gel is very nutritious and contains polysaccharides (55%), sugars (17%), minerals (16%), proteins (7%), lipids (4%) and phenolic compounds (1%). The gel also contains almost all vitamins and minerals. Aloin, Alprogen and emodin are major phytochemicals which have analgesics, anti-inflammatory, antiallergic, hypo-cholesteremic, anticoccidial, antibacterial, antiviral, antifingal activities. In ruminants, the herb has antimethanogenic effect. *Aloe vera* as an additive to livestock and poultry feed has great potentials for improving intestinal health, immune system response, growth performance and reproductive performance.

Keywords: Aloin, Alprogen, Anti-inflammatory, Antibacterial, *Aloe vera*.

21.1 Introduction

Aloe vera is a tropical or subtropical plant with turgid lance shaped leaves with jagged edges and sharp points (Qiao *et al.*, 2013). It is a member of Asphodelaceae (Liliaceae) family. It grows mainly in the dry regions of Africa, Asia, Europe and America. In India, it is found in Rajasthan, Andhra Pradesh, Gujarat, Maharashtra and Tamil Nadu. *Aloe vera* has been used for its medicinal value for several thousand years. Its applications have been recorded in ancient history of India, Egypt, Greece, Rome and China. It has been mentioned throughout recorded history and given a high ranking as an all-purpose herbal plant. In biblical times, the Egyptians hailed *Aloe vera* as the plant of immortality. It has many common names and often referred to as burn plant, first aid plant or medicine plant. Its name is most likely derived from the Arabic word "Alloeh" meaning shining bitter substance. Its botanical name is *Aloe vera* (L.) Burm f. (Bradley, 1992; Newton, 1979; Tucker *et al.*, 1989). There are over 250 species of aloe grown around the world. However, only two species are grown today commercially, with *Aloe barbadensis miller* and *Aloe aborescens* being the most popular. Recently, the ban on the use of antibiotic as a growth promoters in animal feeds, due to their residual effect in animal products as well as development of bacterial resistance in animals and human body, have made a way to look for alternatives of antibiotics in order to eliminate their impact on animals (Yang *et al.*, 2009). A number of feed additives like probiotics, prebiotics, organic acids and plant extracts have been found to have beneficial effects on animal production. Medical herbs properties to improve digestibility, anti-microbial, anti-inflammatory, antioxidant and immune-stimulant activity must be exploited in feeding of animals as well as safe food products for human beings. Recently, the use of *Aloe vera* has gained popularity because of herbal movement initiated by naturopaths, yog gurus, alternative medicine promoters and feed additives.

Animal nutritionist is trying to exploit the potential of *Aloe vera* as a growth promoter and in this connection they have done lots of studies. The most important part of *Aloe vera* is its leaf which is composed of two main sections: latex and gel (Boudreau and Beland, 2006). The gel is composed of about 98.5% to 99.5% water (Femenia *et al.*, 1999), and the remaining dry matter contains more than 75 biologically active ingredients (Boudreau and Beland, 2006) which have medicinal effects that are useful in treating diseases. Major ingredients of *Aloe vera* include anthraquinones, polysaccharides (almost 60 % of DM of gel), vitamins, enzymes, and low-molecular-weight compounds (Chung, 2003) which give *Aloe vera* its anti-inflammatory, immuno-modulatory, wound-healing, anti-viral, anti-fungal, anti-tumour, anti-diabetic, and anti-oxidant effects (Christaki and Florou-Paneri, 2010). Number of studies have suggest that many benefits of *Aloe vera* are due to its polysaccharides contained in gel, which compose a large part of dry matter in this gel (Hamman, 2008). A compound often analysed by researchers is the polysaccharide acemannan which has immuno-modulatory, anti-microbial, and anti-tumour effects (Choi and Chung, 2003). Most of the compounds have various biological activities with potential health benefits such as antibacterial, antiviral, antioxidants, wound healing, immune-modulatory and antidiabetic activites (Pandey *et al.*, 2010). The present chapter aims to review effects of *Aloe vera* as a natural feed additive for livestock and poultry.

21.2 Taxonomy

Kingdom	:	Plantae
Clade	:	Angiosperms
Clade	:	Monocots
Order	:	Asparagales
Family	:	Xanthorrhoeaceae
Subfamily	:	Asphodeloideae
Genus	:	*Aloe*
Species	:	*vera*

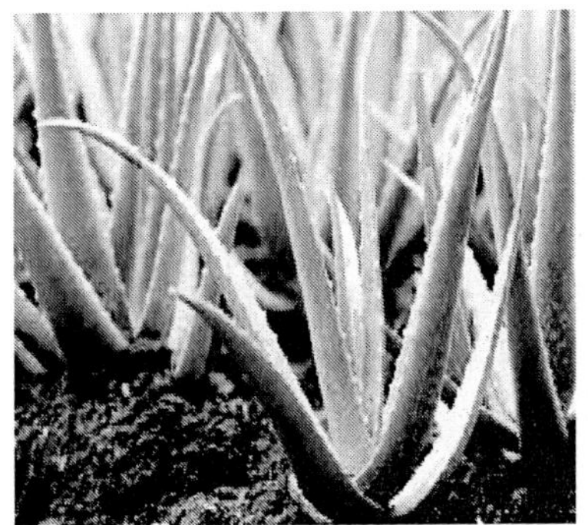

21.3 Chemistry of *Aloe vera*

The chemistry of *Aloe vera* is quite complex and has more than 200 different types of bioactive molecules (Davis, 1997) which is responsible for its medicinal and growth promoting value. The *Aloe vera* leaf gel contains about 98% water (Bozzi *et al.*, 2007). The total solid content of *Aloe vera* gel is 0.66% and soluble solids are 0.56% with some seasonal fluctuation. On dry matter basis aloe gel consists of polysaccharides (55%), sugars (17%), minerals (16%), proteins (7%), lipids (4%) and phenolic compounds (1%). The gel also contains number of vitamins including the important antioxidant vitamins A, C and E. Vitamin B_1 (thiamine), niacin, Vitamin B_2 (riboflavin), choline and folic acid are also present (Lawless and Allen, 2000).The minerals; calcium, magnesium, zinc, manganese, chromium, selenium. Additional minerals found in *Aloe vera* include copper, iron, potassium, phosphorus and sodium, *Aloe vera* also contains the trace minerals of rhodium and iridium used in cancer and tumour research experiments. Many of the medicinal effects of aloe leaf extracts have been attributed to the polysaccharides found in the inner leaf parenchymatous tissue (Davis *et al.*, 1994), but it is believed that these biological activities should be assigned to a synergistic action of the compounds contained therein rather than a single chemical substance (Domkat *et al.*, 2013).

The chemical constituents of *Aloe vera* leaves including the pulp and exudates are given in Table 1.

Table 1: Chemical constituents of *Aloe vera*

Class	*Compounds*	*Properties*
Anthraqu nones/ Anthrones	Aloe-emodin, aloetic-acid, anthranol, aloin A and B, isobarbaloin, emodin, ester of cinnamic acid	Aloin and emodinanalgesics, antibacterials and antivirals.
Carbohydrates	Pure mannan, acetylated mannan, acetylated glucomannan, glucogalactomannan, galactan, galactogalacturan, arabinogalactan, pectic substance, xylan, cellulose	Alprogen- antiallergic, anti-inflammatory.
Chromones	8-C-glucosyl-7-O-methylaloediol A, 8-C-glucosyl-(S)- aloesol, 8-C-glucosyl-7-O-methyl-(S)-aloesol, 8-C-glucosyl-7-O-methylaloediol, 8-C-glucosyl-noreugenin, isoaloeresin D, isorabaichromone, neoaloesin A	Anti-inflammatory
Enzymes	Alkaline phosphatase, amylase, carboxypeptidase, catalase, cyclooxidase, cyclooxygenase, lipase, oxidase, phosphoenolpyruvate carboxylase, superoxide dismutase	Bradykinase-reduce excessive inflammation while others help in thebreakdown of sugars and fats.
Inorganic compounds	Calcium, chlorine, chromium, copper, iron, magnesium, manganese,potassium, phosphorous, sodium, zinc	Essential for proper functioning of various enzymes.
Proteins	Lectins, lectin-like substance	Lignin, - penetrative effect into skin. Saponins- soapy substances, antiseptic properties.
Vitamins	B_1, B_2, B_6, C, β-carotene, choline, folic acid, α-tocopherol	Vitamin A, C and E – antioxidant.
Miscellaneous	Arachidonic acid, γ-linolenic acid, steroids (campestrol, cholesterol, β-sitosterol), triglicerides, triterpenoid, gibberillin, linins, potassium sorbate, salicylic acid, uric acid	
Amino acids	Alanine, arginine, aspartic acid, glutamic acid, glycine, histidine,hydroxyproline, isoleucine, leucine, lysine, methionine, phenylalanine,proline, threonine, tyrosine, valine	

Table 2: Chemical Composition and Bio-chemical activity of *Aloe vera* **leaves** (Ahmeda and Hussainb, 2013)

Nutrients	%	*Biochemical activity*	%
Ash	16.88	Superoxide dismutase (IU/mg)	2830.19
Crude fibre	73.35	Peroxidase (IU/mg)	3.72
Crude protein	6.86	Catalase (IU/mg)	2.8
Crude fat	2.91	Amylase (IU/mg)	24.02
Ascorbic acid	0.004	Reducing sugar (mg/ml)	123.33
-	-	Total soluble sugars (mg/ml)	363.03

21.4 Biological Activities of Aloe vera in Livestock and Poultry

21.4.1 *Growth Performance*

Higher gain in body weight, better feed conversion efficiency (FCE) and production of milk, meat and eggs are important economic goals in livestock and poultry farming. In previous time these goals are achieved by feed additive like antibiotics, but bans on application of AGP have affected this goal, resulting in poor growth performance and production of animals. Many researchers have done to examine potential effects of feed additives, like prebiotics, probiotics, organic acids, and herbs, on growth performance and production compared to those of antibiotics. An experiment conducted by Khan *et al.* (2014) in which they observed that birds fed diet supplemented with 1 % or 2 % *Aloe vera* leaves had greater body weight gain, better feed intake and feed efficiency than those fed diets without *Aloe vera* leaves.

An experiment comparing the effects of *Aloe vera* gel (mixed with feed) and AGP (virginiamycin) indicated that AGP (virginiamycin) resulted in better growth performance compared to the performance of groups that received *Aloe vera* gel (at 1.5%, 2%, and 2.5%), and the control group while no significant difference was observed between the antibiotic group and the 2% *Aloe vera* gel group in terms of body weight gain and feed conversion ratio (Darabighane *et al.*, 2011b). These results are agreed with findings of Mehala and Moorthy (2008). Similar to this Mmereole (2011) also observed that at 1% dietary inclusion of *Aloe vera* leaf powder in broiler diet there was significant difference in body weight gains in birds fed *Aloe vera* supplemented feed as compared to control group. However, Odo *et al.* (2010) reported that the higher weight gain in birds fed 5% level of inclusion *Aloe vera* than those of 10% and explained that *Aloe vera* in large quantitative exerts a powerful purgative effect but in smaller quantity. In an another study Alemi *et al.* (2012) reported a better growth performance in broilers treated with 0.75% and 1% *Aloe vera* gel powder compared to the 0.5% *Aloe vera* gel powder group and the control group. Danhoff and McAnally (1988) observed that the feeding of *Aloe vera* accelerated the growth of new cells, thereby, resulting to increase body weight. Contrary to above studies Hassanbeigy- Lakeh et al (2012) have observed that the supplementation of *Aloe vera* gel (0.6, 1.2, 1.8, 2.4, and 3 ml per liter) in broiler drinking water had no effect on feed intake over the total experiment period, and that the largest body weight gain and the smallest FCR was observed in the

1.8 (ml per liter) *Aloe vera* gel group. Dhurrani *et al.* (2008) stated that the addition of 10 ml aqous extract of aloe gel per litre of drinking water in broiler had beneficial effect on body weight gain and feed conversion efficiency that could be due to diversified antimicrobial activity of *Aloe vera* gel. Actually, polysaccharides of *Aloe vera* (specifically acemannan) has prebiotic like effect that is, they increase the number of lactobacillus colonies and reduce gram negative bacteria (Darabighance *et al.*, 2012). The fermentation product of lactobacillus is short chain fatty acid that will reduce the pH of lower intestine and create anunfavourable environment for gram negative bacteria. Olupona *et al.* (2010) have also observed that supplementation of *Aloe vera* in drinking water had beneficial effect on final body weight, weekly body weight gain, and average feed intake.

There are limited studies on *Aloe vera* as herbal feed additives in pigs. However, in an experiment Qiao *et al.* (2013) found that the 0.05% *Aloe vera* polysaccharide (AVP) had better effect on growth of weaned piglets than 0.02% AVP. They also found the supplementation with higher concentra-tions of AVP not only increased average daily gain, but decreased the incidence of diarrhoea and weaning stress as well.

21.4.2 *Anti-coccidial Activity*

Coccidiosis is one of the dangerous disease in poultry that affects different parts of the intestine, therefore impairs feed utilization, decreases broilers growth and egg production of laying hens and causes death of birds (Lillehoj *et al.*, 2004). Generally, Eimeria (E.) species responsible for coccidiosis in chickens include *E. tenella, E. necatrix, E. acervulina, E. maxima, E. brunetti and E. mitis* (Ayaz *et al.*, 2003; Shah *et al.*, 2009). These species infect epithelial cells of the bird's intestine causing enteritis, bloody diarrhea and immuno-suppression in chickens that paves the way to secondary disease conditions. Therefore, poultry disease management and maintenance of the immune functions for maximum consistent production performance and growth in poultry industry are fundamental requirements for profitable farming. An excellent way to meet these requirements is to use anticoccidial drugs, chemotherapeutic and biological agents including vaccines (Lillehoj and Trout, 1996; Mehala and Moorthy, 2008). Nevertheless, development of resistant pathogenic strains and drug residues in animal products used by the human beingsare the major constraints in this regard (Delespaux and Koning, 2007; Reig and Toldra,

2008).The increasing resistance to avian coccidiosis to anticoccidial drugs currently used by the poultry industry together with the requirement for drug and antibiotic free production systems has meant that it is now important to look for new ways to control the disease. In this regard, *Aloe vera* has been shown to have diverse biological activities. It has been used therapeutically for centuries and is of particular interest due to its historic reputation as a curative agent and dietary supplement (Mehala and Moorthy, 2008).

Researchers have examined potential effects of *Aloe vera* on improving growth performance in broilers with coccidiosis and found that *Aloe vera* powder (0.1%, 0.3%, and 0.5%) added to thefeed of these broilers does not lead to significant difference in terms of body weight gain (Yim *et al.*, 2011). In an another experiments Darabighane and Zarei (2011) adding 1.5%, 2%and 2.5% *Aloe vera* gel to the feed of broilers with coccidiosis and found that improved feed conversion ratio with compared to the control group.According to Dr. Lorenzo, *Aloe vera* leaf extract contains nutrients which enhance the growth of animals and even boost their immunity. It was proven to be more effective in stabilized gel form, he says, which contains upto 75 nutrients, including lignin, saponins, anthraquinones, amino acids, vitamins and minerals among others. In an experiment Akhtar *et al.* (2012) observed that the orally administration of *Aloe vera* extract (ethanol and aqous extract) in the broiler chicken has significantly lowered the oocyst count in faeces with compared to control group. They also found that the broilers that received aqueous extract of *Aloe vera* pulp had the lowest mean scorelesion in caeca and intestine in comparison to the control group and the group that received ethanol extract of *Aloe vera* pulp. Similar to this Mwale *et al.* (2006) also found that the increase in *Aloe vera* and Aloe spicata content significantly decreases coccidian oocyst count. A comparative study has done by Gadzirayi *et al.* (2005) and reported that the anticoccidial effects of *A. excelsa* were comparable with sulphachlopyrazine sodium monohydrate in terms of improved live weight gains and reducing oocyst output in broiler chickens. *A. vera* treatments show tonic effects on the intestinal tract by benefiting microflora and reducing bowel putrefaction as well as reducing inflammation (Bland, 1985). In an *in vitro* trial done by (Marizvikuru *et al.*, 2006) to know the effect of three concentrations (15%, 30%, and 45%) of *A. vera* and *A. spicata* on the inhibition of the sporulation of avian coccidiaoocysts (Marizvikuru *et al.*, 2006). Both aloe extracts showed a concentration-dependant anticoccidial effect, though, *A. spicata* inhibited sporulation to a greater extent than *Aloe vera*. Similar to this Yim *et al.* (2011) have also found that dietary supplementation of *Aloe vera* resulted in significantly lower gut lesion scores and reduced faecal oocyst shedding of *E. maxima* in broiler chickens. They also suggested that reduced faecal oocyst shedding, a protective role against Eimeria infection, in Aloe-based chicken diets could be associated more with cell-mediated responses than antibody responses.In agreement of above studies Darabighane and Zarei (2011) also reported that broilers receiving 2.5% *Aloe vera* gel had the smallest fecal oocyst shedding among all groups when compared to control group.

21.4.3 *Anti-methanogenic Effect*

Rumen is a diverse and unique microbial ecosystem composed of bacteria, protozoa, fungi and bacteriophage. In rumen hydrogen is produced during the anaerobic fermentation of nutrients. This hydrogen can be used during the synthesis of volatile fatty acids (VFAs) and microbial protein synthesis. The excess hydrogen from NADH is eliminated primarily by the formation of methane produced by methanogens. Methane is one of the greenhouse gasses which have 21 times more global warming potential than carbon dioxide (IPCC, 2007). Methane produced in ruminants represents a substantial loss (2–15%) of gross energy intake (Johnson *et al.*, 1991) which reduces the potential conversion of feed energy to metabolizable energy. Hence, the inhibition of methanogenesis has long been considered from nutritional aspects, and more recently from the perspectives on green house gas emissions.

It is a challenging task for the animal nutritionist and rumen microbiologist to make livestock industry economical and eco-friendly by controlling heat production and methane emissions from the ruminants. To combat this problem, many attempts like concentrate supplementation, use of lipid supplementation (Nevel and Demeyer, 1996) antibiotic growth promoters such as monensin and lasalocid, different categories of feed additives like halogenated methane analogues, bacteriocins, propionate enhancers, acetogens, fats, ionophores, defaunating agents, formate etc. (Asanuma *et al.*, 1999; Boadi *et al.*, 2004) had been tried, but the goal could not be successfully achieved either due to some harmful effects on animal itself or due to the presence of their residues in the animal products. Contrary to this, plants containing secondary metabolites are being used in the ethno-veterinary medical practices since long back and have yielded good effects on the animal health.One of the most known therapeutic plants is surely Aloe. The middle part of leaves containing gel, made up of carbohydrates (i.e., acemannan), anthraquinones, enzymes, inorganic compounds, amino acids, vitamins and a miscellaneous (including salicylic acid). These potentially active chemical constituents give Aloe well known therapeutic properties like wound healing, anti-inflammatory, immune-stimulating, etc. Although a lot of works have been carried out on the medicinal uses of *Aloe vera*, there is still little information on the uses of *Aloe arborescence* (syn. Candelabra Aloe; Liliaceae), that as reported by many authors (Di Luccia *et al.*, 2013; Jia *et al.*, 2008) is rich in potential bio-active chemical compounds (i.e., acemannan, amino acids, enzymes).

In an *in-vitro* experiment Calabro *et al.* (2013) observed that a significant effect of *Aloe arborescence* supplementation on the *in vitro* fermentation characteristics of feedstuffs.The supplementation of 120 mg Aloe, higher than that advised for *in vivo*, has beneficial effect on gas production compared to the lowest dosage. The close association between short chain fatty acids and gas production *in vitro* is an indicator of energy availability to the animal (Getachew *et al.*, 2002). Hence, the increased volatile fatty acids production due to the Aloe supplementation probably means higher milk yield and quality, especially in terms of fat. It is possible conclude that *Aloe arborescens* has interesting effect on the rumen microbial *in vitro* activity, stimulating microbial metabolism thereby increasing the volatile fatty acids production in the rumen. These effects may be attributed to the plant extracts rich in some active chemical compounds (i.e., flavonoid) that increase degradation of cell wall constituents, yield and efficiencyof microbial protein synthesis (Sirohi *et al.*, 2009). Similar to this Sachan *et al.* (2014) had supplement five herbs, namely *Trigonella foenum-graecum* (Methi), *Acacia concina* (Shikakai), *Trachyspermum ammi* (Ajwain), *Cinnamomum tamla* (Tejpatta) and *Aloe barbadanis* (*Aloe vera*) at the rate of 1.5%, 2.5% and 4.0% of ration and found that the addition of these herbs had no any adverse effect on rumen pH. There was significant ($P< 0.05$) improvement in *in vitro* dry matter degradability and *in vitro* organic matter degradability % of feed after addition of *Trigonella foenum-graecum* (66.22, 69.63) as compared to control (56.33, 61.37) respectively. Similarly, addition of *Aloe vera* also tended to improve the IVDMD and IVOMD of feed in respect to control. Addition of other herbs *Acacia concina* (Shikakai), *Trachyspermum ammi*

(Ajwain), *Cinnamomum tamla* (Tejpatta) did not show any improvement in the feed digestibility. From the present study, it can be concluded that *Trigonella foenum-graecum,* and *Aloe barbadanis* are the potential fermentation modifier.In agreement of this Sirohi *et al.,* 2009) also reported that among the different extracts tested, IVDMD (%) increased by 15.42% after addition of *Aloe-barbadanis.*

21.4.4 *Anti-fungal Activity*

There are many studies showing that resistance to infections enhanced by *Aloe* either in animals, whether the infective agent is a bacterium, virus or fungus (Plaskett *et al.,* 1997; Fujita *et al.,* 1976). The *Aloe* extract showed the significant antifungal activity against *Aspergillus niger, Crytococcus, neoformans, Penicilliummaneffei, F. oxysporum, Phythium*sp. *Andsolani.* Khaing (2011) Candidiasis infections are mainly caused by*Candida* (fungus) in a variety of places such asoral (thrush), vaginal (yeast infections) andgastrointestinal. These are normally treated with the help of antifungal drugs, but *Aloe vera* can remove Candidiasis infections with its natural antifungal properties. *Aloe vera* shows its antifungal activities against other fungi such as *Candida Paraprilosis, Candida Krusei* and *Candida Albicans* (Das *et al.,* 2011). Saks and Golan (1995) reported that the gel extract from leaves of *Aloe vera* possesses inhibitory action on spore germination and mycelial growth of four common post-harvest fungi: P. *digitatum, A. altemata, B. cinerea,* and P. *expansum.* Fujita *et al.* (1978) also confirmed the anti-fungal properties of Aloe species, *Aloe arborescens* Miller spp. *Natulensis* Berger, active against the human fungal pathogen *Ttichophytonment ugrophytes.*

21.4.5 *Anti-bacterial Activity*

Aloe gel is bacteriostatic or bactericidal against a variety of common wound-infecting bacteria *in vitro*: *Staphylococcus auerus, Streptococcus pyogenes, Serratiamarcescens, Klebsiellapneumoniae, Pseudomonas aeruginosa, E. coli, Salmonella typhosa*and*Mycobacterium tuberculosis.* Aloeemodin also inhibits the growth of *Helicobacter pylori* in a dose dependent fashion. Wound when occurs are more susceptible to exterior infections and other complications, leading to delay in wound healing (Ingold *et al.,* 1993). About 50-75% of the deaths are the result of infection (Mokaddas *et al.,* 1998). It has been found that the antimicrobial are responsible for slowing down the wound healing process. But when *Aloe vera* was applied in combination with an antimicrobial, then the *Aloe vera* have shown to neutralize the effect of antimicrobial and thus improving the healing process. The glycoprotein fraction of the plant is mainly responsible for the beneficial properties of *Aloe vera* of wound healing (Hamman, 2008).

21.4.6 *Anti-parasitic Activity*

Worms are very common in domestic animals, especially in grazing animals, and they cause large economic losses. Alagesan *et al.* (2002) made comparison between the following four sets of Albendazole, Neem oil, Extract of neem seed with bitter gourd, garlic, edible banana stem and *Aloe vera* and reported that the *Aloe vera* has strong antiparasitic activity. In similar to this (Fajimi *et al.*, 2002b) also observed the beneficial effect of *Aloe variegata,* spread over mange lesions.

21.4.7 *Effects on Intestinal Microflora*

The microbial population of the gastro intestinal tract is a very complex, yet stable, ecological community. The colon is populated with more than 400 species of bacteria, with anaerobes outnumbering facultative aerobes by a factor of 10^2–10^4 (Moore and Holdeman, 1975; Simon and Gorbach, 1986). These bacteria are especially important to health because they act as a barrier against the colonization of the intestinal tract with pathogenic bacteria and aid in the normal digestion of food. They also have important roles in the metabolism and toxicity of various endogenous and exogenous compounds (Rowland *et al.*, 1985).

Many studies have been carried out on using additives, including herbs, as alternatives to antibiotics, with direct or indirect effects on intestinal microflora, in poultry products (Taylor, 2001). Many studies have shown antimicrobial properties of herb extracts (Cowan, 1999; Hammer *et al.*, 1999) which can improve intestinal microflora population and enhance health in birds' digestive systems through reduction in number of disease making bacteria (Mitsch *et al.*, 2004). Number of studies have reported anti-bacterial effects of Aloe vera gel (Kwon *et al.*, 2011; He *et al.*, 2011; Pandey and Mishra, 2010; Mbanga *et al.*, 2010; Alemdar and Agaoglu, 2009; Agarry *et al.*, 2005). The studies, indicate that *Aloe vera* supplementation have beneficial effect on improving intestinal microflora, its ecosystem in broilers' intestines and gut morphology; increase in *Aloe vera* gel in broiler feeds

(1.5%, 2%, and 2.5%)led to increased *Lactobacillus* count and decreased *E. coli* count (Darabighane *et al.*, 2012). In addition, Jiang *et al.* (2005) also have reported an increase in *Lactobacillus* count and *Bifidobacteria* count as well as a reduction in *E. coli* count when acemannan (0.1% and 0.05%), polysaccharide (0.1%), and *Aloe vera* gel (0.1%) were added to broiler feed. In the agreement of this, Dai *et al.* (2007) found that herbs and polysaccharide contained in *Aloe vera* can reduce *E. coli* count while increasing the number of *Lactobacillus* and *Bifidobacteria*. Although the exact mechanism by which *Aloe vera* affects intestinal microflora in broilers is unknown, it is likely that this effect is similar to the anti-bacterial effects of some herbs,or likely that the polysaccharide contained in *Aloe vera* (acemannan) has mechanism like that of prebiotics (Guo *et al.*, 2003, 2004b). Some researchers believed that the anti-bacterial effects of *Aloe vera* to its fumaric acid content (He *et al.*, 2011).

21.4.8 *Antioxidant Effect*

The importance of reactive oxygen species (ROS) and free radicals has attracted increasing attention over the past decade. ROS is continuously produced during normal physiologic events and they can easily initiate the peroxidation of membrane lipids, leading to the accumulation of lipid peroxides. Under pathological conditions, ROS is overproduced and results in oxidative stress. Antioxidants are substances that delay or prevent the oxidation of cellular oxidizable substrates. They exert their effect by scavenging reactive oxygen species, activating a buttery of detoxifying proteins or preventing the generation of reactive oxygen species (Halliwell *et al.*, 1992). In recent years, there has been an increasing interest in finding natural antioxidants, which can protect the body from free radicals and retard the progress of many chronic diseases (Kaur *et al.* (2001) and Kinsella *et al.* (1993). Hu *et al.* (2003) have made comparison between the antioxidant activity of polysaccharide and flavonoid concentrations of 2,3,4, years-old *Aloe vera* and BHT and alpha-tocopherol. The results showed that three-years-old *Aloe vera* contained significantly higher levels of polysaccharides and flavonoids than two- and four-years-old Aloe vera, and no significant differences in flavonoid levels were found between three- and four-years-old Aloe vera. All the aloe extracts have significant antioxidant activity. The antioxidant activity of *Aloe vera* extracts & reference compounds followed the order: three-years-old Aloe vera> BHT> four-year-old Aloe vera> alpha-tocopherol> two-years-old Aloe vera. The three-years-old extract exhibited the strongest radical scavenging activity of 72.19%, which is significantly higher than that of BHT at 70.52% and alpha-tocopherol at 65.20%. According to these data, we can say that the *Aloe vera* has a strong antioxidant activity and growth stage plays a vital role in the antioxidant activity of Aloe vera. In an experiment Patel *et al.* (2012) observed excellent anti-oxidant and free radical scavenging activity in *Withania somnifera.* Both the plant possesses almost equivalent hydrogen peroxide scavenging activity while the total antioxidant capacity was found much better in *Withania somnifera* as compared to Aloe vera. The antioxidant activity of both the plant might be attributed to its polyphenolic content and other phytochemicals constituents. The findings of the present study suggested that all extracts could be a potential source of natural antioxidant that could have great importance as therapeutic agents.

21.4.9 *Hypo-cholesterolemic Effect*

High blood cholesterol is a major risk factor for heart disease and stroke. Daily supplementation with *Aloe vera* (L) stimulates immune system and improves wound healing. Iji *et al.* (2010) has conducted an experiment to assess the effect of *Aloe vera* supplementation on cholesterol level, Forty male Wistar rats divided into four groups of ten rats per group were used in the study. Group I which served as the control received 0.9% physiological saline while those in groups II, III and IV received *Aloe vera* gel (100, 250 and 500mg/kg), respectively, for four weeks. There was significant reduction in plasma total cholesterol ($P<0.001$), triglycerides ($P<0.001$) and LDL-cholesterol ratio ($p<0.01$) compared with the control. In a similar manner, those animals that were administered with 500mg/kg gel had significantly higher ($P<0.001$) HDL-cholesterol ratio than those of the control. This study showed that, chronic administration of *Aloe vera* gel extract showed cholesterol lowering action. Similar to this Chandrakar *et al.* (2008) also observed cholesterol lowering action when animals fed. To different doses (3 mg/kg, 4 mg/kg, 5 mg/kg and 6 mg/kg/day) of raw extracts of *Aloe vera* (L.) leaves along with cholesterol, there was significant decrease in serum cholesterol level.

21.4.10 *Immunostimulation/Immunosuppression*

The immuno-modulating effects of Aloe-based carbohydrates are thought to function via activation of macrophage cells and stimulation of the antigen processing. Activated macrophage cells generate nitrous oxide, secrete cytokines, such as TNF-α and IL-6, and present cell surface markers. In a study, aqueous and ethanolic extracts from the *Aloe vera* pulp exerted stimulatory effects on humoral and cellular immune responses in chickens. The higher cellular immune responses in A. vera administered chickens may be due to the Aloe polysaccharides, especially acemannan (ACM), which activated the macrophages to produce inflammatory cytokines such as IL-1, IL-6, and TNF-α (Womble and Helderman, 1988, 1992; Zhang and Tizard, 1996; Tan and Vanitha, 2004; Chow *et al.*, 2005). The ability of *Aloe vera* to stimulate the immune system is attributed to polysaccharides present inthe *Aloe vera* gel. (Davis *et al.*, 1991). Acemannan was found to have immuno-modulatory activity. It activates macrophages; enhance cytokine release; stimulate interactions between macrophages, T lymphocytes and B-lymphocytes; and enhance the generation of cytotoxic T-lymphocytes. Acemannanis potentiateantibodyproduction against coxsackie virus and reduce radiation-induced skin reactions in C3H mice.

Acemannan is also responsible for enhancing the allo-responsiveness of human lymphocytes (Womble and Helderman, 1988) as well as induced the phenotypic and functional maturation of immature dendritic cells 60, It also stimulate the phagocytosis and the candidicidal activity of macrophages (Lee *et al.*, 2001). Alprogen inhibit calcium influx into mast cells, thereby inhibiting the antigen-antibody-mediated release of histamine and leukotriene from mast cells. Ro *et al.* (2000) in a study on mice that had previously been implanted with murine sarcoma cells, acemannan stimulates the synthesis and release of interleukin-1 (IL-1) and tumour necrosis factor from macrophages in mice, which in turn initiated an immune attack that resulted in necrosis and regression of the cancerous cells. Ro *et al.* (2000) also observed that several low-molecular-weight compounds are also capable of inhibiting the release of reactive oxygen free radicals from activated human neutrophils. Recently, there has been an increasing interest of using complementary and alternative medicine. Immuno-modulatory polysaccharide represents one of the many biological response modifiers (BRMs) which can be prepared from bacteria, fungi, and plants. The poly-saccharides are thus very diverse in their components and linkages except those derived from fungi and aloe.An important property of *Aloe vera* that has been the subject of many *in vivo* and *in vitro* experiments is improvement in immune response, probably due to the acemannan contained in *Aloe vera* (Harlev *et al.*, 2012; Djeraba and Quere, 2000; Zhang and Tizard, 1996; Karaca *et al.*, 1995). Acemannan is a â (1-4)-linked acetylated mannan having mannose that can attach to mannose receptors in macrophages (Karaca *et al.*, 1995) and activate these macrophages. In addition, acemannan can stimulate the production of cytokines, release of nitric oxide (Zhang and Tizard, 1996; Karaca *et al.*, 1995). Djeraba and Quere, 2000; Karaca *et al.*, 1995) found promoted macrophage activities in broilers caused by the acemannan contained in Aloe vera. (Djeraba and Quere, 2000; Karaca *et al.*, 1995). In an experiment on *Aloe vera* effects on immunity of broilers, Valle-Paraso *et al.* (2005) who reported that broilers treated with 2% *Aloe vera* gel (in drinking water) showed significant increase in antibody titer against NDV on days 37 and 52, compared to the control group. Similar to this study Darabighane *et al.* (2012) also have reported an increase in antibody titer against Newcastle disease virus(NDV) on days 24 and 38 by adding *Aloe vera* gel to broiler feeds (at 1.5%, 2%,and 2.5%). Alemi *et al.* (2012) added *Aloe vera* gel powder (at 0.5%, 0.75%, and 1%) to broiler feeds and reported an increase in antibody titer against NDV. In agreement of this (Jiang *et al.*, 2005) also have reported an improvement in antibody titer in broilers against NDV as a result of adding acemannan (0.1% and 0.05%), polysaccharide (0.1%), and *Aloe vera* gel (0.1%) to broiler feed (Jiang *et al.*, 2005). In a study on antibody titer against sheep red blood cells (SRBC), Besharatian *et al.* (2012) reported an increase in total immunoglobulin of 35-days-old broilers that received *Aloe vera* leaf powder (0.5% and 1% mixed with feed) and aqueous extract of *Aloe vera* leaf (15 and 30 ml/l, added to drinking water). Similar to this (Mahdavi *et al.*, 2012) found a significant increase in antibody titer for the groups treated with 0.75% and 1% *Aloe vera* gel powder compared to the control group and the group receiving 0.5% *Aloe vera* gel powder.The findings of Besharatian et al. (2012), Akhtar *et al.* (2012), and Darabighane *et al.* (2012) in connection to effects of *Aloe vera* on cellular immunity after PHA-Pinjection indicate improved cellular immune response in broilers that received *Aloevera* : *Aloe vera* leaf powder (0.5% and 1%) and aqueous extract of *Aloe vera* leaf (15 and 30 ml/l) (Besharatian *et al.*, 2012), ethanolic extract of *Aloe vera* pulp (300 mg/kg body weight/day for three consecutive days) (Akhtar *et al.*, 2012), and 2.5% *Aloevera* gel

(Darabighane *et al.*, 2012) showed the best performance compared to other groups. Therefore, *Aloe vera* can affect humoral and cellular immunity as evidenced by those studies that examined *Aloe vera* effects on immune response of broilers. In examining the effects of *Aloe vera* on lymphoid organs, researchers reported relative weight gain in these organs of broilers (Darabighane *et al.*, 2012; Akhtar *et al.*, 2012; Feng *et al.*, 2011; Jiang *et al.*, 2005). Contrary to this Besharatian *et al.* (2012) did not observe a significant difference in weight of lymphoid organs, but reported a weight gain in spleen and bursa. Such relative increase in the weight of lymphoid organs as a result of adding *Aloe vera* to feed or drinking water suggests immune (humoral and cellular) system readiness against antigens.

21.4.11 *Effects on Reproductive Performance*

Estakhr and Javdan (2011) carried an experiment to access the effect of *aloevera* on reproduction, they have administered *Aloe vera* leaf pulp extract, gel extract, and a mixture of both to three groups of 10-weeks old male Wistar rats for 56 consecutive days and found that in all groups except control group the weights of the testes increased. Epididymal sperm counts, sperm motility and testosterone level increased significantly compared to control groups. According to the results of this study, *Aloe vera* has strong spermatogenic activity by increasing sperm parameters. This study strongly proposes that *Aloe ver* a specially its gel fortifies spermatogenesis and can be a good candidate for manufacturing fertility drugs. Contrary to this study Oyewopo *et al.* (2011) suggest that *Aloe vera* has potential antifertility effects in the male rat. In an another study Shima *et al.* (2011) also reported that *Aloe vera* have beneficial and supporting effects on ovarian tissue and folliculogenesis if used as a hypoglycemic agent in diabetes.

21.4.12 *Anti-Tumour Effects*

Polysaccharides isolated from *Aloe vera* have been reported to have anti-tumour activity, and the anti-tumour activity of acemannan has been examined in several animal species. A modified *Aloe vera* polysaccharide, G2E1DS2, isolated from cellulose-treated *Aloe vera* gel was shown to activate macrophages and exhibit potent anti-tumour activity when injected into the peritoneum of mice implanted with sarcoma cells (Im *et al.*, 2005). Similarly, intraperitoneal administration of both enriched and commercial forms acemannan to mice implanted with murine sarcoma cells significantly reduced the tumour burden and increased the survival rate (Peng *et al.*, 1991). Supplementation of the cancer-induced rats with vitamin C or *Aloe vera* gel extract significantly inhibited the development and severity of carcinogenesis, as reflected in the reduction of the percentage surface area of enzyme-positive foci (Shamaan *et al.*, 1998).

21.5 Toxic Effects of *Aloe vera*

Aloe vera latex is known to have toxic effects. Consumption of *Aloe vera* latex is associated with watery diarrhoea leading to electrolyte imbalance and hypokalemia (Cooke *et al.*, 1981). Other side effects include weight loss, central nervous system disturbances, and abnormalities and kidney dysfunction. Compounds in *Aloe vera* latex are also considered genotoxic and may be mutagenic (Mueller *et al.*, 1996). The abuse of *Aloe vera* latex-containing laxatives is associated with melanosis coli, which may play a role in the development of colorectal cancer (Siegers *et al.*, 1993). Intestinal tumors were induced in rats that consumed a diet containing chrysazin, a synthetic anthraquinone with dihydroxy groups like other natural anthraquinones (Mori *et al.*, 1985). In addition, compounds in *Aloe vera* latex are suspected to interact with certain oral conventional drugs, in particular corticosteroids and cardiac glycosides (Abebe, 2003; Mascolo *et al.*, 2004).

21.6 Summary and Conclusions

Keeping farm animals healthy is necessary to obtain healthy animal products. For the last decade the use of additives of natural origin in animal and human nutrition has been encouraged. To gain advantageous effects of herbs and spices, they can be added to feed as dried plants or parts of plants and as extracts. *Aloe vera*, as an additive to livestock and poultry feed, has great potentials for improving intestinal health, immune system response, and growth performance. *Aloe vera* can be used in therapeutic purposes because it contains many physiologically active substances that have effective anti-inflammatory, immunomodulatory, and wound-healing effects. It can also be used in controlling coccidiosis. Advantages of Aloe vera added to livestock and poultry feeds depend on several factors: form of use (powder, gel, extract (ethanolic or aqueous), polysaccharide extracted from gel), dosage, genetics of broilers, ingredients of diet, and farm management. Therefore, further research is required to determine effective dosage and form of use.

References

Abebe W (2000) An overview of herbal supplement utilization with particular emphasis on possible interactions with dental drugs and oral manifestations. J Dental Hygiene 77: 37–46

Agarry OO, Olaleye MT, Michael CO (2005) Comparative antimicrobial activities of Aloe vera gel and leaf. African J Biotechnol 4: 1413–1414

Ahmeda M, Hussain F (2013) Chemical Composition and Bio-chemical Activity of Aloe vera (Aloe barbadensis Miller) Leaves. Int J Chem Bio-chem Sci 3: 29-33

Akhtar M, Hai A, Awais MM, Iqbal Z, Muhammed F, Anwar MI (2012) Immuno-stimulatory and protective effects of Aloe vera against coccidiosis in industrial broiler chickens. Vet Parasitol 186: 170–177

Alemdar S, Agaoglu, S (2009) Investigation of *in vitro* antimicrobial activity of Aloe vera juice. J Anim Vet Adv 8: 99–102

Alemi F, Mahdavi A, Ghazvinian K, Ghaderi M, Darabighane B (2012) The effects of different levels of Aloe vera gel powder on antibody titer against Newcastle disease virus and performance in broilers. Proc. Int Poult Scientific Forum, Georgia World Congress Center, Atlanta, Georgia, 1: 47

Surjushe A, Vasani R, Saple DG (2008) *Aloe vera* : a short review. Indian J Dermatol 53(4): 163–166

Asanuma N, Iwamoto M, Hino T (1999) Effect of the addition of fumarate on methane production by ruminal microorganisms *in vitro*. J Dairy Sci 82: 780–787

Ayaz MM, Akhtar M, Hayat CS, Hafeez MA, Haq AU (2003) Prevalence of coccidiosis in broiler chickens in Faisalabad, Pakistan. Pakistan Vet J 23: 51–52

Besharatian M, Arshami J, Valizade R, Tahmasebi A, Bahari Kashani R (2012) Effects of Aloe vera leaf powder and extract on immune response in broilers. Proc. 5thIranian Congress on Animal Science, Isfahan, Iran, pp. 366–370

Bland J (1985) Effect of orally consumed Aloe vera juice on gastro-intestinal function in normal humans.Preventive Medicine. 14: 152-154

Boadi D, Benchaar C, Chiquette J (2004) Mitigation strategies to reduce enteric methane emission from dairy cows: update review. Canad J Anim Sci 84: 319–335

Boudreau MD, Beland, FA (2006) An evaluation of the biological and toxicological properties of Aloe barbadensis (Miller), Aloe vera. J Environ Sci Health. 24: 103–154

Bozzi A, Perrin C, Austin S, Arce F (2007) Quality and authenticity of commercial aloe vera gel powders. Food Chem 103(1): 22–30

Bradley PR (1992) A handbook of scientific information on widely used plant drugs, British Herbal Compendium. Vol. 1

Kaur C, Kapoor HC (2001) Antioxidants in fruits and vegetables - the millennium's health. J Food Sci Technol 36: 703-710

Choi S, Chung MH (2003) A review on the relationship between Aloe vera components and their biologic effects. Seminars in Integrative Med 1: 53–62

Christaki EV, Florou Paneri PC (2010) Aloe vera: A plant for many uses. J Food Agric Environ 8: 245–249

Cooke WT (1981) Laxative abuse. Acta Gastro-Enterologica Belgica 44: 448–458

Cowan MM (1999) Plant products as antimicrobial agents. Clinical Microbiol Rev 12: 564-582

Dagne E, Bisrat D, Viljoen A, Van Wyk BE (2000) Chemistry of aloe species. Current Organic Chem 4: 1055–1078

Dai B, Jiang L, Chen S (2007) Effects of medicinal herb and polysaccharide from Aloe vera on gut microflora, immune function and growth performance in broiler. China Poultry 29: 21–24

Danhoff IE, McAnally BH (1988) Stabilized *Aloe vera,* its effect on human skin cells. Drugs in the Cosmetic Industry. 133: 52-196

Darabighane B,Zare A,(2011). The effects of the different levels of Aloe vera gel on oocysts shedding in broilers with coccidiosis. Planta Medica 77: 2-10

Darabighane B, Zarei A, Shahneh AZ (2012) The effects of different levels of Aloe vera gel on ileum microflora population and immune response in broilers: a comparison to antibiotic effects. J Applied Anim Res 40: 31–36

Das S, Mishra B, Gill K, Ashraf MS, Singh AK, Sinha M, Sharma S, Xess I, Dalal K, Singh TP, Dey S (2011) Isolation and characterization of novel protein with antifungal and anti-inflammatory properties from Aloe vera leaf gel. Int J Biol Macromol 48(1): 38-43

Davis RH, Donato JJ, Hartman GM, Haas RC (1994) Anti-inflammatory and wound healing activity of a growth substance in Aloe vera. J American Padiatric Medical Assoc 84: 77-81

Davis RH (1997) Aloe vera- A scientific approach. New York: Vantage Press Inc; pp. 290–306

Davis RH, Parker WL, Samson RT (1991) Isolation of a stimulatory system in an aloe vera extract. J Amer Pediatric Med Assoc 81: 473-478

Delespaux V and Koning HD (2007) Drugs and drug resistance in African trypanosomiasis. Drug Resistance Updates 10: 30–50

Di Luccia B, Manzo N, Vivo M, Galan E, Amoresano A, Crescenzi E, Pollice A, Tudisco R, Infascelli F and Calabrò V (2013) A bio-chemical and cellular approach to explore the antiproliferative and prodifferentiative activity of Aloe arborescens leaf extract. Phytother Res 27(12): 1819-28

Diaz A, Avendan OM and Escobar A (1994) Evaluation of *Sapindus saponaria* as a defaunating agent and its effects on different ruminal digestion parameters. Livestock Res Rural Develop. 5: 1–10

Djeraba, A. and Quere, P (2000) *In vivo* macrophage activation in chickens with Acemannan, a complex carbohydrate extracted from Aloe vera. Int J Immunopharmacol 22: 365–372

Domkat LC and Habibu T (2013) Comparative studies of the aqueous extracts of Ocimun gratissmum, Aloe vera, Brassica oleracea and Ipopoea batatas on some bio-chemical parameters in diabetic rats. Int J Pharmacy Biol Sci. 6: 23-29

Estakhr J and Javed N (2011) Spermatogenic activity of aloe vera in adult male rats. Pharmacol online 2: 886-889

Infascelli F, Calabro S, Musco N, Tudisco R, Grossi M, Calabro V, Ferrara M, Cutrignelli MI, Infascelli, F (2013) Effect of Aloe Arborescens on In Vitro Rumen Fermentations. J Nutr Ecology and Food Research, 1(2): 117-123

Fajimi, AK, Ayodeji IO, Ajayi FT, Ogundola FI (2002). Efficacy studies of topically administered aloe-vera in rabbits naturally infested with psoroptic mange mites. Moor J Agric Res 3(2): 199–202

Femenia A, Sanchez ES, Simal S. and Rossello, C. (1999). Compositional features of polysaccharides from Aloe vera (Aloe barbadensisMiller) plant tissues. Carbohydrate Polymers, 39: 109–117

Feng, Y.Z., Gu, F. X., Yuan, Z. X., Zhang. Y. J., Liu, S. H., Hu, L. L. and Xu, L. (2011). Effects of Aloe polysaccharide on immune organ index and immune efficacy of vaccine against Newcastle disease in broiler. J Henan Agric Univ 45: 432–436

Fujita K, Yamada Y, Azuma K, Hirozawa S (1978) Effect of leaf extracts of Aloe arborescens Miller spp. natalensis Berger, active against the human fungal pathogen Trichophyton menta grophytes. Antimicrobial Agents Chemotherap 14: 132–136

Fujita K, Teradaira R, Nagatsu T (1976) Bradykinase activity in Aloeextract. Biocheml Pharmacol 25: 205-210

Gadzirayi CT, Mupangwa, JF, Mutandwa E (2005) Effectiveness of Aloe excelsa in controlling coccidiosis in broilers. Journal of Sustainable Development in Africa. 7: 1-6

Getachew G, Makkar HPS, Becker K (2002) Tropical browses: contents of phenolic compounds, *in vitro* gas production and stoichiometric relationship between short chain fatty acid and in vitro gas production. J Agric Sci 139: 341–352

Harlev E, Nevo E, Lansky EP, Ofir R, Bishayee A (2012) Anti-cancer potential of Aloes: antioxidant, antiproliferative, and immunostimulatory attributes. Planta Medica 78: 843–852

Halliwell B, Aeschbach R, Lo Liger J, Aruoma OI (1995) "The characterization of antioxidant," Food Chem Toxicol 33: 601-617

Hamman JH (2008) Composition and Applications of Aloe vera Leaf Gel. Molecules 13(8): 1599-616

Hammer KA, Carson CF, Riley TV (1999) Antimicrobial activity of essential oils and other plants extracts. J Appl Microbiol 86: 985-990

Hardy B (2002) The issue of antibiotic use in the livestock industry: what have we learned. Animal Bio-technol 13: 129–147

Hassanbeigy Z, Roustaee M, Haghighian M (2012) Effect of Aloe gel on broiler performance. Proc. 5th Iranian Congress on Animal Science

He CL, Fu BD, Shen HQ, Jiang XL, Wei XB (2011)Fumaric acid, an antibacterial component of Aloe vera L. African J Bio-technol 10: 2973–2977

Hess HD, Kreuzer M, Diaz TE, Lascano CE, Carulla JE, Solvia CR, Machmuller A (2003) Saponin rich tropical fruita affect fermentation and methanogenesis in faunated and defaunated rumen fluid. Inter J Biol Sci 109: 79-94

Hosseinifar S, Erfanimajd N, Morovvati H, Najafzadeh H (2011) Aloe vera Gel Protects Ovarian Structure in Diabetic Rat. Amer-Eurasian J Toxicol Sci 3(3): 197-203

Iji OT, Oyagbemi AA, Azeez OI (2010) Assessment of chronic administration of aloe veragel on haematology, plasma bio-chemistry, lipid profiles and erythrocyte osmotic resistance in wistar rats.Nigerian J Physiol Sci 25: 107-113

Im SA, Oh ST, Song S, Kim MR, Kim DS, Woo SS, Jo TH, Park YI, Lee CK (2005) Identification of optimal molecular size of modified Aloe polysaccharides with maximum immunomodulatory activity. Inter Immunopharmacol 5: 271-27

Ingold WM (1993) Wound therapy: growth factors as agents to promote healing, Trends Biotechnol 11: 387-392

IPCC (2007) Guidelines for national greenhouse inventories.Agriculture, forestry and other land use, Emissions from livestock and manure management. Isfahan, Iran, pp. 973–977

Jiang L, Feng Y, Yang X, Zhou X, Yang D (2005) Effects of gel, polysaccharide and acemannan from Aloe vera on broiler gut flora, microvilli density, immune function and growth performance. Chinese J Vet Sci 25: 668–671

Kinsella, J. E., Frankel, E., German, B., and Kanner, J. (1993). Possible mechanism for the protective role of antioxidants in wine and plant foods. Food Technology, 47: 85-89

Qiao, J., Li, H. H., Zheng, C. J., Feng, Z.Y. and Wang. W. (2013). Dietary supplementation with Aloe vera polysaccharide enhances the growth performance and immune function of weaned piglets, Journal of Animal and Feed Sciences, 22: 329–334

Kwon, K. H., Hong, M. K., Hwang, S.Y., Moon, B.Y., Shin, S., Baek, J. H. and Park, Y. H. (2011). Antimicrobial and immuno-modulatory effects of Aloe vera peel extract, Journal of Medicinal Plants Research, 5: 5384–5392

Fujita, K. Teradaira, R. and Nagatsu, T. (1976). Bradykinase activity in Aloe extract", Bio-chemical Pharmacology, 25: 205, 1976.

Karaca, K., Sharma, J. M. and Nordgren, R. (1995). Nitric oxide production by chicken macrophages activated by Acemannan, a complex carbohydrate extracted from Aloe vera. International Journal of Immuno-pharmacology, 17: 183–188

Khaing, T.A. (2011). Evaluation of the Antifungal and Antioxidant Activities of the Leaf Extract of Aloe vera (Aloe barbadensis Miller) World Academy of Science, Engineering and Technology, 75: 2011

Plaskett, L.G. (1997). "Aloe vera against infections", Newsletter 9, Publ. Bio-medical Information Services Ltd., Launceston, Cornwall, UK,

Lee, J.K., Lee, M.K., Yun, Y.P. Kim, Y., Kim, J.S., Kim, Y.S., Kim, K., Han, S.S. and Lee, C.K. (2001). Acemannan purified from Aloe vera induces phenotypic and functional maturation of immature dendritic cells. International Immuno-pharmacology, 1: 1275–1284

Lillehoj, H. S., Min, W. and Dalloul, R. A. (2004). Recent progress on the cytokine regulation of intestinal immune responses to Eimeria. Poultry Science, 83: 611-623

Lillehoj, H.S. and Trout, J. M. (1996). Avian gut-associated lymphoid tissues and intestinal immune responses to Eimeria parasites, Clinical Microbiology Reviews. 9: 349–360

Mahdavi, A., Alemi, F., Ghazvinian, K., Ghaderi, M. and Darabighane, B. (2012). Study of ffects of different levels of Aloe vera gel powder on antibody titre against sheep red blood cells and other blood parameters in broilers. British Poultry Abstracts, 8: 49–50

Makkar, H.P.S., Blummel, M. and Becker, K. (1995). *In vitro* effects of and interactions between tannins and saponins and fate of saponins tannins in the rumen, Journal of the Science of Food and Agriculture. 69: 481–493

Marizvikuru, M., Evison, B., Michael, C. and Tinyiko, E.H. (2006). The in vitro studies on the effect of Aloe vera ((L.) Webb. and Berth.) and Aloe spicata (L.f.) on the control of coccidiosis in chickens. International Journal of Applied Research in Veterinary Medicine. 4: 128-133

Mascolo, N., Izzo, A. A., Borelli, F., Capasso, R., DiCarlo, G., Sautebin, L. and Capasso, F. (2004). Healing powers of aloes. In: T. Reynolds ed. Aloes: The Genus Aloe, 2003 edition, Boca Raton, 38: 209–238

Mbanga, J., Mangoma, N. and Saidi, B. (2010). An evaluation of the antimicrobial activities of Aloe barbadensis, A. chabaudii and A. arborescens leaf extracts used in folklore veterinary medicine in Zimbabwe. Journal of Animal and Veterinary Advances, 9: 2918–2923.

McAnalley, B.H. (1989). Process for preparation of aloe products, Google Patents.

Mehala, C. and Moorthy, M. (2008). Effect of Aloe vera and Curcuma longa (turmeric) on carcass characteristics and bio-chemical parameters of broilers.International Journal of Poultry Science, 7: 857–861

Menke, K. H., Raab, L., Salewski, A., Steingass, H., Fritz, D. and Schneider, W. (1979). The estimation of digestibility and metabolizable energy content of ruminant feedstuffs from the gas production when they incubated withrumen liquor *in vitro*, Journal of Agricultural Science (Camb.), 92: 217-222.

Mitsch, P., Zitterl-Eglseer, K., Kohler, B., Gabler, C., Losa, R. and Zimpernik, I. (2004). The effect of two different blends of essential oil components on the proliferation of Clostridium perfringens in the intestines of broiler chickens. Poultry Science, 83: 669-675

Mmereole, F. (2011). Evaluation of the dietary inclusion of Aloe vera as an alternative to antibiotic growth promoter in broiler production.Pakistan Journal of Nutrition, 10: 1–5

Mokaddas, E., Rotimi, V. O. and Sanyal, S. C. (1998). *In vitro* activity of piperacillin/tazobactam versus other broadspectrum antibiotics against nosocomial gram-negative pathogens isolated from burn patients, Journal of chemotherapy, 10(3): 208-214

Moore, W.E. and Holdeman, L.V. (1975). Some newer concepts of the human intestinal flora.The American journal of medical technology, 41: 427–430

Mori, H., Sugie, S., Niwa, K., Takahashi, M. and Kawai, K. (1985). Induction of intestinal tumours in rats by chrysazin.British Journal of Cancer, 52:781–783

Moss, A. R., Jouany, J. P. and Newbold, J. (2000). Methane production byruminants: Its contribution to global warming, Annales De Zootechnie, 49: 231–253

Ahmeda, M. and Hussain, F. (2013). Chemical Composition and Bio-chemical Activity of Aloe vera (Aloe barbadensis Miller) Leaves, International Journal of Chemical and Bio-chemical Sciences, IJCBS, 3: 29-33

Mueller, S.O., Eckert, I., Lutz, W.K. and Stopper, H. (1996). Genotoxicity of the laxative drug components emodin, aloe-emodin and danthron in mammalian cells: topoisomerase II mediated. Mutation Research, 371: 165–173

Mwale, M., Bhebhe, E., Chimonyo, M. and Halimani, T.E. (2006). The *in vitro* studies on the effect of Aloe vera ((L.) webb. and berth.) and

Aloe spicata (L.f.) on the control of coccidiosis in chickens. The Journal of Applied Research in Veterinary Medicine, 4: 2–5

Newton, L. E. (1979). In defense of the name aloe vera. Cactus and Succulent Journal of Great Britain, 41: 29–30

Ni, Y. and Tizard, I. R. (2004). Analytical methodology: the gel-analysis of aloe pulp and its derivatives. In Aloes the Genus Aloe; Reynolds, T., Ed.; CRC Press: Boca Raton. 111-126

Odo, B. I., Ekenyem, B. U. and Nwamo, A.C. (2010). Effects of Aloe vera as leaf protein concentrate on growth performance of cockerels. International Journal of Poultry Science, 9: 426-28

Olupona, J. A., Omotoso, O. R., Adeyeye, A. A., Kolawole, O.D., Airemionkhale, A. P. and Adejinmi, O. O. (2010). Effect of aloe vera juice application through drinking water on performance, carcass characteristics, haematology and organoleptics properties in broilers. Poultry Science, 88(1): 42

Oyewopo, A. O., Oremosu, A. A., Akang, E. N., Noronha, C. C. and Okanlawon, A. O. (2011). Effects of Aloe vera (Aloe Barbadensis) Aqueous Leaf Extract On Testicular Weight, Sperm Count And Motility of Adult Male Sprague-Dawley Rats. Journal of American Science, 7(4)

Alagesan, P., Alamelu, M. and Suresh. S. (2005). Spreading eco-friendly disease management in sheep – MYRADA KVK's efforts

Pandey, R. and Mishra, A. (2010). Antibacterial activities of crude extract of Aloe barbadensis to clinically isolated bacterial pathogens. Applied Bio-chemistry and Biotechnology, 160: 1356–1361

Peng, S.Y., Norman, J., Curtin, G., Corrier, D., McDaniel, H. R. and Busbee, D. (1991). Decreased mortality of Norman murine sarcoma in mice treated with the immuno-modulator, Acemannan. Molecular bio-therapy, 3: 79–87

Plaskett, L.G. (1976). "Aloe vera against infections", Newsletter , Publ. Bio-medical Information Services Ltd., Launceston, Cornwall, UK

Pogribna, M., Freeman, J.P., Paine, D. and Boudreau, M.D. (2008). Effect of Aloe vera whole leaf extract on short chain fatty acids production by Bacteroides fragilis, Bifidobacterium infantis and Eubacterium limosum. Letters in Applied Microbiology. 46(5): 575-80

Qiao, J., Li, H.H., Zheng, Ch. J., Feng, Z.Y. and Wang, W. (2013). Dietary supplementation with Aloe vera polysaccharide enhances the growth performance and immune function of weaned piglets. Journal of Animal and Feed Sciences, 22: 329-334

Reig, M. and Toldra, F. (2008). Veterinary drug residues in meat: concerns and rapid methods for detection. Meat Science. 78: 60–67

Reynolds, T. and Dweck, A. C. (2001). Aloe vera leaf gel, A review update. Journal of Ethnopharmacology, 1999; 68: 3-37

Kaur, C. and Kapoor, H. C. (2001). Antioxidants in fruits and vegetables– the millennium's health International Journal of Food Science & Technology, 36: 703-725

Ro, J. Y., Lee, B., Kim, J. Y., Chung, Y., Chung, M.H. and Lee, S. K. (2000). Inhibitory mechanism of aloe single component (Alprogen) on mediator release in guinea pig lung mast cells activated with specific antigen-antibody reactions, Journal of Pharmacology and Experimental Therapeutics, 292: 114-21

Rowland, I. R., Mallett, A. K. and Wise, A. (1985). The effect of diet on the mammalian gut flora and its metabolic activities.Critical Reviews in Toxicology, 16: 31–103

Calabro, S., Musco, N., Tudisco, R., Grossi, M., Calabrò, V., Ferrara, M., Cutrignelli, M. I. and Infascelli. F. (2013). Effect of Aloe Arborescens on *In vitro* Rumen Fermentations Journal of Nutritional Ecology and Food Research, 1: 117–123.

Sirohi, S. K., Pandey, N., Goel, N., Singh, B., Mohini, M., Pandey, P. and Chaudhry, P. P. (2009). International Journal of Civil and Environmental Engineering, 1: 1

Jyoti, Sachan, Ravindra, Kumar., Vaswani, S., Kumar, V. and Roy, D. (2010). Effect of addition of herbs on *in vitro* rumen fermentation and digestibility of feed.Indian Journal of Animal Research, 48 (1): 88-90

Saks, Y. and Barkai-Golan, R. (1995). Aloe vera gel activity against plant pathogenic fungi. Post-harvest Bio-technol 6: 159–165

Shah MAA, Song X, Xu L, Yan R, Song H, Ruirui Z, Chengyu L and Li X (2009). The DNA-induced protective immunity with chickens interferon gamma against poultry coccidiosis. Parasitol Res 107: 747–750

Shamaan NA, Kadir KA, Rahmat A and Ngah WZ (1998). Vitamin C and *aloe vera* supplementation protects from chemical hepatocarcinogenesis in the rat. Nutrition. 14: 846–852

Siegers CP, Hertzberg-Lottin E, Otte M and Schneider B (1993) Anthranoid laxative abuse- a risk for colorectal cancer. Gut 34: 1099–1101

Simon GL and Gorbach SL (1986) The human intestinal microflora. Digestive Dis Sci 31: 147–162

Sirohi SK, Pandey N, Goel N, Singh B, Mohini M, Pandey P and Chaudhary PP (2009) Microbial activity and ruminal methanogenesis as affected by plant secondary metabolites in different plant extracts. Int J Civil Environ Eng. 1: 1-5

Surjushe A, Vasani R and Saple DG (2008) *Aloe vera*: A short review. Indian J Dermatol. 53: 163-166

Taylor DJ (2001) Effects of antimicrobials and their alternatives. British Poult Sci. 42: 67-68

Tizard IR and Ni Y (1998) Carbohydrates, immune stimulating. In: Encyclopedia of immunology, Delves P.J., Roitt I.M. (eds). Academic Press Inc., San Diego, CA, 2nd ed., pp. 427–431

Tucker AO and Duke JA (1989) Foster S. Botanical nomenclature of medicinal plants. In: Cracker LE, Simon JE, editors. Herbs, spices, and medicinal plants, vol 4. Phoenix: AR Oryx Press; pp. 169–242

Valle-Paraso M, Vidamo P, Anunciado R and Lapitan A (2005) Effects of Aloe vera *Aloe barbadensis*) on the white blood cell count and antibody titre of broiler chickens vaccinated against Newcastle disease. Philippines J Vety Med 42: 49–52

Verstegen MW and William BA (2002) Alternatives to the use of antibiotics as growth promoters for monogastric animals. Anim Biotechnol. 13: 113–127

Womble DI and Helderman JH (1988) Enhancement of allo-responsiveness of human lymphocytes by acemannan (Carrisyn). Int J Immunopharmacol 10(8): 967-74

Womble D and Helderman JH (1988) The impact of acemannan on the generation and Acemannan, a complex carbohydrate extracted from Aloe vera. International J Immuno-pharmacol 22: 365–372

Hu Y, Xu J and Hu Q (2003) Evaluation of antioxidant potential of aloe vera (Aloe barbadensis miller) extracts. J Agric Food Chem. 51: 77-88

Jia Y, Zhaoa G and Jia J (2008) Preliminary evaluation: the effects of Aloe ferox Miller and Aloe arborescens Miller on wound healing. J Ethnopharmacol 120: 181-186

Yang Y, Iji P and Choct M (2009) Dietary modulation of gut microflora in broiler chickens: a review of the role of six kinds of alternatives to in-feed antibiotics. World's Poult Sci J. 65: 97–114

Yim D, Kang SS, Kim DW, Kim SH, Lillehoj HS and Min W (2011) Protective effects of *Aloe vera* -based diets in Eimeria maxima-infected broiler chickens. Exper Parasitol 127: 322–325

Yimei J, Guodong Z and Jia J (2008) Preliminary evaluation: The effects of Aloe ferox Miller and Aloe arborescens Miller on wound healing. J Ethnopharmacol 120: 181–189

Yolanta S and Barkai-Golan R (1995) Aloe vera gel activity against plant pathogenic fungi. Post-harvest Biol Technol 6: 159-165

Zhang L and Tizard IR (1996) Activation of a mouse macrophage cell line by cemannan: The major carbohydrate fraction from Aloe vera gel. Immuno-pharmacol 35: 119–128.

❏❏❏

Chapter 22

Cumin (*Cuminum cyminum*)

Deepak Upadhyay[1], Ashok Patil[2], Madhu Mishra[3]

[1] Plant Animal Relationship Division, ICAR-Indian Grassland and Fodder Research Institute, Jhansi - 284 003, India, Email: dpkvet@gmail.com

[2] Department of Animal Nutrition, College of Veterinary Science and Animal Husbandry, Nanaji Deshmukh Pashu Veterinary Science University, Jabalpur - 482001, India

[3] Research Scholar, Division of Veterinary Bacteriology, ICAR-Indian Veterinary Research Institute, Izatnagar-243122, India

ABSTRACT

Cumin (*Cuminum cyminum*) is an annual herb and has been used since ancient times as medicine and spices in food. It is considered to be one of the most important spices and ranks second to black pepper. Cumin seed contains several nutrients including carbohydrates, starch, sugars, dietary fibre, protein, amino acids, vitamins, minerals. Cumin oil contain several phytochemicals *viz.* cuminyl alcohol, cumin aldehyde, β-pinene, γ-cymene, α-terpinene, 1,8-cineol, α-pinene, perillaldehyde, limonene, Dipentene and α-terpineol. In Ayurvedic medicine, cumin seeds are considered carminative, eupeptic, antispasmodic, astringent and are often used for treating mild digestive disorders, diarrhoea, dyspepsia, flatulence, colic, abdominal distension, edema, broncho-pulmonary disorders puerperal disorders and as a cough remedy, as well as an analgesic.

Keywords: *Cuminum cyminum*, Cuminyl alcohol, Carminative, Livestock production.

22.1 Introduction

Cumin (*Cuminum cyminum*), commonly known as *zeera* (Hindi), is a annual herb and has been used since ancient times as medicine and spices in food. It is considered to be one of the most important spices and ranks second to black pepper. Cumin plant grows upto 30-50 cm (0.98-1.6 ft) in height. The flowers are small, white or pink and borne in umbels. Worldwide therapeutic uses of cumin have been scientifically validated. In Ayurvedic medicine, cumin seeds are considered carminative, eupeptic, antispasmodic, astringent and are often used for treating mild digestive disorders, diarrhoea, dyspepsia, flatulence, colic, abdominal distension, edema, broncho-pulmonary disorders puerperal disorders and as a cough remedy, as well as an analgesic (Rathore *et al.*, 2013, Joshi, 2000; Mhaskar *et al.*, 2000; Sivarajan and Balachandra, 1994). Actions like enhancing vision, strength, and lactation have also been reported (Rathore *et al.*, 2013). Cumin seeds have been reportedly used for traditional treatment of toothache, dyspepsia, epilepsy and jaundice (Nostro *et al.*, 2005). Pharmacological effects such as anti-diabetic, immunologic, anti-tumour and antimicrobial activities are also reported (Senevirathne *et al.*, 2006). Essential oils of cumin act as powerful external or internal antiseptic, analgesic, anti-inflammatory, hemolytic, or anti-enzymatic action, sedative, stimulants and stomachics (Guenther, 1950). Iranian traditional medicine consider cumin as stimulant, carminative and astringent and its therapeutic effects have been described on gastro-intestinal, gynaecological and respiratory disorders, and also for the treatment of toothache, diarrhea and epilepsy (Zargary, 2001). In traditional medicine of Tunisia, cumin is considered abortive, galactagogue, antiseptic, antihypertensive herb, while in Italy, it is used as bitter tonic, carminative, and purgative (Leporatti and Ghedira, 2009).

22.2 Taxonomy

Kingdom	:	Plantae
Phylum	:	Tracheophyta
Class	:	Magnoliopsida
Order	:	Apiales
Family	:	Apiaceae
Genus	:	*Cuminum*
Species	:	*cyminum*

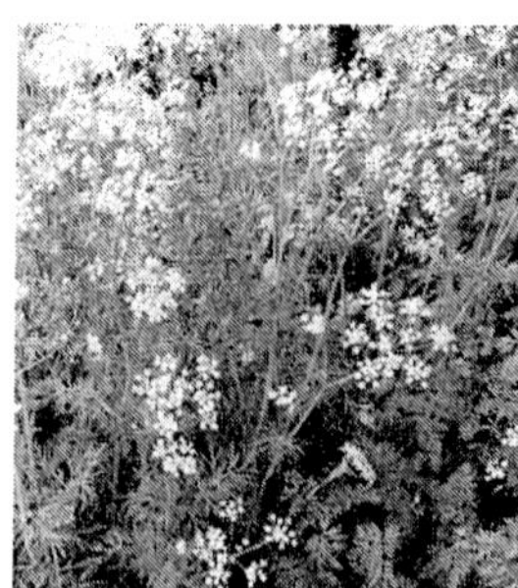

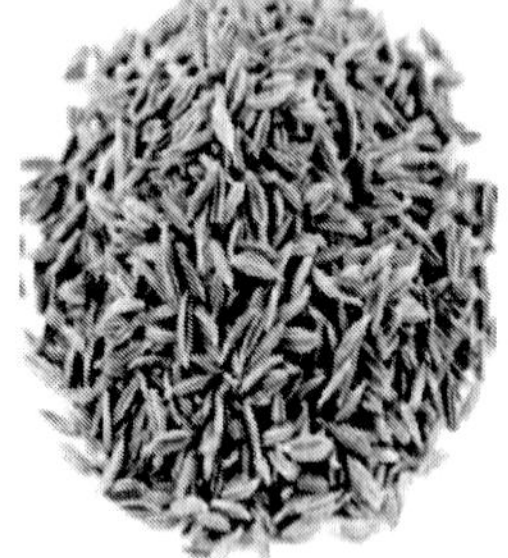

22.3 Chemistry of Cumin Seed

Cumin seed contains several nutrients including carbohydrates, starch, sugars, dietary fibre, protein, amino acids, vitamins, minerals and others (tannins, phytic acid, etc.) (El-Sawi and Mohamed, 2002; Al-Bataina *et al.*, 2003; Maiga *et al.*, 2005; Milan *et al.*, 2008; Toghrol *et al.*, 1974; Uma Pradeep *et al.*, 1993). Cumin seed (100g) contained carbohydrates 44.24g, sugar 2.25g, fiber 10.5g, fat 22.27g, protein 17.81g and water 8.06g (Jonas *et al.*, 2007). The composition of cumin varies based on region and climate where it is grown. Typical cumin ûavor is due to the volatile oil present in the seeds in the range of 3–4% depending on the variety and the origin. The cumin seeds contain 14.5% total lipids on dry weight basis which consists of 84.8% neutral lipid, 10% glycolipids and 5.1% phospholipids. Fatty acid composition of cumin includes both saturated and unsaturated fatty acids, mainly (70% of total) oleic, petroselenic, and linoleic acids (Hemavathy and Prabhakar, 1988).

Cumin essential oil contains several compounds *viz.* cuminyl alcohol (30.02%), cumin aldehyde (25.88%), β-pinene (16.30%), ρ-cymene (15.55%), α-terpinene (5.66%), 1,8-cineol (2.24%), α-pinene (0.98%), perillaldehyde (0.63%), limonene (0.23%), Dipentene (0.21%) and α-terpineol (0.19%) (Chaudhry *et al.*, 2012). Cumin aldehyde, β-pinene, p-cymene and γ-terpinene were the principal compounds (Jirovets *et al.*, 2005; Heri *et al.*, 2003 and Zitao *et al.*, 1993). Good amounts of phenolic compounds show considerable radical scavenging, carotene/linoleic acid chelating and reducing power activities (Rebey *et al.*, 2012).

Table 1: Characteristics of essential oil of cumin

Physical Properties	Values
Colour	Light brownish yellow
Odour	Strong and somewhat disagreeable
Yield	2.8%
Specific Gravity	0.928
Refractive Index	1.503
Acid Value	0.56
Ester Value	5.61

Table 2: Proximate composition of cumin (Miri *et al.*, 2013)

Chemical Properties	Values (%)
Dry matter	94.6
Organic matter	95.1
Crude Protein	6.2
Ether Extract	20
NDF	3.0
ADF	0.6
Ash	4.9
Total Phenol	26.3
Total tannins	13.5
Saponins	5.04

22.4 Different Cumin Preparations

22.4.1 *Cumin seed or Powder*

Cumin is commercially sold as both seeds and powder. Dried cumin is powdered in a hammer mill or a pulverizer, to pass through a mesh size of 30.

22.4.2 *Cumin Essential Oil*

Hydro-distillation and steam distillation are generally used methods of extraction. In hydro-distillation, the seed is powdered and boiled in water and volatile compounds are separated from water by steam condensation and dried over anhydrous sodium sulphate. In steam distillation, the powdered seed is packed loosely without pressure in a distillation unit. From the bottom, steam is let in slowly which passes through the bed of the material and carries along with it, the volatile principles and gets condensed, when it passes through the condenser. When sufficient oil is collected, it is taken out through a trap provided for this purpose. The major flavour components of volatile oil obtained from ground cumin have been reported as β-pinene, p-cymene, γ-terpene, cuminaldehyde, phellandral, cuminyl-alcohol, p-mentha-1-4-dien-7-al, and peril-aldehyde (Eikani *et al.*, 1999; Varo and Heinz, 1970a; 1970b).

22.4.3 *Cumin Oleoresin*

The resin is obtained by solvent extraction of cumin powder. The pooled extract is carefully distilled to remove the solvent to traces. Volatile oil recovered by steam distillation is added back to the resin and blended to obtain oleoresin. Oleoresin, besides containing the flavoring principle of cumin, also contains non-aromatic fat (flxed oil), resin, waxes, pigments, and natural antioxidant which act as a flxative for the volatiles.

22.5 Biological Activity of Cumin in Livestock and Poultry

22.5.1 *Antioxidant Property*

Higher production of free radicals in the body can cause oxidative damage to important biomolecules (*e.g.* lipids, proteins, DNA), leading to many chronic diseases (Poulson *et al.*, 1998). Results of a study conducted in India showed that cumin oils exhibited high antioxidant activity. Cumin seeds contain flavonoids, *viz.*, apigenin and luteolin, which are now generally recognized to have antioxidant activity. The petroleum ether soluble fraction of cumin has been reported to have antioxidant activity (Leung, 1980). In studies in mice, cumin seed elevated levels of glutathione and stimulated other antioxidant systems (Gagandeep, 2003). Cuminaldehyde has been demonstrated to scavenge the superoxide anion (Krishnakantha and Lokesh, 1993). The antioxidant activity of the aqueous extracts of cumin has been reported. The antioxidant activity of the aqueous extracts of cumin has been studied in comparison with the known antioxidant ascorbic acid in *in-vitro* studies. Study has revealed that aqueous extract of cumin exhibits strong antioxidant activity superior to known antioxidant ascorbic acid and indicate that the intake is beneflcial as a food additive (Satyanarayana *et al.*, 2004). The antioxidant activity of cumin seed extracts ranged from 8.25 to 11.24 mg/ml (Juhaimi and Ghafoor, 2013). The antioxidative potential increased with increase of phenolic compounds content of cumin. Cumin seed extracts showed good mean DPPH radical scavenging activities (Juhaimi and Ghafoor, 2013).

Food materials rich in bioactive compounds with higher free radical scavenging abilities are protective against certain types of cancer and may also reduce the risk of cardiovascular and cerebrovascular disorders (Miraliakbari and Shahidi, 2008). Antiradical profile of cumin has been proposed as the underlying mechanism for their multifaceted pharmacological properties such as antimicrobial, antidiabetic, anticarcinogenic/antimutagenic, antistress, antiulcerogenic, etc. as outlined in the succeeding sections.

22.5.2 *Antimicrobial Activity*

Cumin essential oil showed antibacterial activity comparable with standard antibiotics against common pathogens. Cuminaldehyde showed antimicrobial and antifungal properties against *Escherichia coli, Penicillium chrysogenum* (Shetty *et al.*, 1994). *A flavus* and *A niger* (Singh and Upadhyay, 1991). Cumin essential oil showed high antimicrobial activity against molds (*Aspergillus niger*), gram positive bacteria (*Bacillus subtilis, Staphylococcus epidermidis*), gram negative bacteria (*E. coli*) and yeast (*Saccharomyces cerevisiae* and *Candida albicans*) (Jirovets *et al.*, 2005; De *et al.*, 1999). Jazani *et al.* (2008) indicated the potential use of cumin essential oil for the control of some diseases caused by *Pseudomonas aeruginosa* infections. Essential oil and alcoholic extract of cumin has shown antimicrobial activity against *Klebsiella pneumoniae* ATCC 13883 and clinical *Klebsiella pneumoniae* (ceftazidime-resistant strain) (Derakshan, 2007). Cumin oil and cuminaldehyde have been reported to exhibit strong larvicidal and antibacterial activity. At *in vitro* concentrations of 300 or 600 ppm, cumin oil inhibited the growth of *Lactobacillus plantarum* (Kivanc *et al.*, 1991). Biofilm-formation preventive properties were found against *Streptococcus mutans* and *Streptococcus pyogenes* (Derakshan, 2007; Shayegh *et al.*, 2008). Antifungal activity of cumin oil is recorded against soil, food, animal and human pathogens, including dermatophytes, Vibrio *spp.*, yeasts, aflatoxins and mycotoxin producers. (De Martino *et al.*, 2009; Hajlaoui *et al.*, 2010; Mehdi *et al.*, 2009; Boyraz *et al.*, 2005; Farag *et al.*, 1989; Hammad *et al.*, 1995; Razzaghi-Abyaneh *et al.*, 2009; Romagnoli et al. 2010; Skrinjar *et al.*, 2009).

22.5.3 *Immunomodulatory Effect*

Oral treatment with cumin caused modulation of T lymphocytes 2 expression in a dose-dependent manner in normal and immune suppressed animals. It stimulated the T cells (CD4 and CD8) and Th1 cytokines expression in normal and cyclosporine-A induced immuno-suppressed mice. In restraint stress-induced immuno-suppressed animals, the active compound of cumin countered the depleted T lymphocytes, decreased the elevated corticosterone levels and size of adrenal glands and increased the weight of thymus and spleen (Chauhan *et al.*, 2010).

22.5.4 *Effect on Nervous System*

Cumin oil caused suppression of development and expression of morphine tolerance when administered in mice (as measured by tail-flick method) (Haghparast *et al.*, 2008; Khatibi *et al.*, 2008). Cumin oil also showed anti-epileptic activity by decreasing frequency of spontaneous activity induced by pentylenetetrazol (PTZ) (Janahmadi *et al.*, 2006). Cumin oil was found to attenuate seizures induced by maximal electroshock and PTZ in mice (Sayyah *et al.*, 2002a). Significant analgesic action of cumin oil has been documented through chemical model (formalin test) of nociception in rat (Sayyah *et al.*, 2002b). Cuminaldehyde proven to act as tyrosinase inhibitor and prevented the oxidation of l-3.5-dihydroxyphenyklalanine (l-DOPA) (Kubo and Kinst-Hori, 1998).

22.5.5 *Estrogenic/anti-osteoporotic*

Cumin seeds possess estrogenic property (Malini and Vanitha-kumari, 1987). Cumin produced anti-osteoporotic effects due to its phytoestrogens. Administration of cumin extract in animals resulted in reduced urinary calcium excretion and increased calcium content and bone strength. Bone and ash densities and improved micro-architecture with no adverse effects were reported (Shirke *et al.*, 2008).

22.5.6 Body Growth Performance

Supplementing broiler diet with cumin oil has significantly increased body weight as compared with control (Ahmed *et al.*, 2013). Ali *et al.* (2010) reported that negative effects of heat stress can be alleviated and growth performance can be improved by adding 2% cumin in diet of heat stressed broiler. Galib and Al-Kassi (2010) reported that adding cumin and turmeric mixture at levels of 0.75% and 1% in the diets improved body weight gain, feed intake and feed conversion ratio in broilers. Which could be due to role of cumin as a stimulant, carminative, digestion, antimicrobial properties and the prevention of gastric toxicity. Other researchers proved that there is an increase in body weight, feed conversion ratio, with decreasing haematological values of some important blood parameters using 2% of cumin in broiler diets (Ibrahim *et al.*, 2007).

22.5.7 *Gastrointestinal effects*

Stimulation of bile acid secretion and pancreatic enzymes has been demonstrated in rats given a continuous intake of dietary cumin. Perfusion of an aqueous extract of cumin *via* the stomach of pentobarbitone-anesthetized rats under the aspirin-induced gastric mucosal injury showed an increased acid secretion by a cholinergic mechanism (Vasudevan *et al.*, 2009). Aqueous and solvent derived extracts of cumin increased amylase, protease, lipase and phytase activities (Milan *et al.*, 2008).

22.5.8 *Anticarcinogenic / Antimutagenic*

Cumin seeds were able to inhibit the induction of gastric squamous cell carcinomas in mice (Gagandeep *et al.*, 2003). The excretion of fecal bile acids and neutral sterols was significantly increased. In cumin treated rats, the levels of cholesterol, cholesterol/ phospholipid ratio and 3-methylglutaryl COA-reductase activity were reduced (Nalini *et al.*, 2006). In rats fed with cumin, a protective effect against induced colonic cancer, decreased beta-glucuronidase and mucinase activity was demonstrated (Nalini *et al.*, 1998). Histopathological studies also showed lesser infiltration into the submucosa, fewer papillae and lesser changes in the cytoplasm of the cells in the cumin- treated colon. Reverse mutation *Salmonella typhimurium* (TA100) test showed that cumin seeds were not carcinogenic (Al-Batania *et al.*, 1995).

Dietary cumin inhibited benzopyrene-induced fore stomach tumorigenesis, 3-methylcholanthrene induced uterine cervix tumorigenesis, and 3-methyl-4-dimethyaminoazobenzene induced hepatomas in mice. This was attributed to the ability of cumin in modulating carcinogen metabolism via carcinogen/xenobiotic metabolizing phase I and phase II enzymes. Activities of cytochrome (CYP) P-450 reductase and CYP b5 reductase were augmented, whereas phase II enzymes GST and DT-diaphorase were increased (Aruna and Sivaramakrishnan, 1992; Gagandeep *et al.*, 2003).

22.5.9 *Antidiabetic Effect*

The antidiabetic effects of cumin are amply documented (Srinivasan, 2005). In a glucose tolerance test conducted in rabbits, cumin significantly increased the area under the glucose tolerance curve and hyperglycemic peak (Roman-Ramos *et al.*, 1995). Diet containing cumin powder (1.25%) was found to be remarkably beneficial in streptozotocin induced diabetic rats, as indicated by reduction in hyperglycemia and glucosuria, improved body weights, lowered blood urea level and reduced excretions of urea and creatinine by diabetic animals (Willatgamuwa *et al.*, 1998). Cumin at 0.5% g per kg body weight orally administered in rats with induced diabetes, is reported reduce blood glucose levels (Roman- Ramos *et al.*, 1995; Talpur *et al.*, 2005). It might be due to inhibition of aldose reductase and alpha-glucosidase (Lee, 2005). In addition, reduced plasma and tissue cholesterol, phospholipids, free fatty acids, and triglycerides were also reported in another animal study (Dhandapani *et al.*, 2002). Cumin make ingredients of a herbal antidiabetic drug, which was found to be effective in human subjects (Karnick, 1991). Cumin seeds extract found to reduce blood glucose and inhibited glycosylated hemoglobin, creatinine and improved serum insulin and glycogen content in induced diabetic rats (Dhandapani *et al.*, 2002; Jagtap and Patil, 2010). Aqueous cumin extract found to delay the progression and maturation of STZ-induced cataract in rats (Kumar *et al.*, 2009).

22.5.10 *Methane Mitigating Effect*

Recent *in vitro* studies reported inclusion of cumin increase digestibility of dry matter and organic matter in forages and lower methane emission (Khan and Chaudhry, 2010; Kilic *et al.*, 2011; Chaudhry and Khan, 2012). Reduction in methane emission was upto extent of 22% after cumin addition in buffered rumen fluid, *in vitro* (Chaudhry and Khan, 2012). The methane emission in goats which had received diet supplemented with cumin seed extract was found lower (11.8%) (Miri *et al.*, 2013). This effect might be due to inhibitory effect of cumin seed extract on ruminal microbial mass (Lourenco *et al.*, 2010; Ramos Morales *et al.*, 2012). Suppression of ruminal Gram-positive H_2 producing bacteria can reduce the amount of available hydrogen for biohydrogenation as well as methanogensis. The loss of protozoa would be expected to impact positively on the availability of CLA to host animal and negatively on methane emission (Lourenco *et al.*, 2010).

22.5.11 *Milk production*

Bhatt *et al.* (2009) reported that cumin has galactapoiesis property. Cumin is a constituent herbs of Payapro, a known galactagogue. Cumin is known to possess galactopoietics action (ICMR, 1987).

22.5.12 *Other Biodynamic Actions*

Antitussive and relaxant effects of aqueous cumin extract have been reported in guinea pig isolated tracheal chain *via* its beta receptor and/or H_1 receptors stimulation (Boskabady *et al.*, 2005; Boskabady *et al.*, 2006). Anti-aggregatory activity and inhibited eicosanoid synthesis shown by ethereal extract of cumin. Cumin extract also inhibited collagen and adrenaline-induced aggregation (Srivastava, 1989; Srivastava and Mustafa, 1994). Decreased WBC count and increased the haemoglobin concentration, haematocrit, and platelet counts by administration of cumin oil. LDL/HDL ratio was reduced to half (Allaghadri *et al.*, 2010). Anaqueous extract of cumin seeds showed protective action against gentamycin induced nephrotoxicity (Mahesh *et al.*, 2010).

22.6 Summary and Conclusions

Cumin as feed additives may prove beneficial for livestock and poultry owing to its properties *viz.* carminative, eupeptic, antispasmodic, astringent, antiinflammatory, anti-carcinogenic, galactogogue, antimicrobial, methane mitigation, immunomodulatory, antioxidant, growth promoter, *etc.* Apart from this, it also contains nutrients like energy, protein, vitamin, minerals and other essentials to improve animal health. Therefore, it can be recommended that cumin in the form of powder or its essential oils can be used in livestock and poultry feeding.

References

Ahmed A. A, Firas R. Al-Samarai, Jenan S. Al-Shamire and Falah H. Al-Zaidi Al- Anbari, 2013. Effect of using cumin oil (*Cuminum cyminum*) as feed additives on profile analysis and growth curve of broiler. *Eman. H. G.J.B.B.* 2 (3): 326-330.

AL Juhaimi, F. Y., and Ghafoor, K. 2013. Extraction optimization and in vitro antioxidant properties of phenolic compounds from Cumin (*Cuminum cyminum l.*) seed. *Int. Food Res. J.* 20(4): 1669-1675.

Al-Bataina, B.A., Maslat, A.O., and Al-Kofahil, M.M. 2003. Element analysis and biological studies on ten oriental spices using XRF and Ames test. *J. Trace. Elem. Med. Biol.* 17:85–90.

Ali, M. N., Qota, N. M. A. and Hassan, R. A. 2010. Recovery from adverse effects of heat stress on slow growing chicks using natural antioxidant with or without sulfate, *Int. J. Poultry Sci.* 9(2):109-117.

Allaghadri, T., Rasooli, I., Owlia, P., Nadooshan, M.J., Ghanfari, T., Taghizadeh, M. 2010. Antimicrobial property, antioxidant capacity, and cytotoxicity of essential oil from cumin produced in Iran. *J. Food Sci.* 75:H54–61.

Aruna, K., and Sivaramakrishnan, V.M. 1992. Anticarcinogenic effects of some Indian plant products. *Food Chem. Toxicol.* 30:953–6.

Bhatt, N., Singh, M. and Ali, A. 2009. Effect of feeding herbal preparations on milk yield and rumen parameters in lactating crossbred cows. *Int. J. Agric. Biol.,* 11: 721–726.

Boskabady, M.H., Kianai, S., and Azizi, H. 2005. Relaxant effect of *Cuminum cyminum* on guinea pig tracheal chains and its possible mechanism(s) *Indian J. Pharmacol.* 37: 111–5.

Boskabady, M.H., Kianai, S., Azizi, H., and Khatami, T. 2006. Antitussive effect of Cuminum cyminum Linn. in guinea pigs. *Nat. Prod. Rad.* 5:266–9.

Boyraz, N., and Ozcan, M. 2005. Antifungal effect of some spice hydrosols. *Fitoterapia.* 76:661–5.

Chaudhry, A.H., Tanveer, A., Shar, A., Akhtar, M.S., Shahid, M.K., Ashfaq, K.M., Malik, T.A., and Siddiqui, R.H. 2012. Physico-Chemical Investigation and Antimicrobial Activity of Essential Oil of Cuminum cyminum L. *World Appl. Sci. J.* 19 (3): 330-333.

Chaudhry, A.S., and Khan, M.M.H. 2012. Impacts of different spices on in vitro rumen dry matter disappearance, fermentation and methane of wheat or rye grass hay based substrates. *Livest. Sci.* 146:84–90.

Chauhan, P.S., Satti, N.K., Suri, K.A., Amina, M., and Bani, S. 2010. Stimulatory effects of Cuminum cyminum and flavonoid glycoside on cyclosporine-A and restraint stress induced immune- suppression in swiss albino mice. *Chem. Biol. Interac.* 185:66–72.

Cowieson, A. J., Acamovic, T., and Berford, M. R. 2003. Supplementation of diets containing pea meal with exogenous enzymes: Effect on weight gain, feed conversion, nutrient digestability and gross morphology of the gastro-intestinal tract of growing broiler chicks. *Brit. Poul. Sci.* 44:427-437 27.

De Martino, L., De Feo, V., Fratianni, F., and Nazzaro, F. 2009. Chemistry, antioxidant, antibacterial and antifungal activities of volatile oils and their components. *Nat. Prod. Commu.* 4:1741–50.

De, M., De, A.K., and Banerjee A.B. 1999. Antimicrobial screening of some Indian spices. *Phytother Res.* 13: 616-618.

Derakhshan, S., Sattari, and Bigedli, M. 2007. Evaluation of antibacterial activity and bioûlm formation in Klebsiellapneumoniae in contact with essential oil and alcoholic extract of cumin seed (*cuminum cyminum*). 17th European Congress of Clinical Microbiology and Infectious Diseases ICC, Munich, Germany.

Derakhshan, S., Sattari,M., and Bigdeli, M. 2010. Effect of cumin (*Cuminum cyminum*) seed essential oil on biofilm formation and plasmid integrity by *Klebsiella pneumoniae. Pharmacog. Mag.* 6: 57–61.

Dhandapani, S., Subramaniam, V. R., Rajagopal, S., and Namasivayam, N. 2002. Hypolipidemic effect of *cuminum cyminum L* on alloxan induced diabetic rats. *Pharmacol. Res.* 46: 251–255.

Eikani, M. H., Goodarznia, J., and Mirza, M. 1999. Supercritical carbon dioxide extraction of cumin seeds (*Cuminum cyminum L*). *Flav. Frag. J.* 14: 29–31.

El-Sawi, S.A., and Mohamed, M.A. 2002. Cumin herb as a new source of essential oils and its response to foliar spray with some micro-nutrients. *Food Chem.* 77:75–80.

Farag, R.S., Daw, Z.Y., and Abo-Raya, S.H. 1989. Influence of some spice essential oils on Aspergillus parasiticus growth and production of aflatoxins in a synthetic medium. *J. Food Sci.* 54:74–6.

Gagandeep, S., Dhanalakshmi, S., Mendiz, E., Rao, A.R., and Kale, R.K. 2003. Chemopreventive effects of *Cuminum cyminum* in chemically induced forestomach and uterine cervix tumors in murine model systems. *Nutr. Cancer.* 47:171–80.

Galib, A.M. and Al-Kassi, 2010. Effect of feeding cumin (*Cuminum cyminum*) on the performance and some blood traits of broiler chicks. *Pakistan J. Nutri.* 9 (1):72-75.

Ghazalah, A.A., Abd El-Gwad, Soliman, M. S., and Amany Youssef, W. 2005. Effect of enzyme preparation on performance of broiler fed corn- soyabean meal based diets. *Egyptian Poultry Sci.* 25:295-316.

Güenther, E. 1950. The Essential Oils. 3RD Ed. D. Van Nostrand, New York.

Haghparast, A., Shams, J., Khatibi, A., Alizaseh, A.M., and Kamalinejad, M. 2008. Effects of the fruit essential oil of *Cuminum cyminum Linn.* (Apiaceae) on acquisition and expression of morphine tolerance and dependence in mice. *Neurosci. Lett.* 440:134–9.

Hajlaoui, H., Mighri, H., Noumi, E., Snoussi, M., Trabelsi, N., Ksouri, R. 2010. Chemical composition and biological activities of Tunisian *Cuminum cyminum L.* essential oil: A high effectiveness against *Vibrio spp.* strains. *Food Chem. Toxicol.* 48:2186–92.

Hammad, A.A.I., and Youssef, B.M. 1995. Growth inhibition of some pharmacological molds by garlic and cumin essential oils. *Egypt J. Microbiol.* 29:115–20.

Hemavathy, J. and Prabhakar, J. V. 1988. Lipid composition of cumin (*Cuminum cyminum L.*) seeds. *J. Food Sci.* 53(5): 1578–1579.

Heri, Y.J., Wen, T., Ming, Z. and Ninghua, D. 2003. Determination of chemical components of volatile oil from Cuminum cyminum L. by gas chromatography - mass spectrometry." *Peop. Rep.* China, 414000.

I.C.M.R. 1987. Medicinal Plants of India. Indian Council of Medical Research, New Delhi, India. http://www.indiastat.com/agriculture/2/milk and dairy products/167/sta ts.aspx.

Ibrahim, I.A., EIB adwi, S.M.A., Bakhiet, A.O., Abdel Gadir, W.S., and Adam, S.E.I. 2007. A9 -week Feeding Study of *Cuminum cyminum. J. Pharmacol. Toxicol.* 2: 666-671.

Jagtap, A.G. and Patil, P.B. 2010. Anti hyperglycemic activity and inhibition of advanced glycation end product formation by Cuminum cyminum in streptozotocin induced diabetic rats. *Food Chem. Toxicol.* 48: 2030–6.

Janahmadi, M., Niazi, F., Danyali, S. and Kamalinejad, M. 2006. Effects of the fruit essential oil of *Cuminum cyminum Linn.* (Apiaceae) on pentylenetetrazol-induced epileptiform activity in F1 neurones of Helix aspersa. *J. Ethnopharmacol.* 104:278–82.

Jazani, N. H., Zartoshti, M. and Shahabi, S. 2008. Antibacterial Effects of Iranian *Cuminum cyminum* Essential Oil on Burn Isolates of *Pseudomonas aeruginosa. Int. J. Pharmacol.* 4: 157-159.

Jirovets, L., Buchbauer, G., Stoyanova, A.S., Georgiev, E.V. and Damianoga, S.T. 2005. Composition, quality control and antimicrobial activity of the essential oil of Cumin (*Cuminum Cyminum L.*) seeds from Bulgaria that had been stored for up to 36 years. *Int. J. Food Sci. Tech.* 40: 305.

Jonas, D., Skemaite, M., Kirkilaite, G., Vinauskiene, R. and Venskutonis, P.R. 2007. Antioxidant and Antimicrobial properties of caraway (*Carum carvi L.*) and cumin (*Cuminum cyminm*) extracts. *Veterinarija IR Zootechnika T.* 40.

Joshi, S.G.2000. Medicinal plants: Family Apiaceae.1st ed. Delhi: Oxford and IBH Publishing Co. Pvt. Ltd.

Karnick, C. R. 1991. A clinical trial of a composite herbal drug in the treatment of diabetes mellitus. *Aryavaidyan.* 5: 36–46.

Khan, M.M.H. and Chaudhry, A.S. 2010. Chemical composition of selected forages and spices and the effect of these spices on *in vitro* rumen degradability of some forages. *Asian-Aust. J. Anim. Sci.* 23:889–900.

Khatibi, A., Hagrarast, A., Shams, J., Dianati, E., Komaki, A. and Kamalinejad, M. 2008. Effects of the fruit essential oil of *Cuminum cyminum L.* on the acquisition and expression of morphine- induced conditioned place preference in mice. *Neurosci. Lett.* 448:94–8

Kilic, U., Boga, M., Gorgulu, M.S. and Ahan, Z. 2011. The effects of different compounds in some essential oils on in vitro gas production. *J. Anim. Feed Sci.* 20:626–636.

Kivanc, M., Akgul, A. and Dogan, A., 1991. Inhibitory and stimulatory effects of cumin, oregano and their essential oils on growth and acid production of Lactobacillus planatarum and Leuconstoc mesenteroides. *Int. J. Food Microbiol.* 13: 81–85.

Krishnakantha, T. P. and Lokesh, B.R. 1993. Scanvenging of superoxide anions by spice principles. *Indian J. Biochem. Biophys.* 30: 133–134.

Kubo, I. and Kinst-Hori, I. 1998. Tyrosinase inhibitors from cumin. *J. Agric. Food Chem.* 46:5338–41.

Kumar, P.A., Reddy, P.Y., Srinivas, P.N. and Reddy, G.B. 2009. Delay of diabetic cataract in rats by the antiglycating potential of cumin through modulation of α-crystallin chaperone activity. *J. Nut.r Biochem.* 20:553–62.

Lee, H. S. 2005. Cuminaldehyde: Aldose reductase and alpha-glucosidase inhibitor derived from *cuminum cyminum L.* seeds. *J. Agric. Food Chem.* 32: 2446–2450.

Leporatti, M.L. and Ghedira, K. 2009. Comparative analysis of medicinal plants used in traditional medicine in Italy and Tunisia. *J. Ethnobiol. Ethnomed.* 5:31–9.

Leung, A. Y. 1980. Encyclopedia of Common Natural Ingredients used in Foods, Drugs and Cosmetics, John Wiley, Hoboken, NJ.

Lourenco, M., Ramos-Morales, E. and Wallace, R.J., 2010. The role of microbes in rumen lipolysis and bio-hydrogenation and their manipulation. *Animal.* 4:1008–1023.

Mahesh, C.M., Gowda, K.P.S. and Gupta, A.K. 2010. Protective action of *Cuminum cyminum* against gentamicin-induced nephrotoxicity. *J. Pharmacy Res.* 3:753–7.

Maiga, A., Diallo, D., Bye, R. and Paulsen, B.S. 2005. Determination of some toxic and essential metal ions in medicinal and edible plants from Mali. *J. Agric. Food Chem.* 53:2316–21.

Malini, T. and Vanithakumari, G. 1987. Estrogenic activity of *Cuminum cyminum* in rats. *Indian J. Ex.p Biol.* 25:442–4.

Mehdi, R.A., Masoomch, S.G., Mohammad, B.R., Kamkar, J., Soheil, A. and Reza, S. 2009. Chemical composition and antiaflatoxicogenic activity of *Carum carvi L., Thymus vulgaris* and *Citrus aurantifolia* essential oils. *Food Contr.* 20:1018–24.

Mhaskar, K.S., Blatter, E. and Caius, J.F. 2000. In Kiritikar and Basu's Illustrated Indian Medicinal Plants.editors. Vol. 5. New Delhi: Satguru Publications.

Milan, K.S.M., Dholakia, H., Tiku, P.K. and Vishweshwaraiah, P. 2008. Enhancement of digestive enzymatic activity by cumin (*Cuminum cymonum L.*) and role of spent cumin as a bionutrient. *Food Chem.* 110:678–83.

Miraliakbari, H. and Shahidi, F. 2008. Antioxidant activity of minor components of tree nut oils. *Food Chem.*111: 421"427.

Miri, V. H., Tyagi, A. K.; Ebrahimi, S. H. and Mohini, M. 2013. Effect of cumin (*Cuminum cyminum*) seed extract on milk fatty acid profile and methane emission in lactating goat. *Small Rum. Res.* 113:66-72.

Nalini, N., Manju, V. and Menon, V.P. 2006. Effect of spices on lipid metabolism in 1,2- dimethylhydrazine-induced rat colon carcinogenesis. *J. Med. Food.* 9:237–45.

Nalini, N., Sabitha, K., Vishwanathan, P. and Menon, V.P. 1998. Influence of spices on the bacterial (enzyme) activity in experimental colon cancer. *J. Ethnopharmacol.* 62:15–24.

Nostro, A., Cellini, L., Di Bartolomeo, S., Di Campli, E., Grande, R. and Cannatelli, M.A. 2005. Antibacterial effect of plant extracts against Helicobacter pylori. *Phytother. Res.* 19:198–202.

Poulson, H.E., Prieme, H. and Loft, S. 1998. Role of oxidative DNA damage in cancer initiation and promotion. *European J. Cancer Prev.* 7: 9–16.

Ramos Morales, E., Mata Espinosa, M.A., McKain, N. and Wallace, R.J., 2012. Ricinoleic acid inhibits methanogenesis and fatty acid bio-hydrogenation in ruminal digesta from sheep and in bacterial cultures. *J. Anim. Sci.,* http://dx.doi.org/10.2527/jas. 2011-4670.

Rathore, S. S., Saxena, S. N. and Singh, B. 2013. Potential health benefits of major seed spices. *Int. J. of Seed Spices.* 3(2):1-12.

Razzaghi-Abyaneh, M., Shams-Ghahfarokhi, M., Rezaee, M.B., Jimand, K., Alinezahad, S., and Saberi, R. 2009. Chemical composition and antiaflatoxigenic activity of Carum carvi L, Thymus vulgaris and Citrus aurantifolia essential oils. *Food Contr.* 20:1018–24.s

Rebey, I.B., Jabri-Karoui, I., Hamrouni-Sellami, I., Bourgou, S., Limam, F. and Marzouk, B. 2012. Effect of drought on the bio-chemical composition and antioxidant activities of cumin (*Cuminum cyminum L.)* seeds. *Industrial Crops and Products.* 36: 238-245.

Romagnoli, C., Andreotti, E., Maietti, S., Mahendra, R. and Mares, D. 2010. Antifungal activity of essential oil from fruits of Indian *Cuminum cyminum. Pharm Biol.* 48:834–48.

Roman-Ramos, R., Flores-Saenz, J.L. and Alarcon-Aguilar, F.J. 1995. Anti-hyperglycemic effect of some edible plants. *J. Ethnopharmacol.* 48:25–32.

Satyanarayana, S., Sushruta, K., Sarma, G.S., Srinivasn, N. and Subba Raju G.V. 2004. Antioxidant activity of the aqueous extracts of spicy food additives–evaluation and comparison with ascorbic acid in in vitro systems. *J. Herb. Pharmacotherapy.* 4(2):1–10.

Sayyah, M., Mahboubi, A. and Kamalinejad, M. 2002a. Anti-convulsant effect of the fruit essential oil of *Cuminum cyminum* in mice. *Pharmaceut Biol.* 40:478–80.

Sayyah, M., Peirovi, A. and Kamalinejad, M. 2002b. Antinociceptive effect of fruit essential oil of Cuminum cyminum L. in rat. *Iran Biomed. J.* 6:141–5.

Senevirathne, M., Kim, S., Siriwardhana, N., Ha, J., Lee, K. and Jeon, Y. 2006. Antioxidant potential of Ecklonia cava on reactive oxygen species scavenging metal chelating, reducing power and lipid peroxidation inhibition. *Food Sci. Tech. Int.* 12: 27–38.

Shayegh, S., Rasooli, I., Taghizadeh, M and Astaneh, S.D. 2008. Phytotherapeutic inhibition of supragingival dental plaque. *Nat. Prod. Res.* 22:428–39.

Shetty, R.S., Singhal, R.S., and Kulkarni, P.R. 1994. "Antimicrobial properties of cumin". *World J. Microbiol. Biotech.* 10: 232–233.

Shirke, S.S., Jadhav, S.R., and Jagtap, A.G. 2008. Methanolic extract of *Cuminum cyminum* inhibits ovariectomy-induced bone loss in rats. *Exp. Biol. Med.* 233:1403–10.

Singh, G., and Upadhyay. R.K. 1993. Essential oils: a potent source of natural pesticides. *J. Sci. Ind. Res.* 52: 676-683.

Sivarajan, V.V., Balachandran, I. 1994. Ayurvedic Drugs and their Plant Sources. New Delhi: Oxford and IBH Publication.

Skrinjar, M.M., Mandi, AI., Misan, A.C., Sakac, M.B., Saric, L.C. and Zec, M.M. 2009. Effect of mint (*Mentha piperita L.*) and Caraway (*Carum carvi L.*) on the growth of some toxicogenic Aspergillus species and aflatoxin B production. *Proc. Nat. Sci. Matica Srpska Novi Sad.* 116: 131–9.

Srinivasan, K. 2005. Plant foods in the management of diabetes mellitus: Spices as beneficial antidiabetic food adjuncts. *Int. J. Food Sci. Nutr.* 56:399–414.

Srivastava, K.C. 1989. Extracts from two frequently consumed spices-cumin (*Cuminum cyminum*) and turmeric (*Curcuma longa*) inhibit platelet aggregation and alter eicosanoid bio-synthesis in human blood platelets. *Prostaglandins Leukot Essen Fatty Acids.* 37:57–64.

Srivastava, K.C. and Mustafa, T. 1994. Pharmacological effect of spices: Eicosanoid modulating activities and their significance in human health. *Biomed. Rev.* 2:15–29.

Talpur, N., Echard, B., Ingram, C., Bagachi, D., and Preuss, H. 2005. Effects of a novel formulation of essential oils on glucose-insulin metabolism in diabetic and hypertensive rats: a pilot study. *Diabetes Obes Metab.*7: 193–199.

Toghrol, F., and Daneshpejouh, H. 1974. Estimation of free amino acids, protein and amino acid compositions of cumin seed (*Cuminum cyminum*) of Iran. *J Trop Pediatr Environ Child Health.* 20:109–11.

Uma Pradeep, K., Geervani, P. and Eggum, B.O. 1993. Common Indian spices: Nutrient composition, consumption and contribution to dietary value. *Plant Foods Hum. Nutr.* 44:137–48.

Varo, P. T. and Heinz, D. E. 1970a. Identification and characterization of 1,4-p-methadien-7-al isolated from cumin seeds. *J. Agric.Food Chem.* 18 (2):239–242.

Varo, P. T. and Heinz, D. E. 1970b. Volatile components of cumin seed oil. *J.Agric. Food Chem.* 17: 234–238.

Vasudevan, K., Vembar, S., Veeraraghavan, K. and Haranath, P.S. 2000. Influence of intragastric perfusion of aqueous spice extracts on acid secretion in anesthetized albino rats. *Indian J. Gastroenterol.* 19:53–6.

Willatgamuwa, S. A., Platell, K., Saraswathi, G. and Srinivasan, K. 1998. Antidiabetic influence of dietary cumin seeds (*cuminum cyminum*) in streptozotocin induced diabetic rats. *Nutrition Res.* 18(10): 131–142.

Zargary A. 2001. Medicinal Plants.5th Edn. Tehran: Tehran University Publications.

Zitao, J., Yajing, L. and Ximei, N. 1993. Department Food Eng.m Tianjin comer. Coll., Tianjin, Peop. Rep China 300400) *Zhonjjuo Tiaaweipin.* 1: 11-13.

□□□

Chapter 23

Kadipatta (*Murraya koenigii*)

Anshu Rahal

Department of Animal Nutrition, College of Veterinary and Animal Sciences, G B Pant University of Agriculture & Technology, Pantnagar-263145,Uttarakhand, India, E-mail: anshurahal@rediffmail.com

ABSTRACT

Kadipatta (*Murraya koenigii*) commonly known as meetha neem has medicinal value as it possess various pharmaceutical properties. Almost whole plant parts are used in one or the other form for combating infections and other ailments. The medicinal value of the leaf has been reported as antibacterial. Phytoconstituents present in leaves are glycozoline, xanthotoxin and sesquiterpine. The leaves are also used as carminative, antidysentric and for external cures eruptions, anti vomiting, tonic and stomachic purposes. The effects of leaves on blood glucose and plasma insulin levels in alloxan induced diabetic rats have been detected. The fresh kadipatta leaves have chlorophyll, terpenes and anti-oxidants which may also contribute in the hypoglycemic effect and increased insulin secretion. The properties and various method of incorporation of this plant in daily life have been discussed in this chapter.

Keywords: *Murraya koenigii*, Nutritional composition, Glycozoline, Xanthotoxin, Pharmacological properties.

23.1 Introduction

Kadipatta (*Murraya koenigii*) is a multipotential medicinal plant (Kritikar *et al.*, 2004; Aggarwal and Paridhavi, 2007) widely used as aromatic herb, leafy spice or vegetable, condiments and also used to treat various types of ailments in Indian traditional system. Literature reveals notable pharmacological activities of this plant such as activity on heart, anti-diarrhoea activity, phagocytic activity and many more medicinal values. The plant have been reported to possess positive inotropic effect (Rahman and Gray, 2005) antidiabetic and cholesterol reducing property (Ram *et al.*, 2005 ; Kesari *et al.*, 2005), antimicrobial, antibacterial and other microbiological activity (Shrinivasan, 2005; Manfred *et al.*, 1985; Shah *et al.*, 2004), antiulcer activity (Xie Ji *et al.*, 2006), antioxidative property and cytotoxic activity (Shah and Juvekar, 2006). In Ayurveda, along with leaves, whole plant parts have been used to cure diseases. The leaves, bark and the root of the Kadipatta plant are used in indigenous medicine as a tonic and antiflatulent. The leaves of kadipatta have been centre point since its high antioxidant potency has been reported which is mainly due to mahanimbine, murrayanol and mahanine present in *M. koenigii* (Tachibana *et al.*, 2003; Ningappa *et al.*, 2008; Vaijayanthimala *et al.*, 2004). Fresh leaves on steam distillation under pressure yield a volatile oil and residual glucoside named as koenigin. Young leaves have aroma so are mainly used as appetizer but adult have bitter taste due to increased concentration of alkaloids. *Murraya koenigii* is also effective against diabetes Mellitus. If someone is bitten by poisonous animals, local application of the leave paste is effective. The bark and the roots are used as a stimulant by the physicians. The roots are used for treating body aches and the bark for snakebite relief. The leaves and roots are bitter, acrid and antihelminthic. It cures piles, allays heat of the body, and reduces inflammation and itching. It is also useful in leucoderma and blood disorders (Vaibhav *et al.*, 2011). An infusion of the toasted leaves is used to stop vomiting. Crushed leaves are applied externally to cure skin eruption, bruises and burn. It acts as febrifuge, antifungal, depressant, anti-dysentric and used for kidney pain. This bitter herb is a potent blood-purifier and a restorative of the degenerated blood cells. If taken regularly, it builds up and strengthens the liver (Gurgune *et al.*, 2003) and helps in the metabolism of fatty acids. It is a good tonic for the spleen and pancreas and promotes the increase of the cells of the islets of langerhans in the Pancreas. The plant roots and bark are also potent in their health benefit. The bark is acrid, cooling, alexcteric, anathematic and analgesic (Kaur *et al.*, 2011). Kadipatta is also known to strengthen the function of stomach and promote its action. Its leaves are mild laxative in nature.The berries are thirst-quenchers and have a cooling effect on the system. The Indian variety *Murraya koenigii* (L) Spreng and Chinese variety *M. paniculata* are mainly the two species available and both have somewhat common medicinal properties.

Kadipatta is also known as sweet neem due to its medicinal qualities resembling that of Neem. Other Synonyms are Girinimba, Krishnanimba (Sanskrit), Curry leaves (English), Meetha neem, karipatta (Hindi), Karuveppilai, noroxingha (Assamese), Barsunga (Bengali), Limdo or meetholimdo *(Gujarati)*,Karibue (Kannada), Kadhilimbu (Marathi), Karivepku (Telugu), Tamil-Kariveppilai; Malayalam-Kariveppu , Tulu- Bevusoppu; Portuguese- Folhas de caril; Russian-Listya karri; Spanish- Hojas de curry; Italian-Fogli di Cari; French-Feuilles de Cari; German- Curryblatter.

23.2 Taxonomy

Kingdom	:	Plantae
Sub-kingdom	:	Tracheobionta
Superdivision	:	Spermatophyta
Division	:	Magnoliophyta
Class	:	Magnoliospida
Subclass	:	Rosidae
Order	:	Sapindales
Family	:	Rutaceae
Genus	:	*Murraya*
Species	:	*Koenigii*

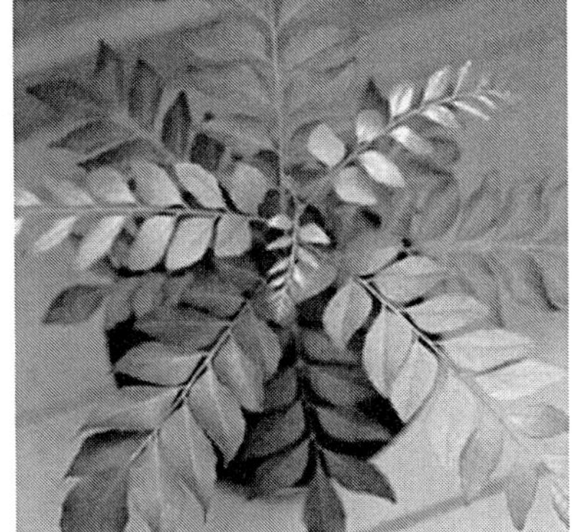

23.3 Distribution

Kadipatta is native of India and Sri Lanka. It grows well in all tropical zones, Asia, South Africa, Malaysia and most parts of India upto an elevation of 1500 m. The plant is also cultivated in Burma, Ceylon, China, Indonesia, Australia and the Pacific Islands. In India, it is found mostly in Sikkim, Garhwal, Bengal, Assam, Western Ghats and Travancore- Cochin. It is also available in other part of Asian region like in moist forests of 500-1600 m height in Guangdong, S Hainan, S Yunnan (Xishuangbanna), Bhutan, Laos, Nepal, Pakistan, Southern California, South Texas and South Florida. In tropical Africa, it is planted in many countries including Nigeria, Kenya, Tanzania and most of the Indian Ocean Islands, where Indian immigrants settled. The species name commemorates the botanist Johann König.

Kadipatta is deciduous, spreading shrub growing upto 6 metres in height and 15 to 40 cms in diameter. The main stem is dark green to brownish, with numerous dots on it; its bark can be peeled off longitudinally, exposing the white wood underneath; the girth of the main stem is 16 cm. Some consider it to be a small tree with pinnate leaves which are used in South Indian curries. It can be grown in pot as well as outdoor. Flowering starts from the middle of April and ends in the middle of May. The peak flowering season under the Sanwara (Himachal Pradesh) conditions is last week of April. The fruiting season continues from the middle of July to the end of August. This plant needs to be fertilized with palm or citrus fertilizer to promote leaf production. It can grow in full sun or light shade but needs to be protected from freezing. It is cultivated extensively for its aromatic leaves and ornamental value throughout India. During the Indian summer, the tree sheds lot of leaves due to the heat but the tree grows gloriously during the monsoon months. Trimming it regularly produces new leaves and keeps the tree healthy.

23.4 Plant Structure

23.4.1 *Leaves*

Leaves are exstipulate bipinnately compound 15-30 cm long having reticulate venation, 2.5-3.5 cm long lanceolate 24 leaflets alternate on rachis, 4.9 cm long,1.8cm broad having 0.5cm long petiole 2-3 mm long with irregularly creatate margins. The stomata are distributed on both the sides. Each leaflet resembles the leaves of the neem tree. The leaves are slightly bitter and aromatic. The leaves of *Murraya koenigii* (L) Spreng are obliquely ovate or somewhat rhomboid with acuminate obtuse or acute apex. The leaves look a bit like bay leaves along a long central stem and are used in a similar fashion.

Under the compound microscope, the stomata can be seen distributed on abaxial surface while the adaxial surface is without stomata. The type of stomata are anomocytic one. The Uniseriate multicellular trichomes are observed on both surfaces, more frequent on upper surface of midrib portion. The wall of trichome is ridged. The transverse section of leaf exposes a layer of epidermis composed of rectangular cells as outermost covering on both upper and lower layer. The upper epidermis is enveloped with deposition of cuticle. In midrib portion, epidermis is followed by 1-4 layers of collenchymatous hypodermis in continuation with 2-5 layers of chlorenchyma cells filled with chlorophyll content. Beneath this, is the ground tissue portion which is composed of oval to polygonal parenchyma cells and is traversed with vascular bundle. This region also consists of calcium oxalate crystals. Towards the vascular bundles, bundle of fibres are present on upper side. Xylem and phloem portion of vascular bundle consist of their basic elements. In lamina portion, upper epidermis is followed by 1-2 layers of palisade parenchyma cells continued with spongy parenchyma cells with intercellular spaces. The whole mesophyll portion is filled with chlorophyll content and spiral type of vessels. Transverse section shows a dorsi ventral structure. Epidermis is composed of cubical to slightly tangentially elongated cells. The upper epidermal cells are polyhedral and straight walled. Trichomes are rarely unicellular and found mainly on midrib. Stomata are anomocytic; with palisade of two layers. Spongy parenchyma is irregular with disodiametrical or rectangular cells. Calcium oxalate crystals are present in the form of prisms. Secretary canals are large and circular. The midrib shows an arc of radiating xylem with phloem below. Pericyclic fibers appear in patches below the phloem. The length of fibers is 2000µ. Collenchyma layers (1-3) are present below lower epidermis. Ground tissue is composed of thin parenchymatous polygonal cells.

The preliminary phytochemical screening of petroleum ether extract, ethyl acetate extract, chloroform extract, ethanol extract and aqueous extract of leaf has indicated the presence of alkaloids, flavonoids, carbohydrates, and sterol in leaf.Other phytochemicals present are tannins, volatile oils, saponins and anthroquinone glycosides. The bio-chemicals found in kadipatta leaves include caryophyllene, cadinene, cadinol, Sabinene, pinene, phellandrene, terpinene, lauric acid, palmitic acid, carbazole alkaloids (Ramsewak *et al.*, 1999; Wang *et al.*, 2003; Ito *et al.*, 1993; Reisch *et al.*, 1994; Reisch *et al.*, 1992), bornyl acetate, humulene, ocimene and bisabolene, etc. Carbazole alkaloids of kadipatta leaves have shown several biological activities such as anticarcinogenic effects in dimethylhydrazine (DMH) treated rats (Farhath-Khanum *et al.*, 2000), antiplatelet activity and vasorelaxing effects (Wu *et al.*, 1998). Chevalier (1996) also reported that kadipatta leaf has medicinal value as traditionally used in eastern Asia. Chowdhury *et al.* (2001) reported that these alkaloids have anti-microbial activity against gram positive and negative bacteria, and fungi. Carbazole derivatives are well known for their various pharmacological activities, including anti-HIV, antibacterial and anti-fungal activities (Tripathi *et al.*, 1982; Adebajo 2000; Ates and Erdognel, 2003). A series of substituted carbazoles, termed N-alkylated

3, 6-dihalogenocarbazoles, exhibit fungicidal activity against *Candida albicans* and the pathogen *Candida glabrata*. The most potent fungicidal compounds of this series are characterized by minimal fungicidal concentration (MFC) between 8.5 and 25 μM. Phytochemically leaves contain alkaloid and volatile oil. Leaves possess anti-inflammatory, anti-feedant activity. The medicinal value of the leaf has been reported as antibacterial. Phytoconstituents present in leaves are Glycozoline, Xanthotoxin and Sesquiterpine. The leaves are also used as carminative, antidysentric and for external cures eruptions, anti-vomiting, tonic and stomachic purposes. The effects of leaves on blood glucose and plasma insulin levels in alloxan induced diabetic rats have been detected. The fresh kadipatta leaves have chlorophyll, terpenes and antioxidants which may also contribute in the hypoglycemic effect and increased insulin secretion. Usually fresh kadipatta leaves are preferred instead of dry powder. Leaves are aromatic and contain proteins, carbohydrates, fiber, minerals, carotene, nicotinic acid and vitamin C. It is rich in vitamin A and calcium but the leaves contain high amount of oxalic acid. Leaves also contain crystalline glycosides, carbazole alkaloids and resin. Fresh leaves contain yellow colour 2.5 % volatile oil. It also contains girinimbin, iso-mahanimbin, koenine, koenigine, koenidine and koenimbine. Mahanimbicine and bicyclomahanimbicine, phebalosin, coumarine as Murrayone imperatoxin, etc. have been also isolated from leaves. The leaves of plant are used as a stimulant, antidysentric and for the management of diabetes mellitus, antihelminthic, analgesic, cures piles, allays heat of the body, thirst, inflammation and itching. The green leaves are stated to be eaten raw for curing dysentry and the infusion of the washed leaves stops vomiting. Steam distillate of the leaves can be used as purgative and antiemetic (Yukari *et al.*, 2001). Leaves are applied externally to bruises and eruption (Kumar *et al.*, 1999; Mohar *et al.*, 2011). The plant's bitterness is about 2.5 unit/gm. The plant possesses haemolytic activity. Leaves contain amino acids viz. phenylalanine and glycine and carbohydrates i.e. galactose, ribose and fructose. Triterpenoid alkaloids like cyclomahanimbine and tetrahydromahanimbine are also present in the leaves. Murrayastine, murrayaline, pypayafolinecarbazole alkaloids and many other chemical compounds have been also reported in the leaves of *M. koenigii*. The gas chromatography-mass spectrometry of volatile oil of fresh leaves of *Murraya Koenigii* has indicated presence of 34 compounds consisting of 97.4% of the oil of which major constituents are alpha-pinene (51.7%), sabinene (10.5%), beta-pinene (9.8%), betacaryophyllene (5.5%), limonene (5.4%), bornyl acetate (1.8%), terpinen-4-ol (1.3%), gamma-terpinene (1.2%) and alpha-humulene (1.2%).The carbazole alkaloids possess anti-oxidant (Patel and Rajorhia, 1979; Nair and Chanda, 2006) properties,insecticidal,anti-microbial specifically mosquitocidal properties and anti-diarrheal properties. The presence of vitamins A,B, C and E help in reducing oxidative stress and free radical scavenging activity.

23.4.2 *Roots*

The root shows tetrarch to pentarch stele. Phelloderm fibres are absent and concentric grains of parenchyma are present. Four carbazole alkaloids, identified as mahanimbine, girinimbine, murrayanine murrayafoline-A and one triterpene (Srivastava and Srivastava, 1993; Prekesh *et al.*, 2006) have been isolated from stem bark and roots of Murraya koenigii.

23.4.3 *Bark*

The bark of *M. koenigii is* grey colour with longitudinal striations on it and beneath it white bark is present. Bark also consists of carbazole alkaloids as murrayacine, murrayazolidine, murrayazoline, mahanimbine, girinimbine, koenioline (Feibigetal, 1985) and xynthyletin. Girinimbine has been shown to possess anti-tumor promoting activity by measuring the percentage inhibition of induced early antigen EA of Epstein Barr virus EBV on the surface of Raji cells. Raji cells are B-human lymphoblastoids latently infected with EBV, in which the early antigen of the virus can be induced by phorbol 12-myristate 13-acetate and n-butyrate to express on the surface of cells which can be detected by immunofluorescence using human antisera of nasopharyngeal carcinoma. Girinimbine strongly inhibited the induction of EA of EBV more than 90 %, when tested at 16.0 and 32.0 μg/ml. The inhibition rate was moderate when tested at 8.0 μg/mL inhibition rate 58% and low at 4.0, 2.0 and 1.0 μg/mL inhibition rates of 46, 35 and 32%, respectively. The inhibition rate at fifty per cent of the compound extrapolated from the dose response curve was 6.0 μg/ml.

23.4.4 *Flowers*

Flowers are bisexual, small,white, funnel-shaped, fragrant, stalked, complete, ebracteate, regular, actinomorphic, pentamerous, hypogynous, the average diameter of a fully opened flower is 1.12 cm; inflorescence, a terminal cyme, each bearing 60-90 flowers; calyx, 5-lobed, pubescent, persistent, inferior, green; corolla, white, polypetalous, inferior, with 5 petals with dotted glands, lanceolate; length, 5 mm; androecium, polyandrous, inferior, with 10 stamens, dorsifixed, arranged into circles of five each; smaller stamens, 4 mm. long, whereas the longer ones, 5-6 mm; gynoecium, 5 to 6 mm long; stigma, bright, sticky; style, short; ovary, superior.

23.4.5 *Fruit*

The small black shiny berries are edible, but their seeds are poisonous. The berries of the plant are green in colour and turn purplish black on ripening. Fruits are ovoid to round, subglobose, wrinkled or rough with glands. It's size of 2.5 cm long and 0.3 cm in diameter and gets purplish black, when ripen. Fruits are generally biseeded. It bears fruits in close clusters/bunches (32-80) glandular, thin pericarp enclosing one or two seeds which generally occur in spinach green colour, 11 mm long, 8 mm in diameter and weighs upto 445 mg. Seeds are fragile so need to be handle with care. Seeds are shipped in moist peat moss/coir mix and should be planted immediately.

Seeds must be ripe and fresh to plant; dried or shrivelled fruits are not viable. One can plant the whole fruit, but it is best to remove the pulp before planting in the potting mix which is kept moist. Stem cuttings can also be used for propagation.

23.5 Nutritional Significance of Kadipatta

As indicated in Table 1, Kadipatta leaves are rich in vitamin A, phosphorus, iron, nicotinic acid, vitamin C and calcium. Mature leaves contains 63.2% moisture, 1.15% total nitrogen, 6.15% fat, 18.92% total sugars, 14.6% starch, 6.8% crude fiber, 13.06% ash, 1.35% acid insoluble ash, 1.82% alcohol soluble extractive, 27.33% cold water (20°C) extractive and a maximum of hot water soluble extractive 33.45%. The pulp of fruits generally contain 64.9% moisture, 9.76% total sugar, 9.58% reducing sugar, 0.17% non-reducing sugar, 13.35%vitamin C and negligible amount of tannin and acids. The pulp of fruits contain trace amount of minerals like 1.97% phosphorus,

0.082% potassium, 0.811% calcium, 0.166% magnesium and 0.007% iron. Fresh leaves on steam distillation under pressure yield 206% of volatile oil that may find use as a fixative. The fruit yields 0.76% of a yellow volatile oil with neroli like odour and also contain markable amount of protein.

Table 1: Nutritional value of Kadipatta (Spices Board of India, the Ministry of Commerce and Industry, Government of India)

Nutrition	Value per 100 g	Nutrition	Value per 100 g
Moisture	63 g	Protein	6.1 g
Fat	1 g	Minerals	4 g
Fiber	6 g	Carbohydrates	18 g
Energy	108 kcal	Calcium	830 mg
Phosphorus	57 mg	Iron	0.93 mg
Magnesium	44 mg	Copper	0.1 mg
Manganese	0.15 mg	Zinc	0.2 mg
Chromium	0.006 mg	Vitamin A(carotene)	7560 µg
Thiamine	0.08 mg	Riboflavin	0.21 mg
Niacin	2.3 mg	Folic Acid(total) Folic acid (free)	93.9 µg 23.5 µg
Vitamin C Sulphur Chlorine	4 mg 81mg 198 mg	Riboflavin Oxalic acid Phytin Phosphorus	0.21mg 132mg 35mg

Amino acids such as alanine, tryptophan and tyrosine are found in the leaves. Carbazole alkaloids such as koenigine, mahanimbine, muconicine have been found to demonstrate anticancer properties and antioxidant properties. Kadipatta leaves have both hypoglycemic effect and also help in reducing triglycerides count in animals and human beings. The essential constituents of Kadipatta leaf are monoterpenes including phellandrene, a-pinene, and pinene. In some species, sesquiterpenes is the main constituent. The plant is highly valued for its leaves as important ingredient in an Indian cuisine to promote appetite and digestion. The leaves, root and bark are tonic, stomachic and carminative. Fruits are also considered as astringent in Indo-China. The plant is credited with tonic and stomachic property. The fruits are known to have very high nutritional values with many medicinal properties. The branches of *M. koenigii* are very popular for cleaning the teeth so used as datun. It is also said that the branches of *M. koenigii* are used to strengthen gums and teeth's. It has also been used as an anti-periodic and many times the powdered dry leaf, mixed with honey and juice of betel nut, is recommended in the Ayurvedic system of medicine. It is good herbal tonic for kidney problems; prevent early development of cataracts and treatment for weight loss. They have the ability to prevent diabetes whether it is hereditary or due to obesity. They can be used for eye disorders as well for kidney failure. They are recommended for anaemia due to high iron content. They are helpful to reduce premature hair graying /falling, ease constipation, asthama and blood pressure. They are used in the treatment of more than 18 maladies. Unique leaf therapy indicates that if one eats about 300 leaves of kadipatta, person can live disease -free life. It is a good digestive, especially after fatty and fried food consumption. Indigestion, nausea, sour belching, heartburn, morning sickness and other digestive disorders such as diarrhoea, dysentery, bilious vomiting and haemorrhoids also respond well to treatment with kadipatta leaves. It is an essential ingredient of almost all traditional medicine systems of peninsular India. Unani, Ayurveda and other systems use it to cure ailments such as piles, to allay heat of the body and are useful in leucoderma and blood disorders, and this has been proven by experts of western medicine also.

Curry leaves improve functioning of the stomach and small intestine and promote their action. They improve the quality of digestive juices secreted during digestion. Their action starts with intake. Their smell, taste and visual impression initiates salivary secretion and initiates the peristaltic wave, which is the first step in good digestion. They are mildly laxative and thus, can tackle multiple digestive problems caused by food intake. The vitamins and minerals contained in curry leaves such as folic acid, calcium, beta carotene, riboflavin, zinc, etc. promotes oral health.

The health of the infants and growing animals and human beings is stimulated as kadipatta supplies essential vitamins, minerals and antioxidants. It is good for eyesight, effective against gastro-intestinal disorders, remedy for diarrhoea and dysentery, offer liver protection, has neuroprotective properties and helps in building the immune system.

23.6 Kadipatta Powder Characteristic

Powdered leaf material when analyzed for its fluorescence with chemical reagents such as alcohol, sulphuric acid, sodium hydroxide and nitric acid shows following specific colours as indicated below:

Treatment	Day light	UV light
Powder as such	Pale Green	Fluorescent Pale Green
Power in distilled water	Bluish-Green	Fluorescent Bluish-Green
Powder in absolute alcohol	Olive-Green	Fluorescent Orange
Powder in 10% NaOH	Light-Brown	Fluorescent Dark Brown
Powder in 50% HNO3	Yellow	Fluorescent Black
Powder in 50% H2SO4	Dark Green	Fluorescent Yellowish- Green

Green colour with no distinct odour or taste, unicellular, bent or curved trichomes, two layered palisade, portion of secretory canals, well developed pericyclic fibers and a few prismatic crystals of calcium oxalate are the important identifying characters of Kadipatta leaf powder. The powder when treated with 1 N methanolic sodium hydroxide shows yellowish white colour and when mounted in nitrocellulose emits chocolate fluorescence. The higher percentage of total ash and acid insoluble ash in powder is due to presence of calcium oxalate crystals or other inorganic salts present in various metabolites. The presence of the phytochemicals make the plant useful for treating different ailments and have a potential of providing useful drugs of human use. The quantitative determination of pharmacognostic parameters help in setting standards for crude drugs. The total ash is particularly important in evaluating the purity of drugs.

23.7 Pharmacological Properties of Kadipatta

23.7.1 *Gastro-intestinal Protection*

Kadipatta leaves have a natural mild laxative effect. Soaking Kadipatta leaves in warm water for two hours and drinking the water with a teaspoon of honey early in the morning helps to cleanse the system, constipation and improve appetite. Alternatively, fresh kadipatta leaves juice can be mixed with buttermilk and consumed three times in a day for effective results. The presence of antioxidants, vitamins and alkaloids in kadipatta leaves helps in promoting health of digestive system. A glass of buttermilk with a pinch of salt and a spoonful of grounded kadipatta leaf paste, taken on an empty stomach, relieves stomachache. Usually for digestive upset, buttermilk enriched with the paste of kadipatta leaves, common salt and cumin seed powder is recommended. This combination is also useful in problems such as loss of appetite, tastelessness of mouth as in case of fever, etc. where food intake is a problem. Kadipatta leaves are one of the important ingredients of herbal tonics and are parallel to digestive enzymatic tonics in allopathy. Kadipatta leaves and black pepper beaten with sour curd is beneficial to those suffering from gas formation due to indigestion.

The carbazole alkaloids present in kadipatta leaves play an important role in controlling diarrhoea. For this purpose, kadipatta leaves can be taken either as juice or as a freshly ground paste. Chewing the tender leaf helps control loose motions. Bio-active alkaloids, kurryam and koenimbine obtained from fractionated n-hexane extract of the seeds of *M. koenigii* were found to exhibit inhibitory activity against castor oil-induced diarrhoea and prostaglandin E2-induced enteropooling in rats in charcoal meal test in Wister rats. These compounds were found to exhibit significant reduction in gastro-intestinal motility. Kadipatta leaves improve the quality of digestive juices. Fresh Kadipatta leaves can stimulate salivary secretions which in turn initiate the secretion of digestive juices. To control indigestion and flatulence, add a spoonful of dried and ground mixture of Kadipatta leaves, jeera, black salt and dried ginger in warm water or one can take a glass of fresh juice made from Kadipatta, coriander and mint leaves. Kadipatta leaves mixed with ginger and rice and consumed in the morning along with water will reduce stomach disorders, dizziness and constipation.

Decoction of powdered bark of kadipatta tree made in cold water or few leaves added in buttermilk or roasted curry leaves can be taken daily (Mhaskar *et al.*, 2000) to get remedy of vomition. Fresh juice of kadipatta leaves, with lime juice and sugar, is an effective medicine in the treatment of morning sickness, nausea and vomiting due to indigestion and excessive use of fats. A paste of these leaves with limejuice and honey/sugar/crystal sugar powder is a time-tested medicine in the treatment of hyperemesis graviderum. Nausea, dry vomiting, vomiting and food intolerance are few other conditions where this paste is used as a remedy. Fresh juice/a paste of fresh leaves/a teaspoonful of powdered dried leaves / a mixture of Kadipatta leaves, coriander, mint leaves, etc. is a commonly known home-made remedy. A decoction of the leaves and even of the roots or bark can be used to combat the vomiting associated with cholera. To control morning sickness, especially during pregnancy, decoction can be prepared with one teaspoon of kadipatta leaves juice, one tablespoon of lime juice and one teaspoon of honey and consumed early in the morning or add few kadipatta leaves while brewing tea. Roasted curry leaves also prevent nausea. The tannins and carbazole alkaloids (Gurgune *et al.*, 2003) present in Kadipatta exhibit hepato-protective properties from various diseases such as hepatitis and cirrhosis as discussed above.

23.7.2 *Antimicrobial/Antibacterial / Antifungal Activity*

Kadipatta leaves are effective in fighting bacterial and fungal infections (Tripathi *et al.*, 1982; Darvekar, 2011). The essential oil from *M. koenigii* leaves showed antibacterial effect against *B. subtilis, Staph. aureus, C. pyogenes, P. vulgaris and Pasteurella multicida.* The pure oil is active against the first three organisms even at a dilution of 1: 500. Acetone extract of *M. koenigii* is active against *Aspergillus niger,* benzene extract is most active against *Alternaria solani* and *Helmintho-sporium solani* and ethanol extract is active against *Penicillum notatum.*Benzoisofuranone derivatives along with six known carbazole alkaloids and three known steroids were isolated from stem bark of *M. Koenigii* to study antimicrobial activity of Kadipatta (Shan *et al.*, 2007; Kumar 2013; Bonde *et al.*, 2017). These compounds were found to be effective in range 3.13-100 µg/ml concentration. Methanolic extract of 21 plant species were screened for *in vitro* anti-bacterial activity against multi-resistant bacterial isolates including Gram positive and Gram negative strains. Study showed that *M. koenigii had* maximum antibacterial activity. Staphylococcus *epidermidis* was significantly inhibited by *M. koenigii.* Mahanimbine, murrayanol and mahanine are three carbazole alkaloids isolated from the acetone extract of the fresh leaves of *M. Koenigii.* Of these three, murrayanol showed an IC50 of 109 µg/mL against hPGHS-1 and an IC50 of 218 µg/mL against hPGHS-2 in anti-inflammatory assays, while mahanimbine displayed anti-oxidant activity at 33.1 µg/ml. All these three carbazole alkaloids were mosquitocidal and anti-microbial and exhibited topoisomerase I and II inhibition activities and anti-bacterial activity against *S. typhi* and *E. coli.*

23.7.3 *Antioxidative Property*

An aryl hydroxyl substituent on the carbazole ring plays a role in stabilizing the thermal oxidation and rate of reaction against DPPH radicals. The antioxidative properties of the leaf extracts of *Murraya Koenigii* using different solvents were evaluated based on the oil stability index (OSI) together with their radical scavenging ability against 1, 1-diphenyl-2-picrylhydrazyl (DPPH). The methylene chloride (CH2Cl2) extract and the ethyl acetate (EtOAc) soluble fraction of the 70 % acetone extract prolonged the OSI values significantly compared to alpha-tocopherol and BHT. Five carbazole alkaloids were isolated from the CH2Cl2 extract and their structures were identified to be euchrestine, bi-smurrayafoline, mahanine, mahanimbicine and mahanimbine based on 1H and 13C NMR and mass (MS) spectral data. Mahanimbine and koenigine, two carbazole alkaloids, isolated from the leaves of *M. koenigii* showed antioxidant activity. Koenigine also showed a high degree of radical scavenging properties.

Kadipatta leaves boiled in milk are used for treating heat rashes and bruises. It can be used with turmeric for treatment of acne. It's paste also helps in healing wounds, treating burn wounds and skin eruptions (Kesari *et al.*, 2005; Satyavathi *et al.*, 1983). Leaves have antioxidant & microbial properties so help in blood purification and provide beautiful radiance to the skin. Kadipatta leaves are also used as a cure to skin rashes and allergies. Along with mint leaves and coriander leaves, Kadipatta leaves can be used in treating excessive pitta conditions. The formulation of cream of essential oil of leaf of *M. koenigii* has been found to have sun protection factor. The cream has been found useful in maintaining the natural skin pigmentation. It can be used as additives in other formulations to enhance the activity. Kadipatta leaves ground with turmeric and taken daily is an effective remedy for allergic reactions.

23.7.4 *Anti-inflammatory Activity*

The alcohol extract of stem bark (1 gm/kg body weight) is effective against carrageenan-induced inflammation (Gahlawat, 2014). Crude root extract also showed anti-inflammatory activity. Ethanolic extract of *M. koenigii* (EEMK) (300 and 400 mg/kg) showed anti-histaminic actions in the histamine-aerosol protocol. The mast cell stabilization and anti-histaminic effects of EEMK were suggested to be the probable mechanisms for its anti-inflammatory action.

23.7.5 *Anti-diabetic*

Chewing fresh Kadipatta leaves continuously for 3 months help to control blood sugar in non-insulin dependent diabetics. Intake of Kadipatta leaves stop the production of digestive enzyme pancreatic alpha–amylase which convert starch to sugar and release it in blood. In diabetes, the body has high level of sugars in the blood which are not being regulated by insulin which is due to the (diabetesI or diabtesII) inability of pancreas to produce sufficient amounts of insulin to curb the sugar production. By reducing the availability of the pancreatic alpha-amylase enzyme, the leaves are able to inhibit the conversion of starches to sugar which can help treat diabetes effectively. Kadipatta leaves help reduce the blood sugar level in the human body. M. koenigii possessed statistically significant hypoglycemic (Yadav *et al.*, 2002; Handral *et al.*, 2010; Handral *et al.*, 2012) potential in STZ-induced diabetic rats. The M. koenigii extract is more effective than glibenclamide, a known antidiabetic drug. Research conducted at University of Madras, Chennai in Department of Biochemistry and Molecular Biology indicated that anti-hyperglycemic property of Kadipatta leaves is beneficial in controlling blood glucose level in diabetic rats. Mahanimbine a chemical constituent of *M. koenigii* was isolated from column chromatography of the petroleum ether extract of dried plant. The anti-diabetic activity was performed on the streptrozotocin induced wistar rats by using pure compound at a dose of 50 mg/kg and 100 mg/kg. The possible mechanism by which the mahanimbine decreases blood sugar level may be by potentiating insulin effect either by increasing the pancreatic secretion of insulin from beta cells of islets of langerhans or by increasing the peripheral glucose uptake. Mahanimbine showed appreciable alpha amylase inhibitory effect compared with acarbose.

23.7.6 *Anti-ulcer Activity*

Anti-ulcer activity of aqueous and ether extracts of *M. koenigii* has been studied in reserpine induced gastric ulcer model in albino rats. Extracts were effective in gastric ulceration and suggested as protective as ranitidine. Crude aqueous extract of leaves showed anti-ulcer activity which was evaluated by using models of acute gastric lesions induced by ethanol induced, aspirin induced, cold restrain stress and pylorus ligation in rats. Animals were pretreated with doses of 200 mg/kg and 400 mg/kg of aqueous extract which showed efficient reduction in lesion index, total affected area and percentage of lesion in comparison with control group in the ethanol induced, aspirin induced, cold restrain stress induced ulcer and pylorus ligation models. The observations indicated that aqueous extract of leaves of *M. koenigii* can act as good anti-ulcer drug.

23.7.8 *Antihelminthic Effect*

Kadipatta leaves methanolic extract can kill roundworm parasites in the intestine.The antihelminthic activity was performed on adult Indian earth worm 'Pheretima posthuma'. The organism was chosen due to its resemblance with the intestine round worm parasites of human beings (Sindhu and Arora, 2014; Jain *et al.*, 2012). Petroleum ether and alcoholic extracts were selected for the activity and Piperazine citrate as standard. Ether and methanolic extracts were taken at 25 mg/ml, 50mg/ml and 100 mg/ml concentrations. Worms were kept under observation to notice the time taken to paralysis and death in individual worms. Paralysis was said to occur, when the worms do not revive even in normal saline. Death was concluded when the worms lost their motility followed by the fading of body color. Among them alcoholic extract of plant leaves at a dose of 100 mg/ml had significant antihelminthic activity, whereas petroleum ether showed moderate activity.

23.7.9 *Hypocholesterolemic Activity*

Hypocholesterolemic activity was checked in aged mice using crude ethanol extract of plant leaves of *M. Koenigii*. The experiment was confirmed by observing decrease in cholesterol level in dose dependent manner in aged mice. The dose of 500 mg/kg was found more efficient than the 300 mg/kg and was comparable with the standard cholesterol reducing agent, Simvastatin. Carbazole alkaloids a major phytochemical constituent of plant was found to have various biological activities like anti-oxidant, anti-diabetic, anti-microbial, lipid lowering, etc. The antioxidants present in curry leaves help in controlling/reducing the Low Density Lipoprotein or bad cholesterol and aid in increasing the High Density Lipoprotein or good cholesterol levels. Consuming ground leaves mixed with curd helps to reduce cholesterol levels and aid in weight loss.

The status of lipid peroxidation was investigated in rats fed with *M. Koenigii*. The concentration of melondialdehyde showed a significant decrease, while hydroperoxides and conjugated dienes were significantly increased in liver and heart (Saini and Reddy, 2015). Glutathione levels in liver, heart and kidney were lowered in rats after administering this plant. Glutathione reductase, Glutathione peroxidase, Glutathione-STransferase, SOD and catalase activity showed a sharp increase.

23.7.10 *Wound Healing Effect*

Male albino rats were used to check the wound healing activity by screening with ethanolic extract of leaves of *M. Koenigii.* In the excision, wound healing model revealed that three groups which were taken for wound healing activity showed a decrease in wound area from day-to-day. Incision model showed a significant increase in tensile strength of the 12-days old wound due to treatment with *M. koenigii.* Thus, the leaves of *Murraya koenigii* were proved to possess significant wound healing capacity. When ground with raw turmeric to a paste and applied on the foot, it also prevents cracking.

23.7.11 *Phagocytic Activity*

The methanol extract of *M. koenigii* leaves was evaluated on human oral and cell mediated immune response to ovalbumin, phagocytic activity by carbon clearance test, nitric oxide (NO) release from murine peritoneal macrophages and cyclophosphamide induced myclosuppression. Phagocytic nature of macrophages was increased by the increase in production of Nitrite. Extract showed significant increase in NO production from peritoneal macrophage at 416 μg/ml and 834 μg/ml with 24% and 56%, respectively. This activity was evidenced by increase in Phagocytic index in carbon clearance test.

23.7.12 *Cytotoxic Activity*

The isolated carbazole alkaloid as Koenoline from root bark of *M. koenigii* exhibited the cytotoxic activity against KB cell culture system. Carbazole alkaloids isolated from the stems of *M. koenigii* have effects on the growth of the human leukemia cell line HL-60. Also, the carbazole alkaloids, mahanine, Pyrafoline-D and murrafoline-I showed significant cytotoxicity against HL-60 cells and induced the loss of mitochondrial membrane potential.

23.7.13 *Vasodilating Activity*

Crude aqueous leaf extract of *M. koenigii* was prepared which showed a dose dependent negative chronotropic effect on cardiovascular system of frog heart preparations which might be due to its direct actions on the heart and blood vessels. Potassium ion concentration was also found to be very negligible by flame photometry, indicating no involvement of potassium ions. The aqueous leaf extract possesses vasodilatory effect which is independent of muscarinic, histaminergic and β-adrenergic receptor as it increased the number of drops/minute in frog hind limb perfusion experiment and also does not possess α-adrenergic receptor antagonistic activity. The aqueous leaf extract showed significant effect at concentration of 1 mg/ml. Crude ethanolic extract of fresh leaves of *M. koenigii* showed dose dependent positive ionotropic effect on an isolated frog heart. The response to *M. koenigii* 62.5-1000 μg was not affected in either way by theophylline, imidazole, propanolol and sildenafil. The changes in potassium and sodium concentration did not alter. The result suggested that *M. koenigii* induced positive ionotropic effect possibly by increasing availability of calcium from extra cellular sites.

23.7.14 *Radioprotective and Chemoprotective Activity*

Research on the extracts of Kadipatta leaves has shown a reduction in the side effects of both chemotherapy and radiation therapy .The study was done to investigate the radioprotective and chemoprotective effect of *M. koenigii* methanolic extract after irradiation. It has demonstrated protection against radiation RT & cyclophosphamide CP induced chromosomal damage *in vivo*. Gama Radiation 4Gy produced a significant increase in the per cent aberrant metaphases and different types of aberrations compared to same treated control. Radiation increased all types of aberrations like fragment chromatid and chromosome breaks, rings and dicentrics. Quantitatively, methanolic extract pretreated group showed similar aberrations only in one group. But treatment with methanolic extract of *M. koenigii* before radiation significantly reduced percentage aberrant metaphases and different types of aberrations. The study on leaf extract revealed that a single dose of 100 mg/kg methanolic extract of *M. koenigii* can significantly decrease the chromosomal damage caused by irradiation and cyclophosphamide and also showed bone marrow protection and prevention of free radicals becoming active in the body.

Table 2. Pharmacological Activities of Kadipatta Plant

Pharmacological Activity	Plant part	Extract
Anti-inflammatory	Leaf	Ethanol, Petroleum ether, Chloform, Methanol
Anti-amnesic	Leaf	Petroleum ether
Hypocholesterolemic	Leaf	Ethanol
Memory enhancer	Leaf	petroleum ether
Anti-helminthic	Leaf	Alcoholic
Anti-bacterial	Bark, Leaf	Petroleum ether, Alcohol
Anti-cancer	Stem bark	Petroleum ether
Anti-diabetic	Whole plant, fresh leaf, fruit.	Aqueous, methanol
Antidiarrhoeal	Seeds	n-hexane
Anti-fungal	Leaf	Petroleum ether, alcohol and actone
Radioprotective and Chemoprotective	Leaf	Methanol
Analgesic and Antinociceptive	Leaf	Methanol
Anti-oxidant	Leaf	Methanol and Aqueous
Cardiovascular	Leaf	Aqueous
Anti-lipid peroxidative	Leaf	Methanol
Anti-tumor	Leaf	Petroleum ether
Anti-ulcer	Leaf	Aqueous
Cytotoxicity	Roots, stem	Aqueous
Wound healing activity	Leaf	Ethanol
Phagocytic activity	Leaf	Methanol

23.8 Research Trials conducted on Use of Kadipatta Livestock and Poultry

In albino rats (150-200gm), 2500 mg/kg dose was found to be the lethal dose (LD50). 1/10th of the LD50 is considered as an effective dose i.e. 250 mg/kg. The Carrageenan induced rat paw oedema has been a popular inflammatory model to investigate the anti inflammatory effect of compounds. It has a biphasic effect. The first phase is due to release of histamine and serotonin (5HT) (0-2hr), plateau phase is maintained by kinin like substance (3hr) and second accelerating phase of swelling is attributed to P.G. release (>4hr). The ethanolic extract of *Murraya koenigii* (250mg/kg, p. o.) significantly reduces oedema induced by carrageenan in all the phases as ethanolic extract of *Murraya koenigii* possess anti-inflammatory activity that may be mediated by alkaloids, flavonoids and triterpenoids. Kadipatta leaf (*Murraya koenigii*) extract possesses the property to decrease blood cholesterol and blood glucose levels in diabetic mice. Mice received daily intraperitoneal injections of 80 mg/kg Kadipatta leaf extract for 10 consecutive days. The extract significantly decreased blood cholesterol level from 277.6 ± 16.6 mg/d (day 0) to 182.0 ± 15.3 mg/

d (day 10, p < 0.01 compared with the change in vehicle group). The extract also significantly decreased blood glucose level from 387.0 ± 15.6 mg/dl (day 0) to 214.0 ± 26.6 mg/dl (day 10, p < 0.01). In addition, body weight was reduced after extract treatment. Kadipatta leaf may be of clinical importance in improving the management of high cholesterol level and type 2 diabetes (Xie JT *et al.,* 2006).

The antioxidant effect of curry leaf powder (CLP) was determined by assessing the formation of lipid peroxides, free fatty acids (FFA) and thiobarbituric acid substances (TBARS) in raw ground and cooked goat meat patties during refrigerated storage. pH, water holding capacity and cooking loss per cent were not affected by curry leaf powder, when added in raw ground goat meat. Fresh goat meat with CLP had acceptable odour upto 5 days, whereas in control sample it was up to 3 days. Raw goat meat with CLP had significantly lower free fatty acids content than control during 9 days refrigerated storage. CLP significantly inhibited the rate of lipid peroxides and TBARS formation in raw meat than control. CLP in cooked goat meat patties showed significant antioxidant effect as indicated by TBARS values measured by distillation as well as extraction method. CLP did not affect microbial population in raw and cooked goat meat during entire storage period. These results show that CLP at concentrations as low as 0.2% is a very effective inhibitor of primary and secondary oxidation products in raw ground and cooked goat meat patties and has potential as a natural antioxidant in raw and cooked meat systems.(Das *et al.,* 2011).

A research trial was conducted in broilers by including dried ginger, pepper and curry leaf powders as feed additive at different levels in broiler diet. The feed conversion ratio was significantly (p<0.01) superior in ginger-curry leaf (T6) and pepper-curry leaf powder (T7) fed groups compared to control. Dressed, eviscerated weights, ready-to-cook percentage, abdominal fat percentage and giblets weight did not differ significantly between the treatment groups fed different levels of dried ginger, pepper and curry leaf powder from 1-6 weeks of age (Moorthy *et al.,* 2009). There was a proportionate increase in body weight in groups fed with graded levels of dried ginger powder either alone or in combination with curry leaf when compared to control which might be due to the anti-oxidant property of curry leaf powder and increased digestibility property of ginger included in the broiler diet, The feed conversion ratio was significantly (p<0.01) superior in ginger-curry leaf (T6) and pepper-curry leaf powder (T7) fed groups. An experiment was conducted on 120 white leghorn layers (22 weeks age) to discern the effect of supplementation of neem *(Azadirachta indica)* and kadipatta *(Murraya koeinigii)* leaf powder on production performance, feed nutrient utilization, egg composition and haemato-biochemical parameters (Rishishwar, 2014). Supplementation of *neem* and *kadipatta* leaf powder in layer diet resulted in more of HDL cholesterol with subsequent fall in LDL cholesterol and triglyceride contents. Another feeding trial was conducted to study the effect of dietary incorporation of neem and kadipatta leaf powder on growth performance, nutrient utilization, carcass traits and haemato-biochemical parameters in commercial broilers (Khulbey, 2015). Nutrient utilization in terms of dry matter,crude protein,crude fat and crude fibre was significantly ($P<0.05$) improved in broilers fed diet supplemented with 0.2% kadipatta+0.2%neem leaf powder.

23.9 Future Concept

It is a best classical approach in search of new lead molecules for management of various diseases. Usually Kadipatta is available in markets as dried curry leaves/curry leaf powder in packing of 10g, 25g, 500g or 3Kg.In near future it is hoped that Kadipatta will occupy prominent position in list of useful herbs. These can be included in baby diet (6-8 months age) by either boiling or steaming them, turn it into fine paste along with other vegetables and lentils. Vitamin C (immune system) vitamin A (eyesight), folic acid, niacin (brain development), thiamin (organ and nervous development), riboflavin, calcium (bone development) and iron (anaemia & haemoglobulin) plays an important role in baby's development.

References

Adebajo AC, Reisch J (2000) Minor furocoumarins of Murraya Koenigii.Fitoterapia 71(3): 334-337

Aggarwal SS,Paridhavi M(2007)Herbal Drug Technology,University Press(India)Pvt. Ltd.,Hyderabad. p. 326

Ates DA,Erdogrul OT(2003) Antimicrobial activity of various medicinal and commercial plants extracts.Turkish Journal of Biology 27: 157-162

Bonde SD,Nemade LS,Patel MR,Patel AA(2017)Murraya Koenigii(curry leaf): Ethnobotany, phytochemistry and pharmacology-A review. International Journal of Pharmaceutical and Phytopharmacological Research 1(1): 23-27

Chevallier A (1996) The encyclopedia of medicinal plants.Darling Kindersley, London, UK.

Chowdhury BK, Jha S, Bhattacharyya P, Mukherjee J(2001) Two new carbazole alkaloids from *Murraya koenigii*. Indian Journal of Chemistry 40: 490-494

Darvekar VM,Patil VR,Choudhari AB(2011)Anti-inflammatory activity of Murraya Koenigii Spreng on experimental animals.J Nat Prod Plant Resour 1(1):65-69

Das AK, Rajkumar V, Dwivedi DK (2011) Antioxidant effect of curry leaf (*Murraya koenigii*) powder on quality of ground and cooked goat meat. International Food Research Journal 18: 563-569

Farhath-Khanum KRA, Sudarshana-Krishna KR, Vishwanathan KR, Santhanam K (2000) Anticarcinogenic effects of curry leaves in dimethylhydrazine treated rats. Plant Food and Human Nutrition 55: 347-355

Feibig M,Pezzuto JM,Seojarto DD,Kinghorn AD(1985)Koenoline-a further cytotoxic carbazole alkaloid from Murraya Koenigii. Phytochemistry 24(12):3041-3043

Gahlawat, D. K., Jakhar, S., & Dahiya, P. (2014). Murraya koenigii (L.) Spreng: An ethnobotanical, phytochemical and pharmacological review. *Journal of Pharmacognosy and Phytochemistry*, 3(3), 109-119.

Gurgune VJ,Pande MS,Jain DK(2003) Hepatoprotective activity of Murraya Koenigii leaves against carbon tetrachloride induced hepatotoxicity in rats.Antiseptic 100(12):493-496

Handral HK, Pandith A, Shruthi SD (2012) A review on M*urraya Koenigii*: multi-potential medicinal plant. Asian Journal of Pharmaceutical and Clinical Research, 5(4)5-14

Handral HK, Jha PK, Shruthi SD (2010) Pharmacognostic and phytochemical studies on the leaves of *murraya koenigii* (l) spreng. *Pharmacophore* 1 (3): 231-238

Ito C,Thoyama Y,Omura M,Kajiura I,Furukawa H(1993)Alkaloidal constituents of Murraya Koenigii,Isolation and structural elucidation of novel binary carbazolequinones and carbazole alkaloids. Chem. Pharm. Bull41(12):2096-2100

Jain V, Momin M, Laddha K (2012) Murraya koenigii: An updated review. *International Journal of Ayurvedic and Herbal Medicine*, 2(04): 607-627.

Kaur K,Gupta AK,Ahmad S,Alam P(2011)Pharmacognostic studies on bark of Murraya Koenigii Spreng International Journal of Research in Pharmaceutical and Bio-medical SciencesVol2(4):1670-1677. ISSN:2229-3701

Kesari AN, Gupta RK, Watal G (2005) Hypoglycemic Effects of Murraya koenigii on Normal and Alloxan-Diabetic Rabbits. Journal of Ethno pharmacology Vol. 97: 247-251

Khulbey R (2015) Effect of feeding dried neem Azadirachta indica) and Kadipatta (Murraya Koenigii) leaf powder on growth performance, nutrient utilization, carcass traits and haemato-biochemical parameters in broiler chicken. MVSc. Thesis submitted to G.B. Pant University of Agriculture and Technology, Pantnagar.

Kumar SR, Loveleena D, Godwin S (2013) Medicinal property of Murraya Koenigii-a review. International Research Journal of Biological Sciences 2(9):80-83

Kumar VS, Sharma A, Tiwari R, Kumar S (1999) Murraya Koenigii: A review. *J. of Med. and Aromat. Plant Sci* 21: 1139-1144.

Kritikar KR, Basu BD (2004) Indian Medicinal Plants, International Book Distributors, Dehradun. p. 472-479.

Moorthy M, Ravi S, Ravikumar M, Viswanathan K, Edwin SC (2009) Ginger, Pepper and Curry Leaf Powder as Feed Additives in Broiler Diet. International Journal of Poultry Science 8(8): 779-782.

Manfred F. John MP, Dajaja DS, Douglas AK (1985) A further cytotoxic carbazole alkaloid from Murraya Koenigii.*Phytochem.* 24(12): 3041-3043

Mhaskar KS, Blatter E. Caius JF, Kirtikar, Basu (2000) Illustrated Indian Medicinal Plants Their Usage in Ayurveda and Unani Medicine, Vol. 3, Shri Satguru Publication, Delhi. pp. 656-65

Mohar SA,Sanjay K,Hotam SC,Ravindra MT,Santosh KV,Chandrabhan S (2011) The efficacy of Murraya Koenigii leaf extract on some bacterial and a fungal strain by disc diffusion method.Journal of chemical and Pharmaceutical Research 3(5):697-704

Nair R, Chanda S (2006) Activity of some medicinal plants against certain pathogenic bacterial strains. Indian Journal of Pharmacology 38: 142-144

Ningappa, MB, Dinesha R, Srinivas L (2008) Antioxidant and free radical scavenging activities of polyphenol-enriched curry leaf (*Murraya koenigii* L.) extracts. Food Chemistry 106: 720-728

Patel RS,Rajorhia (1979)Antioxidative role of curry (Murraya Koenigii) and betal(Piper betel) leaves in ghee.J.Food Sci.Tech,16(4):158-160

Prekesh M,Ananda-Kumar S,Karmegam N(2006) Synergistic effect of selected medicinal plant extracts against bacteria.Indian Journal of Applied Microbiology 6:52-53

Rahman, MM, Gray AI (2005) A benzoisofuranone derivative and carbazole alkaloids from Murraya koenigii and their anti-microbial activity. Antimicrobial and *Phytochemistry*, 66(13): 1601-1606

Ram HNA,Hatapakki BC,Hukkeri IVJ(2002) Antiulcer activity of Murraya Koenigii.Aryavaidyan 16(1):40-44

Ramsewak RS,Nair MG,Strasburg GM,Dewitt DL,Nitiss JL(1999) Biologically active carbazole alkaloids from Murraya Koenigii. J.Agri.Food Sci 47(2):444-447

Reisch J, Goi O, Wickramasinghe A, Herath HMT, Henkel G (1992) Carbazole alkaloids from seeds of Murraya Koenigii. Phyto-chemistry, 31(8):2877-2879

Reisch J, Adebajo AC, Vijaya Kumar, Aladesanmi AJ (1994) Two carbazole alkaloids from Murraya Koenigii. Phytochemistry 36(4):1073-1076

Rishishwar K (2014) Effect of feeding dried Neem (Azadirachta indica) and Kadipatta (Murraya Koenigii) leaf powder on nutrient utilization, production performance and haemato-biochemical parameters in layers. MVSc. Thesis submitted to G.B.Pant University of Agriculture and Technology, Pantnagar.

Saini SC, Reddy GBS (2015) A review on curry leaves (Murraya koenigii): versatile multi-potential medicinal plant. *American Journal of Phytomedicine and Clinical Therapeutics* 3(04): 363-368

Satyavathi GV, Raina MK., Sharma M (1983) Medicinal plants of India. Indian Medicinal Plants 2: 289-299.

Shah KJ, Juvekar AR (2006) Positive inotropic effect of Murraya Koenigii (Linn.)Spreng extract on an isolated perfused frog heart. Ind. J. of Exp. Bio. 44: 481-484

Shah AS, Wadake AS, Juvekar AR (2004) Immuno-modulatory activity of methanolic extract of Murraya Koenigii (L.) Spreng Leaves.Ind.J. Exp. Biol. 46(7): 505-509

Shah Rajesh Kumar, Das Loveleena, Sangma Godwin (2013) Medicinal Property of *Murraya Koenigii*- A Review. *International Research Journal of Biological Sciences Vol.* 2(9): 80-83

Shan B, Cai Y, Brooks JD, Corke H (2007)The *in vitro* anti-bacterial activity of dietary spice and medicinal herb extracts. International Journal of Food Microbiology 117(1): 112-119.

Sindhu RK, Arora S (2014) Anti-inflammatory potential of different extracts isolated from the roots of Ficus lacor buch. Hum and Murraya koenigii L. spreng. *Archives of Biological Sciences*, 66(3): 1261-1270.

Srinivasan K (2005) Plant foods in the management of diabetes mellitus: spices as beneficial antidiabetic food adjuncts. *International journal of food sciences and nutrition* 56(6): 399-414

Sinha Parul, Akhtar Javed, Batra Neha, Jain Honey, Bhardwaj Anuj (2012) Curry Leaves-A Medicinal Herb. Asian J. Pharm. Res. Vol. 2(2): 51-53

Srivastava SK, Srivastava SD (1993) New constituents and biological activity of the roots of Murraya Koenigii. J. Ind. Chem. Soc 70(7): 655-659

TachibanaY, Kikuzaki H, Lajis NH, Nakatani N (2003) Comparison of anti-oxidative properties of carbazole alkaloids from *Murraya koenigii* leaves.Journal of Agriculture and Food Chemistry 51: 6461-6467

Tripathi RN, Pandey DK, Tripathi NN, Dixit SN (1982) Antifungal activity of pollens of some higher plants.Ind. Phytopathol 35(2): 346-348

Vaibhav M, Darvekar Vijay, Patil R, Choudhari AB (2011) Anti-inflammatory activity of *Murraya koenigii* Spreng on experimental animals. *J. Nat. Prod. Plant Resour.* 1(1): 65-69

Vaijayanthimala J,Rajendra Prasad N, Anand C,Pugalendi KV(2004) Anti-dermatophytic activity of some Indian medicinal plant.J.Nat. Remedies 4(1): 26-31

Wang YS, He HP, Shen YM, Hong X, Hao XJ (2003) Two new carbazole alkaloids from Murraya Koenigii.Phytochemistry 66(3): 416-418

Wu TS, Chan YY, Liou MJ, Lin FW, Shi LS Chen K T(1998) Platelet aggregation inhibitor from *Murraya keonigii*. Phytotherapy Research 12: 380-382

Xie JT, Chang WT, Wang CZ, Mehendale SR, Li J, Ambihaipahar R, Ambihaipahar U, Yukari T, Hiroe K, Nordin HL, Nobuji N(2001) Antioxidative. Activity of Carbazoles from Murraya koenigii leaves *J. Agri. Food Chem* 49; 5589-5594.

Xie JT, Chang WT, Wang C Z, Mehendale SR, Li J, Ambihaipahar R, Fong HH, Yuan CS (2006) Curry leaf (Murraya koenigii Spreng.) reduces blood cholesterol and glucose levels in ob/ob mice. *Am. J. Chin. Med* 34(02): 279-284

Yadav S, Vats V, Dhunnoo Y, Grover JK (2002) Hypoglycemic and anti-hyperglycaemic activity of Murraya Koenigii leaves in diabetic rats.J. Ethanopharmacol 82(2-3): 111-116.

❑❑❑

Chapter 24

Coriander (*Coriandrum sativum*)

Brishketu Kumar[1], Anamika[2] and Dinesh Kumar[3]

[1] Department of Animal Science, College of Agriculture, Nevsari Agricultural University, Bharuch-392011, Gujarat, India, E.mail : brishketuk@gmail.com

[2] Department of Animal Nutrition, Khalsa College of Veterinary and Animal Sciences, Amritsar-143001, Punjab, India, E-mail : dranamika80@gmail.com

[3] Department of Veterinary Science & Animal Husbandry, College of Agriculture, Jawahar Lal Nehru Krishi Vishwavidyalaya, Tikamgarh-472001, Madhya Pradesh, India, E-mail: kr.dinesh7@gmail.com

ABSTRACT

Coriander (*Coriandrum sativum* L.) is an annual herb, most commonly used for seasoning purpose and is also called as 'herb of happiness'. Whole plant of coriander, mainly fresh leaves and ripe fruits are used for culinary purposes. Coriander plant is a rich reservoir of micronutrients and nutritional elements and is very low in saturated fat. Coriander leaves are rich in proteins, vitamins and minerals like calcium, phosphorus, and iron while seeds are rich in polyphenols and essential oils. Coiander seeds contain linalool, limonene, pyrazine, pyridine, thiazole, furan, phenolic acids and sterols, flavonoids. Coriander is well known for its anti-oxidant, anti-diabetic, anti-mutagenic, anti-anxiety and anti-microbial activity along with analgesic and hormone balancing effect that promotes its use in foods due to numerous health benefits and its protective effect to preserve the food for longer period. Some other health benefits of coriander include treatment of swellings, high cholesterol levels, diarrhoea, mouth ulcers, anaemia, indigestion, menstrual disorders, small pox, eye care, conjunctivitis, skin disorders, blood sugar disorders, etc. Supplementation of the coriander seed meal to broiler diet had shown beneficial effects on growth performance and carcass yield as well as its effect as immune enhancer and stress removal. Other than this coriander has shown its beneficial effect on methane mitigation in livestock. Thus, coriander is one of miraculous herb that functions as spice as well as herbal medicine and feed additive.

Keywords: Coriander. Anti-diabetic, Livestock, Linalool Methane.

24.1 Introduction

Coriander (*Coriandrum sativum* L.) is an annual herb, most commonly used for seasoning purpose. Its plant, seeds, leaves and roots are edible, although they have very distinct flavours and uses. The herb has a light and fresh flavour. Whole plant of coriander, mainly fresh leaves and ripe fruits are used for culinary purposes. Coriander leaves have different taste than its seeds, with citrus overtones. Coriander plant is a rich reservoir of micronutrients and nutritional elements and is very low in saturated fat. It also contains good amount of linoleic acid which is a good source of á-tocopherol and vitamin K. All parts of coriander plant are edible; however, its fresh leaves and dried seeds are most frequently used. Its green foliage, containing proteins, vitamins and minerals (like calcium, phosphorus, and iron), fibres and carbohydrates, is used as vegetable, and in salads, while both the leaves and seeds contain essential oil, rich in varying components, which provides typical flavour, when added to the food products and acts as preservative (Kalemba and Kunicka, 2003). The coriander seed essential oil (CSEO) is triglyceride oil; petroselinic acid, a monounsaturated fatty acid, is the major fatty acid in CSEO. Thus, the plant is a potential source of lipids (rich in petroselinic acid) and essential oil (high in linalool) isolated from the seeds and the aerial parts. Leaves of plant are rich source of vitamins while seeds are rich in polyphenols and essential oils. Coriander taste is devoted to its essential oil comprising a significant content of linoleic and furanocoumarins (coriandrine and dihydrocoriandrine). Coriander is also well known for its anti-oxidant, anti-diabetic, anti-mutagenic, anti-anxiety and anti-microbial activity along with analgesic and hormone balancing effect that promotes its use in foods due to numerous health benefits and its protective effect to preserve the food for longer period.

The *C. sativum* (family *Umbelliferae/ Apiaceae*) is an erect annual herb with pronounced taproot, and slender branching stems up to 20–70 cm in height. There are two varieties of *C. sativum*: vulgare and microcarpum; the former has larger fruits (3–5 mm diameter) with essential oil yields of 0.1%–0.35% (v/w) while the latter has smaller fruits (1.5–3 mm diameter) with essential oil yields of 0.8%–1.8% (v/w) (Burdock and Carabin, 2009). India is the biggest producer, consumer and exporter of coriander in the world. Coriander EO also has a long history of use as a traditional medicine. Coriander was used in time-honoured Greek medicines by Hippocrates (460-377 BC).

Decoction and tincture of powdered seeds of C. *sativum* alone or in combination with other herbal agents are recommended for dyspeptic complaints, loss of appetite, convulsion, insomnia and anxiety (Grieve, 1971). This CSEO was also found to improve blood glucose control and thus, it held promise for use as an antihyperglycemic agent (Gallagher *et al.*, 2003).

Taxonomy of Coriander

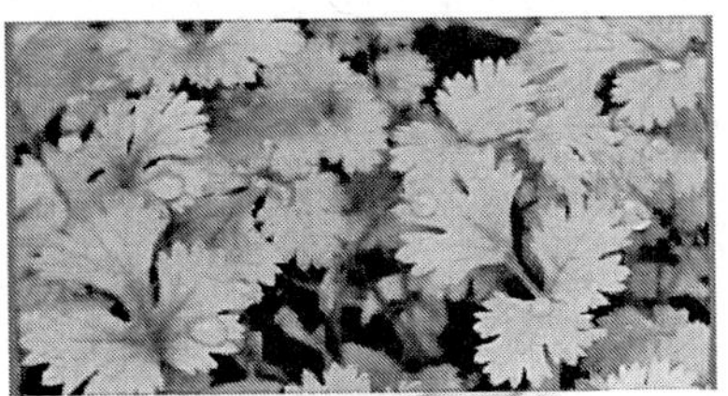

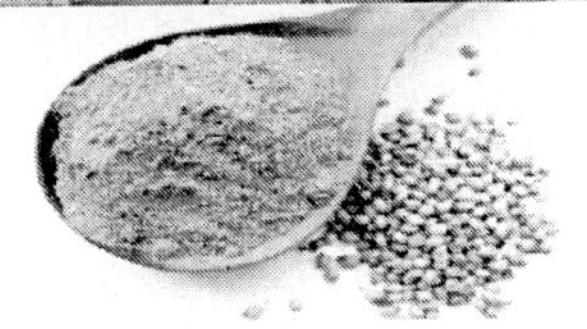

Kingdom	:	Plantae
Subkingdom	:	Viridoplantae
Division	:	Tracheophyta
Class	:	Magnolipsida
Order	:	Apiale
Family	:	Apiaceae
Genus	:	Coriandrum
Species	:	*Coriandrum sativum*

24.2 Chemical composition

A range of aldehyde compounds are largely responsible for the aroma of coriander leaves. The largest proportion of these are those aldehydes with 6-10 carbon atoms, particularly decyl and nonyl aldehydes. Other major constituents of the leaves are 2-decenoic acid, decanoic acid (also known as capric acid) and tetradecenoic acid. The chemical composition of coriander seeds is slightly different, with the alcohol linalool being the major constituent. Coriander leaves contain high levels of organic compounds called aldehydes. The same aldehydes, or similar, are often commonly found in soaps and lotions. However, perception of this facet of coriander's taste isn't purely chemical. Scientists have discovered that dislike of the taste of coriander may also be influenced, to an extent, by genetic factors. Studies have also suggested that crushing coriander leaves may lead to faster breakdown of aldehydes, diminishing the soapy taste.

Coriander nutrition is basically due to its green leaves and dried fruits. Like all other green leafy vegetables, its leaves are a rich source of vitamins, minerals and iron. Its leaves contain high amount of vitamin A (β-carotene) and vitamin C. The green herbs contain vitamin C upto 160 mg/100 g and vitamin A upto 12 mg/100 g (Girenko,

1982). It is very low in saturated fat and cholesterol and a very good source of thiamine, zinc and dietary fiber. Green coriander contains 84% water. All parts of coriander plant are edible; however, its fresh leaves and dried seeds are most frequently used. Its green foliage, containing proteins, vitamins and minerals (like calcium, phosphorus, and iron), fibres and carbohydrates, is used as vegetable, and in salads, while both the leaves and seeds contain EO, rich in varying components, which provides typical flavour, when added to the food products and acts as preservative.

The various nutrients present in coriander leaf and seeds are shown in Table 1. The characteristic aromatic flavour of its seeds comes from many fatty acids and essential volatile oils. According to USDA (2013), cholesterol content of its seeds is nil. Its seeds are considered as an important source of vitamins, minerals and lipids. Among minerals, potassium is present in high amount (1267 mg/100 g) followed by calcium (709 mg/100 g), phosphorus (409 mg/100 g), magnesium (330 mg /100 g), sodium (35 mg/100 g), zinc (4.70 mg/ 100 g). The folate content in coriander seed is 200 μg/ 100 g (fresh weight) (Iwatani *et al.*, 2003).

Table 1: Nutrient composition of coriander leaf and seeds (per 100 g)

Nutrient	Coriander leaf	Coriander seed
Water	7.30 g	8.86 g
Protein	21.93 g	12.37 g
Total lipid (fat)	4.78 g	17.77 g
Carbohydrate	52.10 g	54.99 g
Fiber, total dietary	10.40 g	41.9 g
Calcium, Ca	1246 mg	709 mg
Iron, Fe	42.46 mg	16.32 mg
Magnesium, Mg	694 mg	330 mg
Phosphorus, P	481 mg	409 mg
Potassium, K	4466 mg	1267 mg
Sodium, Na	211 mg	35 mg
Zinc, Zn	4.72 mg	4.70 mg
Vitamin C	566.7 mg	21.0 mg
Thiamin	1.252 mg	0.239 mg
Riboflavin	1.500 mg	0.290 mg
Niacin	10.707 mg	2.130 mg
Vitamin B_{12}	0.00 μg	0.00 μg

Vitamin A, RAE	293 µg	0.00µg
Vitamin A, IU	5850 IU	0 IU
Vitamin D ($D_2 + D_3$)	0.00µg	0.0 µg
Vitamin D	0 IU	0 IU
Total saturated fatty acids	0.115 g	0.990 g
Total monounsaturated fatty acids	2.232 g	13.580 g
Total polyunsaturated fatty acids	0.328 g	1.750 g
Cholesterol	0.00 mg	0 mg
Energy	279 kcal	298 kcal

Coriander contains high amount of essential oils that are very important for growth and for proper functioning of brain. The main essential fatty acids present in coriander include linoleic and linolenic acids. Linoleic acids belong to PUFA (polyunsaturated fatty acid) group. Dietary supplementation of coriander seed greatly affects the lipid composition of carcass by decreasing saturated fatty acid (SFA) contents (palmitic and stearic acids) and by increasing monounsaturated and polyunsaturated fatty acid (MUFA and PUFA) (Ertas *et al.,* 2005).

This plant is a potential source of lipids (rich in petroselinic acid) and an essential oil (high in linalool) isolated from the seeds and the aerial parts (Sahib *et al.,* 2012). The high content of fats and protein in the fruits make distillation residues suitable for animal feed. Coriander fruits yield 5 to 7% of ash, 13% resin, astringent principle, malic acid and alkaloids. Coriander oil contains coriandrol, jireniol and vebriniol (Rao *et al.,* 2012).

24.3 Phytochemical Constituents of Coriander

Coiander seeds contain up to 1.8% volatile oil according to origin. The distilled oil (coriander oil BP) contains 65 to 70% of linalool (coriandrol), depending on the source. It includes: Monoterpene hydrocarbons viz α- pinene, β-pinene, limonene, γ-terpinene, ρ-lymene, borneol, citron wllol, Xmphoe, Geraniol and Geranylacetate; Hetero-cyclic compounds *viz.* pyrazine, pyridine, thiazole, furan, tetrahydrofuran derivatives; Isocoumacin *viz.* coriandrin, dihydrocoriandrin, coriandrones A-E, glazonoids; Phtha-lides viz - neochidilide, Z-digustilide; Phenolic acids and sterols, flavonoids (Wallis, 2005). Carotenoids are of ubiquitous occurrence in all plants with higher concentrations in reproductive organs. In green leafy vegetables, carotenoids, particularly β-carotene is deposited mainly in leaves. Carotenoids can also be processed and used as colouring agents as well as good source of antioxidants. Besides other roles, carotenoids chiefly function as scavengers of the free radicals produced by chlorophylls during photo-oxidation.

Its leaves being good source of β-carotene serve as a precursor of vitamin A. In coriander, β-carotene content, 160 μg/100 g is present, whereas total carotenoid content is 1010 μg/100 g (Kandlakunta *et al.*, 2008). Its foliage is used in various types of foods especially in diets of people facing vitamin A deficiency. Green foliage contains anthocyanin (Omidbaigi, 2005). Anthocyanins are bioactive flavonoid compounds that prevent body from various chronic diseases. Anthocyanin in foliage acts as antioxidants which are very useful in improvement of nutritional value as well as maintenance of health and well being (Rahimi *et al.*, 2013).

24.4 Different Coriander Preparations

The complex chemistry of coriander makes it plausible that variations in processing can yield quite different preparations, i.e. dehydrated coriander powder, essential oil, coriander purees, pastes and other by-products.

24.4.1 *Coriander Powder*

Green coriander fruits have sharper and more pronounced flavour than ripe seeds. Mature brown seeds can be used and grind to form powder. Seed heads are cut along with certain inches of stalk or plant may be pulled out with roots and hang in bags upside down, when seeds are fully dry these tend to detach from stalk, collected and store in cool, dry location or ground to obtain a fine powder. In order to remove field heat and prolong shelf life after harvesting, it is necessary to pre-cool harvested coriander before transportation. This can be done by vacuum cooling. Vacuum cooling is achieved through boiling part of the moisture of the product under vacuum conditions. This cooling has a significant effect on amount of vitamin C and shelf life (Apichart *et al.*, 2012).

24.4.2 *Coriander Seed Essential Oil*

The *C. sativum* essential oil and extracts possess promising anti-bacterial, anti-fungal and anti-oxidative activities as various chemical components in different parts of the plant, which thus, play a great role in maintaining the shelf-life of foods by preventing their spoilage. This edible plant is non-toxic to humans, and the *C. sativum* essential oil is thus, used in different ways, *viz.*, in foods (like flavouring and preservatives) and in pharmaceutical products (therapeutic action) as well as in perfumes (fragrances and lotions). Ripe seeds of coriander may be sometimes processed to obtain essential oil. This oil is mainly obtained by steam distillation, super critical CO_2 extraction, etc. Oil extraction from its seeds was studied with carbon dioxide and propane as solvents, under sub and supercritical conditions. The ratio of solvent to seed (g/g) required to achieve a complete oil extraction was between 20 and 40 using CO_2 at pressures of 200 and 300 bar and temperature of 35°C. A complete oil recovery was attained with propane or propane-rich solvents at 25°C and 50, 80 and 100 bar. The solvating power of propane and propane-containing solvents was proved to be much higher than that of CO_2 (Illes *et al.*, 2000). Its oil has a characteristic odour of linalool and warm aromatic flavour. This oil is approved for food use by FDA (Food and Drug Administration), FEMA (Foreign Exchange Management Act) and Council of Europe (Silva *et al.*, 2011).

24.4.3 *Coriander Leaves*

Coriander leaves may also be processed to form various products like purees and pastes which are tremendously used now-a-days in fast food industries. After harvesting of fresh mature plant, degradation of its components starts. Such degradations may be prevented by processing and converting harvested leaves into product formulation like purees, pastes, sauces, salsas, etc. Coriander sauce gives an intense flavour and deep green colour but is not spicy. In case of powder formation, freshly harvested leaves are blanched at 90°C for at least 2 min. so as to inactivate peroxidase enzyme, dried and then ground to uniform size and preserved for further use (Ahmed *et al.*, 2003). Fresh coriander leaves were steam and water blanched at 100°C and at 90 and 100°C, respectively, for one to ten minutes, and subsequently comminuted to form a paste. Pasty products obtained from its fruits were processed after water-blanching applying the same time-temperature regimes.

24.5 Functional Properties of Coriander

The functional properties of coriander cannot be underestimated. Besides nutritional benefits, it is well known for its health or medicinal benefits as well as for additional benefits like it acts as antimicrobial agent. The type of meat and temperature did not influence the antimicrobial activity of the oil; indicating the potential of coriander oil to serve as a natural antimicrobial compound against Campylobacter jejuni in food (Rattanachaikunsopon and Phumkhachorn, 2010). The most important and well Characterized functional aspect involves antioxidant activity.

24.5.1 *Antioxidant Activity*

Antioxidants are used in the food industry to increase the shelf-life of the foods. Coriander, like many spices, contains antioxidants, which can delay or prevent the spoilage of food seasoned with this spice. Coriander is a good source of polyphenols and phyto-chemicals which are reasons for its high antioxidant activity. Reactive species of oxygen can cause oxidative stress and consequently, the damage of tissues and biomolecules (Barros *et al.*, 2012). Both leaves and seeds of coriander contain antioxidants but leaves contain more amounts of antioxidants than seeds (Wangensteen *et al.*, 2004). Its antioxidant content is attributed to its high content of pigments particularly carotenoids. The carotenoids of its extract were found to show higher hydroxyl radicals scavenging potential thereby protecting cells from oxidative damage (Peethambaran *et al.*, 2012). Among secondary metabolites, phenolic compounds are considered as one of the most important and largest group. Phenolic groups may be categorized into four main groups depending upon number of phenol rings and structural elements that bind these rings. These groups include: flavonoids (anthocyanins, flavones and isoflavones), tannins, stilbenes and lignans (Balasundram *et al.*, 2006).

In recent years, essential oils have been qualified as natural antioxidants. Coriander essential oils serve as potential antioxidants. Main components of its essential oil are: camphor (44.99%), cyclohexanol acetate (cis-2-tert.butyl) (14.45%), limonene (7.17%), α-pinene (6.37%). This essential oil at percentage of 0.05, 0.10 and 0.15 is very much effective in inhabiting primary and secondary oxidation products. It was found that at the proportion of 0.02%, its effects were almost equal to BHA (butylated hydroxyanisole) (Darughe *et al.*, 2012). One of the major problems in high lipid product in food industry is rancidity resulting in undesirable flavour changes and decline in nutrients (vitamins) leading to change in their texture and appearance. Use of antioxidants reduces oxidative rancidity (Bhanger et al. 2007). Addition of coriander essential oil may greatly serve the purpose. Darughe *et al.* (2012) studied the antioxidant effects of CEO (coriander essential oils) in cake. It was found that antioxidant effect of CEO may be due to the presence of terpenoid components (camphor, limonene, α-pinene and geraniol). This essential oil due to its radical scavenging activity can be used as natural antioxidant to enhance the shelf stability of many foods (Ramadan *et al.*, 2003).

24.5.2 *Anti-hyperglycemic Activity*

Its seed extract is used as a traditional medicine for diabetic patients. Incorporation of ground coriander seed extract in diet led to marked decline in blood glucose and rise in levels of insulin in diabetic rats. Besides peroxidative damage inhibition, addition of its seed extract reactivated antioxidant enzymes and antioxidant levels in diabetic rats (Deepa and Anuradha, 2011). Gray and Flatt (1999) studied insulin releasing and insulin like activity of coriander. It was observed that its aqueous consumption evoked 1.3-5.7 fold stimulation of insulin secretion from colon B-cell line. An aqueous extract of coriander (1 mg/ml) increased the 2-deoxyglucose transport by 1.6 folds, glucose oxidation by 1.4 folds and incorporation of glucose into glycogen of isolated murine abdominal muscle by 1.7 folds.

24.5.3 *Hypolipidimic Effect*

Hyperlipidemia increases the risk for generation of lipid oxidation products, which accumulate in the subendothelial spaces of vasculature and bone. Atherogenic high-fat diets increase serum levels of oxidized lipids, which are known to attenuate osteogenesis in culture and to promote bone loss (Pirih *et al.*, 2012). Lal *et al.* (2004) studied the hypolipidemic effect of coriander (*Coriandrum sativum* L.). Coriander was given at a dose of 1g/kg to triton induced hyperlipidemic rats. It was found that coriander decreases the uptake and enhances the breakdown of lipids. Results were compared with commercially available herbal drug for hypolipidemia. From these findings, it was assumed that coriander can be used as preventive and curative herbal against hyperlipidemia.

24.5.4 *Anthelmintic Activity*

In vitro anthelminthic activities of crude aqueous and hydro-alcoholic extracts of the seeds of Coriander were investigated on the egg and adult nematode parasite Haemonchus contortus. Its aqueous extract was also investigated for in vivo anthelminthic activity in sheep infected with H. contortus. Both extract types of coriander inhibited hatching of eggs completely at a concentration less than 0.5 mg/ml (Debella *et al.*, 2007).

24.5.5 *Ant- anxiety Effect*

An internal turmoil often accompanied by various diseases like stomach ache, nervous behaviour, anxiety may sometimes be uncontrollable and irritating. Coriander has been used as folk medicine in Iran for treatment of insomnia. Mahendra and Bisht (2011) studied anti-anxiety activity of hydro alcoholic extract of coriander in mice using diazepam as standard. It was observed that the extract of 100 and 200 mg/kg produced anti-anxiety effects similar to diazepam. Its aqueous extract causes anxiolytic effect and was studied by using extract (10, 25, 50, 100 mg/kg) in male albino mice using elevated plus-maze as an animal model of anxiety. It was found that aqueous extract at 50, 100 and 500 mg/kg significantly reduced spontaneous activity and neuromuscular coordination, compared to control group. All these results led to conclusion that coriander extract can be used as potential sedative and muscle relaxant (Masoumeh *et al.*, 2005).

24.5.6 Diuretic Activity

Jabeen *et al.* (2009) studied the diuretic activity of the plant extracts on wistar rats of either sex (200 to 250 g). Negative and positive control group comprising of five animals, each received saline and standard diuretic drug: furosemide (10 mg/kg), while rest of the groups with similar number of animals, were given different doses of the plant extracts dissolved in saline (50 ml/kg). The results concluded that the diuretic effect of coriander was confirmed due to significant increase in urine output (diuresis) in rats, similar to furosemide, a standard diuretic. Therefore, diuretic is considered as one of the best choices for the treatment and management of uncomplicated hypertension.

24.5.7 *Metal Detoxification*

Coriander can be used as a natural cleansing agent as it has potential to remove toxic metals from body. Chemical compounds present in coriander attach to toxic metals and remove them from cells (Abidhusen, 2012). Arunasagar *et al.* (2005) observed that this plant is very effective to remove inorganic (Hg^{2+}) and methyl mercury

($CHHg^+$) from aqueous solutions. This effect was due to the binding effect of carboxylic group to mercury. These results clearly showed that sorbent can be used to remove inorganic and methyl mercury from contaminated water. Kansal *et al.* (2011) found that coriander led to marked decline in oxidative stress caused by lead nitrate.

24.5.8 *Anti-bacterial Activity*

Delaquis *et al.* (2002) examined the antibacterial activity of crude oil and the distilled fractions of coriander (seeds of C. sativum L.) and cilantro (leaves of immature C. sativum) against some Gram-positive and Gram-negative food spoilage bacteria (Salmonella typhimurium, Listeria monocytogenes, Staphylococcus aureus, Serratia grimesii, Enterobacter agglomerans, Yersinia enterocolitica, Bacillus cereus). The inhibitory effect of C. sativum on potential spoilage bacteria such as Klebsiella neumonia, Bacillus megaterium, Pseudomonas aeruginosa, S. aureus, Escherichia coli, Escherichia cloaca, Enterococcus faecalis, has been reported (Keskin and Toroglu, 2011). The C. sativum fruit EO (15 mL/disc) exhibited antibacterial effect against *E. coli, P. aeruginosa* and *Salmonella typhi*. Linalool, the major component of the oil, which was reported to have antibacterial effect against many bacterial strains (Ates and Erdogrul, 2003), could be responsible for antibacterial activity. Aliphatic (2E)-alkenals and alkanals characterized from the fresh leaves of the coriander were found to possess bactericidal activity against Salmonella choleraesuis spp.

24.5.9 *Anti-fungal Activity*

Moisture content and pH of the foodstuffs have been reported as the main biotic factors affecting the fungal deterioration, especially in high moisture foods. Common moulds found in cakes and bakery products are Penicillium expansum, Penicillium stoloniferum, Rhizopus stolonifer, Aspergillus niger, Monilia sitophila and species of Mucor and Geotrichum. Among these moulds, Penicillium expansum, Penicillium stoloniferum and Mucor are mycotoxins producers. Darughe *et al.* (2012) studied the antifungal activity of coriander essential oil in cakes having moisture content and pH ranges between 13 to 15.5% and 6.64 to 7.81%, respectively. After 30 days, it was found that percentage of moulds in cakes containing coriander essential oil at 0.05% did not differ from cakes containing 0.01% BHA and both concentration were not able to control mould growth in cakes but increasing concentration of CEO up to 0.15%, anti-fungal activity of CEO showed better control on mould growth in cakes than control sample and BHA samples.

24.6 Methane Mitigation in Livestock

Researchers at Newcastle University in the United Kingdom tested five spices found in common curries on bacteria from sheep stomach and found upto a 40 per cent reduction in the production of methane (CH_4). Methane is about 20 times more noxious at affecting global warming than carbon dioxide (CO_2). One sheep can produce over 0.7 cubic feet of methane per day, while a single cow can belch out about 18 cubic feet per day, according to popsci.com. Abdul Shakoor Chaudhry from the School of Agriculture, Food and Rural Development investigated that the spices like coriander, turmeric, cumin, clove and cinnamon, act as natural antibiotics, killing off "bad," methane-producing bacteria while allowing "good" bacteria to act in its place. Introducing spices to livestock feed could be an effective natural means of reducing methane production. The European Union banned the addition of antibiotics to livestock feed in 2006. Coriander was found as the most effective in methane reduction upto 40 per cent. Turmeric came in second at 30 per cent and cumin third at 22 per cent. The researchers found that cinnamon and cloves were less effective in methane reduction. The research group tested the spices *in-vitro* on sheep gut bacteria, but they said the effect should be the same on cows and goats. Plants like coriander are an ideal solution, especially in the parts of the world where expensive treatments are not an option.

24.7 Effect on Meat yield and Meat quality in Broiler Chicken

In a study conducted by Rashid et al. (2014), a total of 72 as hatched Cobb 500 broilers were fed ad libitum on a diet with 0%, 0.5%, 1.0% and 1.5% of coriander seed meal (CSM) to assess its feeding value. Treatment group with 1.5% of CSM significantly ($p<0.05$) affected live weight of broilers at the age of 28 and 35 days. Among the dietary groups, there was no significant difference in feed intake and feed efficiency. Meat yield characteristics especially abdominal fat level decreased significantly ($p<0.01$) at 1.5% level of CSM. Cost of production per kg live broiler decreased, when dietary inclusion level was increased. Profit per kg of live broiler was significantly ($p<0.05$) increased with the increase levels of dietary CSM. These results suggest that the CSM could be considered as a potential natural growth promoter for poultry, and showed the best responses at 1.5 % level of inclusion. It was concluded that the supplementation of the coriander seed meal to broiler diet had beneficial effects on body weight gain, feed conversion ratio and carcass yield.

24.8 Immune Enhancer and Stress Removal in Broiler Chicken

In a study conducted by Al-Jaff *et al.* (2011) to investigate the potential effect of coriander seeds on physiological traits. One hundred and eighty days-old Arbor Acer broiler chick were randomly assigned to four dietary treatments with three replicate pens (15 birds/pen). Birds were fed experimental diets containing 0% (T1), 1% (T2), 2% (T3) and 3% (T4) coriander seed. Feed and water were provided ad libitum during the experiment. Performance and physiological parameters were monitored at the end of the study (6 weeks of age) which includes live body weight, feed conversion ratio (g. Feed gain/g. Gain) total protein, albumin, globulin, A/G ratio, GTP, GOT, alkaline phosphatase, glucose, cholesterol, LDL, HDL, triglycerides, phospholipids, uric acid, creatinine and antibody titer (ND). Results showed that final body weight was higher in 2% coriander seed (T3) than all other groups and feed conversion ratio was significantly better for birds that were fed 2% (T3) and (T4) coriander seed than all other groups. Serum protein and albumin were higher in 2% (T3), while serum globulin lower in 2% coriander seed (T3), when compared with other groups. GOT and GPT were lower for 2% (T3) and 3% (T4) coriander seed, while alkaline phosphatase was lower in 2% (T3) group. Serum glucose lower in 2% (T3) coriander seed than all other group, Serum cholesterol was lower in 2% (T3) and 3% (T4) compared with other groups. LDL was lower in (T3) group, while HDL was lower in T3 and T4 groups, when compared with the control. Serum triglycerides and antibody titers were higher in 2% and 3% coriander seed when compared with other groups. It could be concluded from this study that the inclusion of coriander seeds at levels of 2% have a positive effect on blood pictures, broiler performance and immune system during heat stress (high ambient temperature).

24.9 Some other Benefits of Coriander

Coriander seeds have a health-supporting reputation that is high on the list of the healing spices. In parts of Europe, coriander has traditionally been referred to as an "anti-diabetic" plant. In parts of

India, it has traditionally been used for its anti-inflammatory properties. In the United States, coriander has recently been studied for its cholesterol-lowering effects. The health benefits of coriander include treatment of swellings, high cholesterol levels, diarrhoea, mouth ulcers, anaemia, indigestion, menstrual disorders, small pox, eye care, conjunctivitis, skin disorders, blood sugar disorders, etc.

24.9.1 *Anti-inflammatory Activity*

Cineole, one of the 11 components of the essential oils, and linoleic acid, present in coriander, possess anti-rheumatic and anti-arthritic properties, which are very beneficial for swelling caused due to these two reasons. For others, such as swelling due to malfunctioning of kidney or anaemia, it is seen to be effective to some extent, as some of the components help excretion of extra water from the body as a whole.

24.9.2 *Anti-diarrhoeal Activity*

Some of the components of essential oils in coriander such as Borneol and Linalool, aid digestion, proper functioning of liver and bonding of bowels, helping cure diarrhoea. It is also helpful in diarrhoea caused by microbial and fungal action, since components like Cineole, Borneol, Limonene, Alpha-pinene & beta-phelandrene have anti-bacterial effects. In addition, the fresh coriander leaves are excellent appetizers.

24.9.3 *Anti-anaemic Activity*

Coriander is good in iron content which directly helps curing anaemia.

24.9.4 *Appetizing Activity*

Coriander, due to its rich aroma because of its essential oils, apart from being an excellent appetizer, helps in proper secretion of enzymes and digestive juices in the stomach, stimulates digestion and peristaltic motion. It is helpful in treating problems like anorexia.

24.9.5 *Expectorant Activity*

The fresh and strong aroma gives the Coriander its role as an expectorant. In cases where cold is blocking nasal passage, taking in some *Coriandrum sativum* by boiling it into water and taken as the extract, will surely act as reliever from blocked noses or chest congestion.

24.9.6 *Small Pox* Treatment

The essential oils in coriander are rich in anti-microbial, anti oxidant, anti-infectious and detoxifying components and acids. The presence of vitamin-C and iron strengthen the immune system too. These properties help prevent and cure small pox. They also reduce the pain and have a soothing effect on pox patients.

24.9.7 *Menstruation Regulatory Activity*

Being stimulating in nature and helping proper secretion from the endocrine glands, it also helps proper secretion of the hormones and thereby inducing proper menstrual cycles and reducing pains, etc. during periods.

24.9.8 *Eye Caring Activity*

Coriander has lots of anti oxidants, vitamin-A, vitamin-C and minerals like phosphorus in the essential oils in it which prevents ageing of eye, macular degeneration and soothes eyes against stress.

24.9.9 *Cure Skin Disorders*

The disinfectant, detoxifying, anti-septic, anti-fungal and anti-oxidant properties of coriander are ideal for curing skin disorders such as eczema, dryness and fungal infections.

24.10 Summary and Conclusions

Herbs and spices are processed in foods from early times for seasoning as well as to increase shelf life of food and to restore health. Coriander is one of miraculous herb that functions as both, spice as well as herbal medicine. Although plant can be grown throughout the year, it is processed to increase its palatability, profitability and facilitate international trade. The leaves and fruits are highly fragrant and contain nutrients like fat, proteins, vitamins, minerals, etc. Its health benefits activities ranging from antibacterial to anticancer activities. Most important and well characterized property of coriander is its use as antioxidant. Numerous phytochemical and pharmacological studies have been conducted on different parts of Coriander which supports the potential of *Coriander sativum* as a nutritional and medicinal plant. More research can be done to explore the unexplored and idle potential of this plant. Considering these potentials, coriander functional ingredients possess a tremendous prospect in the health associated industries. Due to its multifunctional uses and protective and preventive action against various chronic diseases, this herb is righty called as "herb of happiness".

References

Abidhusen HM, Sawapnil SA Amit VG (2012) *Coriandrum sativum*: Review of advances in psychopharmacology. Int J Res Pharm Sci 3(5): 1233-1239

Ahmed J, Shivhare US Singh P (2003) Colour kinetics and rheology of coriander leaf puree and storage characteristics of paste. Food Chem 84: 605-611

Al-Jaff FK (2011) Effect of coriander seeds as diet ingredient on blood parameters of broiler chicks raised under high ambient temperature. Int J Poultry Sci 10 (2): 82-86

Apichart S, Danai B, Pichaya B (2012) Effect of vacuum cooling on physico-chemical properties of organic coriander. Asian J Food Ag-Ind 5(2): 96-103

Arunasagar D, Balarama KMV, Rao SV, Arunachalam J (2005) Removal and pre concentration of inorganic and methyl mercury from aqueous media using a sorbent prepared from plant *coriander sativum*. J Hazard Mat 118: 133-39

Ates DA, Erdogrul OT (2003) Antimicrobial activities of various medicinal and commercial plant extracts. Turk J Biol 27: 157-62

Balasundram N, Sundram K, Samman S (2006) Phenolic compounds in plants and agri-industrial by-products, antioxidant activity, occurrence, and potential and uses. Food Chem 99: 191-203

Barros L, Duenas M, Dias MI, Sousa MJ, Santos-Buelga C (2012) Phenolic profile of *in vivo* and *in vitro* grown *coriander sativum L.* Food Chem 132(2): 841-848

Bhanger MI, Iqbal S, Anwar F, Imran M, Akhtar M, Zia-ul-Haq M (2007) Antioxidant potential of rice bran extracts and its effects on stabilization of cookies under ambient storage. Int J Food Sci Technol 43(5): 779-786

Burdock GA, Carabin IG (2009) Safety assessment of coriander (*Coriandrum sativum L.*) essential oil as a food ingredient. Food Chem Toxicol 47: 22-34

Darughe F, Barzegar M, Sahari MA (2012) Antioxidant and antifungal activity of Coriander (*Coriandrum sativum* L.) essential oil in cake. Int Food Res J 19(3): 1253-1260

Debella A, Feleke A, Makonnen E, Tilahun G, Eguale T (2007) *In vitro* and *in vivo* antihelminthic activity of crude extracts of *Coriandrum sativum* against *Haemonchus contortus*. J Ethnopharmacol 110: 428-433

Deepa B, Anuradha CV (2011) Antioxidant potential of *coriander sativum L* seed extract. J Exp Biol 49: 30-38

Delaquis RJ, Stanich K, Girard B, Massa G (2002) Antimicrobial activity of individual and mixed fractions of dill, cilantro, coriander and eucalyptus essential oils. Int J Food Microbiol 74: 101-109

Ertas ON, Guler IT, Ciftcvi DMB, Yilmaz O (2005) The Effect of a Dietary Supplement coriander seeds on the fatty acid composition of breast muscle in Japanese quail. J Revuede Med Vet 156(10): 514-518

Gallagher AM, Flatt PR., Duffy G, Abdel-Wahab YHA (2003) The effects of traditional antidiabetic plants on *in vitro* glucose diffusion. Nutr Res 23: 413-24

Girenko MM (1982) Initial material and basic trends in breeding of some uncommon species of vegetables. J Bull VIR im Vavilova 120: 33-37

Gray AM, Flatt PR (1999) Insulin-releasing and insulin-like activity of the traditional anti-diabetic plant *Coriandrum sativum* (coriander). J Nutr 81(3): 203-209

Grieve M (1971) A modern herbal New York: Dover Publications.

Illes V, Daood HG, Perneczki S, Szokonya L, Then M (2000) Extraction of coriander seed oil by CO_2 and propane at super- and subcritical conditions. J Supercritical Fluids 17: 177-186

Iwatani Y, Arcot J, Shreshtha AK (2003) Determination of folate contents in some Australian vegetables. J Food Compos Anal 16: 37-48

Jabeen Q, Bashir S, Lyoussi B, Gilani A (2009) Coriander fruit exhibits gut modulatory, blood pressure lowering and diuretic activities. J Ethno Pharmacol 122(1): 123-130

Kalemba D, Kunicka A (2003) Antibacterial and antifungal properties of essential oils. Curr Med Chem 10: 813-29

Kandlakunta B, Rajendran A, Thingnganing L (2008) Carotene content of some common (cereals, pulses, vegetables, spices and condiments) and unconventional sources of plant origin. Food Chem 106: 85-89

Kansal L, Sharma V, Sharma A, Lodi S, Sharma H (2011) Protective role of *Coriandrum sativum* (coriander) extracts against lead nitrate induced oxidative stress and tissue damage in the liver and kidney in male mice. Int J Appl Pharmaceut Technol 2(3): 65-83.

Keskin D, Toroglu S (2011) Studies on antimicrobial activities of solvent extracts of different spices. J Environ Biol 32: 251-6

Lal AA, Kumar T, Murthy PB, Pillai KS (2004) Hypolipidemic effect of *Coriandrum sativum* in triton-induced hyperlipidemic rats. J Exp Biol 42(9): 909-912

Mahendra P. and Bisht S. (2011) Anti-anxiety activity of *Coriandrum sativum* assessed using different experimental anxiety models. J. Pharmacol 43(5): 574-577

Masoumeh E., Mohammad K. and Maryam F.A. (2005) *Coriandrum sativum* evaluation of its anxiolytic effect in the elevated plus-maze. J. Ethnopharmacol 96(3): 365-337

Omidbaigi R (2005) Production and processing of medicinal plants. Astan Quds Publication, Tehran 2: 397.

Peethambaran D., Bijesh P. and Bhagyalakshmi N. (2012) Carotenoid content, its stability during drying and the antioxidant activity of commercial coriander (*Coriandrum sativum L.*) varieties. Int J Food Res 45(1): 342-350

Pirih F, Lu J, Ye F, Bezouglaia O, Atti E, Ascenzi MG, Tetradis S, Demer L, Aghaloo T, Tintut Y (2012) Adverse effects of hyperlipidemia on bone regeneration and strength. J Bone Miner Res 27(2): 309-318

Rahimi AR, Babaei S, Kambiz M, Asad R, Sheno A (2013) Anthocyanin content of coriander leaves as affected by salicylic acid and nutrients application. Int J Biosci 3(2): 141-145

Ramadan MF, Kroh LW, Mo Rsel JT (2003) Radical scavenging activity of black cumin (*Nigella sativa L.*), coriander (*Coriandrum sativum L.*), and niger (*Guizotia abyssinica Cass.*) crude seed oils and oil fractions. J Agric Food Chem 51: 6961-6969

Rao AS, Ahmed MF, Ibrahim M (2012) Hepatoprotective activity of Melia azed arach leaf extract against simvastatin induced hepatotoxicity in rats. J Appl Pharm Sci 2(7): 144-148

Rashid MM, Ahammad MU, Ali MS, Rana MS, Ali MY, Sakib N (2014) Effect of different levels of Dhania seed (*Coriandrum sativum*) on the performance of broiler. Bang J Anim Sci 43(1): 38-44

Rattanachaikunsopon P, Phumkhachorn P (2010) Potential of coriander (*Coriandrum sativum*) oil as a natural antimicrobial compound in controlling *Campylobacter jejuni* in raw meat. J Biosci Biotechnol Biochem 74(1): 31-35

Sahib NG, Anwar F, Gilani AH, Hamid AA, Saari A, Alkharfy KM (2012) Coriander (*Coriandrum sativum L.*): A potential source of high-value components for functional foods and nutraceuticals- A Review. J Phytother Res 27(9): doi10.1002/ptr. 4897

Silva F, Ferreira S, Queiroz JA, Fernanda C.D. (2011) Coriander *(Coriandrum sativum L.)* essential oil, its antibacterial activity and mode of action evaluated by flow cytometry. J. Med. Microbiol 60: 1479-1486

USDA (2013) National Nutrient Database for Standard Reference Release 26 Full Report (All Nutrients) Spices, coriander seed

Wallis TE (2005) Textbook of Pharmacognosy; 5th edn, S. K. Jain for CBS publishers and distibuters; New Delhi (India). pp. 125-126

Wangensteen H, Samuelsen AB, Malterud KE (2004) Antioxidant activity in extracts from coriander. Food Chem 88: 293-297.

□□□

Chapter 25

Ajwain (*Trachyspermum ammi*)

Avinash Kumar[1], Shalu Kumari Pathak[2] and Pankaj Kumar Singh[3]

[1] Department of Animal Nutrition, College of Veterinary Sciences & Animal Husbandry, DUVASU, Mathura-281001, India, *E-mail: avinashbvc04@gmail.com*

[2] Research Scholar, Division of Animal Genetics and Breeding, Indian Veterinary Research Institute, Izatnagar-243122, India

[3] Department of Animal Nutrition, Bihar Veterinary College, Bihar Animal Sciences University, Patna-800014, India

ABSTRACT

Trachyspermum ammi (Linn.), commonly known as ajwain is an annual herbaceous plant which belongs to medicinally important family Apiaceae. Fruits and seeds of ajwain were traditionally used for healing of different ailments. The seeds of ajwain are bitter in taste with pungent aroma and it acts as anthelmintic, carminative, laxative and stomachic. The fruits and seeds contain brown coloured oil known as ajwain oil. The main component of this oil is thymol, which is used in curing gastro-intestinal ailments, lack of appetite and bronchial problems. The oil exhibits anti-inflammatory, analgesic, antibacterial, antihelmintic, antihypertensive, antiflatulent, antispasmodic, antidiarrhoeal, bronchodilator, hepatoprotective, antiplatelet, insecticidal and spermicidal activities. The non-thymol fraction called as thymene constituents mainly saponins, glycosides, phenolic compounds, volatile oil (thymol, ãterpinene, para-cymene, and α- and β-pinene). The present chapter summarizes the information concerning the pharmacognostic, phytochemistry and pharmacological studies of *Trachyspermum ammi*.

Keywords: Ajwain, Essential oil, Thymol, Antibacterial, Anti-inflammatory, Antispasmodic.

25.1 Introduction

Since the beginning of human civilization, plants are being used as medicine. People of all ages in both developing and developed countries have utilized many plants to cure various diseases and to get relief from physical sufferings. *Trachyspermum ammi* (Linn.), commonly known as ajwain is an annual herbaceous plant which belongs to medicinally important family, Apiaceae (Gersbach and Reddy, 2002). The Plant is a native of Egypt and is being cultivated in Iraq, Iran, Afghanistan, Pakistan, and India. In India, it is cultivated in Madhya Pradesh, Uttar Pradesh, Gujarat, Rajasthan, Maharashtra, Bihar and West Bengal. It is widely grown in soil containing high amount of salts of arid and semi-arid regions (Joshi, 2000). Ajwain is a profusely branched annual herb and about 60-90 cm in length. It has an erect and striated stem with compound umbel inflorescence and pinnate leaves. Flowers are actinomorphic, white, male, bisexual and fruits are aromatic, ovoid, cordate, cremocarp with a persistent stylopodium. Fruit, consists of two mericarps which are greyish brown, ovoid, compressed, about 2 mm long and usually separate. The herb is generally grown in October–November and harvested in May–June (Chauhan *et al.*, 2012; Ranjan *et al.*, 2012).

The most utilized part of ajwain is the small caraway like fruit. Greyish brown seeds or fruits of ajwain are utilized for medical and nutritional purposes (Chauhan *et al.*, 2012). Ajwain is famous for its brownish essential oil. Fruits of Ajwain accumulate upto 5% essential oil in its compartments (Minija and Thoppil, 2002). The seeds contain 2–4.4% brown coloured oil known as ajwain oil. The main component of this oil is thymol, which is used in curing gastro-intestinal ailments, lack of appetite and bronchial problems. The oil exhibits anti-inflammatory, analgesic, antibacterial, antihelminthic, antihypertensive, antiflatulent, antispasmodic, bronchodilator, hepatoprotective, antiplatelet, insecticidal and spermicidal activities. It is an important remedial agent for flatulence, atonic dyspepsia and diarrhoea. The seeds of ajwain are bitter in taste with pungent aroma and it acts as antihelminthic, carminative, laxative and stomachic. It also cures abdominal tumours, abdominal pains, piles and bears anti-inflammatory and antioxidant activity. Usually, Thymol is the main constituent of ajwain essential oil and its yield may vary from from 35% to 60% (Ishikawa *et al.*, 2001; Zarshenas *et al.*, 2014). Thymol acts as a strong germicide, anti-spasmodic and fungicide. Thymol is also used in toothpaste and perfumery. In ayurvedic medicines, it is used as a medicinal plant for its antispasmodic, stimulant, tonic, and carminative properties. In traditional Persian medicine, it was used for therapeutic effects on rheumatic and neuralgic pain (Dashti-Rahmatabadi *et al.*, 2007) as well as for providing relief from diarrhea, dyspepsia, colic and indigestion (Hejazian, 2006; Mohagheghzadeh *et al.*, 2007). Besides, the herb has exhibited the antilithiatic activity in animal models (Kaur *et al.*, 2009).

25. 2 Classification

Kingdom	:	*Plantae*
Division	:	*Magnoliophyta*
Class	:	*Magnoliopsida*
Order	:	*Apiales*
Family	:	*Apiaceae*
Genus	:	*Trachyspermum*
Species	:	*ammi*

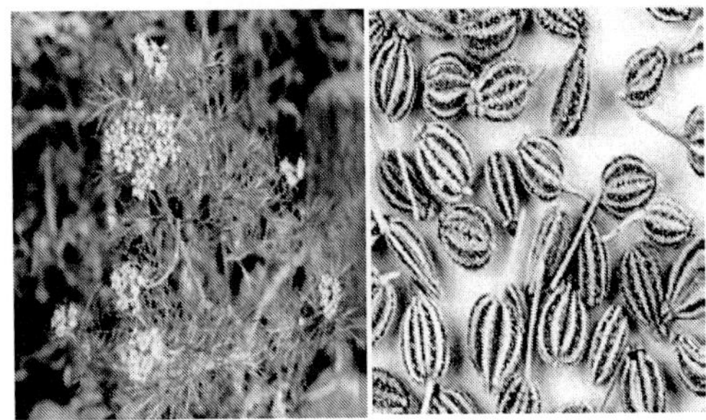

25.3 Chemistry of Ajwain

A number of chemical constituents have been studied and reported for the herb. Quantitative phytochemistry revealed that phytochemical constituents of ajwain comprises fiber (11.9%), carbohydrates (24.6%), tannins, glycosides, moisture (8.9%), protein (17.1%), fat (21.1%), saponins, flavones and other components (7.1%) including calcium, phosphorous, iron, cobalt, copper, iodine, manganese, thiamine, riboflavin and nicotinic acid (Duke, 1992; Qureshi and Kumar, 2010; Ranjan *et al.*, 2012). Similar to the most species of the family Apiaceae, ajwain is famous for its brownish essential oil which is responsible for its odor and taste. The ajwain fruits yield 2% to 4% brownish essential oil, with thymol as the major constituent varying from 35% to 60% (Ishikawa *et al.*, 2001). The non-thymol fraction called as thymene comprises para-cymene, γ-terpenine, α- and β-pinenes, dipentene, α-terpinene, and carvacrol (Chopra, 1982). Little amounts of camphene, myrcene, and α-3-carene also have been found in the plant. Saponin, a highly hygroscopic constituent occurs in alcoholic extracts (Ranjan *et al.*, 2012).

In an investigation, carvone (46.2%), limonene (38.1%) and dillapiole (8.9%) were identified as principal oil constituents

(Choudhury *et al.*, 1998). Also oleic, linoleic, palmitic, petroselinic acid and resin acids are isolated from fruits of ajwain (Qureshi and Kumar, 2010). Glycosyl constituents such as 6-hydroxycarvacrol 2-O-β-D-Glucopyranoside and 3, 5-Dihydroxytoluene 3-O-β-D-Galacto-pyranoside have been recently reported from fruits of ajwain (Gang *et al.*, 1980). Also, a steroid like compound known as 6-O-β- Gluco pyranosyloxythymol has been isolated from the fruits (Garg 1998). Water-soluble extract of ajwain fruit revealed many compounds such as monoterpenoid, glucosides and also nucleosides.

25.4 Different Preparations

25.4.1. *Essential Oil*

According to European pharmacopeia procedure, fruits of ajwain are powdered using domestic model mixi and are subjected to hydrodistillation in a Clevenger type apparatus for 6 h. Yellow-colored oil with characterstic odour and sharp taste is obtained. Further, It is dried over anhydrous sodium sulphate to remove traces of moisture and stored in refrigerator in dark at 4°C until use.

25.4.2 *Acetone Extract*

After the isolation of the essential oil, the powdered fruits are dried at 25 °C. Extract is obtained by extracting 20 g of dried fruits with 900 mL of acetone for 6 h in a Soxhlet apparatus. The extract is concentrated upto 20 mL by evaporating the remaining acetone in a vacuum drier under reduced pressure. The viscous extract, known as oleoresin is stored in a freezer at 4°C until use.

22.5 Biological Activities of Ajwain in Livestock and Poultry

25.5.1 *Antimicrobial Actions*

Ajwain helps in the protection of foodstuffs against microbial spoilage due to its antimicrobial action. The active principles considered to be responsible for the antimicrobial activity of ajwain are carvacol and thymol (Saxena and Vyas, 1986). Thymol kills the bacteria resistant to even prevalent third generation antibiotics as well as multi-drug resistant microbial pathogens and thus can be used as a plant based 4th generation herbal antibiotic formulation (Khanuja, 2004). Antifungal action of volatile constituents of *Trachyspermum ammi* seeds on ten fungi (*Acrophialophora fusispora, Curvularia lunata, Fusarium chlamydosporum, F. poae, Myrothecium roridum, Papulaspora sp., Alternaria grisea, A. tenuissima, Drechslera tetramera,* and *Rhizoctonia solani*) have been tested. Ajwain seeds were found to inhibit the growth of all test fungi by 72-90% (Singh *et al.*, 1979). Phenolic compounds, such as thymol and carvacol, are known to be either bacteriostatic or bactericidal agents depending on the concentration used (Caccioni *et al.*, 2000). An *in vitro* assay was carried out for the evaluation of ajwain antiviral activity. The methanolic extract of the herb showed significant inhibitory effects on Hepatitis C Virus (HCV) protease (Hussein *et al.*, 2000).

25.5.2 *Digestive Stimulant Actions*

Ajwain has been reported to increase the secretion of gastric acid. The addition of ajwain to the infusion increases the amount of gastric acid. The gastric acid secretion gets increased by nearly four-fold. Effect of ajwain on the food transit time has been studied in experimental rats *in vivo*. The addition of ajwain to the diet reduced food transit time and also enhanced the activity of digestive enzymes and augmented secretion of bile acids (Platel and Srinivasan, 2002).

Ajwain fruit exhibit antiulcer activity by using different ulcer models. Decreased ulcer index has been found in animals pre-treated with ethanolic extract in all models. The extract has shown significant protection ($p<0.001$) by reducing ulcerative lesions in comparison to control group of animals (Ramaswamy *et al.*, 2010). The hepato-protective actions *in vivo* showed that *T. ammi* was 80% protective in mice against a normally-lethal dose of paracetamol (1 g/kg). It prevented the CCl_4-induced prolongation of pentobarbital sleeping time in mice. It tended to normalize the high serum levels of liver enzymes caused by CCl_4-induced liver damage in rats (Ahsan *et al.*, 1990).

25.5.3 *Effect on Reproduction*

Spermicidal activities of ajwain essential oil was determined by an *in vitro* study. It was revealed that the volatile oil possessed potent spermicidal action (Buch *et al.*, 1988). Therefore, the oil may be used as a natural contraceptive agent. The total phytoestrogen content of dry ajwain seed has been determined as 473 ppm. The herb ranks second highest in the list of plants tested for total phytoestrogen content (Aghili-Shirazi and Makhzan ol Advieh, 1992). Traditionally, the herb has been used as a galactagogue also (Harjit, 1998). Ajwain has been listed in 14 indigenous medicinal plants which are used for abortion in some districts of Uttar Pradesh (India) from ancient time. The herb is not 100% effective so the possibility of causing congenital defects is one of the major concern in this regard. A high risk of potential human foeto-toxicity of ten plants including *T. ammi,* based on teratogenicity has been observed in rat fetuses (Nath *et al.*, 1997). The National Dairy Research Institute in India investigated the oestrogenic content of some herbs (including ajwain) that are traditionally used to increase milk yield in dairy cattle. Ajwain has also been traditionally used as a galactogogue in humans (Kaur, 1998).

25.5.4 *Analgesic and Antinociceptive Effects*

Analgesic and antinociceptive activity of ajwain was evaluated by using a Tail-flick Analgesiometer Device (Chaubey, 2008). The study revealed that the ethanolic extract significantly increased Tail-Flick Latency (TFL) within 2 hours postdrug administration. An experimental trial study was also carried out to compare the antinociceptive effect of the hydroalcoholic extract of ajwain with morphine sulphate using formalin test.

25.5.5 *Antioxidant Effect*

In an *in vivo* investigation in rats, antioxidant and ameliorative property of ajwain extract on hexachlorocyclohexane induced oxidative stress and toxicity has been evaluated. Pre-feeding of ajwain extract increased GSH, GSH-peroxidase, G-6-PDH, SOD, catalase, glutathione S-transferase (GST) activities and decreased hepatic levels of lipid peroxides. It was concluded that HCH administration caused hepatic free radical stress, resulting in toxicity which could be ameliorated by the dietary ajwain extract (Anilakumar *et al.*, 2009).

25.5.6 *Detoxification of Aflatoxins*

Aqueous extract of ajwain seeds has been found to contain an aflatoxin inactivation factor (IF). Thin layer chromatography analysis of the aflatoxins after treatment with IF has showed relative reduction of aflatoxin G1 > G2 > B1 > B2. These findings are confirmed by quantification of toxin using a fluorotoxin meter as well as the Enzyme Linked Immuno-sorbent Assay (ELISA). An approximate 80% reduction in total aflatoxin content over the controls has been observed.

This observed phenomenon of reduction in total toxins referred as toxin inactivation. Temperature also influences the rate of toxin inactivation. At 45°C, toxin inactivation occurs rapidly during the initial 5 h and slows later. The IF has been found to retain considerable activity even after boiling and autoclaving, indicating partial heat stability. The activity is also influenced by pH. Above pH 4.0, it has been found to be increased gradually, reaching the maximum at pH 10.0 and lost below pH 4.0. Also, IF activity has been found to be stable to gamma irradiation which emphasizes the potential of ajwain IF in aflatoxin removal from contaminated food commodities (Velazhahan *et al.*, 2010).

25.5.7 *Hypolipidaemic Action*

Antihyperlipidaemic effect of ajwain seed has been observed in albino rabbits. It was assessed that *Trachyspermum ammi* powder at dose rate of 2 g/kg body weight and its equivalent methanol extract were extensively effective in lipid lowering action by decreasing total cholesterol cholesterol, LDL-cholesterol, triglycerides and total lipids (Javed *et al.*, 2002).

25.5.8 *Anti-inflammatory Activity*

Anti-inflammatory principles have been found in the total alcoholic extract (TAE) and total aqueous extract (TAQ) of the ajwain seeds.TAE and TAQ exhibits significant ($P<0.001$) anti-inflammatory activity in animal models. The weight of the adrenal glands gets significantly increased in TAE and TAQ treated animals. TAE and TAQ extracts from the ajwain seeds exhibit significant anti-inflammatory potential (Thangam *et al.*, 2003).

25.5.9 *Insecticidal Activity*

Essential oil extracted from the seeds of ajwain can exhibit insecticidal activity in the oviposition step as well as egg hatching stage. It also inhibits developmental activities of *Callosobruchus chinensis* (Kostyukovsky *et al.*, 2002; Dashti-Rahmatabadi *et al.*, 2007).

22.5.10 *Antihelminthic Activity*

Antihelminthic activity of *Trachyspermum ammi* has been observed against specific helminths, e.g. *Ascaris lumbricoides* in humans and *Haemonchus contortus* in sheep (Kwon Park *et al.*, 2007). *Trachyspermum ammi* exert anthelmintic activity by interferring with the energy metabolism of parasites through augmentation of ATPase activity resulting in loss of energy reserves (Kostyukovsky *et al.*, 2002). The plant also increases peristaltic movements of the gut through its cholinergic activity, thus helping in expulsion of intestinal parasites contributing to its anti-helminthic activity (Tamurab and Iwamoto, 2004; Jabbar *et al.*, 2006). Constituents of ajwain oil (camphene, pinene, myrcene, limonene, terpinene, terpinen-4-ol, thymol and carvacrol) have shown nematicidal activity against pinewood nematode *Bursaphelenchus xylophilus*. Thymol and carvacrol have been reported to interfere with the neuromodulator octopamine (Choi *et al.*, 2007) or GABA-gated chloride channels of insect pests (Kong *et al.*, 2006). These studies confirm that the nematicidal activity of ajwain oil was mainly attributed to the activity of thymol and carvacrol (Wright 1981). LC_{50} (Lethal Concentration) values for nematicidal activity of ajwain essential oils was 0.431 mg/mL (Kwon *et al.*, 2007).

22.5.11 *Antifilarial Activity*

The effect of methanolic extract of fruits of *T. ammi* (Apiaceae) on *Setaria digitata* worms has been investigated. The crude extract as well as active fraction showed significant activity against the adult *S. digitata* by both worm motility and MTT [3-(4, 5- dimethylthiazol-2-yl)-2, 5- diphenyltetrazolium bromide] reduction assays. The isolated active principle "phenolic monoterpene" was screened for *in vivo* antifilarial activity against the human filarial worm *B. malayi* in *Mastomys coucha*, showing macrofilaricidal activity and female worm sterility. *Trachyspermum ammi* crude extract exhibited only macrofilaricidal activity (Mathew *et al.*, 2008).

22.5.12 Antiplatelet-aggregatory

In vitro experiments with blood from human volunteers showed that a dried real extract of ajwain seeds inhibited aggregation of platelets induced by arachidonic acid, collagen and epinephrine. Experimental study supported the traditional use of ajwain in women post-parturition (Srivastava, 1988).

22.5.13 *Antitussive Effects*

Different concentrations of aqueous and macerated extracts and carvacrol, codeine, and saline were tested for the antitussive effects by counting the number of coughs produced. Significant reduction of cough number was reported in the presence of both concentrations of aqueous and macerated extracts and codeine (p < 0.001 for extracts and p < 0.01 for codeine (Boskabady *et al.*, 2005).

22.5.14 *Antihypertensive and Broncho-dilating Activity*

Ajwain has been reported to have antihypertensive effect *in vivo* and the antisplasmodic and broncho-dilating actions *in vitro*. It has been reported that calcium channel blockade mediate the spasmolytic effects of plant materials and supported the use of ajwain in hyperactive disease states of the gut such as colic, diarrhoea as well as in hypertension (Gilani *et al.*, 2005).

25.5.15 *Antilithiasis and Diuretic Activity*

The roots of ajwain are diuretic in nature. Antilithiasis and diuretic actions *in vivo* of *T. ammi* on inhibiting oxalate urolithiasis induced in rats. In a further study of a possible diuretic effect the results found that ajwain was not effective in increasing the 24 hours urine production. The results concluded that the traditional use of ajwain in the treatment of kidney stones was not supported by their experimental evidence (Ahsan *et al.*, 1990).

25.6 Adverse Reactions

Ajwain (carom seeds) are likely safe in food amounts. Ajwain seeds are also possibly safe in therapeutic dosage. The excess amount can cause nausea, acidity, mouth ulcer, stomach ulcer, internal bleeding, ulcerative colitis and headache. It is contraindicated in hyperacidity. It may worsen liver function in people with liver disease particularly when combined with herbs and supplements that can cause hepatotoxicity (destructive effects on the liver), such as Borage, Chaparral, Uva-Ursi, and others. It also increases the risk of bleeding when used in combination with herbs and supplements that might affect platelet aggregation such as Angelica, Danshen, Garlic, Ginger, Ginkgo, etc. It may have additive effects when used with herbs and substances that increase photosensitivity, such as St. John's Wort. It has been reported that ajwain shows teratogenicity in rat fetuses. Therefore, its ingestion may be harmful during pregnancy (Nath *et al.*, 1997).

25.7 Summary and Conclusions

Trachyspermum ammi (ajwain) is an important herbal plant, which has both nutritional as well as medicinal uses. This particular plant has a wide therapeutic use which needs scientific research to explore the hidden curative and therapeutic potential.

References

Aghili-Shirazi S, Makhzan ol Advieh (1992) 1st ed. Tehran: Intisharat va Amoozesh enghelab Islami Press

Ahsan SK, Shah AH, Tanira MOM, Ahmad MS, Tariq M, Ageel AM (1990) Studies on some herbal drugs used against kidney stones in Saudi folk medicine. Fitoterapia. 61(05): 435-458

Anilakumar KR, Saritha V, Khanum F, Bawa AS (2009) Ameliorative effect of ajwain extract on hexachlorocyclohexane-induced lipid peroxidation in rat liver. ýFood Chem Toxicol. 47: 279-282

Boskabady MH, Jandaghi P, Kiani S, Hasanzadeh L (2005) Antitussive effect of *Carum copticum* in guinea pigs. J Ethnopharmacol. 97: 79-82

Buch JG, Dikshit RK, Mansuri SM (1988) Effect of certain volatile oils on ejaculated human spermatozoa. Indian J Med Res. 1988 Apr; 87: 361–363

Caccioni DLR, Guizzardi M, Biondi DM (2000) Relationships between volatile components of citrus fruit essential oil and antimicrobial action on *Penicillium digitatum* and *Penicillium italicum*. Int J Food Microbiol. 88: 170-175

Chaubey MK (2008) Fumigant toxicity of essential oils from some common spices against pulse beetle, *Callosobruchus chinensis* (Coleoptera: Bruchidae). J Oleo Sci. 57(3): 171–179

Chauhan B, Kumar G, Ali M (2012) A Review on phytochemical constituents and activities of *Trachyspermum ammi* (L.) sprague fruits. Am J Pharmtech Res. 2(4): 329–340

Choi IH, Shin SC, Park IK (2007) Nematicidal activity of onion (*Allium cepa*) oil and its components against the pine wood nematode (*Bursaphelenchus xylophilus*). Nematol. 09: 231–235

Chopra RN (1982) Chopra's Indigenous Drug of India, 2nd ed. Calcutta (INDIA): Academic Publishers

Choudhury S, Ahmed R, Kanjilal PB, Leclercq PA (1998) Composition of the seed oil of *Trachyspermum ammi* (L.) Sprague from Northeast India. J Essent Oil Res: JEOR. 10(5): 588–590

Dashti-Rahmatabadi M.H., Hejazian S.H., Morshedi A. and Rafati A (2007) The analgesic effect of *Carum copticum* extract and morphine on phasic pain in mice. J Ethnopharmacol. 109(2): 226–228

Duke J (1992) Handbook of phytochemical constituents of GRAS herbs and other economic plants. 1st ed. Boca Raton: CRC Press

Gang SK, Sharma ND, Gupta SR (1980) A phenolic glucoside from the seeds of *Carum copticum*. Phytochem. 9(10): 2215–2216

Garg S (1998) A new glucoside from *Trachyspermum ammi*. Fitoterapia. 69(6): 511–512

Gersbach PV, Reddy N (2002) Non-invasive localization of thymol accumulation in *Carum copticum* (Apiaceae) fruits by chemical shift selective magnetic resonance imaging. Ann Bot 90(2): 253–257

Gilani AH, Jabeen Q, Ghayur MN, Janbaz KH, Akhtar MS (2005) Studies on the antihypertensive, antispasmodic, bronchodilator and hepato protective activities of the *Carum copticum* seed extract. J Ethnopharmacol. 98(12): 127-135

Harjit K (1998) Estrogenic activity of some herbal galactogogue constituents. Indian J Anim Nutr. 15(3): 232–234

Hejazian S (2006) Analgesic Effect of essential oil (EO) from *Carum copticum* in mice. World J Med Sci. 1: 95–99

Hussein G, Miyashiro H, Nakamura N, Hattori M, Kakiuchi N, Shimotohno K (2000) Inhibitory effects of Sudanese medicinal plant extracts on Hepatitis C Virus (HCV) protease. Phytother Res. 14(7): 510–516

Ishikawa T, Sega Y, Kitajima J (2001) Water-soluble constituents of Ajowan. Chem Pharmaceut Bull. 49(7): 840–844

Jabbar A, Iqbal Z, and Khan MN (2006) *In vitro* antihelminthic activity of *Trachyspermum ammi* seeds. Pharmacogn Mag. 2: 126-129

Javed IMS, Akhtar T, Khaliq MZ, Khan G, Muhammad M (2002) Antihyperlipidaemic effect of *Trachyspermum ammi* (Ajwain) in rabbits, In: Proc 33rd All Pak Sci Conf Univ Agri Faisalabad, 2002

Joshi S (2000) Medicinal plants. 1st ed. Delhi: Oxford and IBH Publisher. p. 47

Kaur H (1998) Estrogenic activity of some herbal galactogogue constituents, Indian J Anim Nutr. 15(03): 232-234

Kaur T, Bijarnia RK, Singla SK, Tandon C (2009) *In vivo* efficacy of *Trachyspermum ammi* anticalcifying protein in urolithiatic rat model. J Ethnopharmacol. 126: 459–462

Khanuja SPS (2004) Formulation Comprising Thymol useful in the Treatment of Drug Resistance Bacterial infection, CCIR, New Delhi (INDIA): United state patent 6824795(2): 2004

Kong J, Lee SM, Moon YS, Lee SG, Ahn YJ (2006) Nematicidal activity of plant essential oils against *Bursaphelenchus xylophilus*. J Asia Pac Entomol. 09: 173-178

Kostyukovsky M, Rafaeli A, Gileadi C, Demchenko N, Shaaya E (2002) Activation of octopaminergic receptors by essential oil constituents isolated from aromatic plants: possible mode of action against insect pests. Pest Manag Sci. 58(11): 1101–1106

Kwon Park I, Junheon K, Sang-Gil L (2007) Nematicidal Activity of Plant Essential Oils and Components From Ajwain (*Trachyspermum ammi*), Allspice (*Pimentadioica*) and Litsea (*Litseacubeba*) Essential Oils Against Pine Wood Nematode (*Bursaphelenchus Xylophilus*). J Nematol. 39(03): 275-279

Mathew N, Bhattacharya SM, Perumal V, Muthuswamy K (2008) Antifilarial Lead Molecules Isolated from *Trachyspermum ammi*. Molecules. 13: 2156-2168

Minija J, Thoppil JE (2002) Essential oil composition of *Trachyspermum ammi* (L.) sprague from South India. Indian J Pharmaceut Sci. 64(3): 250–251

Mohagheghzadeh A, Faridi P, Ghasemi Y (2007) *Carum copticum* Benth and amp; Hook., essential oil chemotypes. Food Chem. 100: 1217–1219

Nath D, Sethi N, Srivastava S, Jain AK, and Srivastava R (1997) Survey on indigenous medicinal plants used for abortion in some districts of Uttar Pradesh, Fitoterapia. 68(3): 223-225

Platel K, Srinivasan K (2001) Studies on the influence of dietary spices on food transit time in experimental rats, Nutr Res. 21(9): 1309-1314

Qureshi AA, Kumar KE (2010) Phytochemical constituents and pharmacological activities of *Trachyspermum ammi*. Plant Archives. 10(2): 955–959

Ramaswamy S, Sengottuvelu S, Haja SS, Jaikumar S, Saravanan R, Prasadkumar C, Sivakumar T (2010) Gastroprotective Activity of Ethanolic Extract of *Trachyspermum ammi* Fruit. Int J Pharma Bio Sci. 01(01): 01-15

Ranjan B, Manmohan S, Singh SR, Singh RB (2012) Medicinal uses of *Trachyspermum ammi*: a review. Pharmacogn Rev. 6(11): 56–60

Saxena AP, Vyas KM (1986) Antimicrobial activity of seeds of some ethnomedicinal plants. J Econ Taxon Bot. 08(2): 291-300

Singh DB, Singh SP, Gupta RC (1979) Anti fungal effect of volatiles from seeds of some Umbelliferae. Trans Br Mycol Soc. 73(2): 349-350

Srivastava KC (1988) Extract of a spice-omum (*Trachyspermum ammi*)- shows antiaggregatory effects and alters arachidonic acid metabolism in human platelets. Prostaglandins Leukot Essent Fatty Acids. 33(01): 16

Tamurab T, Iwamoto H (2004) Thymol - a classical small molecule compound that has a dual effect (potentiating and inhibitory) on myosin. Biochem Biophys Res Commun. 18: 786-789

Thangam C, Dhananjayan R (2003) Antiinflammatory Potential of the Seeds of *Carum Copticum* Linn. Indian J Pharmacol. 35: 388-391

Velazhahan R, Vijayanandraj S, Vijayasamundeeswari A, Paranidharan V, Samiyappan R, Iwamoto T (2010) Detoxification of aflatoxins by seed extracts of the medicinal plant, *Trachyspermum ammi* (L.) Sprague ex Turrill Structural analysis and biological toxicity of degradation product of aflatoxin G1. Food Control. 21: 719–725

Wright DJ (1981) Nematicides: Mode of action and new approaches to chemical control, Vol 3. New York (USA): Zukerman & Rhode Publisher. pp. 421–49

Zarshenas MM, Petramfar P, Semani SM, Moein M (2014) Analysis of the essential oil components from different *Carum copticum* (L.) samples from Iran. Pharmacognosy Res. 6(1):62-66. doi: 10.4103/0974-8490.122920

❑❑❑

Chapter 26

Wormwood (*Artemisia absinthium*)

Yasir Afzal Beigh

Division of Animal Nutrition, Faculty of Veterinary Sciences & Animal Husbandry, Sher-e-Kashmir University of Agricultural Sciences and Technology of Kashmir, Srinagar- 190006, India, E-mail: vetyasir1@gmail.com

ABSTRACT

Artemisia absinthium Linn. (Wormwood) is an important perennial shrubby plant, distributed in the temperate areas across the globe and within India has been recorded in the Himalayan region. It is used as herbal medicine in Ayurveda, Homeopathy, Unani and Siddha; besides, has been incorporated as feed additive in livestock nutrition for augmenting nutrient utilization and animal performance. The plant contains phytochemicals such as absinthin, anabsinthin, anabsin, artabsin, absintholide, artabin, matricin, beta-santonin and ketopepenolid. It has a great importance in folk medicine during ancient times as an antiseptic, antihelminithic, antipyretic, antimalarial, antioxidant, hepatoprotective and neuroprotective. Improving the feeding value of animal diets using bioactive and highly nutritious medicinal plants such as wormwood can be an important factor not only to enhance animal production, product quality but also to lower feed cost in developing nations especially in temperate zones.This review provides information on the phytochemistry, medicinal uses and pharmacological evaluation studies along with preliminary investigations in the direction for use of *A. absinthium* L. in animal nutrition.

Keywords: *Artemisia absinthium*, Absinthin, Livestock, Nutrition, Properties.

26.1 Introduction

Wormwood (*Artemisia absinthium* L.) is a highly medicinal plant and almost mentioned in all the books of herbal medicine, distributed mainly in the temperate zones of Asia, Europe and North America.

A. absinthium is one of the important specie among the 45 members represented by genus Artemisia in the Indian flora, and is naturally distributed in the Himalayan region across Jammu and Kashmir at an altitude range of 1500-2700 m (Chopra *et al.*, 1956). *A. absinthium* L. is a hardy perennial sub-shrub. Erect, woody stems (over 1 m) bear alternate, much divided, silvery ovate to obovate leaves with silky soft hairs on each side. Tiny, rayless yellowish-green flowers occur in late summer in loose panicles which arise from the woody stems. It has a distinctive fragrance, thrives in sunny positions in poor soils and can become very woody.

26.2 Taxonomy

Artemisia absinthium L. belongs to the genus Artemisia, which is one of the largest and most widely distributed genera of the family Asteraceae (Compositae). It is a heterogenous genus, consisting over 500 diverse species. The species are perennial, biennial and annual herbs or small shrubs (Mehrdad *et al.*, 2007). Asteraceae is the largest family of angiosperms.

Kingdom	:	Plantae
Sub-kingdom	:	Tracheobionta
Super division	:	Spermatophyta
Division	:	Magnoliophyta
Class	:	Magnoliopsida
Sub-class	:	Asteridae
Order	:	Asterales
Family	:	Asteraceae
Genus	:	*Artemisia*
Species	:	*absinthium*

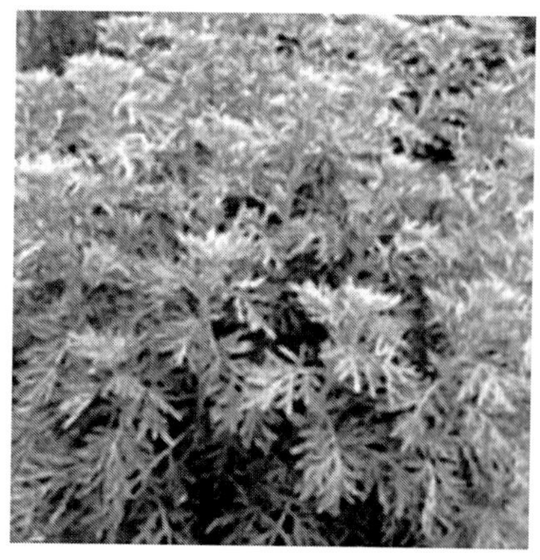

Artemisia absinthium L. is known by different vernacular names. Afsantin (Urdu); green ginger, absinthe, absinthium, wormwood (English); Apsinthion (Greek); *A. absinthium* (Latin); Afsanteen, Damseeh (Arabic); Ku ai, Yang ai (Chinese); Vermouth, Genepi (French); Wermut, Absinth (German); Afsantine (Iran); Anjenjo (Mexican); Majri, Karmala, Majtari, Mastiyarah (Hindi); Afsanteen (Unani), Absinthium (Hemopathy) (Ahmad *et al.*, 2010), and locally known as 'Tethwen' in Kashmir.

A similar specie, native to Britain, is sea wormwood *Artemisia maritima* L. which is widespread on coasts in Britain and northern Europe. It is smaller (to 60 cm) with strongly scented woolly divided leaves with blunt, narrow segments. Oval yellow-orange florets occur in late summer season. Other resembling species includes mugwort (*Artemisia vulgaris* L.), Roman wormwood (*Artemisia pontica* L.), tarragon (*Artemisia dracunculus* L.) and southernwood (*Artemisia abrotanum* L.) (Bown, 1995).

26.3 Phytochemical Constituents

The active constituents present in *A. absinthium* L. are the bitter substances, essential oils and other compounds. Bitter constituents (0.15-0.4%) consists of sesquiterpene lactones, a class of natural compounds with several proved medicinal effects and includes guanolide dimmers as absinthin (0.2–0.28%) and its isomers anabsinthin, anabsin, artabsin (0.04–0.16%), and absintholide (Beauhaire *et al.*, 1984); germacrene type as artabin (Akhmedov *et al.*, 1970); matricin (0.007% in the drug); beta-santonin and ketopepenolid-A (Perez-Souto *et al.*, 1992).

Essential oils (EO), mixtures of natural volatile compounds isolated by steam distillation from *A. absinthium* vary qualitatively and quantitatively according to geographical location and environmental conditions (Bakkali *et al.*, 2008). The yield of essential/wormwood oil (max. 0.2-1.5% in the drug) increases from arid to humid climate (Riahi *et al.*, 2015). The 4 main components described are: α-thujone, (Z)-epoxy-ocimene, trans-sabinylacetat and chrysanthenyl-acetate (HagerROM, 2006). α-thujone is typical for plants grown in areas below 1,000 m above mean sea level and is present at levels of approximately 40-70% of the wormwood oil (Tucker *et al.*, 1993). (Z)-epoxy-ocimene is the main component in plants grown in Europe at altitudes higher 1,000 m above mean sea level. In France, there are different chemotypes with trans-sabinyl-acetate and chrysanthenyl-acetate as main components, while plants from eastern Europe are mostly mixed types (Chialva *et al.*, 1983). Other constituents present at significant levels include myrcene (Â 35%), α-pinene (6%) and nerol (3%) in wormwood oil of Russian origin (Goraev *et al.*, 1962); p-cymene (16.5%), β-pinene (7.3%) and 7-ethyl-5,6-dihydro-1,4-dimethylazulene (5.5%) in Iranian wormwood oil (Semnani and Akbarzadeh 2005); cis-chrysanthenyl acetate (7.7-17.9%), a dihydrochamazulene isomer (5.5-11.6%), germacrene D (2.4-8.0%), linalool acetate (trace-7.0%), α-phellandrene (1.0-5.3%, and linalool (5.3-7.0%) in Tajikistanish wormwood oil (Sharopov *et al.*, 2012). High levels of thujanol and thujyi acetate (60-70%), myrcene (35%), camphor and 1,8-cineole were also determined in the wormwood oil (Wright, 2002). Thujones, trans-sabinyl acetate, cis-chrysanthenyl acetate and cis-epoxyimene are the most common constituents in wormwood oils (Juteau *et al.*, 2003). Other compounds present in *A. absinthium* L. are phenolic acids (2.6%) including chlorogenic, caffeic, syringic, coumaric, salicylic and vanillic acids; flavonoids (1.3%) including quercetin, rutin and glycosides (Canadanovic-Brunet *et al.*, 2005), tannins (Slepetys, 1975); lignans (Greger and Hofer, 1980), carotenoids, coumarins, homo-diterpen peroxides and thiophene (Canadanovic-Brunet *et al.*, 2005).

26.4 Medicinal Uses

The herb has always been of a great botanical and pharmaceutical interest and is used in indigenous systems of medicine as a vermifuge (Tariq *et al.*, 2009), an insecticide (Kordali *et al.*, 2005), acaricide (Chiasson *et al.*, 2001), cardiac stimulant (Guarrera, 2005), antispasmodic, antiseptic and diuretic, and for the treatment of chronic fevers and hepatitis (Gilani and Janbaz, 1995), stomach aches (Baytop 1984; Koul, 1997), restoration of declining mental function and to improve memory (Wake *et al.*, 2000). Its essential oil has antimicrobial (Juteau *et al.*, 2003), antifungal (Saban *et al.*, 2005), neuroprotective (Bora and Sharma, 2010) and antimalarial (Irshad *et al.*, 2011) activity. Volatile oil of *A. absinthium* is rich in thujone (α and β) having anthelmintic activity (Meschler and Howlett, 1999). In addition, the herb is used to make a tea for helping pregnant women during pain of labour and in treating leukaemia and sclerosis (Canadanovic-Brunet *et al.*, 2005). Moreover, the organic extract of this herb revealed toxic and anti-feedant effects (Erturk and Uslu, 2007). Recently, the aerial part of *A. absinthium* L. has shown to possess anti-snake venom activity (Nalbantsoy *et al.*, 2013). Anticancer activities are among the prominent biological effects reported for different species of the genus Artemisia (Irshad *et al.*, 2011). It is commonly used in food industry in the preparation of aperitifs, bitters and spirits (Basta *et al.*, 2007). *A. absinthium* is used as whole plant in ruminant feeding.

26.5 Biological Activities of Wormwood in Animal Production

26.5.1 Digestive Effects

26.5.1.1 *Enhance Palatability*

A. absinthium has strong flavour, which may alter feed sensory characteristics and therefore, affect feed intake. Constituent phytochemicals impart strong flavours to wormwood that may increase palatability and feed intake of diets in animals. Although, the freshly cut wormwood is typically distasteful to ruminants; however, drying the plant increases its attractiveness to ruminants. Kim *et al.* (2002) reported 18% increase in dry matter and organic matter intake in sheep fed diets containing wormwood relative to those fed the diet without wormwood. Also, Kim *et al.* (2006) reported higher intake of diets containing wormwood silage compared to the control diet in sheep, which was partly attributable to the lower fibre and higher protein concentration and higher digestibility of diets that contained wormwood silage. Replacing rice straw with wormwood silage in ruminant diets can improve dietary nutrient supply and digestion, and enhance the content of health-promoting compounds in beef (Kim *et al.*, 2012).

26.5.1.2 *Hyper-secretary Activity*

Bitter constituents of wormwood stimulate the gustatory nerves in the mouth and increase the secretion of gastric juice and bile (Blumberger and Glatzel, 1966), thereby promote appetite and digestion. An intra-venous injection of decoctions of *A. absinthium* (equal to 5 g herbal substance) caused a threefold increase of bile secretion in dogs (Kreitmair, 1951). Liquid preparations of *A. absinthium* stimulated gastric secretion in humans when it was given orally five minutes before meal (Mills and Bone, 2000). Again, Bone (2003) reported dramatic increase in duodenal levels of pancreatic enzymes and bile by oral dosing of liquid *A. absinthium*. The essential oil of wormwood acts antispasmodic in small amounts; however, at high dosages or after longer-lasting intake the essential oil acts as a convulsant poison.

26.5.1.3 *Digestibility Enhancement Activity*

Improvement in the secretion of gastric juice and bile by supplementation of *A. absinthium* or its extracts result in enhanced digestibility of feed in animal system. Kim *et al.* (2002) reported that digestibility of DM and TDN value were significantly increased ($p<0.05$) in sheep fed diets containing the three levels (@ 3, 5 and 10% substitution of rice straw) of dried wormwood inclusion compared with the un-supplemented control. Digestibilities of crude protein and fibre in the 5% dried wormwood inclusion highly increased ($p<0.05$) upto 8.2 and 5.5% respectively relative to the control treatment. Ko *et al.* (2006) reported that substituting wormwood for rice straw in the sheep diets increased *in vivo* nutrient digestibility, N retention and microbial N yield, particularly at the medium and high levels of wormwood inclusion. The reason for higher digestibility of the diets might be related to the presence of 6,7-dimethylesculetin, capillarisin and coumarin in wormwood, which stimulate the secretion of bile salts and lipolytic enzymes in the small intestine (Hahn, 1966).

26.5.1.4 *Improve Rumen Fermentation*

A. absinthium have potential benefits of using as a forage/feed additive source for ruminants, particularly in promoting the rumen fermentation pattern for efficient utilization of diets. Previous studies have shown that feeding dried wormwood, instead of rice straw, did not affect rumen pH (Kim *et al.*, 2002). However, Kim *et al.* (2006) reported that ruminal fermentation characteristics were improved by substituting wormwood silage for rice straw in sheep diets with decreased ruminal pH. This decreases ruminal biohydrogenation of poly-unsaturated fatty acids (PUFA), and increase transfer of 18:3 and 18:2 PUFA from the diet to muscle tissue, thereby enhancing concentration of health-promoting fatty acids in the muscle of the steers (Kim *et al.*, 2012).

26.5.2 Hepatic Effects

Hepatic ailments are one of the major serious health issues throughout world now-a-days, but regardless of remarkable advances in the modern medicine, their prevention options and treatments still remain inadequate. The blockage or retardation of the chain reactions of inflammatory process and oxidation is considered as efficient therapeutic approach for prevention as well as treatment of hepatic injuries. In recent times, the most frequent and well recognized *in vivo* model used for the investigation of novel hepatoprotective agents is rodent model of hepatic disorders induced *via* carbon tertrachloride (CCl_4) which is a hepatotoxin that triggers hepato-cellular damage mediated by free radicals (Jung *et al.*, 2015). Phytochemicals (sesquiterpene lactones, flavonoids, phenolic acids and tannins) present in *A. absinthium* L. and its extracts reveal strong antioxidant and/or immune modulatory potential, and thus, exhibit hepato-protective activity in animal based models. Furthermore, caffeoyl and dicaffeoylquinic acids present in *A. absinthium* are hepatoprotective in nature.

Aqueous-methanolic extract of *A. absinthium* exhibited hepatoprotective effect against acetaminophen and CCl_4 induced hepatic damage (Gilani and Janbaz, 1995), and thereby scientifically support its traditional usage against various liver diseases like hepatitis and other hepatobiliary ailments (Said, 1982). The mechanism of action may be associated with inhibition of hepatic microsomal drug metabolizing enzymes, antioxidant activity, and/or blocking calcium channels. *Mohammadian et al.* (2016) reported that administration of hydroalcoholic extract of *A. absinthium* would improve the liver function and the level of oxidative stress parameters such as total thiol groups in blood. *A. absinthium* extract seems to be able to preserve the structural integrity of the hepatocellular membrane leading to reduction of serum aspartate aminotransferase and alanine aminotransferase activities. Beigh *et al.* (2017) reported that supplementation of *A. absinthium* L. herb alone or in combination with exogenous fibrolytic enzymes cocktail as feed additive to complete feed is possible for intensive rearing of lambs without any adverse effect on hepato-renal functioning. However, hepatoprotective effects of wormwood is possible at doses lower than 200 mg/kg (Amat *et al.*, 2010), but at high doses *A. absinthium* plays a prooxidant and inflammatory role such as gallic acid (Dianat *et al.*, 2014), thereby induce hepatotoxicity by inflammation and oxidation depending on its thujone content, drying and harvesting conditions or climate that the plant was growing in (Lachenmeier *et al.*, 2010).

26.5.3 Neurologic Effect

A. absinthium has both neuroprotective as well as neurotoxic effects depending upon the intake amount of the active phytoconstituent into the animal system.

26.5.3.1 *Neuroprotective Activity*

A. absinthium has a long history of use as restorative of lost or declining cognitive functions in traditional medicine. It has shown cognitive enhancement because of its nicotinic and muscarinic receptor activity, which was studied and reported in homogenates of human cerebral cortical membranes by Wake *et al.* (2000). Moreover, it has been reported that ethanolic extract of *A. absinthium* enhanced neurite outgrowth by potentiating nerve growth factor and PC12D cells (Li and Ohizumi, 2004). *A. absinthium* exhibited neuroprotective eûects against focal ischemia and reperfusion-induced cerebral injury in rats (Adams and Garcia, 2006). Neuroprotection is also exhibited by its extract as it is evident from the reduction of brain infarct volume and oxidative stress, restoration of endogenous antioxidants, and also significant improvement in behavioural outcome during cerebral ischemia and reperfusion injury. The mechanism by which *A. absinthium* normalized the damage, inhibited lipid peroxidation and neurological deficits, and restored the endogenous antioxidant defense enzymes, is probably by its antioxidant properties, suggesting that *A. absinthium* may prove to be useful adjunct in the treatment of stroke (Bora and Sharma, 2010). Also, Zeng *et al.* (2015) reported that a natural sesquiterpene dimer Caruifolin D from *A. absinthium* L. considerably suppressed the production of intracellular reactive oxygen species that displayed its neuroprotective mechanism.

Conventional Chinese medicine practitioners utilize *A. absinthium* to deal with neurodegenerative disorders (Parekh *et al.*, 2009). The herb might be beneficial for the treatment of the glial and neuronal alterations observed during chronic lead intoxication in adult rat (Sansar and Gamrani, 2013). Hallal *et al.* (2016) reported that treatment with *A. absinthium* L. show a significant amelioration in activity of antioxidant enzymes (superoxide dismutase, catalase and glutathione peroxidase), which may be associated with the level of non-enzymatic antioxidants than the activity of enzymatic antioxidants and protects brain dysfunction induced by mercuric chloride ($HgCl_2$), suggesting that this molecular approach can be a strategy to a possibly therapeutic action of *A. absinthium* in the treatment of neurodegeneration produced by $HgCl_2$.

26.5.3.2 *Neurotoxic Activity*

Chronic use of *A. absinthium* has been reported to have some neurotoxic effect due to presence of thujone and its derivatives (Donald 1981). Thujone is a $GABA_A$ receptor antagonist that can cause epileptic-like convulsions (Behrens *et al.*, 2004) by rapidly modulating the GABA-gated chloride channel. The effect appears to be due to the parent compound, while metabolism leads to detoxification. Intraperitoneal injection of thujone was convulsant in mice (Hold *et al.*, 2000) and the action was blocked by earlier intraperitoneal administration of diazepam or phenobarbital.

26.5.4 Anti-parasitic Effect

Till such time that immunization procedures could be developed against major parasitic diseases, a renewal of interest in the safe, sustainable and effective (yet relatively inexpensive) resource, that is, medicinally active plants/herbs, seems a viable option. There has been resurgence in the use of medicinal plants to treat cases of parasitism in livestock and much of the success has been achieved in this direction against a variety of parasites.

26.5.4.1 *Antihelminthic Activity*

In indigenous systems of medicine, *A. absinthium* has been used as a vermifuge, and is considered to be an effective natural alternative remedy for parasite control both in humans as well as in animals. Volatile oil rich in thujone (α and β) from *A. absinthium* has been earlier reported to have an antihelminthic activity (Meschler and Howlett, 1999). The genus is a rich source of sesquiterpene lactones (like artemisinin) and flavonoids that also might have anthelmintic activity with low risk of mammalian toxicity (Kerboeuf *et al.*, 2008). Singh *et al.* (1994) reported that an aqueous extract of fresh leaves of *A. absinthium* L. given with sugar solution on empty stomach for 8-10 days, expelled out round worms completely. Also, it has been reported that crude aqueous and ethanol extracts of the aerial parts of *A. absinthium* exhibit significant antihelminthic activity in comparison to albendazole against the gastrointestinal nematodes in sheep, without apparent toxicity to the animals. *In vitro*, both extracts reduced the motility of *Haemonchus contortus* at 25 mg/mL, and both aqueous and ethanolic extracts were effective *in vitro* and *in vivo*, but ethanolic outperformed the aqueous extracts (Tariq *et al.*, 2009). These results agree with others (Urban *et al.*, 2008) who found that ethanolic extracts of *A. absinthium* significantly reduced egg development and juvenile (L3) larval motility of *Ascaris suum in vitro*. In contrast, Worku *et al.* (2009) did not observed gastrointestinal nematicidal activity *of A. absinthium* aqueous extract in goats. Also, Squires *et al.* (2011) reported that crude ethanolic extract of *A. absinthium* did not have antihelminthic activity against *H. contortus* in gerbils. While, methanol extract of the aerial parts of *A. absinthium* at a dose of 300 mg/kg reduced numbers of *Trichinella spiralis* larvae in the muscle of rats (Caner *et al.*, 2008) as well as its essential oils caused 66% reduction of intestinal *T. spiralis* adult parasites in mice (Garcia-Rodriguez *et al.*, 2015). These discrepancies in results emphasize the difficulties associated with efforts to evaluate and standardize antiparasitic effects of the plant and plant-derived products. Studies have reported that polar extracts obtained with water or ethanol have a greater anthelmintic activity than non-polar extracts obtained with hexane, which usually have low or no anthelmintic activity.

26.5.4.2 *Antiprotozoal Activity*

The antiparasitic drugs which have been evaluated against the pathogenic protozoa often have severe side effects. In this context, medicinal plants as a source have attracted a considerable attention in the development of new antiprotozoal drugs. *A. absinthium* and its extracts besides anthelmintic properties have antiprotozoal activities too. *A. absinthium* extracts have been reported as exhibiting antiprotozoal potential against *Trypanosoma brucei, T. cruzi* and *Leishmania infantum* (Valdes *et al.*, 2008). The antileishmanial activity is due to its constituent flavonids whose action depends on the presence of two hydroxyl groups in the molecule at C-3 and C-4 and that activity is lost with a methoxy at C-3 (Taleb-Continil *et al.*, 2004). Besides, the oxygenated monoterpene camphor present in *A. Absinthium* shows antileishmanial activity against promastigote and axenic amastigote forms of two *Leishmania* strains (*L. aethiopica* and *L. donovani*) (Tariku *et al.*, 2011). Also, Bailen *et al.* (2013) reported that the essential oils of *A. absinthium* showed antiparasitic effects against *Leishmania infantum* at all the lowest dose tested, while these essential oils were active against *Trypanosoma cruzi* at 800 and 400 μg/mL under *in vitro* experimentation. Leishmanicidal and trypanocidal activities of *A. absinthium* essential oils have also been reported by Martinez-Diaz *et al.* (2015). A constituent sesquiterpene lactone-artemetin has been described as a synergist for the trypanocidal effects of other flavones (Hoet *et al.*, 2004). Ethanol and aqueous extract of *A. absinthium* showed growth inhibitory effects against brain-eating amoeba *Naegleria fowleri* due to its constituent sesquiterpene lactone-artemisin (Mendiola *et al.*, 1991). *A. absinthium* also shows antimalarial activity. The aqueous and alcoholic leaf extracts of *A. absinthium* showed antimalarial activity against a strain of *Plasmodium berghei* in mice (Zafar *et al.*, 1990). While the aqueous extract as well as a sesquiterpene lactone fraction of *A. absinthium* has inhibited the growth of *P. falciparum* known to cause malaria in humans (Valdes *et al.*, 2008). Maximum percentage of inhibition of growth (89.9%) was shown by aqueous extract at a dilution of 1:35. The LD_{50} value of the sesquiterpene lactone fraction was 31.4 µg/ml (Ramazani *et al.*, 2010). The constituent sesquiterpene lactones- artemetin and casticin enhanced the antiplasmodial action of artemisinin. Both the flavones showed *in vitro* antimalarial effects against *P. falciparum* (Liu *et al.*, 1992).

Coccidiosis is one of the most important infections in livestock caused by Eimeria species and is of greater economic importance due to high morbidity. In order to develop alternative, safer and environmental friendly anti-coccidial agent, potent medicinal benefits for *Artemisia* species have been reported. Anticoccidian activity of *A. absinthium* and its extracts have been reported in ruminants as well as in poultry; however, the activity depends on the number of oocysts and the type of *Eimeria*. Aqueous extract *A. absinthium* at a dose of 3 mg/kg of feed per day reduces the number of oocysts in broiler chicken infected with *E. tenella* and can be used for the prophylaxis of moderate coccidiosis (Kostadinovic *et al.*, 2012). Tests have been conducted on different breeds of chickens, using different concentrations of extracts in correlation to the number of artificially entered Eimeria oocysts (Allen *et al.*, 1997; Arab *et al.*, 2006; Dragan *et al.*, 2010). However, Iqbal *et al.* (2013) observed that *A. absinthium* was not effective against coccidian infection in goats & recommended further studies with different dosages, concentrations and solvent preparations of *A. absinthium* extracts to arrive at a certain conclusion about its efficacy against goat coccidian.

26.5.4.3 *Anti-feedant Activity*

Arthropod parasites such as mosquitoes, fleas, flies and ticks, apart from their direct ill-effects of discomfort, blood loss and dermatitis to their hosts, are highly important vectors of a variety of disease-agents affecting both human and animals. The active ingredients of several plants and herbs are known to possess insect repellent, insecticidal, growth inhibitory and anti-moulting activities. *A. absinthium* is famous for its anti-feedant properties (Nin *et al.*, 1997). Ethnobotanical studies refer to its insect repellent properties and external use of its aerial parts in cattle skin disorders (Jaric *et al.*, 2007). The activities of *A. absinthium* is due to its essential oil that has been shown to have acaricidal (Chiasson *et al.*, 2001), insecticidal (Kaul *et al.*, 1978) and repellent effects against fleas, flies, mosquitoes (Erichsen-Brown, 1979) and ticks (Jaenson *et al.*, 2005). Parveen *et al.* (2014) reported that 5, 10 and 20% concentrations of *A. absinthium* ethanolic extracts showed 100% inhibition for hatching of cattle tick (*Rhipicephalus microplus*) eggs *in vitro*, suggesting that *A. absinthium* could form alternatives to commercially available synthetic acaricides. Additionally, its organic extracts exhibited anti-feedant effects and were toxic to *Leptinotarsa decemnlineata* (Erturk and Uslu, 2007), and *Rhopalosiphum padi* (Halbert *et al.*, 2009); however, the extraction method play an important role when evaluating the potential anti-feedant applications of *A. absinthium* extracts (Martín *et al.*, 2012).

26.5.5 Anti-inflammatory Effect

A. absinthium has a rational basis for its traditional use in some painful and inflammatory conditions. *A. absinthium* and its extracts have been demonstrated to possess a strong anti-inflammatory activity in animal model. Its phytoconstituents *viz.* flavonoids (Yin *et al.*, 2008) and sesquiterpene type molecules (Ruikar *et al.*, 2011) are well known to possess anti-inflammatory activity through the mechanism associated with synthesis or release of inflammatory mediators such as the histamine, serotonin, bradykinins and prostaglandins. Ahmad *et al.* (1992) have evaluated the analgesic and anti-inflammatory activities of alcoholic extracts of *A. absinthium*. Hadi *et al.* (2014) reported that the essential oil and aqueous extract of *A. absinthium* possess significant anti-inflammatory effect in laboratory animals at the doses investigated with more activity for the essential oil compared to the aqueous extract. Zeng *et al.* (2015) reported that natural sesquiterpene dimer caruifolin D was a major anti-inflammatory component from *A. absinthium* L. which has potent anti-neuroinflammatory effects and suggested that caruifolin D might be developed as a drug candidate for neuro-inflammation-related diseases. Nalbantsoy *et al.* (2013) studied the anti-snake venom activities of *A. absinthium* L. in comparison with carrageenan-induced acute inflammation model in rats and reported for the first time the toxicity and inflammatory actions and cytotoxic actions of crude *Montivipera xanthina* venom as well as inhibition of venom-induced inflammation by methanolic extract of *A. absinthium*

26.5.6 Anti-oxidant Effect

The conventional therapeutic approaches for different chronic diseases caused by oxidative damage of reactive oxygen species often have severe side effects that impresses for requirement of antioxidants, which are considered as chemical substances that lessen and prevent oxidation. Antioxidants have the ability to protect from the damaging effects of radicals in tissue. In this context, the use of plants and herbs as a source of natural antioxidant and biologically active compounds has attracted a great deal of scientific interest. The anti-oxidant properties of these medicinal plants are mainly attributed to their constituent phytochemicals produced as part of their normal metabolic activities. Among different classes of secondary metabolites, plant polyphenols constitute the largest group of natural antioxidants (Ciesla *et al.*, 2012). Antioxidant activity have been reported for essential oil of *A. absinthium* L. (Kordali *et al.*, 2005) and its extracts (Canadanovic-Brunet *et al.*, 2005), which is possibly due to its constituent flavonoids (rutin and quercetin), thymol and carvacrol as well as other phenolic compounds (Bora and Sharma, 2011a). Artemetin (flavone) has been described as an antioxidant that neutralizes peroxide radicals (Dugas *et al.*, 2000). Some researchers have even reported that essential oils rich in non-phenolic compounds also have antioxidant potential (Juteau *et al.*, 2003).

The antioxidative activity of *A. absinthium* extracts have been tested by measuring their ability to scavenge stable 2,2-diphenyl-1-picrylhydrazyl (DPPH) free radical and reactive hydroxyl radical during the Fenton reaction trapped by 5,5-dimethyl-1-pyrroline-N-oxide, using electron spin resonance spectroscopy (Bora and Sharma, 2011b). The DPPH free radical scavenging activity of *A. absinthium* in callus cultures has been found to be independent on biomass accumulation, but it is dependent on secondary metabolites production during the culture growth. Highest antioxidant activity (63.3%) and maximum accumulation of total phenolics (1.48 mg GAE/g DW) and total flavonoids (0.48 mg QE/g DW) were recorded in 35 days old calli which declined thereafter representing a positive correlation of phenolic compounds and antioxidant activity in callus cultures of *A. absinthium* L. (Ali *et al.*, 2013).

26.5.7 Anti-microbial Effect

26.5.7.1 *Anti-bacterial Activity*

In recent decades, antimicrobial herbal products have received considerable attention because of a rapid increase in antibiotic resistance in microorganisms (Essawi and Srour, 2000). *A. absinthium* have been reported to have a broad spectrum of inhibitory activity against a variety of micro-organisms due to presence of essential oil for which the herb is most likely still used as a cure for gastro-intestinal disorders and the treatment of wound infections as an antiseptic. Extracts of *A. absinthium* have been shown to exhibit strong antimicrobial activity, especially against gram positive pathogenic bacteria (Fiamegos *et al.*, 2011) which could be attributed to the presence of the major (camphor, p-cymene, caryophyllene) or minor (α-pinene, β-pinene) components of the plant or synergy between these compounds (Moslemi *et al.*, 2012). These pinene-type monoterpenes (α-pinene, β-pinene) are well-known chemicals having antimicrobial potentials; besides enantiomers of α-pinene and β-pinene have a strong antibacterial activity (Leite *et al.*, 2007). Camphor, as the major constituent of *A. absinthium*, has been reported to have a strong antibacterial activity against gram positive bacteria (Jeong-Dan, 2007). Essential oils can also inhibit the synthesis of DNA, RNA, protein, and polysaccharide in bacterial cells (Abad *et al.*, 2012).

Ethanol extracts of *A. absinthium* possess same effects against different specific bacterial strain with inhibition zones of 10-15 mm in diameter for *Staphylococcus aureus* (Dulger *et al.*, 1999). Habibipour and Rajabi (2015) also reported higher effect of extract of *A. absinthium* on *Haemophilus influenza* which was even better than Ofloxacin. Likewise, Moslemi *et al.* (2012) reported that topical application of *A. absinthium* extract on the infected wound sites produced significant antibacterial activity against *S. aureus*. Significant antibacterial activity of *A. absinthium* essential oil and its extract also suggest its capacity as a natural food preservative in the food industry for preservation of food material from degradation mainly by micro-organism activity during production, storage, and marketing as an alternative to synthetic antibiotics that has lead to an increase of some pathogens' resistance and uncomfortability to patients due to their adverse drug reactions (Msaada *et al.*, 2015). These plants based secondary metabolites such as essential oil and extracts are widely used in the food industry and are considered Generally Recognized as Safe (GRAS).

26.5.7.2 *Anti-fungal Activity*

The emerging resistance of microbes to synthetic antifungal agents has serious implications in the management of infections; besides, these antifungal compounds also act on targets found in mammalian cells which may result in toxicity or adverse drug interactions, thereby necessitating the discovery of novel antifungals. Herbs/botanicals could be a better source of medicine as compared to synthetically produced drugs. *A. absinthium* have been reported to have inhibitory activity against a variety of fungi which could be attributed to the major component of essential oil. The anti-fungal activity of essential oils of wormwood gives it an important role in the field of food, cosmetics, and pharmaceutical industries. The essential oils containing (Z)-epoxyocimene and chrysanthenyl acetate as major components distilled from the aerial parts of *A. absinthium* from France inhibited *in vitro* growth of *Candida albicans* and *Saccharomyces cerevisiae* var. chevalieri (Juteau *et al.*, 2003). Wormwood essential oil from a Turkish population, whose main components are camphor, 1,8-cineole and chamazulene, has been described as fungicidal at a dose of 20μL against 34 species of fungi including *Fusarium solani* and *Fusarium oxysporum* (Kordali *et al.*, 2005). *F. oxysporum* and *F. solani* were affected by essential oils (cis-epoxyocimene, chrysanthenol, and chrysanthenyl acetate) from cultivated as well as commercial oil samples of *A. absinthium* has also been reported by Bailen *et al.* (2013). Significant inhibitory activity of wormwood essential oils against the three phytopathogenic fungi *viz. F. graminearum, F. culmorum* and *F. oxysporum* has been observed by Msaada *et al.* (2015). Furthermore, *A. absinthium* essential oil from Uruguay rich in thujone showed anti-fungal effects against *Alternaria* sp. and *Botrytis cinerea* (Umpierrez *et al.*, 2012).

26.5.8 Other Effects

26.5.8.1 *Antipyretic Activity*

In Turkish folk medicine, *A. absinthium* has been used as an antipyretic herbal drug (Baytop, 1984). Khattak *et al.* (1985) reported that hexane-, chloroform-, and water-soluble extracts of *A. absinthium* exhibit antipyretic activity comparable to potency of aspirin against subcutaneous yeast injections in rabbits. No toxic effects were documented for the plant extract at doses up to 1.6 g/kg. In another study with the ethanolic extract of *A. absinthium* which contains

24-β-ethyl p-cholesta-7, 22-dien-3 Bat, shows antipyretic activity in rats with least side effects (Carner *et al.*, 2008).

26.5.8.2 *Hypolipidemic Activity*

Hyperlipidemia is considered to be a major risk factor for cardiovascular diseases including atherosclerosis, myocardial infarction, heart attacks and cerebrovascular diseases (Na *et al.*, 2008), which can be treated with *A. absinthium* extract that has been reported to reduces serum cholesterol and triglyceride by 8 and 3.5 times, respectively in rabbits (Daradka *et al.*, 2014). *A. absinthium* ethanolic extract (500, 1000 mg/kg) have potent antihyperlipidemic activity in high cholesterol diet induced hyperlipidemia models. The possible mechanism of lipid alteration might be cholestatic effect of *A. absinthium* in liver by enhanced removal or catabolism of lipoproteins (Brattsand, 1975) and/or inhibition of lysosomal lipid hydrolytic enzymes secreted by the liver (Sherlock, 1998).

26.5.8.3 *Immuno-modulatory Activity*

In traditional medicine, worldwide, herbal drugs are used to treat immune disorders, such as inflammatory and autoimmune diseases. *A. absinthium* is commonly used to modulate immune-mediated disorders in indigenous system of medicine. It has been reported that polysaccharides isolated from *A. absinthium* have immuno-modulatory eûects by induction of a Th1 response and stimulation of nitric oxide production (Danilets *et al.*, 2010). In addition, *in vivo* studies indicated that *A. absinthium* suppressed tumour necrosis factor alpha (TNF-α) and accelerated healing in patients with Crohn's disease (Krebs *et al.*, 2010). *A. absinthium* extract, at concentrations below 100 μg/mL can modulate the immune response towards a Th1 pattern, by induction of CD40 expression on dendritic cells and cytokine production with inhibition of dendritic T cell stimulating activity at high concentrations (Shahnazi *et al.*, 2015).

26.5.9 Adverse Reactions

Thujone, a characteristic component of essential oil of the *A. absinthium* L., is a known central nervous system toxin; however, the toxicological risk from use of conventional wormwood preparations is very low and aqueous extracts contain little thujone. Excessive dosing, long-term use or use of the essential oil could lead to toxicity "absinthism" -mental disorder in humans (Mc Guffin, 1997) with the symptoms of hallucinations, sleeplessness and convulsions. The side effects may include brain damage and even death, insomnia, intestinal cramps, nausea, restlessness, seizures, stomach cramps, tremors, urine retention, vertigo and vomiting (Duke, 2002). Several animal experiments conducted with pure thujone have confirmed its properties to cause dose-dependent tonic-clonic seizures (Lachenmeier, 2010). The no-effect level (NOEL) has been reported to be in the range between 5 and 12.5 mg/kg bodyweight/day (SCF, 2003).

26.6 Summary and Conclusions

The present review emphasizes the traditional uses, phytochemistry, ethnopharmacological and toxicological information on *A. absinthium* L. in animal and human studies. In recent years, phytochemical studies have received considerable attention to know about numerous known and unknown constituent compounds of medicinal value that can be screened for their beneficial purpose in animal and/or human system. Ethano-veterinary medicinal studies on *A. absinthium* have revealed its pharmacological potential, which is essential for its further consideration and standardization as a medicine or feed additive at safer level. *A. absinthium* have strong flavours, thus have very powerful actions in animals including ruminants, and should be used with care because elevated doses can stimulate undesirable side effects. Improving the feeding value of animal diets through supplementation of bio-active and high nutritional herbal plants such as wormwood is a viable proposition to enhance the nutrient utilization efficiency for augmenting productivity as well as product quality to have sustainable livestock production, particularly where feeding of low grade roughages is indispensable. However, it is more essential to evaluate its potential on modern scientific lines through phytochemical, pharmacological studies, and clinical and nutritional trials.

References

Abad MJ, Bedoya LM, Apaza L, Bermejo P (2012) The *Artemisia* L. genus: a review of bio-active essential oil. Molecules 17: 2542-2566

Adams JD, Garcia C (2006) Women's health among the Chumash. E CAM, pp. 1-7

Ahmad F, Khan RA, Rasheed S (1992) Study of analgesic and anti-inflammatory activity from plant extracts of *Lactuca scariola* and *Artemisia absinthium*. J Islam Acad Sci 5: 111-114

Ahmad W, Hasan A, Adullah A, Tarannum T (2010) Medicinal importance of *Artemisia absinthium* Linn (Afsanteen) in Unani medicine: a review. Hippoc J Unani Med 5(4): 117-125

Akhmedov IS, Kasymov SZ, Sidyakin GP (1970) Artabin- a new lactone from *Artemisia absinthium.* Chemist Nat Comp 6: 634

Ali M, Abbasi BH, Ihsan-ul-haq (2013) Production of commercially important secondary metabolites and antioxidant activity in cell suspension cultures of *Artemisia absinthium* L. Indust Crop Prod 49: 400-406

Allen PC, Lydon J, Danforth HD (1997) Effects of components of *Artemisia annua* on coccidia infections in chickens. Poult Sci 76(8): 1156-1163

Amat N, Upur H, Blazekovic B (2010) *In vivo* hepatoprotective activity of the aqueous extract of *Artemisia absinthium* L. against chemically and immunologically induced liver injuries in mice. J Ethnopharm 131(2): 478-484

Arab HA, Rahbari S, Rassouli A, Moslemi MH, Khosravirad F (2006) Determination of artemisinin in *Artemisia sieberi* and anticoccidial effects of the plant extract in broiler chickens. Trop Anim Healt Prod 38: 497-503

Bailen M, Julio LF, Diaz CE, Sanz J, Martinez-Diaz RA, Cabrera R, Burillo J, Gonzalez-Coloma A (2013) Chemical composition and biological effects of essential oils from *Artemisia absinthium* L. cultivated under different environmental conditions. Industr Crop Prod 49: 102-107

Bakkali F, Averbeck S, Averbeck D, Idaomar M (2008) Biological effects of essential oils-a review. Food Chem Toxicol 46: 446-475

Basta A, Tzakou O, Couladis M, Pavlovic M (2007) Chemical composition of *Artemisia absinthium* L. from Greece. J Essent Oil Res 19: 316-319

Baytop T (1984) *Therapy with Medicinal Plants in Turkey*. Istambul University Press, Istambul, Turkey, pp 166-167

Beauhaire J, Fourrey JL, Guittet E (1984) Structure of absintholide a new guaianolide dimer of *Artemisia absinthium* L. Tetrahedron Letters 25: 2751-2754

Behrens M, Brockhoff A, Kuhn C, Bufe B, Winnig M, Meyerhof W (2004) The human taste receptor hTAS2R14 responds to a variety of different bitter compounds. Biochem Biophy Res Commun 319(2): 479-485

Beigh YA, Ganai AM, Sheikh GG, Ahmad HA, Bilal S, Amin U, Mir MS (2017) Effect of feeding complete diet supplemented with feed additives alone and in combination on nutritional and hepatorenal function test profile in crossbred lambs. Haryana Vet 56(1): 58-62

Blumberger W, Glatzel H (1966) Contributions to the physiology of spices and condiments. VII. Research on the mechanism of action on salivary gland function. European Rev Nutr Diet 8(2): 145-160

Bone K (2003) *A Clinical Guide to Blending Liquid Herbs*. St Louis, Missouri: Churchill Livingstone

Bora KS, Sharma A (2010) Neuroprotective effect of *Artemisia absinthium* L. on focal ischemia and reperfusion induced cerebral injury. J Ethnopharmacol 129: 403-409

Bora KS, Sharma A (2011a) Evaluation of antioxidant and free-radical scavenging potential of *Artemisia absinthium*. Pharmaceu Bio 49(12): 1216-1223

Bora KS, Sharma A (2011b) The genus Artemisia: a comprehensive review. Pharmaceut Bio 49(1): 101-109

Bown D (1995) Encyclopedia of Herbs. Dorling Kindersley, London

Brattsand R (1975) Actions of vitamins A and E and some nicotinic acid derivatives on plasma lipids and on lipid infiltration of aorta in cholesterol-fed rabbits. Atherosclerosis 22: 47-61

Canadanovic-Brunet JM, Djilas SM, Cetkovic GS, Tumbas VT (2005) Free-radical scavenging activity of wormwood (*Artemisia absinthium* L) extracts. J Sci Food Agri 85(2): 265-272

Caner A, Doskaya M, Degirmenci A, Can H, Baykan S, Uner A, Basdemir G, Zeybek U, Guruz Y (2008) Comparison of the effects of *Artemisia vulgaris* and *Artemisia absinthium* growing in western Anatolia against trichinellosis (*Trichinella spiralis*) in rats. Exper Parasitol 119: 173-179

Chialva F, Liddle PAP, Doglia G (1983) Chemotaxonomy of wormwood (*Artemisia absinthum* L.) - I. Composition of the essential oil of several chemotypes. Zeitschrift für Lebensmittel-Untersuchung und Forschung 176(5): 363-366

Chiasson H, Belanger A, Bostanian N, Vincent C, Poliquin A (2001) Acaricidal properties of *Artemisia absinthium* and *Tanacetum vulgare* (Asteraceae) essential oils obtained by three methods of extraction. J Econ Entomol 94: 167-171

Chopra RN, Nayar SL, Chopra IC (1956) Glossary of Indian Medicinal Plants, NISCIAR, CSIR, New Delhi, pp. 25

Ciesla L, Kowalska I, Oleszek W, Stochmal A (2012) Free radical scavenging activities of polyphenolic compounds isolated from M*edicago sativa* and M*edicago truncatula* assessed by means of thin-layer chromatography DPPH rapid test. Phytochem Analy (http://dx.doi.org/10.1002/pca.2379)

Danilets MG, Belskii IP, Gurev AM, Belousov MV, Belskaia NV, Trofmova ES, Uchasova EG, Alhmedzhanov RR, Ligacheva AA, Iusbov MS, Agefonov VI (2010) Eûect of plant polysaccharides on TH1-dependent immune response: screening investigation. Eksp Klin Farmakol J 73(6): 19-22

Daradka HM, Badawneh M, Al-Jamal JA, Bataineh Y (2014) Hypolipidemic efficacy of *Artemisia absinthium* extracts in rabbits. World Appl Sci J 31(8): 1415-1421

Dianat M, Sadeghi N, Badavi M, Panahi M, Moghadam MT (2014) Protective effects of co-administration of gallic acid and cyclosporine on rat myocardial morphology against ischemia reperfusion. Jundishapur J Nat Pharma Prod 9(4): e17186

Donald DV (1981) Absinthium: a nineteenth-century drug of abuse. J Ethnopharmacol 4: 337-343

Dragan L, Titilincu A, Dan I, Dunca I, Dragan M, Mircean V (2010) Effects of *Artemisia annua* and *Pimpinella anisum* on *Eimeria tenella* (Phylum Apicomplexa) low infection in chickens. Scientia Parasitologica 11(2): 77-82

Dugas AJ, Castaneda-Acosta J, Bonin GC, Price KL, Fischer NH, Winston GW (2000) Evaluation of the total peroxyl radical-scavenging capacity of flavonoids: structure-activity relationships. J Nat Product 63: 327-331

Duke JA (2002) Handbook of Medicinal Herbs, 2nd edition. Boca Raton, Florida, CRC Press

Dulger B, Ceylan M, Alitsaous M, Ugurlu E (1999) Anti-microbial activity of *Artemisia absinthium* L. Turkish J Bio 23: 377-384

Erichsen-Brown C (1979) Use of Plants for the Past 500 Years. Aurora, Ontario, Canada

Erturk O, Uslu U (2007) Antifeedant, growth and toxic effects of some plant extracts on *Leptinotarsa decemlineata* (Say.) (Coleoptera, Chrysomelidae). Fresenius Environ Bulle 16(6): 601-607

Essawi T, Srour M (2000) Screening of some Palestinian medicinal plants for antibacterial activity. J Ethnopharmacol 70: 343-349

Fiamegos YC, Kastritis PL, Exarchou V, Han H, Bonvin AM, Vervoort J, Lewis K, Hamblin MR, Tegos GP (2011) Antimicrobial and efflux pump inhibitory activity of caffeoylquinic acids from *Artemisia absinthium* against Gram-positive pathogenic bacteria. PLOS ONE 6: 1-12

Garcia-Rodriguez JJ, Andres MF, Nez-Escribano AI, Julio LF, Burillo J, Bolas-Fernandez F, Gonzalez-Coloma A (2015) Selective nematocidal effects of essential oils from two cultivated *Artemisia absinthium* populations. Zeitschrift fur Naturforschung 70: 275-280

Gilani AUH, Janbaz KH (1995) Preventive and curative eûects of *Artemisia absinthium* on acetaminophen and CCl4-induced hepatotoxicity. Gen Pharmacol 26(2): 309-315

Goraev MI, Bazalitskaya US, Lishtvanova LN (1962) The terpene portion of the essential oil of *Artemisia absinthium*. Zeitschrift fur Naturforschung 35: 2799-2802

Greger H, Hofer O (1980) New unsymmetrical substituted tetrahydrofurofuran lignans from *Artemisia absinthium*. Assignment of the relative stereochemistry by lanthanide induced chemical shift. Tetrahedron 36: 3551-3558

Guarrera PM (2005) Traditional phytotherapy in central Italy (Marche, Abruzzo, and Latium). Fitoterapia 76: 1-25

Habibipour R, Rajabi M (2015) Antibacterial effects of Arctium lappa and Artemesia absinthium extracts in laboratory conditions. J HerbMed Pharmacol 4(4): 133-137

Hadi A, Hossein N, Shirin P, Najmeh N, Abolfazl M (2014) Anti-inflammatory and analgesic activities of *Artemisia absinthium* and chemical composition of its essential oil. Intern J Pharma Sci Rev Res 24(2): 237-244

HagerROM (2006) Absinthii herba. In Blaschek W, Ebel S, Hackenthal E, Holzgrabe U, Keller K, Reichling J, Schulz V, editors. Hagers Handbuch der Drogen und Arzneistoffe. Springer Medizin Verlag, Heidelberg

Hahn DY (1966) Biochemical studies on the constituents of *Artemisia masser-*schmidtiana Besser var. viridis Besser need to italicize some of these names and their derivatives. J Pharma Soc, Korea 10: 25-29

Halbert SE, Corsini D, Wiebe M, Vaughn SF (2009) Plant-derived compounds and extracts with potential as aphid repellents. Annal Appl Bio 154: 303-307

Hallal N, Kharoubi O, Benyettou I, Tair K, Ozaslan M, Aoues AEK (2016) *In vivo* amelioration of oxidative stress by *Artemisia absinthium* L. administration on mercuric chloride toxicity in brain regions. J Bio Sci 16: 167-177

Hoet S, Opperdoes F, Brun R, Quetin-Leclercq J (2004) Natural products active against African trypanosomes: a step towards new drugs. Nat Prod Rep 21: 353-364

Hold KM, Sirisoma NS, Ikeda T (2000) Alpha-thujone (the active component of absinthe): gammaaminobutyric acid type A receptor modulation and metabolic detoxifcation. Proc Nation Acad Sci United States of America 97: 3826-3831

Iqbal A, Tariq KA, Wazir VS, Singh R (2013) Antiparasitic efficacy of *Artemisia absinthium*, toltrazuril and amprolium against intestinal coccidiosis in goats. J Para Disea 37(1): 88-93

Irshad S, Butt M, Hira Y (2011) *In-vitro* antibacterial activity of two medicinal plants neem (*Azadirachta indica*) and peppermint. Intern Res J Pharma 1(1): 9-14

Jaenson TGT, Palsson K, Borg-Karlson AK (2005) Evaluation of extracts and oils of tick-repellent plants from Sweden. Med Vet Entomol 19: 345-352

Jaric S, Popovic Z, Macukanovic-Jocic M, Djurdjevic L, Mijatovic M, Karadzic B, Mitrovic M, Pavlovic P (2007) An ethnobotanical study on the usage of wild medicinal herbs from Kopaonik mountain (Central Serbia). J Ethnopharmacol 111: 160-175

Jeong-Dan C (2007) Chemical composition and antibacterial activity against oral bacteria by the essential oil of *Artemisia iwayomogi*. J Bacteriol Virol 37: 129-136

Jung EH, Lee JH, Kim SC, Kim YW (2015) AMPK activation by liquiritigenin inhibited oxidative hepatic injury and mitochondrial dysfunction induced by nutrition deprivation as mediated with induction of farnesoid X receptor. European J Nutr (doi: 10.1007/ s00394-015-1107-7)

Juteau F, Jerkovic I, Masotti V, Milos M, Mastelic J, Bessiere JM, Viano J (2003) Composition and antimicrobial activity of the essential oil of *Artemisia absinthium* from Croatia and France. Planta Medica 69(2): 158-161

Kaul VK, Nigam SS, Banerjee AK (1978) Insecticidal activity of some essential oils. Ind J Pharm Sci 40: 22

Kerboeuf D, Riou M, Guegnard F (2008) Flavonoids and related compounds in parasitic disease control. Mini-Rev Med Chem 8: 116-128

Khattak SG, Gilama SN, Ikram M (1985) Antipyretic studies on some indigenous Pakistani medicinal plants. J Ethnopharmacol 14: 45-51

Kim JH, Kim CH, Ko YD (2002) Influence of dietary addition of dried wormwood (*Artemisia* sp.) on the performance and carcass characteristics of Hanwoo steers and the nutrient digestibility of sheep. Asian-Australasian J Anim Sci 15: 390-395

Kim SC, Adesogan AT, Shin JH (2012) Effects of dietary addition of wormwood (*Artemisia montana* Pampan) silage on growth performance, carcass characteristics, and muscle fatty acid profiles of beef cattle. Anim Feed Sci Tech 177: 15-22

Kim SC, Adesogan AT, Kim, JH, Ko YD (2006) Influence of replacing rice straw with wormwood (*Artemisia montana*) silage on feed intake, digestibility and ruminal fermentation characteristics of sheep. Anim Feed Sci Tech 128: 1-13

KoYD, Kim JH, Adesogan AT, Ha HM, Kim SC (2006) The effect of replacing rice straw with dry wormwood (*Artemisia* sp.) on intake, digestibility, nitrogen balance and ruminal fermentation characteristics in sheep. Anim Feed Sci Tech 125: 99-110

Kordali S, Kotan R, Mavi A, Cakir A, Ala A, Yildirim A (2005) Determination of the chemical composition and antioxidant activity of the essential oil of *Artemisia dracunculus* and of the antifungal and antibacterial activities of Turkish *Artemisia absinthium*, *A. dracunculus*, *Artemisia santonicum*, and *Artemisia spicigera* essential oils. J Agri Food Chem 53(24): 9452-9458

Kostadinovic L, Levic J, Galonja-Coghill T, Ruzicic L (2012) Anticoccidian effects of the *Artemisia absinthium* L. extracts in broiler chickens. Archiva Zootechnica 15(2): 69-77

Koul MK (1997) Medicinal plants of Kashmir and Laddakh, Temperate and Cold arid Himalaya, Indus publishing company, FS-5, Tagore Garden, New Delhi, India.

Krebs S, Omer TN, Omer B (2010) Wormwood (*Artemisia absinthium*) suppresses tumour necrosis factor alpha and accelerates healing in patients with Crohn's disease - A controlled clinical trial. Phytomedicine 17(5): 305-309

Kreitmair H (1951) *Artemisia absinthium* L., the true wormwood. Die Pharmazie 6(1): 27-28

Lachenmeier DW (2010) Wormwood (*Artemisia absinthium* L.)-a curious plant with both neurotoxic and neuroprotective properties. J Ethnopharmacol 31(1): 224-277

Leite AM, Lima EO, de Souza EL, Diniz MF, Trajano VN, de Medeiros IA (2007) Inhibitory effect of â-pinene, á-pinene and eugenol on the growth of potential infectious endocarditis causing Gram-positive bacteria. Revista Brasileira de Ciencias Farmaceuticas 43: 121-126

Li Y, Ohizumi Y (2004) Search for constituents with neurotrophic factor-potentiating activity from the medicinal plants of paraguay and Thailand. J Pharma Soc Japan 124: 417-424

Liu KCSC, Yang SL, Roberts MF, Elford BC, Phillipson JD (1992) Antimalarial activity of *Artemisia annua* flavonoids from whole plants and cell cultures. Plant Cell Rep 11: 637-640

Martinez-Diaz R, Nez-Escribano AI, Burillo J, De Las Heras L, Del Prado G, Agullo-Ortuno MT, Julio LF, Gonzalez-Coloma A (2015) Trypanocidal, trichomonacidal and cytotoxic components of cultivated *Artemisia absinthium* Linnaeus (Asteraceae) essential oil. Memorias do Institute Oswaldo Cruz 110(5): 693-699

Mc Guffin M, Hobbs C, Upton R, Goldberg A (1997) American Herbal Products Association Botanical Safety Handbook, Boston, CRC Press

Mehrdad I, Seyed EA, Meysam MS (2007) Detection of sesquiterpene lactones in ten Artemisia species population of Khorasan provinces. Iranian J Basic Med Sci 10: 183-188

Mendiola J, Bousa M, Perez N, Hernandez H, Torres D (1991) Extracts of *Artemisia abrotanum* and *Artemisia absinthium* inhibit growth of *Naegleria fowleri in vitro*. Transac Royal Soc Tropical Med Hygiene 85: 78-79

Meschler JP, Howlett AC (1999) Thujone exhibits low affinity for cannabinoid receptors but fails to evoke cannabimimetic responses. Pharmacol Biochem Behav 62: 413-480

Mills S, Bone K (2000) Principles and Practice of Phytotherapy: Modern Herbal Medicine. London, Churchill Livingstone

Mohammadian A, Moradkhani S, Ataie S, Shayesteh TH, Sedaghat M, Kheiripour N, Ranjbar A (2016) Antioxidative and hepatoprotective effects of hydroalcoholic extract of *Artemisia absinthium* L. in rat. J Herbmed Pharmacol 5(1): 29-32

Moslemi HR, Hoseinzadeh H, Badouei MA, Kafshdouzan K, Fard RMN (2012) Antimicrobial activity of *Artemisia absinthium* against surgical wounds infected by *Staphylococcus aureus* in a rat model. Ind J Microbio 52(4): 601-604

Msaada K, Salem N, Bachrouch O, Bousselmi S, Tammar S, Alfaify A, Al-Sane K, Ammar WB, Azeiz S, Brahim AH, Hammami M, Selmi S, Limam F, Marzouk B (2015) Chemical composition and antioxidant and antimicrobial activities of Wormwood (*Artemisia absinthium* L.) essential oils and phenolics. J Chem article ID 804658:1-12

Na YY, Hyeung RK, Hae YC, Jae SC (2008) Antihyperlipidemic effect of edible brown algae, *Eclonia stolonifera* and its constituents on Poloxamer 407-Induced hyperlipidemic and cholesterol-fed rats. Archies Pharma Res 31(12): 1564-1571

Nalbantsoy A, Erel SB, Koksal C, Gocmen B, Yýldýz MZ, Karabay YN (2013) Viper venom induced inflammation with *Montivipera xanth*ina (Gray, 1849) and the anti-snake venom activities of *Artemisia absinthium* L. in Rat. Toxicon 65: 34–40

Nin S, Bennici A, Roselli G, Mariotti D, Schiff S, Magherini R (1997) Agrobacterium-mediated transformation of *Artemisia absinthium* L. (wormwood) and production of secondary metabolites. Plant Cell Rep 16(10): 725-730

Parekh HS, Liu G, Wei MQ (2009) A new dawn for the use of traditional Chinese medicine in cancer therapy. Molecular Cancer 8: 21

Parveen S, Godara R, Katoch R, Yadav A, Verma PK, Katoch M, Singh NK (2014) *In vitro* evaluation of ethanolic extracts of *Ageratum conyzoides* and *Artemisia absinthium* against cattle tick, *Rhipicephalus microplus*. The Scientific World J Article ID 858973 (http://dx.doi.org/10.1155/2014/858973)

Perez-Souto N, Lynch RJ, Measures G, Hann JT (1992) Use of high-performance liquid chromatographic peak deconvolution and peak labelling to identify antiparasitic components in plant extracts. J Chromatography 593: 209-215

Ramazani A, Sardari S, Zakeri S, Vaziri B (2010) *In vitro* antiplasmodial and phytochemical study of five Artemisia species from Iran and *in vivo* activity of two species. Parasitol Res 107(3): 593-599

Riahi L, Ghazghazi H, Ayari B, Aouadhi C, Klay I, Chograni H, Cherif A, Zoghlami N (2015) Effect of environmental conditions on chemical polymorphism and biological activities among *Artemisia absinthium* L. essential oil provenances grown in Tunisia. Ind Crop Prod 66: 96-102

Ruikar AD, Misar AV, Jadhav RB, Rojatkar SR, Mujumdar AM, Puranik VG, Deshpande NR (2011) Sesquiterpene lactone, a potent drug molecule from *Artemisia pallens* wall with anti-inflammatory activity. Arzneimittelforschung 61(9): 510-514

Saban K, Recep K, Ahmet M, Ahmet CAA, Ali Y (2005) Determination of the chemical composition and antioxidant activity of the essential oil of *Artemisia dracunculus* and of the anti-fungal and anti-bacterial activities of Turkish *Artemisia absinthium*, *Artemisia dracunculus*, *Artemisia santonicum*, and *Artemisia spicigera* essential oils. J Agri Food Chem 53: 9452-9458

Said HM (1982) Drugs used in liver diseases since ancient times. In: Diseases of the Liver: Greco-Arab Concepts, Hamdard Foundation Press, Karachi, pp. 100-131

Sansar W, Gamrani H (2013) The pharmacological effect of *Artemisia absinthium* extract in protecting adult rats against lead neurotoxicity. J Neurol Sci 333: e598

SCF (2003) Opinion of the Scientific Committee on Food (SCF) on thujone. <http://ec.europa.eu/food/fs/sc/scf/out162 en.pdf> (accessed 08.02.10)

Semnani KM, Akbarzadeh M (2005) Essential Oils Composition of Iranian *Artemisia absinthium* L. and *Artemisia scoparia* Waldst. J Essential Oil Res 17: 321-322

Shahnazi M, Azadmehr A, Hajiaghaee R, Mosalla S, Latif R (2015) Eûects of *Artemisia absinthium* L. extract on the maturation and function of dendritic cells. Jundishapur J Nat Pharm Prod 10(2): e20163

Sharopov FS, Sulaimonova VA, Setzer WN (2012) Composition of the Essential oil of *Artemisia absinthium* from Tajikistan. Rec Nat Prod 6(2): 127-134

Sherlock S (1998) Overview of chronic cholestatic conditions in adults: Terminology and definitions. Clin Liver Dis 2: 217-233

Singh OP, Tiwari SK, Ojha D (1994) Pilyriasis versicolor vis-a-vis sidhma and its ayurvedic management. Sadvitra Ayurveda 46(12): 920

Slepetys J (1975) Biology and biochemistry of wormwood: Accumulation dynamics of tannins, ascorbic acid, and carotene. Liet. TSR Mokslu Akad Darb, Ser C 1: 143-148

Squires JM, Ferreira JFS, Lindsay DS, Zajac AM (2011) Effects of artemisinin and Artemisia extracts on *Haemonchus contortus* in gerbils (*Meriones unguiculatus*). Vet Parasitol 175: 103-108

Taleb-Continil SH, Salvador MJ, Balanco JMF, Albuquerque S, De Oliveira DCR (2004) Antiprotozoal effect of crude extracts and flavonoids isolated from *Chromolaena hirsuta* (Asteraceae). Phytother Res 18: 250-254

Tariku Y, Hymete A, Hailu A, Rohloff J (2011) *In vitro* evaluation of antileishmanial activity and toxicity of essential oils of *Artemisia absinthium* and *Echinops kebericho*. Chem Biodivers 8(4): 614-623

Tariq KA, Chishti MZ, Ahmad F, Shawl AS (2009) Anthelmintic activity of extracts of *Artemisia absinthium* against ovine nematodes. Vet Parasitol 160(1-2): 83-88

Tucker O, Maciarello MJ, Sturtz G (1993) The essential oils of Artemisia ''Powis Castle'' and its putative parents, *A. absinthium* and *A. arborescens*. J Essential Oil Res 5: 239-242

Umpierrez ML, Lagreca ME, Cabrera R, Grille G, Rossini C (2012) Essential oils from Asteraceae as potential biocontrol tools for tomato pests and diseases. Phytochem Rev 1-12

Urban J, Kokoska L, Langrova I, Matejkova J (2008) *In vitro* anthelmintic effects of medicinal plants used in Czech Republic. Pharma Bio 46: 808-813

Valdes AFC, Martínez JM, Lizama RS, Vermeersch M, Cos P, Maes L (2008). *In vitro* anti-microbial activity of the Cuban medicinal plants *Simarouba glauca* DC, *Melaleuca leucadendron* L. and *Artemisia absinthium* L. Memorias do Instituto Oswaldo Cruz 103: 615-618

Wake G, Court J, Pickering A, Lewis R, Wilkins R, Perry E (2000) CNS acetylcholine receptor activity in European medicinal plants traditionally used to improve failing memory. J Ethnopharmacol 69: 105-114

Worku M, Franco R, Miller JH (2009) Evaluation of the activity of plant extracts in Boer goats. American J Anim Vet Sci 4: 72-79

Wright CW (2002) Artemisia. Taylor and Francis Inc., New York

Yin Y, Gong FY, Wu XX, Sun Y, Li YH, Chen T, Xu Q (2008) Anti-inflammatory and immuno-suppressive effect of flavones isolated from *Artemisia vestita*. J Ethnopharmacol 120: 1-6

Zafar MM, Hamdard ME, Hameed A (1990) Screening of *Artemisia absinthium* for anti-malarial effects on *Plasmodium berghei* in mice: a preliminary report. J Ethnopharmacol 30(2): 223-226

Zeng KW, Liao LX, Song XM, Lv HN, Song FJ, Yu Q, Dong X, Jiang Y, Tu PF (2015) Caruifolin D from *Artemisia absinthium* L. inhibits neuroinflammation via reactive oxygen species-dependent c-jun N-terminal kinase and protein kinase c/NF-êB signaling pathways. European J Pharm 767: 82-93.

□□□

Chapter 27

Herbal Galactogogues

Debashis Roy
Department of Animal Nutrition, College of Veterinary Science and Animal Husbandry, DUVASU, Mathura-281001, Uttar Pradesh, India, E-mail: debashis2k4@gmail.com

ABSTRACT

Galactogogues are the substances which augment established lactation. Effective use of single or combination of herbal galactogogue can improve the milk production without causing any toxic effect in animals. Many herbal plants like shatavari (*Asparagus racemosus*), ashwagandha *(Eutharia somnifera)*, fenugreek (*Trigonella foenumgraecum*), alfalfa (*Medicago sativa*), chaste berry (*Vitex agnus-castus*), dill (*Anethum graveolens*), goat's rue (*Galega officinalis*), milk thistle (*Silybumm arianum*), ashok *(Saraca indicalinn),* fennel (*Foeniculum vulgare*), nettle (*Urtica diotica*) and jivanti (*Leptadenia reticulata*) are mostly used as galactogouge in dairy animals alone or in combination. Main constraint of using these herbal preparation is the cost which limit their use in low producing animals. With progress in mentality of farmers and strategies of the Government, herbal preparation will get their market in near future.

Keywords: Galactogougues, Dairy animals, *Asparagus racemosus, Eutharia somnifera, Trigonella foenumgraecum.*

27.1 Introduction

The terms 'galactopoietics' or 'galactogogues' refers to the substances which augment established lactation. Medication or supplements exerting their effects through antagonism of dopamine receptors resulting in increased prolactin are galactogogues which are assisting initiation, maintenance and augmentation of maternal milk production. They act either by blocking hypothalamic dopaminergic receptors or by inhibiting dopamine producing neurons.

Progesterone falls and a full milk supply (lactogenesis) is initiated during parturition. An increase in prolactin level is needed to increase production. Herbal galactogogues are originated from medicinal plants that are used to augment milk production in animals as well as nursing mothers. Several herbal galactogogues have galactogenic effect. Effective feed management along with use of herbal agents to potentiate milk production would prompt a good augment in production potential in dairy herd. Several indigenous herbs possess galactoogenic properties and can safely be used to enhance milk production. These herbal agents have been tested in human medicine and also have proven ayurvedic strategies (Pattnaik, 2003). They are believed to exert action through the adreno-hypothalamo-hypophyseal-gonadal axis. Though the exact pharmacodynamics of mammogenic effects of these plants have not been authenticated, these have been used since long in human medicine. After the bitter experience of antibiotic and chemotherapeutic agents by the scientists'worldwide, now it is the turn of Ayurveda again to restore tissue functions in a natural way within the micro-environment of body physiology. There are many plants available with galactogenic and progenic properties.

27.2 Different Herbal Galactogogues

A wide variety of herbal plants contain good number of chemical active principles including alkaloids are having galactogenic property which helps the milking animals for augmenting milk production. Among these herbal plants; shatavari (*Asparagus racemosus*), ashwagandha *(Eutharia somnifera)*,fenugreek (*Trigonella foenum-graecum*), alfalfa (*Medicago sativa*), chaste berry (*Vitex agnus-castus*), dill (*Anethum graveolens*), goat's rue (*Galega officinalis*), milk thistle (*Silybumm arianum*), ashok *(Saraca indicalinn)*, fennel (*Foeniculum vulgare*), nettle (*Urtica diotica*) and jivanti (*Leptadenia reticulata*) are mostly used as galactogouge in human being while few of them are used in dairy animals alone or in combination. Effects of herbal galactogogues are discussed in details.

27.2.1 Shatavari *(Asparagus racemoscisliliaceac)*

The tuber root of shatavari is generally used in ayurvedic medicines. The root contains four steroids (saponin and shatavarin). It is generally recommended as nerve tonic, debilitation, and vitalizer. Significant increase in milk yield was observed by the use of herbal preparations containing Shatavari plant ingredients (Chopra *et al.*, 1956).Studies on the effect of herbal preparation on hypogalactic-crossbred cows revealed that the milk yield in treated group increased which might be due to Shatavari (Kirtikar and Basu, 1975). Studies on the effect of ayurvedic formulation containing Shatavari discerned improved appetite, digestion and resistance in the patients. There was marked effect on glucose level. The elevated glucose level helps in synthesis of milk in mammary gland (Vaidya and Kulkarni, 1991). This herb is seen in tropical and subtropical countries. Tanwar *et al.* (2008) reported overall increase in milk production by 1.06±0.17 kg daily in cattle and buffalo and increase in average milk production in buffaloes and cattle by 0.8±0.34 kg, 1.32±0.15 kg, respectively as compared to their previous production when fed with 50 gm shatavari root powder daily. Though its precise action as galactogogue has not been recommended, it is definite that the tuberous root has rejuvenation actions in the body and thus, can augment mammary gland proliferation and production potential.

27.2.2 Ashwagandha/ Winter Cherry *(Eutharia somnifera)*

This herb has been in ayurveda since 1000 A.D. The root has a strong pungent smell and bitter to taste and contains several alkaloids (0.13% to 4.30%), which offer medicinal usages. The root contains plenty of protein, calcium and phosphorus and iron i.e., every 100g of Ashwagandha carries 789.4 mg of iron. In addition, it also contains amino acids, like proline, tyrosine, tryptophan, alanine and lysine. The root, stem and fruits contain tannin and flabiroids. It has been recommended as a nerve tonic, heamatinic, and analgesic. Significant increase in milk yield was observed by the use of herbal preparations containing Ashwagandha plant ingredients (Chopra *et al.*, 1956). Studies on the effect of herbal preparation on hypogalactic-cross bred cows revealed that the milk yield in treated group increased which might be due to Ashwagandha (Kirtikar and Basu, 1975). There was markedeffect on glucose level. The elevated glucose level helps in synthesis of milk in mammary gland (Vaidya and Kulkarni, 1991). It increases vigour and vitality as it retards the geriatric changes in the body.

27.2.3 Fenugreek *(Trigonella foenumgraecum)*

Fenugreek is an important medicine in India's Ayurvedic tradition, where it is used to treat a variety of digestive and mucosal conditions (Passano, 1995; Escot 1994). Fenugreek supports the production of milk because it is rich source of essential fatty acids (Mowrey, 1986). Fenugreek seed contain saponins and protein (Mir *et al.*, 1997; Rao and Sharma, 1987). Saponin has been shown to decrease circulating cholesterol concentrations in many species, including rats (Petit *et al.*, 1993) and humans (Al-Habori and Raman, 1998; Sharma *et al.*, 1990). But its evaluation in dairy cows in scanty. Shah and Mir (2004) reported that feeding fenugreek seed improved profile of functional fatty acids ($P < 0.05$) in the milk, reduced blood cholesterol concentration (by 4% units more than the control diet) and produced lower concentrations in milk (1.48 vs. 1.83 mg/g milk lipid) in a 3-wk study with dairy cows, without altering milk flavour or taste and concluded that fenugreek seed could be used in dairy rations to improve milk characteristics.

27.2.4 Goat's Rue *(Galega officinalis)*

The legume genus Galega (tribe Galegeae) is generally considered to consist of six species distributed in Eurasia and North Africa. The geographical origin of the genus is not clear, but it seems to be located in Western Asia, and from there it was carried to Europe by Arabians or Hungarians, and later to the rest of the world (Heywood and Ball, 1968; Milne Redhead and Polhill, 1971). The species of agronomic importance are *Galega orientalis Lam.* and *Galega officinalis L.* The first is sometimes called "fodder galega", and the second "goat's rue", although some authors use "goat's rue" for both species. From ancient times it was known that *G. officinalis* forage increased the milk production of goats and other mammals (Castroviejo, 1999), and it is considered a medicinal herb (Duke, 1987). The lactogenic value attributed to *G. officinalis* makes it potentially interesting for animal production. Few studies have been found on its effects on milk production in cattle. Kudrna *et al.* (1992), Sharifyanov *et al.* (1996), and Bikbulatov *et al.* (1997) demonstrated an increase in milk production of cows when *G. officinalis* was included in their daily diet. Latvietis *et al.* (2002) described a higher production of milk in cows fed with *G. orientalis*. However, species of the genus *Galega* have been included in lists of poisonous plants for livestock in New Zealand (Parton and Bruere, 2002) and the United States (Di Tomaso, 1994). It stimulates the production performance of mammary gland. Animal studies show that this herb can increase milk supply upto 50%. French dairy farmers noted a 35-50% increase in their cow milk output when fed with it as a galactogogue. It reduces blood glucose level and can replace insulin therapy. Consumption in excess can cause nausea, vomition, irritation and inflammation of stomach and bowels. As it reduces blood glucose level, the herb should be used with caution.

27.2.5 Milk Thistle *(Silbanumm arianum)*

Milk thistle has been used historically to increase milk supply. The leaves are used to increase milk supply and build moderate estrogen levels. Vojtísek *et al.* (1991) reported increase in milk production by 7.7% in cows fed with milk thistle. The entire plant is edible and aids in digestion. It contains active principles like silydianin and silychristin, which are believed to have liver protective properties and also protects the heart. It should be given in the treatment of jaundice. One of its constituents does stimulate liver and gallbladder activity. It has a mild transient laxative effect in some individuals, which usually ceases within two to three days. Allergic reactions have not been reported for this herbal galactogogue.

27.2.5 Fennel *(Foeniculum vulgare)*

Ayurveda recommends this drug as a galactogogue. Fennel is a common herbal galactogogue and is used in promoting milk ejection reflex. The seeds of fennel are related to improve milk supply. Although clinical evidence for its efficacy is lacking, Till date its mechanism of action is not clear (Weed, 1986). It has mild estrogenic properties (Bingel and Farnsworth, 1991). Fennel contains essential fatty acids, flavonoids, vitamins, minerals and volatile oils. Fennel is bitter to taste. Seeds and herbs are important for stimulating the release of digestive juices for improving digestibility of nutrients (Bove and Romm, 1997; Gladstar, 1993). Fennel seed or fennel oil has no known adverse effects but it is recommended for use not more than a few weeks at a time (Blumenthal *et al.*, 2000). In case of women the fennel is a commonly used galactogogue. It promotes the milk ejection reflex, rather than actually increasing milk supply. In one study, Torabi Gudarzi *et al.* (2008) found that average daily milk yield in Holstein Friesian cows were increased by 15.4 % litre compared to control group when fed with herbal mixture containing funnel and concluded that medicinal plants mixture was effective in galactopoesis of dairy cows.

27.2.6 Nettles *(Urtica diotica)*

Nettles include two families of the herb i.e., Stinging nettle (Utica dioica) and Nettle leaf (Urticaurens). Stinging nettle leaf is one of the less used herbal galactogogue among the community participant in Africa. Though stinging nettle has a long standing reputation for enriching milk (Gladstar, 1993; Weed, 1986; Yarnell, 1998). The herb is believed to be completely non-toxic (Yarnell, 1998). It is rich in trace minerals like iron, calcium and vitamins like A, C and K including phosphorus, potassium, sulphur and vitamin-D, and promotes milk production (Weed, 1986; Lieberman, 1995). It also contains B-complex vitamins and appreciable amounts of magnesium. It contains up to 20% mineral salts, mainly calcium, potassium, silicon and niyrates (Blumenthal *et al.*, 2000). Nettle extracts contain all of the essential amino acids. Nettle is believed to support lactation by providing essential nutrients (Weed, 1986). It has no medicinal action apart from being mildly diuretic and haemostatic (Bradley, 1992). Dried nettle mixed into cattle fodder are known to boost milk production in cows (Grieve, 1971; Phillips and Fov, 1990). Nettle is used to support lactation and nettle leaves are typically brewed as a tea, often in combination with raspberry leaf.

27.2.7 Jivanti (*Leptadenia reticulata*)

Jivanti (*Leptadenia reticulata*), belonging to family Asclepiadaceae is well known for its tonic, restorative and stimulant property in the Indian system of medicine. This plant is distributed in the Southern parts of India. *L. reticulata* is a much branched twining shrub. The bark is yellowish brown, corky, deeply cracked; the leaves are ovate-cordate, coriaceous glabrous above, more or less finely pubescent beneath; the flowers are in many-flowered cymes, greenish yellow; the follicles are sub-woody and turgid. The main constituents reported are stigmasterol, β – itosterol, flavonoids, pregnane glycosides and proteins. Presence of triterpenes and steroids were also reported. Aerial parts of *Leptadenia reticulata* is reported to contain tocopherol and possess several pharmacological activities such as galactogogue, antimicrobial and anti-inflammatory activity (Sathiyanarayanan *et al.*, 2007).

Jivanti is considered a stimulant and tonic in Ayurvedic literature. Its medicinal use dates back to 4500 to 1600 B.C, as mentioned in the Atharvaveda. Its lactogenic effect has been reported in various domestic animals (Dadarkar *et al.*, 2005). *Leptadenia reticulata* has been shown to increase milk production without affecting milk composition (Anjuaria and Gupta, 1967). Galog is a herbal preparation which contain *Leptadenia reticulate* as the main component and it may be attributed to certain metabolic changes in their body tissues and the mammary gland, where the absorbed nutrients are utilized more effectively (Thakur 1977).

27.2.8 Ashok *(Saraca indicalinn)*

This herb is very common in tropical region. Active principles like haemato-quiline, tannin, glycosides, saponins, pegenin, sayanidin, calcium, iron are enriched in the seed, bark, root and flowers of the herb. In human medicine all the parts of the herb are used to tune the cyclic activity of ovary and to maintain tonicity of uterus and breast. Thus, the herb is a best female vitalizer.

27.2.9 Alfalfa *(Medicago sativa)*

Alfalfa is generally used as high quality fodder to dairy animal. Alfalfa is used to increase appetite, vitality and helps in water retention and can reduce cholesterol level in animals with high fat diets. It also boost milk production as it is high in various nutrients, high in protein and contains vitamins like A, B_1, B_{12}, B_6, C, E, K_1 along with minerals like calcium, potassium, phosphorus, iron and zinc. This is a valuable and effective pregnancy herb and great blood builder.

27.2.10 Chaste Berry *(Vitex agnus-castus)*

Vitex is a small shrub native to Greece and Italy. Chaste berry has a normalizing effect on the progesterone function of the pituitary gland. Vitex stimulates prolactin production and is used for nursing mothers to increase milk supply (Tierra, 1983; Gladstar, 1993; Bove and Romm, 1997; Crawfrod, 1997; Hobbs, 1997). Some study also reported that vitex has negative impact on milk production and hence, it should not be recommended as a galactogogue (Bone, 1994; Harrar and Altshul, 1999; Presser, 2000). Most of the reported studies are on human being. Animal trials may be done to see their effects of milk production performance in animals.

27.2.11 Dill *(Anethum graveolens)*

Dill is a well-known galactogogue in human being and it has the properties of antispasmodic, diuretic, antiflatulentand is used in colic. The oil and tea are used for their antifoaming action and appetite stimulant. It is contraindicated in low salt diet, as it is high in sodium.

27.3 Combination of Herbal Mixture

In present days different combinations of herbal preparation are in use to stimulate milk production and overall activities of dairy animals. Several studies were conducted to see their potentiality. Ruchamax is one of the herbal formulations, which contains 28 different herbs and some minerals. The ingredients of Ruchamax include *Allium sativum, Azadirachta indica, Calotrophis orocera, Centratherum anthelmenticum, Commiphoramukul, Ecliptaelba, Embelicaribes, Picorrhiza kurora, Zinziber officinale and Piper longum*, etc. It is used as an appetizer, restorative, carminative, stomachic and tonic. Payapro is another herbal preparation which is a combination of *Leptadeniareticulata, Nigella sativa, Foeniculam vulgare, Pueraria tuberosa, Glycerrizag lobra, Cuminum cyminum and Asparagus racemosus* etc. All these herbs are known to possess galactopoietics action (ICMR, 1987). Bhatt *et al.* (2009) reported that the use of herbal preparations increased the average milk production in lactating cows, which was highest (11.8 L/day) in ruchamax supplemented and moderate (9.3 L/day) in payapro supplemented as compared to control animals (7.1 L/day). They concluded that herbal preparations can increase milk yield in lactating dairy cows through improving their rumen environment. In another study, a significant higher ($P<0.05$) total milk yield (14.24 %) of treatment group was recorded in lactating surti buffalo which was supplemented with a poly-herbal galactogogue biscuits without altering on milk compositions (Patel *et al.*, 2013).

References

Al-Habori M, Raman A (1998) Antidiabetic and hypocholesterolaemic effects of fenugreek: Review. Phytother Res 12: 233–242

Anjaria JV, Gupta I (1967) Studies on lactogenic properties of Leptadeniareticulata and Leptaden tablets in goats, sheep, cows and buffaloes. Indian Vet J 44: 967-974

Bhatt N, M Singh and A Ali (2009) Effect of feeding herbal preparations on milk yield and rumen parameters in lactating crossbred cows. Int J Agric Biol 11: 721–726

Bikbulatov ZG, Zainutdinov FA, Sharifyanov BG (1997) Feeds from goats' rue in diets for cows. Kormoporizvodstvo 7: 28-31

Bingel AS, Farmsworth MR (1991) Higher plants as potential sources of galactagogues. Econ Med Plant Res 6: 1-14

Blumenthal M, A Goldberg, A Brinkmann, J Eds (2000) Herbal medicine: Expanded commission E monographs. Austin, Tex : American Council

Bone K (1994) VitexAgnusCastus. Eu J Herbal Med. 1: 2

Bove M, Romm A (1997) Herbs for pregnant and lactating women.8th annual AHG symposium, Oct. 17-20

Bradley PR (1992) British Herbal compendium.Vol.1.Borhe Mouth, British Herbal Medicine Association

Castroviejo S (1999) Flora Iberica. Vol. VII Leguminosae. Madrid, Real JardínBotánico, CSIC. 578 p

Chopra RN, Nayar SL Chopra IC (1956) Effect of some herbal preparations as galactogogue in milch animals. Glossary of Indian Medicinal Plants, CSIR Publication, New Delhi

Crawford AM (1997) Herbal Remedies for Women, MNIMH California Prima publishing

Dadarkar SS, Deore MD, Gatne M (2005) Preliminary Evaluation of a Polyherbal Formulation for Its Galactogogue Properties in PrimiparousWistar Rats. J Bombay Vet Coll 13 (1&2): 50-53

Di Tomaso, JM (1994) Plants reported to be poisonous to animals in the United States. Vet Human Toxicol 36: 49-52

Duke JA (1987) CRC Handbook of medicinal herbs. Boca Ratón, CRC Press

Duke JA (1992) Handbook of Phytochemical Constituents of GRAS Herbs and Other Economic Plants. Florida: CRC Press, Florida

Escot N (1994) Fenugreek. Atoms: 7-12

Gladstar R (1993) Herbal healing for women, New York, NY: Simon Schuster

Grieve M (1971) A Modern Herbal [reproduction of the 1931 original]. New York, NY, Dover

Harrar S, Altshul ODS (1999) The Women's Book of Healing Herbs. Rodale Press

Heywood VH, Ball, PW (1968) Leguminosae. In: Tutin, T., V. Heywood, N. Burges, D. Moore, D. Valentine, S. Walters, D. Webb. ed. Flora Europaea, Vol. 2. Cambridge, Cambridge University Press. Pp. 86-93

Hobbs C (1997)The Women's Herb, California Botanica University

ICMR (1987) *Medicinal Plants of India*. Indian Council of Medical Research, New Delhi, India.Indiastat.com:http://www.indiastat.com/agriculture/2/milkanddairyproducts/167/sta ts.aspx (accessed on 13/05/2017)

Kirtikar KP, Basu BD (1975) Effect of herbal preparation on hypogalactic cross breed cows. In: Indian Medicinal Plants, 2nd Edn., Periodical Express, New Delhi

Kudrna V, Rendla J, Markalous E (1992) Stimulation of milk production by feeding with Galegaofficinalis L Fytotechnicka Rada 9: 254

Ladstar R (1993) Herbal healing for women., Simon and Schuster, New York

Latvietis J, Drikis J, Auzins V, Trupa A, Kaldmae H (2002) Some types of grass silage used in feeding cows. Proceedings of the Animal Nutritions Conference, Tartu, Estonia. Pp. 7-15

Lieberman, L (1995) Remedies to file for future reference. Birth kit, 5 (spring): 1

Milne-Redhead, E, Polhill RM (1971) Flora of tropical East Africa. Part 4. London. Pp. 505-1108

Mir Z, Acharya SN, Mir PS, Taylor WG, Zaman MS, Mears GJ., Goonewardene LA (1997) Nutrient composition, in vitro gas production and digestibility of fenugreek (*Trigonellafoenum-graecum*) and alfalfa forages. Can J Anim. Sci 77: 119–124

Mishra, UK, Kanesh JS, Mandal AK, Das RK, Rayaguru K, Parija SC (2006) Potentials of herbal galactogogues in milk production in ruminants. The Indian Cow. July to Sep. Pp. 44-52

Mowrey, DB (1986) The scientific validation of herbal medicine. New camaan, Keats, pp: 276-293

Parton K, Bruere AN (2002) Plant poisoning of livestock in New Zealand. New Zealand Vet J 50(3): Suppl. 22-27

Passano, P (1995) The many uses of methi. Namushi 3: 31-34

Patel MD, Tyagi KK, Sorathiya LM, Fulsoundar AB (2013) Effect of polyherbal galactogogue supplementation on milk yield and quality as well as general health of Surti buffaloes of south Gujarat. Vet World 6(4): 214- 218, doi:10.5455/vetworld. 2013. 214-218

Pattnaik AK (2003) Effect of herbal additives on lactating ruminants with or without subclinical mastitis, Thesis submitted to Orissa university of Agriculture and Technology, Bhubaneswar (Orissa) India.

Petit P, Sauvaire Y, Ponsin G, Manteghetti M, Fave A, Ribes G (1993) Effects of a fenugreek seed extract on feeding behaviour in the rat: Metabolic-endocrine correlates. Pharmacol Biochem Behav 45: 369–374

Phillips R, Fov N (1990) The Random House Book of Herbs. Random House, New York.

Presser K (2000) Arthur M.D. Pharmacists Guide to Medicinal Herbs. Smart Publications.

Rao, R. U. and R. D. Sharma. 1987. An evaluation of protein quality of fenugreek seeds (*Trigonellafoenumgraecum*) and their supplementary effects. Food Chem 24: 1–7

Sathiyanarayanan L, Arulmozhi S, Chidanbaranathan N (2007) Anticarcinogenic activity of Leptadeniareticulata against Dalton's Ascitic Lymphoma. Iranian J Pharmacol. & Therapeutics 6: 133-135

Shah MA, Mir PS (2004) Effect of dietary fenugreek seed on dairy cow performance and milk characteristics. Can J Anim Sci 84(4): 725-729

Sharif yanov BG, Kharrasov R. M, Khaziakhmetov FS (1996) Goat's rue (*Galega officinalis*) in rations for cows. Zootekhniya 5: 15-16

Sharma RD, Raghuram TC, Sudhakar RN (1990) Effect of fenugreek seeds in blood glucose and serum lipids in type I diabetes. Eur J Clin Nutr 44: 301–306

Tanwar PS, Rathore SS, Kumar Y (2008) Effect of shatavari (*Asparagus recemosus*) on milk production in dairy animals. Indian J Anim Res 42(3):232-233

Thakur, SS (1977) Effect of Galog on milk production and feed intake, M. Sc dissertation, Kurukshetra University, published by NDRI.

Tierra M (1983) The Way of Herbs. Washington Square Press, C.A.M.D., New York.

TorabiGudarzi M, Qarah GL, Faramarz Y, Abu A, Akbari H (2008) Investigation on to the effect of fennel (*Foeniculum vulgare*) and nigella (*Nigella sativa*) on production in milking cow. http://agris.fao.org/agris-search/search.do? Record ID= IR2010000035

Vaidya K, Kulkarni PH (1991) A study of an Ayurvedic formula. Jivak. J. Beorghaya Int., 7(1): 20

Vojtísek B, Hronová B, Hamrík J, Janková B (1991) Milk thistle (*Silybumm arianumi, L., Gaertn.*) in the feed of ketotic cows.Vet Med (Praha) 36(6): 321-330

Weed S (1986) Wise Woman Herbal for the Child Bearing Year. New York, Ash Tree, pp. 128-276

Yarnell E (1998) Stinging nettle: A modern view of our ancient healing plant. Alter. Complther 4: 180-186.

□□□

Chapter 28

Mojave Yucca (*Yucca schidigera*)

Ravindra Kumar[1] and Pankaj Kumar Singh[2]

[1] Division of Animal Nutrition and Product Technology, ICAR-Central Institute for Research on Goats, Makhdoom -281122, India, E-mail: ravindra.srivastava@gmail.com

[2] Department of Animal Nutrition, Bihar Animal Sciences University, Patna - 800014, India

ABSTRACT

Yucca schidigera (YS), also named as yucca, is a tropical plant which has been used to treat inflammatory illnesses effectively since long time. *Yucca schidigera* is a rich source of saponin and phytochemicals such as steroidal saponins, polyphenolics *viz.* resveratrol and some other stilbenes including yuccaols A, B, C, D and E. Extract of the plant has potential of improving feed conversion efficiency thus enhancing animal growth, ameliorating the environmental pollution and participating in microbial activity modification. Yucca has been claimed to reduce the methane and ammonia emission during enteric fermentation of feeds during rumen digestion process.

Keywords: *Yucca schidigera*, Saponin, Yuccaols, Methane, Livestock.

28.1 Introduction

Plants containing saponins have been widely used as feed additives in the animal feeding system. A desert plant from Mexico *Yucca schidigera* and its extract (Yucca extract, YE) have been used commercially as a source of saponins. *Yucca* genus of perennial shrubs and trees in the family Asparagaceae, subfamily Agavoideae. Its 40-50 species are notable for their rosettes of evergreen, tough, sword-shaped leaves and large terminal panicles of white or whitish flowers. They are native to the hot and dry (arid) parts of the Americas and the Caribbean. *Yucca schidigera* is native to the southwestern United States and Mexico. Currently, most commercial production of yucca products takes place in Mexico where the plants are harvested by farmers and transported to processing plants. The succulent trunk (yucca logs) is the part used. The logs are mechanically macerated, and either dried and ground to produce 100% yucca powder, or the macerated material is subjected to mechanical squeezing in a press, producing yucca juice. The juice is concentrated by evaporation, and the concentrated product referred to as YE. Yucca extract (YE) is used as a feed additive to reduce ammonia and faecal odours in animal excreta. Saponins, by virtue of their surfactant properties, have anti-protozoal activity, and they have membranolytic properties; they complex with cholesterol in protozoal cell membranes, causing celllysis. They have antibacterial activity, and modify ruminal fermentation by suppressing ruminal protozoa and selectively inhibiting some bacteria. Ruminal ammonia concentrations are reduced. YE is used for prevention and treatment of arthritis in horses, although convincing evidence of its efficacy has not been reported. Saponins influence absorption of lipids, through formation of micelles with bile salts and cholesterol in the intestine.

Yucca schidigera (YS), also named as yucca, is valued since long as it was used to treat inflammatory illnesses effectively (Cheeke 2000). Being a tropical plant, YS originally grows in North America, especially in arid Mexican dessert (Cheeke *et al.*, 2006). With regard to nutritional beneficial effects, *Yucca schidigera* extracts (YSE) has potential of improving feed conversion efficiency thus enhancing animal growth, ameliorating the environmental pollution and participating in microbial activity modification (e.g., anti-protozoal activity) (Piacente *et al.*, 2005 and Cheeke *et al.*, 2006).

28.2 Taxonomy

Kingdom	:	Plantae
Phylum	:	Tracheophyta
Class	:	Liliopsida
Order	:	Asparagales
Family	:	Asparagaceae
Genus	:	Yucca
Species	:	*Yucca schidigera*

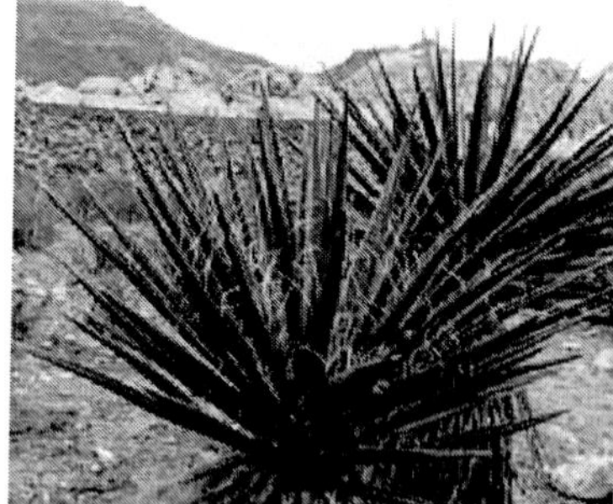

28.3 Chemical Composition of *Yucca schidigera*

Yuccas are widely grown as ornamental plants in gardens. Many species also bear edible parts, including fruits, seeds, flowers, flowering stems, and more rarely roots. Roots of soap tree yucca (*Yucca elata*) are high in saponins and are used as a shampoo in Native American rituals. Dried yucca leaves and trunk fibers have a low ignition temperature, making the plant desirable for use in starting fires via friction. In rural Appalachian areas, species such as *Yucca filamentosa* are referred to as "meat hangers". The tough, fibrous leaves with their sharp-spined tips were used to puncture meat and knotted to form a loop with which to hang meat for salt curing or in smoke houses. The flower petals are eaten. The petals are blanched for just 5 minutes, and then cooked *a la mexicana* (with tomato, onion, chile) or in *tortitas con salsa* (egg-battered patties with green or red sauce).

Yucca (*Yucca schidigera*) is a rich source of phytochemicals with promising bioactive functions (Francis *et al.*, 2006), YS has several components such as steroidal saponins, polyphenolics (e.g., resveratrol and some other stilbenes including yuccaols A, B, C, D and E) (Cheeke *et al.*, 2006; Headon *et al.*, 1991; Patel, 2012). With 10% of steroidal saponins in its stem dry matter (Kaneda *et al.*, 1987) YS has been perceived as one of the two major commercial saponin sources, the other one is *Quillaia saponaria*. Saponins have been considered to be vital components of YS in odor control in intensive farming industry (Matusiak *et al.*, 2016; Xu *et al.*, 2010). The 3-dimensional spatial orientation, its lipophilic aglycon, and the sugar composition all together contribute to the biological properties of YS (Miyakoshi *et al.*, 2000). In addition, new steroidal saponins with different structures included in YS have been detected continuously (Miyakoshi *et al.*, 2000; Oleszek *et al.*, 2001 and Kowalczyk *et al.*, 2011).

28.4 Application of Yucca in Ruminant's Ration

Yucca has been claimed to reduce the methane and ammonia emission during enteric fermentation of feeds during rumen digestion process. Methane suppressing effects of steroidal saponins containing plants like YSE specifically is through the inhibition of the growth of H_2-producing bacteria (Wallace *et al.*, 1994; Wang *et al.*, 1998). Ciliate protozoa, which provides substrate (H_2) for methanogens (Stumm *et al.*, 1986; Ushida *et al.*, 1997) is associated with 9-25% of ruminal methanogens (Newbold *et al.*, 1995). Reduced methane emission due to saponin addition is regarded as the result of its toxicities towards protozoa population (Holtshausen *et al.*, 2009; Guo *et al.*, 2008). The symbiotic relationship between methanogens and protozoa in the ruminal environment accounts at least partially for decrease in methane production due to YSE inclusion in diets (Zijderveld *et al.*, 2011). When YSE is added in diets, the balance between meth-anogens and protozoa would be broken which will lead to meth-anogens reduction, and eventually influence the production of the emitting methane (Lila *et al.*, 2005). During the process of feed fermentation if there is more production of propionic acid there is reduction in methane production (Pen *et al.*, 2006). *S. ruminantium*, the most predominant bacterium in the process of succinate decarboxylation, accounts for the majority of propionate yield in the rumen (Wolin *et al.*, 1988). Strobel *et al.* (1989) and Narvaez *et al.* (2013) further noticed that *S. ruminantium* were significantly increased with YSE supplementation, indicating a positive transaction of microbial population towards those propionate-producing bacteria. According to Lila *et al.* (2003), YSE addition can only decrease protozoal populations at 6 h of fermentation in *in vitro* batch cultures since samples collected at 24 h had no detectable protozoa. It seems that YSE has a short lived effect on protozoa *in vitro*, which gives us a partly explanation about reduction of methane with YSE addition.

Table 1: Effect of YSE addition on methane production and rumen fermentation in ruminants

Animals	Dose	Results	Reference
***In vitro* studies**			
Dairy Cows	0 or 110 g/kg	CH_4 production at 24 h was reduced	Xu *et al.* (2010)
Dairy Cows	0, 5, 10 or 15 g cow/d (Sarsaponin)	Rumen NH_3-N levels tended (P=0.06) to decrease with increased YSE level.	Singer *et al.* (2008)
Dairy Cows	0, 1.2, 1.8, 2.4, 3.2 g/L (Sarsaponin)	Fermentation of soluble potato starch (P<0.05) corn starch (P<0.05), or hay plus concentrate (P<0.05) decreased CH_4 production with the concentration of sarsaponin increased.	Lila *et al.* (2003)
Dairy Cows	0, 2, 4, and 6 mL/L	Rate and extent of CH_4 production were reduced (P<0.001) by YSE addition in a	Pen *et al.* (2006)

	(80-100 g/kg saponin)	dose-dependent manner by up to 42% and up to 32%.	
Dairy Cows	650 µg/ml (100 µg/mL steroidal sapogenin)	YSE treatments decreased CH_4 production when measured as per unit of DM (P<0.05).	Narvaez *et al.* (2013)
Dairy Cows	1, 20 and 100 mg/kg DM (sarsaponin)	Substantive effects of the saponin-rich products on ruminal nitrogen metabolism (CH_4, ruminal NH_3 level) were observed only at doses exceeding those recommended by the manufacturers.	Sliwinski *et al.* (2002a)
Dairy Cows	15, 30, 45 g/kg DM	Methane production *in vitro* was lowered (P<0.05)	Holtshausen *et al.* (2009)
Sheep	0, 2, 4, 6, 8 mg/mL (saponins: 44 g/kg DM)	CH_4 production was reduced (P<0.05).	Rira *et al.* (2015)
***In vivo* studies**			
Dairy Cows	10 g/kg of DM (6.0% saponin)	Methane *in vivo* was not affected either at low or high supplementations.	Holtshausen *et al.* (2009)
Steers	0, 11.2, 22.4 g (sarsaponin)	Approximately 12.7% of CH_4 was inhibited (P<0.05).	Lila *et al.* (2005)
Lambs	2 and 30 mg/kg DM (sarsaponin)	CH_4 production was not affected (P>0.05).	Sliwinski *et al.* (2002b)
Lambs	120 ppm	NH_3-N was not affected (P>0.05).	Santoso *et al.* (2004)
Lambs	240 ppm	Ruminal NH_3 concentration was decreased (P<0.05), urinary N was lowered (P<0.01).	Santoso *et al.* (2006)
Lambs	14 mL (1.31-1.64 g of saponins /wether/d)	NH_3-N and total VFA concentrations declined (P<0.001) with administration YSE.	Pen *et al.* (2007)
Lambs	100, 200, 300 mg/kg	Ruminal NH_3 concentration was decreased (P<0.05).	Liu *et al.* (2007)
Sheep	170 mg/d	NH_3-N concentrations was lowered (P<0.05).	Wang *et al.* (2009)
Sheep	0, 100, 200, 300 mg/kg	The 200 and 300 mg/kg YSE groups have a suppressing effect on ruminal NH_3 concentration (P<0.05) than control.	Liu *et al.* (2011)
Sheep	0, 1.5, 3.0, 4.5, 6.0 g/d of saponins	CH_4 emissions were not affected (P>0.05).	Canul-Solis *et al.* (2014)

(Adopted from Sun *et al.*, 2017)

The pH value is another factor that has an impact on YSE function on the reduction of methane production in rumen. In general, reduction of methane production entails an alteration in total VFA concentration (Cieslak *et al.*, 2012)which relates strongly with the acetate/propionate ratio, and this ratio is dependent partly on pH (Rira *et al.*, 2015). Cardozo *et al.* (2005) observed that YSE increased the proportion of propionate at pH 5.5, but not at pH 7.0 in *in vitro* rumen environment. CO_2, an end product of lactate fermentation to propionate, may contribute to the increasing of total gas production. It is suggested that with the increasing of sarsaponin levels in rumen, CO_2 would be generated through succinate:propionate pathway (Lila *et al.*, 2003).

Effect of YSE supplementation on methane and rumen fermentation is presented in table 1. A number of studies have been conducted both *in vitro* as well as *in vivo* involving cattle and sheep. Results were quite variable depending upon dose of YSE, feed substrate, animal species, etc. Singer *et al.* (2008) reported that with increased feeding of YSE to lactating dairy cows, 4 h and 24 h gas production generated through these collected rumen fluids were increased, exhibiting a strong linear effect ($P<0.05$). A similar result was observed in another *in vitro* experiment which involved different ruminal substrates including soluble potato starch, cornstarch, or hay plus concentrate (1.5:1) in the incubation process (Lila *et al.*, 2003). Total gas productions at 6 h and 24 h were increased as dietary sarsaponin increased from 1.2 to 3.2 g/L, and the methane reduction rate was statistically upto different substrates. Methane production was decreased ($P<0.05$) by YSE addition in both gas production rate (mL/min) and extent (L) (Pen *et al.*, 2006). Xu *et al.* (2010) reported that methane production at 24 h was decreased ($P<0.05$) by 110 g/kg of YSE addition, although *in vitro* gas production was not affected. Holtshausen *et al.* (2009) reported that in order to avoid the potential side effects of YSE on ruminal fermentation and feed digestion, saponin levels were reduced (10 g/kg of DM) that resulted in a non-significant difference of methane production *in vitro* among different treatments. However, when sarsaponin concentration was 1% of DM (22.4 g), YSE addition in diets resulted gas reduction in steers effectively, in which methane was inhibited by approximately 12.7% ($P<0.05$) from day 6 to day 9 of the 10 days feeding period without impairing animal performance (Lila *et al.*, 2005).

Zijderveld *et al.* (2011) reported that YSE supplementation of 3 g/kg of DM did not reduce methane production in lactating dairy cows. Similar results were also observed by Li and Powers, 2012 reported that even the 1.5% YSE inclusion groups failed to alter either methane, or ammonia, or nitrous oxide emissions on a daily basis (per unit DMI) in steers. Methanol extract of YSE was used in an experiment *in vitro*, and YSE decreased ($P<0.05$) methane production when calculated by per unit of dry matter, but not by per unit of true digested dry matter (Narvaez *et al.*, 2013).

Results of YSE supplementation were also variable when sheep was used as experimental animal. *In vitro* supplementation of sarsaponin (100 mg/kg dietary of DM) showed reduction in the ruminal ammonia over 21% throughout the measurements from day 5 to day 10 (Sliwinski *et al.*, 2002a). In the subsequent *in vivo* study, addition of 2 and 30 mg/kg of DM YSE in the diets resulted in to slight trends to reduced gas emission without statistical effect over a 15 days period (Sliwinski *et al.*, 2002b). Feeding the diets with 120 ppm YSE in sheep resulted into reduced N losses in urine and total N losses, leading to a 50% higher retained N, and ammonia N concentration was lowered by 11.9% although not significant (Santoso *et al.*, 2004). In the subsequent experiment supplementation of YSE in the basal diet (240 ppm DM per day) with 14 days dietary YSE feeding, YSE reduced rumen ammonia N concentrations ($P<0.05$) in Cheviot wethers in comparison to the control diet (Santoso *et al.*, 2006). Liu et al.(2007) reported that at 4 h and 6 h after feeding YSE-containing diets (300 mg/kg) in sheep, propionate concentration was increased and acetic concentration was lowered, but neither of them changed significantly. Liu *et al.* (2007) reported that at 2 h after feeding YSE-containing diets (300 mg/kg), protozoan population was decreased ($P<0.05$) and ammonia concentration increased. When supplementing 170 mg/d YSE with two other additives (flavomycin and ropadiar) in sheep diets, rumen liquor samples were taken on the day 9 and day 11, and gas production from the sheep was measured from day 12 to day 14. Results indicated an increase in VFA concentration and a decrease in acetate: propionate ratio ($P<0.05$), while ammonia N concentration ($P<0.05$) and average methane production ($P<0.05$) were reduced compared to the control (Wang *et al.*, 2009). A later experiment *in vivo* reported that ruminal ammonia concentration, ammonia N concentration and protozoa population in sheep were suppressed especially by the 200 and 300 mg/kg YSE treatment groups in the experimental conditions where dietary YSE levels were 100, 200, 300 mg/kg (Liu *et al.*, 2011).

Canul-Solis et al. (2014) reported that methane production was not affected (*P*>0.05) by YSE-contained diets, even at highest levels (6 g/d saponins). However, Rira *et al.* (2015) reported that YSE reduced methane significantly (*P*<0.05) in a dose dependent manner, with dates byproducts and the vetch-oat as substrates. When saponin levels were over 8 mg/mL, the decreasing percentages of methane can be as high as 60% (Rira *et al.*, 2015). Pen *et al.* (2006) reported decreased methane production (11%) in wether sheep by YSE (14 mL) in two 23 h runs (day 16 to day 17 of the 18 days period). Ammonia reduction inside the rumen is caused by the two components of *Yucca schidigera*, one is glycocomponent and other one is saponin fraction that act differently in binding ammonia (Headon *et al.*, 1991). The glyco-component has an ability to bind ammonia directly, while saponin fraction may inhibit ammonia concentrations by membranolytic properties through altering rumen ciliate protozoa, as it (saponin fraction) can cause cell lysis by acting with cholesterol in membranes of protozoal cell (Cheeke *et al.*, 2006). However, the indirect way to reduce ammonia concentration through saponin may contribute most to ammonia reduction since the suppressing potential of glycocomponent is limited (Wallace *et al.*, 1994). Lila *et al.* (2005) pointed out that the lowering of ruminal ammonia concentration in response to YSE to a less extent could be attributed to an inhibited deaminative activity. Gram-positive bacteria and protozoa may be inhibited due to the sarsaponin inclusion which resulted in the falling of ruminal ammonia concentration (Lila *et al.*, 2003). Although both experiments *in vitro* and *in vivo* have demonstrated the decreasing of ammonia (Newbold *et al.*, 1997, Teferedegne, 2000), the effects could only be observed when at higher application rates of YSE (Wallace *et al.*, 2002). When at low application rates, YSE processed little biological effects on ruminal ammonia utilization (Hristov *et al.*, 2004). When high levels of YSE (i.e., > 5 mg/mL) were added in diets, protease activity may be increased, while deaminase activity was unchanged to avoid dietary protein degrade to ammonia (Wang *et al.*, 1998). Rumen ammonia N levels tended to reduce with the increasing levels of YSE at high application rates (Singer et al 2008, Hristov *et al.*, 1999).

28.5 Application of Yucca in Poultry Ration

A number of studies have been carried out to determine the effects of YSE on reducing ammonia in poultry farms. According to Liang et al. (2009), urease activity might be inhibited efficiently with YSE inclusion, which would decrease the speed of ammonia N formation from urea, so the increasing trends of ammonia N concentrations would be reduced. The dynamic balance of N would be broken in this moderate manner, hence ammonia emission rate would be lowered down. As for hydrogen disulfide reduction, it is hypothesized that YSE may decompose the generation of dissolvable sulfide by inhibiting sulphate reducing bacteria or involves in the process where sulfate reductase participate. It is speculated that antimicrobial abilities of saponins may also accounted for the high efficiency of YSE in dealing with odor from poultry feces (Matusiak *et al.*, 2016). The positive effect of YSE on ammonia reduction may also due to the readily volatilized ability of urinary ammonium which is part of ammonia emitted from manure (Panetta *et al.*, 2006).

Cabuk *et al.* (2004) reported that feeding of 120 mg/kg dietary YSE resulted in a decreased ammonia concentration of broiler houses at day 19 without impairing broiler performance. But Corzo *et al.* (2007) reported no effect of supplementation of 100 ppm of YSE and *Quillaja saponaria* in a corn-soybean control diet on ammonia emission of broiler chicken litters in 42 days experimental period. Inclusion of 100 ppm YSE in layers diet significantly reduced ammonia emission by 44% and 28% for the first two days of manure storage (Chepete *et al.*, 2012). However, an experiment showed that ammonia N concentrations and micro-organism levels of litter materials (half was wood shavings, the other was rice hull) among examined groups did not show statistical difference when pulverized YSE was applied to different litter materials at the level of 0, 4% and 8%. This show that efficiency of YSE could be amplified if litter was used in farming houses under bad situations (Onbasilar *et al.*, 2013). YSE showed highest potentials in reducing volatile odorous compounds such as ammonia, trimethylamine, dimethylamine, isobutyric acid and hydrogen sulfide concentrations after 96 h of the process (Matusiak *et al.*, 2016).

28.6 Application of Yucca in Swine Ration

Addition of Yucca in the ration of swine has been claimed to reduce the still birth in the pigs. Cline *et al.* (1996) found that giving a commercial feed additive containing YE to sows prior to farrowing resulted in a significant reduction in numbers of pigs born dead (stillbirths). They found that blood oxygen levels were higher in piglets at birth from sows fed the YE, and suggested that the reduction in stillbirths was a result of improved blood oxygen supply to the fetuses during birth. Pre–weaning mortality was also reduced; piglets suffering from oxygen deprivation during birth are less viable and more likely to succumb to stresses of post uterine life (Herpin *et al.*, 2001). The results of Cline *et al.* (1996) were later confirmed by Herpin *et al.* (2001) who observed that the inclusion of whole yucca plant powder in sow diets caused a reduction in stillbirths and increased viability of neonatal pigs although there were no differences in blood oxygenation between control and yucca–fed pigs. Litters with stillbirths have a higher pre weaning mortality than litters without (Leenhouwers *et al.*, 1999).With regard to reduction of ammonia emission few studies in swine have been carried out. Panetta *et al.* (2006) observed no significant effect of dietary YSE (0, 62.5, 125 mg/kg) on ammonia emission during 72 h of consecutive measurement after 4 days dietary adjustment. Hong *et al.* (2001) reported a decreasing tendency ($P>0.05$) in ammonia gas production of fecal samples during a 30 days experiment period. However, Liang *et al.* (2009) indicated that YSE added in the feed (125 mg/kg) decreased the emission of ammonia and hydrogen disulphide in the 35 days trials.

28.7 Summary and Conclusions

Yucca schidigera has potential to be used as feed additive in case of ruminants with regard to its application in methane mitigation. This can also be used in the ration of swine and poultry to reduce the ammonia. Although conflicting results are reported but many positive effects of YSE on methane/ammonia mitigation show it as a novel feed additive due to its saponin contents.

References

Cabuk M, Alcicek A, Bozkurt M, Akkan S(2004) Effect of Yucca schidigera and natural zeolite on broiler performance. Int J Poultry Sci 3(10): 651-654

Canul-Solis JR, Piñeiro-Vázquez AT, Briceño-Poot EG, Chay-Canul AJ, Alayón-Gamboa JA, Ayala-Burgos AJ, *et al.* (2014) Effect of supplementation with saponins from Yucca schidigera on ruminal methane production by Pelibuey sheep fed Pennisetumpurpureum grass. Anim Prod Sci 54(10): 1834-1837

Cardozo PW, Calsamiglia S, Ferret A, Kamel C (2005) Screening for the effects of natural plant extracts at two pH levels on *in vitro* rumen microbial fermentation of a high-concentrate diet for beef cattle. J AnimSci 83(11): 2572-2579

Cheeke PR, Piacente S, Oleszek W (2006) Anti-inflammatory and anti-arthritic effects of *Yucca schidigera*: A review. J Inflamm 3: 6

Cheeke, PR (2000) Actual and potential applications of *Yucca schidigera* and *Quillajasaponaria* saponins in human and animal nutrition. J AnimSci 77(E-Suppl): 1-10

Chepete HJ, Xin H, Mendes LB, Li H, Bailey TB (2012) Ammonia emission and performance of laying hens as affected by different dosages of Yucca schidigera in the diet. J Appl. Poultry Res 21(3): 522-530

Cieslak A, Zmora P, Pers-Kamczyc E, Szumacher-Strabel M (2012) Effects of tannins source (Vaccinium vitisidaea L.) on rumen microbial fermentation *in vivo*. Anim Feed Sci Tech 176(1-4): 102-106

Corzo A, Kidd MT, Miles DM, Dozier WA, Cheeke PR (2007) Yucca schidigera and Quillajasaponaria supplementation in broiler diets abstract. International Poultry Scientific Forum 64 p

Francis G, Kerem Z, Makkar HP, Becker K (2002) The biological action of saponins in animal systems: a review. Brit J Nutr 88(6): 587-605

Goel G, Makkar HPS (2012)Methane mitigation from ruminants using tannins and saponins. Trop Anim Health Pro 44(4): 729-739

Guo YQ, Liu JX, Lu Y, Zhu WY, Denman SE, McSweeney CS(2008)Effect of tea saponin on methanogenesis, microbial community structure and expression of mcrA gene, in cultures of rumen microorganisms. LettApplMicrobiol 47(5): 421-426

Headon DR, Buggle KA, Nelson AB, Killeen GF (1991) Glycofractions of the Yucca plant and their role in ammonia control. In: Lyons TP, editor. Biotechnology in the Feed Industry. Nicholasville, KY: Alltech Technical Publications. p. 95-108

Holtshausen L, Chaves AV, Beauchemin KA, McGinn SM, McAllister TA, Odongo NE, *et al.* (2009) Feeding saponin-containing Yucca schidigera and Quillaja saponaria to decrease enteric methane production in dairy cows. J Dairy Sci 92(6): 2809-2821

Hong JW, Kim IH, Moon TH, Kwon OS, Lee SH, Kim YG(2001)Effects of yucca extract and (or) far infrared emitted materials supplementation on the growth performance, serum characteristics and ammonia production of growing and finishing pigs. Asian Austral J Anim 14(9): 1299-1303

Hristov AN, Grandeen KL, Ropp JK, Greer D (2004)Effect of Yucca schidigera-based surfactant on ammonia utilization in vitro, and in situ degradability of corn grain. Anim Feed Sci Tech 115(3-4): 341-355

Hristov AN, McAllister TA, Herk FHV, Cheng KJ, Newbold CJ, Cheeke PR(1999)Effect of *Yucca schidigera* on ruminal fermentation and nutrient digestion in heifers. J AnimSci 77(9): 2554-2563

Kaneda N, Nakanishi H, Staba EJ (1987) Steroidal constituents of Yucca schidigera plants and tissue cultures. Phytochemistry 26(5): 1425-1429

Kowalczyk M, Pecio L, Stochmal A, Oleszek W (2011) Qualitative and quantitative analysis of steroidal saponins in crude extract and bark powder of Yucca schidigera. Roezl. J Agric Food Chem 59(15): 8058-8064

Li W, Powers W(2012)Effects of saponin extracts on air emissions from steers. J AnimSci 90(11): 4001-4013

Liang GQ, Wang XP, Wang XM, Li CP, Chen AG (2009)Effects of camphor familiar plant extract and *Yucca* extracts on emission of NH_3 and H_2S in slurry of weaned pigs. Chinese J AnimSci 45(13): 22-26

Lila ZA, Mohammed N, Kanda S, Kamada T, Itabashi H (2003)Effect of sarsaponin on ruminal fermentation with particular reference to methane production *in vitro*. J Dairy Sci 86(10): 3330-3336

Lila ZA, Mohammed N, Kanda S, Kurihara M, Itabashi H (2005)Sarsaponin effects on ruminal fermentation and microbes, methane production, digestibility and blood metabolites in steers. Asian Austral J Anim 18(12): 1746-1751

Liu CL, Li ZQ, Du J, Shan AS (2007) The effect of *Yucca schidigera* extract on ruminal fermentation and parameters traits in sheep. AgrSci China 6(1): 121-128

Liu CL, Li ZQ (2011) Effect of levels of *Yucca schidigera* extract on ruminal fermentation parameters, digestibility of nutrients and growth performance in sheep. Adv Mater 343-344: 655-660

Lundeen T (2000) Yucca extract improves feed efficiency, decreases abdominal fat in broilers. Feedstuffs 72(33): 9

Mackie RI, Gilcrist FMC, Heath S (1984)An *in vitro* study of ruminal micro-organisms influencing lactate turnover and its contribution to volatile fatty acid production. J Agric Sci 103(1): 37-51

Matusiak K, Oleksy M, Borowski S, Nowak A, Korczynski M, Dobrzanski Z, *et al.* (2016) The use of Yucca schidigera and microbial preparation for poultry manure deodorization and hygienization. J Environ Manage 170: 50-59

Miyakoshi M, Tamura Y, Masuda H, Mizutani K, Tanaka O, Ikeda T, *et al.* (2000)Antiyeast steroidal saponins from Yucca schidigera (Mohave Yucca), a new anti-food-deteriorating agent. J Nat Prod 63(3): 332-338

Moss AR, Jouany JP, Newbold J (2000) Methane production by ruminants: its contribution to global warming. Ann Zootech 49(3): 231-253

Nahm KH (2003) Evaluation of the nitrogen content in poultry manure. World Poultry Sci J 59(1): 77-88

Narvaez N, Wang YX, McAllister T (2013) Effects of extracts of Humuluslupulus (hops) and Yucca schidigera applied alone or in combination with monensin on rumen fermentation and microbial populations in vitro. J Sci Food Agric 93(10): 2517-2522

Newbold CJ, EL Hassan SM, Wang J, Ortega ME, Wallace RJ (1997) Influence of foliage from African multipurpose trees on activity of rumen protozoa and bacteria. Brit J Nutr 78(2): 237-249

Newbold CJ, Lassalas B, Jouany JP (1995)The importance of methanogens associated with ciliate protozoa in ruminal methane production in vitro. LettApplMicrobiol 21(4): 230-234

Oleszek W, Sitek M, Stochmal A, Piacente S, Pizza C, Cheeke P (2001) Steroidal saponins of Yucca schidigeraRoezl. J Agric Food Chem 49: 4392-4396

Onbasilar EE, Erdem E, Ünal N, Kocakaya A, Torlak E (2013) Effect of *Yucca schidigera* spraying in different litter materials on some litter traits and breast burn of broilers at the fifth week of production. KafkasUniv Vet FakDerg 19(5): 749-753

Panetta DM, Powers WJ, Xin H, Kerr BJ, Stalder KJ (2006) Nitrogen excretion and ammonia emissions from pigs fed modified diets. J Environ Qual 35(4): 1297-1308

Patel S (2012) Yucca: A medicinally significant genus with manifold therapeutic attributes. Nat Prod Bioprospect 2(6): 231-234

Pen B, Sar C, Mwenya B, Kuwaki K, Morikawa R, Takahashi J (2006) Effects of Yuccaschidigera and Quillajasaponaria extracts on in vitro ruminal fermentation and methane emission. Anim Feed Sci Tech 129(3-4): 175-186

Pen B, Takaura K, Yamaguchi S, Asa R, Takahashi J (2007) Effects of Yuccaschidigera and Quillajasaponaria with or without 1-4 galacto-oligosaccharides on ruminal fermentation, methane production and nitrogen utilization in sheep. Anim Feed Sci Tech 138(1): 75-88

Piacente S, Pizza1 C, Oleszek W (2005) Saponins and phenolics of Yucca schidigeraRoezl: Chemistry and bioactivity. Phytochem Rev 4(2-3): 177-190

Pratt EV, Rose SP, Keeling AA (2002) Effect of ambient temperature on losses of volatile nitrogen compounds from stored laying hen manure. BioresourceTechnol 84(2): 203-205

Rira M, Chentli A, Boufenera S, Bousseboua H (2015) Effects of plants containing secondary metabolites on ruminal methanogenesis of sheep *in vitro*. Energy Procedia 74: 15-24

Santoso B, Mwenya B, Sar C, Gamo Y, Kobayashi T, Morikawa R, *et al.* (2004) Effects of supplementing galacto-oligosaccharides, *Yucca schidigera* or nisin on rumen methanogenesis, nitrogen and energy metabolism in sheep. Livest Prod Sci 91(3): 209-217

Santoso B, Mwenya B, Sar C, Takahashi J (2006) Ruminal fermentation and nitrogen metabolism in sheep fed a silage-based diet supplemented with Yucca schidigera or Y. schidigera and nisin. Anim Feed Sci Tech 129(3-4): 187-195

Singer MD, Robinson PH, Salem AZM, DePeters EJ (2008) Impacts of rumen fluid modified by feeding *Yucca schidigera* to lactating dairy cows on *in vitro* gas production of 11 common dairy feedstuffs, as well as animal performance. Anim Feed Sci Tech 146(3-4): 242-258

Sliwinski BJ, Kreuzer M, Wettstein HR, Machmuller A (2002b) Rumen fermentation and nitrogen balance of lambs fed diets containing plant extracts rich in tannins and saponins, and associated emissions of nitrogen and methane. Arch AnimNutr 56(6): 397-392

Sliwinski BJ, Soliva CR, Machmuller A, Kreuzer M(2002a)Efficacy of plant extracts rich in secondary constituents to modify rumen fermentation. Anim Feed Sci Tech 101(1): 101-114

Strobel HJ, Russell JB (1989)Non-proton-motive-force-dependent sodium efflux from the ruminal bacterium Streptococcus bovis: bound versus free pools. Appl Environ Microbiol 55(10): 2664-2668

Stumm CK, Zwart KB (1986) Symbiosis of protozoa with hydrogen utilizing methanogens. MicrobiolSci 3(4): 100-105

Sun DS, Jin X, Shi B, Xu Y, Yan S (2017)Effects of *Yuccaschidigera* on gas mitigation in livestock production: A review. Braz. Arch. Biol. Technol.http://dx.doi.org/10.1590/1678-4324-2017160359 ISSN 1678-4324 Online Edition

Teferedegne B (2000) New perspectives on the use of tropical plants to improve ruminant nutrition. P NutrSoc 59(2): 209-214

Ushida K, Tokura M, Takenaka A, Itabashi H (1997) Ciliate protozoa and ruminal methanogenesis. In: Onodera R, Itabashi H, Ushida K, Yano H, Sasaki Y, eds. Rumen Microbes and Digestive Physiology in Ruminants. Tokyo: Japan Scientific Societies Press & S. Karger AG Basel p. 209-220

Wallace RJ, Arthaud L, Newbold CJ (1994) Influence of *Yucca shidigera* extract on ruminal ammonia concentrations and ruminal micro-organisms. Appl Environ Microbiol 60(6): 1762-1767

Wallace RJ, McEwan NR, McIntosh FM, Teferedegne B, Newbold CJ (2002)Natural products as manipulators of rumen fermentation. Asian Austral J Anim 15(10): 1458-1468

Wang CJ, Wang SP, Zhou H (2009) Influences of flavomycin, ropadiar, and saponin on nutrient digestibility, rumen fermentation, and methane emission from sheep. Anim Feed Sci Tech 148(2-4): 157-166

Wang Y, McAllister TA, Newbold CJ, Rode LM, Cheeke PR, Cheng KJ (1998) Effect of Yucca schidigera extract on fermentation and degradation of steroidal saponins in rumen simulation technique (RUSITEC). Anim Feed Sci Tech 74(2): 143-153

Wolin MJ, Miller TL (1988) Microbe-microbe interactions. In: The Rumen Microbial Ecosystem. London: Elsevier Applied Science. p. 343-359

Xu M, Rinker M, McLeod KR, Harmon DL (2010) *Yucca schidigera* extract decreases *in vitro* methane production in a variety of forages and diets. Anim Feed Sci Tech 159(1-2): 18-26

Zijderveld SMV, Dijkstra J, Perdok HB, Newbold JR, Gerrits WJJ (2011) Dietary inclusion of diallyl disulfide, yucca powder, calcium fumarate, an extruded linseed product, or medium-chain fatty acids does not affect methane production in lactating dairy cows. J Dairy Sci 94(6): 3094-3104.

□□□

Chapter 29

Shatavari (*Asparagus racemosus*)

Jaya Bharati[1] and Satish Kumar[2]

[1] Department of Veterinary Physiology and Biochemistry, Faculty of Veterinary and Animal Sciences, Banaras Hindu University, Varanasi-221005, India e-mail: jayabvc07@gmail.com

[2] Research Scholar, Division of Animal Genetics and Breeding, Indian Veterinary Research Institute, Izatnagar-243122, India e-mail: hilsa.satis2007@gmail.com

ABSTRACT

Shatavari (*Asparagus racemosus*) the "Queen of Herbs" in Ayurveda occupies the reputation of a rasayana herb and is the most commonly used species of *Asparagus* in traditional medicine. The therapeutic applications of this plant have been reported in Indian and British Pharmacopoeias and in traditional system of medicine, such as Ayurveda, Unani and Siddha. It occupies an important position in Indian system of medicine as a bitter-sweet, emollient, cooling, nervine tonic, antisplasmodic, constipating, aphrodisiac, antacid, diuretic, rejuvenating, carminative, stomachic, tonic, anabolic, appetizer and nutritive herbal plant. The crude, semi-purified and purified extracts obtained from different parts of this plant are rich in bioactive phytochemicals, saponins and flavonoids which alone or in combination mediate various pharmacological activities and have been widely used in therapeutic applications. Shatavari is well acclaimed for its adaptogenic, antioxidant, antimicrobial, immuno-stimulatory properties and have stimulatory role in growth, reproduction, milk yield and composition of livestock. It exerts cytoprotective effect on gastric mucosa and estrogenic effect on female reproductive system and mammary gland. Considering its nutritional benefits, Shatavari root powder is used as a herbal feed additive/supplement in poultry feed. Shatavri has been regarded as completely safe for long-term use, even during pregnancy and lactation. There is a need of further research regarding the mode of action and role of the various active principles to exploit the potential of Satavari in the areas of female and male reproduction, milk yield and composition in livestock and poultry meat and egg yield. No doubt utilization of phytomedicine Shatavari as a feed additive in livestock and poultry warrants increased efficiency and production potential of livestock, in safest and most economic way.

Keywords: Shatavari, Saponins, Immunomodulator, Adaptogenic, Galactogogue, Phytoestrogens.

29.1 Introduction

Shatavari (*Asparagus racemosus*), is an ethno-pharmacologically acclaimed ayurvedic medicinal plant of Asparagaceae family, and is called as 'Queen of Herbs' in Ayurveda. Its medicinal usage has been reported in the Indian and British Pharmacopoeias and in the traditional systems of medicine such as Ayurveda, Unani and Siddha. Ancient ayurvedic texts like Charak Samhita, Susruta Samhita and Astanga Samhita has also mentioned its beneficial effects.

The genus *Asparagus* includes about 300 species around the world, out of which 22 species of *Asparagus* are recorded in India. Shatavari (*Asparagus racemosus)* is the most commonly used species of *Asparagus* in traditional medicine. It is commonly called wild asparagus in English, other common names of this plant in different Indian languages are Satawar or Satmuli in Hindi; Satavari in Sanskrit; Shatavari or Shatmuli in Marathi; Shimai-Shadavari, Ammaikodi, Inli-chedi, Kilwari in Tamil; Challagadda, Toala-gaddalu, Pilligadalu in Telgu; Majjige-gedde, Aheru-balli in Kannada; Saatawari, Ekalakanto in gujarathi, shatawarmul, Shatamuli in Bengali; Shatavali; Kairuwa in Kumaon; Narbodh or Satmooli in Madhya Pradesh; Norkanto or Satawar in Rajasthan and Chatavali in Malayalam (Anonymous, 1987). Shatavari is found throughout tropical and subtropical parts of India and in the Himalayas upto an altitude of 1,500 m elevation (Mazumdar and Mukhopadhyay, 2006). It is also found in parts of Sri Lanka, Indonesia, Australia and tropical Africa (Chauhan *et al.*, 2011). The plant is a spinous under-shrub, with tuberous, short rootstock bearing numerous succulent tuberous roots (30–100 cm long and 1–2 cm thick) that are silvery white or ash coloured externally and white internally (Chauhan *et al.*, 2011). The stems are armed with numerous recurved spines, sickle-shaped cladodes with scale leaves, small white flowers and fruits can be seen with attractive globose red berries. The stem is woody, climbing, whitish grey or brown coloured with small spines (Anonymous, 1987). The crude, semi-purified and purified extracts obtained from different parts of this plant have been widely used in therapeutic applications. Shatavari occupies the reputation of a rasayana herb in Ayurveda i.e. plant drugs promoting general well being by increasing cellular vitality and resistance (Goyal *et al.*, 2003), and has been used extensively as an adaptogenic drug (Bhattacharya *et al.*, 2000) to increase the non-specific resistance of organisms against a variety of stresses. It occupies an important position in Indian system of medicine as a bitter-sweet, emollient, cooling, nervine tonic, antispasmodic, constipating, aphrodisiac, antacid, diuretic, rejuvenating, carminative, stomachic, tonic, anabolic, appetizer and nutritive herbal plant. The studies on the total extracts and the isolated principles have revealed a wide range of biological activities. These includes anti-anaphylactic (Padmalatha *et al.*, 2002), anti-stress (Kamat *et al.*, 2000; Bhattacharya *et al.*, 2002; Murugan-andam *et al.*, 2002), anti-ulcer (Datta *et al.*, 2002; Goel and Sairam 2002; Sairam *et al.*, 2003), anti-diarrhoeal (Venkatesan *et al.*, 2005), antitussive (Mandal *et al.*, 2000), astringent, antiseptic (Seena and Kuttan, 1993), anticancer (Diwanay *et al.*, 2004), immuno-modulator (Gautam *et al.*, 2004), antioxidant (Parihar and Hemnani, 2004), antibacterial (Mandal *et al.*, 2000) and radioprotective (Arora *et al.*, 2005) properties. Formulations from Shatavari have been used traditionally for the treatment of many diseases (Jetmalani *et al.*, 1967). Its beneficial effects are suggested in nervous disorders, dyspepsia, diarrhoea, dysentry, tumors, inflammations, hyperdipsia, neuropathy, hepatopathy, cough, bronchitis, hyperacidity, gonorrhoea, piles, diabetes, rheumatism, gastric troubles, headache, for increasing lactation and certain infectious diseases (Goyal *et al.*, 2003; Chauhan *et al.*, 2011).

29.2 Taxonomy of Shatavari

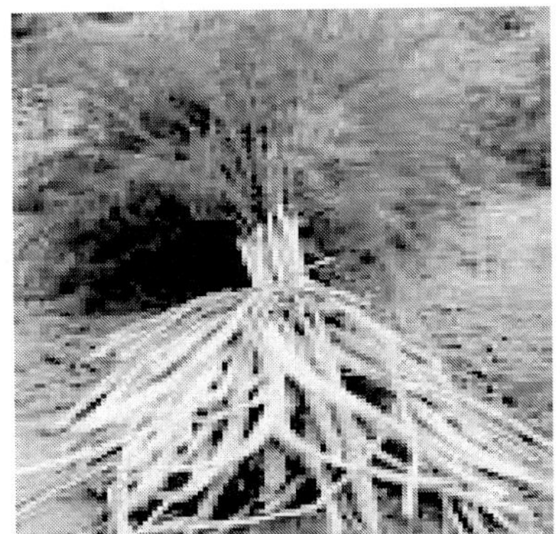

Kingdom	:	Plantae
Clade	:	Angiosperms
Clade	:	Monocots
Order	:	Asparagales
Family	:	Asparagaceae
Subfamily	:	Asparagoideae
Genus	:	*Asparagus*
Species	:	*Racemosus*

29.3 Chemical Composition of Shatavari

Shatavari is rich in non-nutrient bioactive principles which are essentially the secondary metabolites in addition to different types of ubiquitous primary metabolites (e.g. carbohydrates, proteins, fats and nucleic acids). The composition of Shatavari is root is shown in Table 1. It also contains saccharine, polysaccharides and mucilaginous substances in large proportion. Roots are rich in trace minerals namely zinc (53.15), manganese (19.98 mg/g), copper (5.29 mg/g), cobalt (22.00 mg/g) along with calcium, magnesium, potassium, zinc and selenium (Mohanta *et al.*, 2003; Choudhary and Kar, 1992). High content of NFE indicates that Shatavari is a rich source of energy.

Table 1: Composition of Shatavari root

Components	Quantity	Reference
Dry matter	91%	Mirzaei (2012)
Crude protein	4.6 to 6.1%	Mishra et al. (2005)
Crude fibre	8.32%	Mirzaei (2012)
Ether extract	0.66%	Mirzaei (2012)
Nitrogen free extract	74.02%	Mirzaei (2012)
Total ash	13.15%	Mirzaei (2012)
Phenols	3.1 to 5.2 mg/g	Mishra *et al.* (2005)
Phytosterols	0.79%	Visavadiya and Narasimhacharya (2007)
Tannins	4.8 to 5.1 mg/g 88.2 mg/100ml	Mishra *et al.* (2005) Velavan *et al.* (2007)
Saponin	4.1%	Mishra *et al.* (2005)
Carbohydrates	36.8 to 47.5%	Mishra *et al.* (2005)
Galactose	54%	Kamat and Venkatachalam (2004)
Glucose	28%	Kamat and Venkatachalam (2004)
Rhamnose	4%	Kamat and Venkatachalam (2004
Xylose	5%	Kamat and Venkatachalam (2004)
Arabinose	8%	Kamat and Venkatachalam (2004)
Flavonoids	6.7 mg/100ml	Velavan *et al.* 2007)
Vitamin-C	42.4 mg/100ml	Velavan *et al.* (2007)

29.4 Active Principles in Shatavari

The genus *Asparagus* is a rich source of sapogenins and saponins, known as Shatavaris from various parts of the plant (Table 2), which contributes to its medicinal value. It has been shown to contain steroidal saponins (Hayes *et al.*, 2006) and racemofuran (Ahmad and Jain, 1991;

Wiboonpun *et al.*, 2004). Shatavari root is rich in steroidal saponins, such as Shatavarin VI, Shatavarin VII, Shatavarin VIII, Shatavarin IX and Shatavarin X, together with other saponin-like Shatavarin I (Asparoside B), Shatavarin IV (Asparinin B), Shatavarin V, Immunoside and Schidigerasaponin d5 (Asparanin A). They have been isolated from the roots by RP-HPLC and characterised by spectroscopic and spectrometric methods (Hayes *et al.*, 2008). The other three steroidal saponins, such as Racemoside A, Racemoside B and Racemoside C have been isolated from the methanolic extract of the Shatavari fruits (Mandal *et al.*, 2006). Kaepfrol along with sarsapogenin from woody portions of tuberous roots could be isolated (Ahmed *et al.*, 1991). Besides saponins root extract of Shatavari also contains other phytocomponents such as alkaloids, phytosterols, polyphenols, tannins, flavonoids and essential fatty acids like gamma linoleinic acids, vitamin A, total ascorbic acid, thus making it a rich source of secondary plant metabolites (Subramanian and Nair, 1968).

Table 2: Active principles odiffferent parts of Shatavari plant

	Synonym	Part of Plant	References
Steroidal Saponins			
Shatavarin VI		Roots	Hayes *et al.* (2006)
Shatavarin VII		Roots	Hayes *et al.* (2006)
Shatavarin VIII		Roots	Hayes *et al.* (2006)
Shatavarin IX		Roots	Hayes *et al.* (2006)
Shatavarin X		Roots	Hayes *et al.* (2006)
Shatavaroside A		Roots	Sharma *et al.* (2009)
Shatavaroside B		Roots	Sharma *et al.* (2009)
(25*S*)-5*β*-spirostan-3*β*-ol-3-O-{*β*-d-glucopyranosyl(1→6) -[*a*-l-rhamnopyranosyl (glucopyranosyl(1→4)] -*β*-d-gluco-pyranoside}	Racemoside A	Fruits	Mandal *et al.* (2006)
(25*S*)-5*β*-spirostan-3*β*-ol-3-O-*a*-l-rhamnopyranosyl(1→6)] -*β*-d-glucopyranosyl(1→6) -*β*-d-glucopyrano-side	Racemoside B	Fruits	Mandal *et al.* (2006)
(25*S*)-5*β*-spirostan-3*β*-ol-3-O-{*a*-lrhamnopyranosyl-(1→6) -[*a*-l-rhamnopyranosyl(1→4)] -*β*-d-glucopyranoside	Racemoside C	Fruits	Mandal *et al.* (2006)
Saponins			
Shatavarin I	Asparoside B	Roots	Joshi (1988); Hayes *et al.* (2006)
Shatavarin IV	Asparinin B	Roots	Joshi (1988); Hayes *et al.* (2006)

Shatavarin V,		Roots	Hayes *et al.* (2 008)
Oligospirostanoside	Immunoside	Roots	Handa *et al.* (2003); Hayes *et al.* (2008)
Schidigerasaponin d5	Asparanin A	Roots	Hayes *et al.* (2008)
Filiasparoside C		Roots	Sharma *et al.* (2009)
Isoflavone,			
8-methoxy-5,6,4'-trihydroxyisoflavone-7-O-β-d-Glucopyranoside		Roots	Saxena and Chourasia (2001)
9,10-dihydro-1,5-dimethoxy-8-methyl-2,7-phenanthrenediol		Roots	Sekine *et al.* (1997)
Alkaloid			
Asparagamine A	Pyrrolizidine alkaloid	Ethanol extract of the roots	Sekine *et al.* (1995)
Quercetin		Roots, fruits and flowers	Mazumdar and Mukhopadhyay (2006)
Glycosides of quercetin			
Quercetin-3-O-rutinoside	Rutin	Roots, fruits and flowers	Mazumdar and Mukhopadhyay (2006)
Quercetin 3-O-galactoside **20**)	Hyperoside	Roots, fruits and flowers	Mazumdar and Mukhopadhyay (2006)
Quercetin 3-glucuronide		Leaves	Mazumdar and Mukhopadhyay (2006)
Sapogenin			
Diosgenin		Leaves	Mazumdar and Mukhopadhyay (2006)

29.5 Use of Shatavari and their Effects on Livestock

29.5.1 *Adaptogenic Activity*

Shatavari is an Ayurvedic rasayana used as an adaptogen. Adaptogenic substances are drugs which function as anti-stress agents by promoting non-specific resistance of the body and thus, help to counteract any type of physical, chemical or biological stress. An aqueous extract of the whole plant of Shatavari was administered orally to animals and then exposed them to biological, physical and chemical stress. It was concluded that Shatavari extract offered protection against these stressors, as judged by using markers of stress responses and objective parameters for stress manifestations (Rege *et al.*, 1999). Shatavari supplementation was able to reverse chronic stress-induced bio-chemical, physiological and behavioural perturbations (Bhattacharya *et al.*, 2000). The active principle, 2'!1 linked fructo-oligosaccharides (FOS) found in Shatavari potentiates the natural killer (NK) cell activity and this could be an important mechanism underpinning the '*Rasayana*' properties of this plant (Thakur *et al.*, 2012).

29.5.2 *Gastro-intestinal Effects*

Shatavari is used in Ayurveda as a treatment for dyspepsia (*amlapitta*) and has also been mentioned for the treatment of ulcerative disorders of stomach. Shatavari promptly and persistently relieves pain and burning sensation as well as other dyspeptic symptoms due to duodenal ulcer (Singh and Singh, 1986). Dalvi *et al.* (1990) used the powdered dried root of Shatavari for dyspepsia and found that oral administration of formulation promoted gastric emptying. Its action can be compared with that of the synthetic dopamine antagonist metoclopromide. Dahanukar *et al.* (1983) reported that Shatavari protected gastric mucosa against pentagastrin and carbachol induced ulcers, by significantly reducing both the severity of ulceration and ulcer index. It decreased the volume and increased the pH of the secretions, thus suggesting a reduced responsiveness of the gastric parietal cells to secretogogues and narcotizing agents. The cytoprotective effect is due to increased output of mucus. Other possible mechanism may be by deactivation and binding of pepsin and/or bile salts.

Since Shatavari did not have either antacid or antisecretory properties, thus the observed mild reduction in acid secretion may be due to some changes in the gastric mucosa. It has been suggested to heal the ulcers by potentiating defensive factors and many hypotheses have been put forward for its possible mechanism.

i) It may prolong the life span of mucosal cells, increase the secretion and viscosity of mucus and strengthen the mucosal barrier and thus reduces H^+ ion diffusion back into the mucosa.

ii) Shatavari may form a complex with the mucus of other substances at the base of ulcer which may protect the ulcer from the corrosive and proteolytic effects of acid-pepsin.

iii) It may have cytoprotective action like that of prostaglandins.

29.5.3. *Effect on Growth*

Supplementation of Shatavari in complete feed led to positive effect on digestible energy availability from feed and increased intake of digestible crude protein (DCP) and total digestible nutrient (TDN) owing to increased intake and digestibility of nutrients (Barhane and Singh, 2002). Higher DCP and TDN intake and nutrient digestibility particularly of dry matter (DM) and crude protein (CP0 and its high content of calcium, zinc and vitamins B may be the reason for significant difference in weight gain in animals receiving Shatavari herb as feed additive (Amanullah *et al.*, 2009). Supplementation of Shatavari significantly increases rumen volatile fatty acid (VFA) profile, microbial efficiency, propionate, glucose and glucose-6-phosphate in ruminants. It also reduces protein degradation and ammonia nitrogen production in rumen and causes increased nitrogen intake and balance (Pattanaik *et al.*, 2009). Calves supplemented with Shatavari root decoction at the rate of 100 mg/kg for a varying period of 4 weeks to 8 months showed 81.19% weight gain as compared to 67.9% in non-suplemented group (Sharma *et al.*, 1996). It did not have any adverse effect on the progeny of the treated animals. The growth promoting effect can be ascribed to its adaptogenic property.

29.5.4 *Effect on Reproduction*

Shatavari is well known for its phytoestrogenic properties and use as a hormone modulator (Mayo, 1998). Phytoestrogens are defined as any plant compound structurally and/or functionally similar to ovarian and placental oestrogens and their active metabolites (Whitten and Patisaul, 2001). Phytoestrogens affect the regulation of ovarian and oestrous cycles in female mammals and the promotion of growth, differentiation and physiological functions of the female genital tract, pituitary, mammary gland and several other organs and tissues in both the sexes. Shatavari root extract exerted a mammotropic and/or lactogenic influence on normal as well as on oestrogen-primed animals (Rao, 1981). The aqueous extract of Shatavari roots increase the weight of mammary glands in postpartum and oestrogen-primed rats and the uterine weight in the oestrogen-primed group (Sabnis *et al.*, 1968). This effect is attributed to the action of released corticoids or prolactin. The oral administration of the alcoholic extract of Shatavari root in the dose of 30 mg/100 g body weight, daily for 15 days to adult pregnant female albino rats had an oestrogenic effect on the female mammary glands and genital organs (Pandey *et al.*, 2005). It also caused an increase in uterine weight and uterine glycogen without altering serum oestrogen and progesterone levels in immature rats as against ovariectomised rats used as control (Gopumadhavan *et al.*, 2005). Thus the phytoestrogen in Shatavari performs its function by binding directly to the oestrogen receptor without enhancing the endogenous oestrogen levels.

Shatavari is believed to increase fertility in females and helps in conception by restoring hormonal balance in body of females which is important for conception. It also balances the pH levels in vagina, which increases chance of pregnancy by creating a proper environment for sperm motility. During gestation, it helps in maintaining the health of foetus and also reduces chances of abortion. Barhane and Singh, (2002) reported that supplementation of Shatavari (100 g on alternate day) post-partum alone led to 100% estrus and 75% conception in treatment group as compared to 50% in control crossbred cow within 90 days of calving. Hegde *et al.* (2002) reported that supplementation of Shatavari root powder 100g + 10g Aloe dried pulp powder to cows following artificial insemination per animal/day improved conception rate. Improvement of reproduction performance in supplemented groups of does was also reported by Mirzaei and Prasad (2011).

Enhanced reproductive performance may be through correction in the nutritional deficiency disorders involving mineral and vitamin deficiency. It has an immune-modulation and immune-potentiation effect in late gestation and has been shown to shortening the uterine involution period (Hussein and Badr, 2008). The estrogenic property of Shatavari, stimulates the ovarian function, improves uterine tonicity thus helps in early uterine involution which consequently results into early initiation of the estrus cycle (Pandey *et al.*, 2005). Additionally, resumption of ovarian cyclicity after parturition depends on the nutritional status, body energy reserves and blood glucose levels of the animal, which is maintained by Shatavari.

29.5.5 *Antimicrobial Activity*

A crude methanol extract of the Shatavari roots showed *in vitro* antibacterial efficacy against *Escherichia coli, Shigella dysenteriae, Shigella sonnei, Shigella flexneri, Vibrio cholerae, Salmonella typhi, Salmonella typhimurium, Pseudomonas putida, Bacillus subtilis* and *Staphylococcus aureus* (Mandal *et al.*, 2000b). The extracts obtained from the roots have also been evaluated for antifungal activities against

Candida (Uma *et al.*, 2009), *Malassezia furfur* and *M. globosa* (Onlom *et al.*, 2014). These studies revealed the antifungal potential of *A. racemosus* root extracts. In another study from leaves, the crude extracts obtained using different solvents like petroleum ether, methanol, chloroform, acetone, ethyl acetate and water were tested on Gram-positive bacteria like *B. subtilis, S. aureus* and Gram-negative bacteria *E coli, Pseudomonas* and the yeast *Candida utilis* by *in vitro* agar well diffusion method. The study revealed that the methanolic extract can be effectively used for curing the bacterial diseases (Patel and Patel, 2013).

29.5.6 *Antioxidant Activity*

Shatavari is also reputed for its antioxidant activity. The methanolic root extract with daily dose of 100 mg/kg/body weight increased superoxide dismutase (SOD), catalase and ascorbic acid levels appreciably, while decreasing lipid peroxidise products in indomethacin-treated rats (20 mg/kg/body weight) (Bhatnagar *et al.*, 2005). Crude extract of Shatavari has potent antioxidant properties against damage induced by gamma radiation in rat liver mitochondria (Kamat *et al.*, 2000). In the study done with both crude and purified aqueous fraction in terms of protection against lipid peroxidation, protein oxidation, depletion of protein thiols and the levels of the antioxidant enzyme SOD. The crude extract at 10 ìg/ml gave 94% protection and at 50 μg/ml showed complete protection (100%) against lipid peroxidation and the purified fraction showed complete inhibition at both concentrations (Kamat *et al.*, 2000). Moreover, alcoholic extract of root of *A. racemosus* has been shown to significantly reduce the enhanced levels of SGOT and SGPT in carbon chloride induced hepatic damage in rats (Acharya *et al.*, 2012).

Supplementation of SRP at 5 and 10 % level reduces the plasma and hepatic lipid (cholesterol) levels and also decreases lipid peroxidation. The inhibitory effects of active principles consisting of polysaccharide component rich in galactose, glucose and smaller amount of arabinose at the concentration of 10 ìg/ml, are comparable to that of the established antioxidants glutathione (GSH) and ascorbic acid (Kamat *et al.*, 2000). GSH is an important antioxidant which acts as a nucleophilic scavenger of toxic compounds and as a substrate in the GPx-mediated destruction of hydroperoxides which would otherwise accumulate to toxic levels in tissues (Parihar and Hemnani, 2004). The mice treated with Shatavari extract showed an enhancement in GPx activity and GSH content, and reduction in membranal lipid peroxidation and protein carbonyl content. The plant extract plays the role of an antioxidant by attenuating free radical-induced oxidative damage (Parihar and Hemnani, 2004). This attribute of Shatavari make it an ideal herb for use as feed additive in livestock.

29.5.7 *Effect on Immunomodulation*

Various studies have indicated immunomodulatory properties of Shatavari root extracts and formulations. It has been reported that shatavari supplementation induces leucocytosis with predominant neutrophila, associated with stimulation of phagocytic and bactericidal capacity of neutrophils and macrophages (Thatte and Dhanukar, 1989). Shatavari root extract was shown to restore lymphocyte and neutrophils counts in myelosuppressed animals (Thatte and Dahanukar, 1988) and it modulates macrophage functions resulting in significant reduction in severity of peritoneal adhesions (Rege *et al.*, 1989). Hydro-alcoholic extract of Shatavri induces lag in tumor development in experimental animals (Seena *et al.*, 1993). Crude and hydro-alcoholic extracts of Shatavari have modulatory effect on TNF-alpha secretion, phagocytosis and neuro-endocrinal secretions (Bhatnagar *et al.*, 2005; Parihar and Hemnani, 2004; Dalvi *et al.*, 1990; Dhuley, 1997).

Immunoadjuvant activity of Shatavri aqueous root extract has been established. It upregulates Th1 and Th2 cytokines, significantly increases in delayed type hypersensitivity response, antibody titres and CD3+, CD4+/CD8+ percentages indicating towards its effect on T cell activation, hence suggesting Th1/Th2 adjuvant activity (Gautam et al. 2004). It enhances immunity through T-cells and resulted in a significant increase in antibody titers showing appreciable humoral response (Gautam *et al.*, 2009). Steroidal sapogenins and steroidal saponins (shatavaroside A and shatavaroside B) are major secondary metabolites present in Shatavri that might be attributed to show immunomodulatory effects (Sharma *et al.*, 2010) and boosted as well as restored both cellular and humoral immunity. Oral administration of decoction of powdered root has been found to enhance the immunomodulatory effect (Uma *et al.*, 2009). It not only provides enhanced protective immune response but also improves kidney and liver function tests as manifested by normal levels of SGOT, SGPT, alkaline phosphatase, creatinine and urea in blood plasma with normal histological observations (Sachdeva *et al.*, 2014). Shatavarin

IV has been reported to display significant activity as an inhibitor of core Golgi enzymes transferase in cell free assays and exhibit immunomodulation activity against specific T-dependent antigens in immuno compromised animals (Alok *et al.*, 2013). Dhuley (1997) has reported the revival of macrophage chemotaxis and interleukin-I (IL-I) and tumour necrosis factor α (TNF α) production by the oral treatment of Shatavari root extract in ochratoxin A treated mice. Thus, immunostimulation property of Shatavari can be utilized for enhancing the immune status of livestock by including it as a feed additive.

29.5.8 *Effect on Milk Production*

Shatavari has lactogenic/galactagogue properties to improve the milk production (Tanwar *et al.*, 2008). The aqueous extract of the root of this plant at 250 mg/kg has been shown to increase both the weight of mammary lobulo-aveolar tissue and the milk yield of oestrogen-primed rats. This effect was attributed to the action of released corticosteroids or an increase in prolactin (Joglekar *et al.*, 1967; Narendranath *et al.*, 1986). The active principles, Shatavarin-I, II, III and IV stimulates the hypothalamus or directly pituitary gland and is antagonist to dopamine receptors, which in turn increases the prolactin secretion (Baig and Bhagwat, 2009) resulting in increased milk yield. Shatavari root supplementation increases milk yield after calving, help mammary gland development, hastens letting down time, stimulate lactiferous tissues and keeps udder and treats in smooth condition (Somkuwar *et al.*, 2005). It causes proliferation in the lumen of the duct of mammary gland due to hypertrophy of ductal and glandular cells (Pandey *et al.*, 2005). When it is supplemented with the fodder, it increases the GPT (Glutamic Pyruvate Transminase) and GOT (Glutamic Oxaloacetate Transminase) activities which increases the digestibility and nutrient assimilation resulting in the improved galactogogue activity in lactating animals (Patel and Kanitkar, 1969). This may be due to stimulation of more feed intake and better digestibility contributing to increased milk. It increases weight of mammary glands and adrenal glands with release of pituitary ACTH, resulting into well-developed lobulo-alveolar tissues in mammary gland by a direct action through pituitary or pituitary adrenal axis resulting in the secretion of prolactin and ACTH (Somkuwar *et al.*, 2005). Systemic administration of the alcoholic extract of Shatavari in weaning rats increased weight of the mammary glands, inhibited involution of lobulo-alveolar tissue and maintained milk secretion (Sabins *et al.*,

1968). The same extract in estrogen-primed rats showed well developed lobulo-alveolar tissue and lactation.

The dose of Shatavari in dairy animal is based on body weight or dry matter intake and is not well standardized. Supplementation of SRP 100 g/day/animal and 50 g/day/animal irrespective of body weight have been found to increase milk production in crossbred cows (Tanwar *et al.*, 2008). Feeding herbal formulation containing 25% SRP enhanced milk production (25.1%) in lactating animals over control group. It increased daily milk yield and overall average milk production in buffaloes and crossbred cows, but the response in buffaloes was higher than cows but the reason was not explained (Tanwar et al. 2008). Supplementation of fresh root at the rate of 500 g per day with concentrate at the time of milking significantly increased milk yield of buffaloes (Patel and Kanitkar, 1969). However, it was found that supplementation of SRP (100 g on alternate day/animal) in freshly calved crossbred cows did not improved milk production. Similar result was also observed in lactating goats. Thus, Shatavari can be used as an alternative for lactogenic hormones for inducing and enhancing milk yield in lactating animals.

29.5.9 *Effect on Milk Composition*

Herbs and their metabolites modify the rumen ecosystem and their supplementation can change the normal composition of milk. Shatavari supplementation significantly increases milk fat, total solid content and protein; and decreases lactose content of milk in lactating cows and buffaloes. Since, Shatavari root is a rich source of minerals and trace elements such as calcium, copper, magnesium, iron, manganese, nickel, and zinc (Lohar *et al.*, 1991), the sufficient supply of the mineral nutrition to lactating cows is also a reason behind increase in milk yield. Shatavari by virtue of its hypocholesterolemic effect significantly reduces blood cholesterol level and thereby milk fat cholesterol is diminished.

The improvement in fat content may be due to increased ruminal activity and stimulation of high amount of acetic acid production and increased acetate propionate ratio in rumen, which are precursors of fatty acids of upto 16 carbon atoms in length. Also, the lipogenic activity of Shatavari may synergize the effect. The possible mechanism involved may be acetyl-CoA translocation and direct fusion of acetate across mitochondrial membrane. This could be involved in hydrolysis of acetyl-CoA in mitochondria via acetyl-CoA hydrolysis through rumen lipolysis and bio-rumenhydrolization process. There is subsequent regeneration of acetyl-CoA in cystol via. lipogenic enzyme acetyl thio kinase and malate dehydrogenase in mammary tissue and approximately 100 folds increase in the rate of fatty acid synthesis. Shatavari stimulates the peptidase enzymes, thus increasing the digestibility of crude protein and resulting into higher protein in milk. SRP causes decrease in serum glucose, since glucose and galactose is the precursors of lactose in milk, thus resulting in decreased lactose content in milk (Moran *et al.*, 1994).

29.5 Use of Shatavari as Feed Additive in Poultry

Considering the nutritional benefits, SRP is used as a herbal feed additive/supplement in poultry feed. It increased weekly gain in body weight and feed conversion ratio of broilers. The inclusion of SRP at 1 per cent in broiler ration as a herbel feed supplement was found to be better in terms of overall performance of broiler and net profit (Mane *et al.*, 2012). The feed conversion efficiency improved better as the level of SRP increased, the higher inclusion level showed better protein digestibility resulting in higher body weight. SRP at 0.5, 1.0 and 1.5 per cent of broiler diet enhances growth performance and stimulate immune system of birds and increased feed consumption, body weight gain, feed conversion ratio, performance efficiency, dressing percentage, mortality, and sensory characteristics in broilers with respect to all the attributes, *viz.*, appearance, flavour, tenderness, stickiness to mouth, juiciness and overall acceptability along with economic efficiency. Herbal formulations containing extracts of shatavari is recommended for use as positive immuno-modulator in normal and immuno-compromized broiler chicks. It also indicated the determinative roles of herbal feed additives in effective augmentation of humoral and cell mediated immune responses providing better protection level against infections (Kumari *et al.*, 2012a). It can also be used potentially before mass vaccination of the chicks for its property of immuno-modulation like levamisole. (Kumari *et al.*, 2012b). beneficially used as an effective feed supplement in poultry for its encouraging results in relation to total body weight gain and feed conversion efficiency. The better performance was likely to be due to higher immuno-modulatory, antioxidant and anti-stress effects of SRP. Supplementation of SRP along with vitamin E supplementation removed cold stress and improved immune status of broilers (Kant *et al.*, 2014). Shatavari can thus be incorporated into poultry feed for obtaining increased efficiency of production.

29.7 Adverse Effect and Toxicological Reports

In Ayurveda, Shatavri has been regarded as completely safe for long-term use, even during pregnancy and lactation (Goyal *et al.*, 2003). Appropriate amount of any feed additive depends on several factors like age, stage of lactation, health status, etc. This implies equally to natural products also. The aqueous extract of the roots studied for the acute toxicity with the high dose of 3200 mg/kg showed no fatality (Kumar *et al.*, 2010). Long-term administration of root extracts did not show any toxicity in animals (Sharma *et al.*, 1985). The methanol extract did not show any acute toxicity or subacute toxicity even at high dose of 2000 mg/kg or 1000 mg/kg, respectively (Goel *et al.*, 2006). There were no changes observed in terms of mortality, physiological and biological parameters, haemorrhage or necrosis in the tissues of treated rats. The ethanolic and aqueous extracts have also not shown any toxic effect with doses ranging from 50 mg/kg to 1 g/kg body weight for four weeks in Wistar albino rats (Devi and Divya, 2013). Thus, Shatavari can be included easily as feed additive in livestock and poultry feed formulations with high safety margin.

29.8 Future Aspect of Shatavari

However, Shatavari has been a part of ethno-veterinary practices, but only a few studies regarding its effects have been scientifically evaluated and documented in livestock and poultry. There are also several gaps in the existing literature with regard to the pharmacological actions of Shatavari. There is an incomplete understanding about the interaction/synergy between Shatavari and other plant constituents in polyherbal formulations; scanty information regarding the mode of action of the various active principles, etc. Consequently, a 'systems biology' approach has been suggested that includes metabolite profiling, metabolic fingerprinting, metabolite target analysis and metabonomics to enable further research and document its crucial role in animal production.

With the growing human awareness and demand of chemical residues free animal products, there is a need to carry bio-chemical work and more detailed studies on safety and efficacy of Shatavari being used as feed additive in livestock and poultry. With the demand of organic food and ban on the use of antibiotics in the livestock and poultry feed, the search for alternative feed additives has become the necessity of the day and thus, inclusion of Shatavari in feed of livestock and poultry can eliminate the use of non-plant xenobiotic agents from the diets of animals. Furthermore, its use as feed additive will need to be sanctioned by the registration authorities within the countries in which they will be used or in which the products from livestock will be sold and consumed. The use of Shatavari as immuno-modulators in combination with conventional chemotherapy to enhance host immune responses can have several advantages as a means to improving current therapeutic regimens. Saponins have been long recognized to show cytotoxic activity in various cancerous cell lines. Immunoside, the saponin from Shatavari induces strong cytotoxicity towards tumours. Hence, further isolation and characterization of compounds from Shatavari that induce apoptosis are more likely to show a therapeutic window in future (Bhutani *et al.*, 2010). With an increasing realization that hormone replacement therapy with synthetic oestrogens is neither as safe nor as effective as previously envisaged, the interest in plant-derived oestrogens has increased tremendously making Shatavari particularly important. More research is needed to define the effect of phytoestrogens from this plant on different species of livestock and poultry. Studies are required to exploit the potential of Satavari in the areas of female and male reproduction, milk yield and composition in livestock. This is because, reproductive performance and milk yield account for an index of profitability of a livestock enterprise.

Due to its multiple uses, the demand for Shatavari is constantly on the rise. Keeping in mind the fact that it is the active principle that imparts medicinal value to a plant; consistency in quality and quantity needs to be maintained to ensure uniform drug efficacy. Also, deliberate or inadvertent adulteration needs to be dealt with at an early stage. To overcome these prevalent problems, the availability of genetically superior and uniform planting material is essential. Destructive harvesting, combined with habitat destruction and deforestation, the plant is now considered endangered in its natural habitat. Therefore, the need for conservation of this plant is crucial. This can be obtained by a combination of various bio-technological tools involving chemoprofiling, tissue culture and use of molecular markers. Along with the application of these methods, proper agro-techniques and adequate marketing opportunities would encourage cultivation of Shatavari and thereby contribute to its conservation.

29.9 Summary and Conclusions

Shatavari as an ingredient of Ayurvedic preparations has been in practice for thousands of years in India and its use for human being is already well-documented and support its therapeutic use as a multi-purpose medicinal agent and has shown huge medicinal potential in modern pharmacology as well. The inclusion of Shatavari extracts/ formulations in livestock and poultry ration as a herbal feed supplement can increase overall performance. However, there is still a need to fill gaps between traditional knowledge and modern pharmacology with respect to its use as feed additive in livestock and poultry.

Shatavari, well known for its adaptogenic, galactogogue, anabolic, diuretic, rejuvenating, carminative, stomachic, antiseptic, emollient, cooling, nervine tonic activity antimicrobial, antioxidant, antiulcer, phytoestrogenic effects, neuroprotective effect, etc. As a growth promoter and immuno-stimulant, it can enhance nutrient utilization efficiency and performance of livestock and poultry. The utility of this plant is constrained due to the inadequate understanding and insufficient evidence regarding its potential health effects in different species of livestock and poultry. It is obvious that Shatavari with its several therapeutic attributes have a wide range of biological activities and have enormous potential as a feed additive in context of the preservation of livestock health. A holistic approach making use of Shatavari as feed additive in livestock and poultry production could help in amelioration of excessive stress on production capacity of livestock and poultry.

References

Acharya SR, Acharya NS, Bhangale JO, Shah SK, Pandya SS (2012) Antioxidant and hepatoprotective action of *Asparagus racemosus*wild root extracts. Indian J Exp Biol 50: 795–801

Ahmad S, Jain PC (1991) Chemical examination of shatavari (*A. racemosus*). Bull Med Ethnobot Res 12: 157–160

Alok S, Jain SK, Verma A, Kumar M, Mahor A, Sabharwal M (2013) Plant profile, phytochemistry and pharmacology of *Asparagus racemosus* (Shatavari): A review. Asian Pac J Trop Dis 3(3): 242-51

Amanullah SM, Haque KS, Sultana N (2009) Evaluation of some plant sources as herbal feed additive for Boosting growth in cattle. Proc. Anim. Nutr. Assoc. World Conf., 14-17 Feb., New Delhi, India. p.28

Anonymous (1987) The Wealth of India, Raw materials. Publication and Information Directorate, CSIR, N. Delhi, pp. 468–472

Arora R, Gupta D, Chawla R, Sagar R, Sharma A, Kumar R, Prasad J, Singh S, Samanta N, Sharma RK (2005) Radioprotection by plant products: present status and future prospects. Phytother Res. 19: 1–22

Baig MI, Bhagwat VG (2009) Study the efficacy of Galactin Vet Bolus on milk yield in dairy cows. Veterinary World 2: 140-142

Barhane M, Singh VP (2002) Effect of feeding indigenous galactopoietics feed supplements on milk production in crossbred cows. Indian J Anim Sci 72: 609–611

Bhatnagar M, Sisodia SS, Bhatnagar R (2005) Antiulcer and antioxidant activity of *Asparagus racemosus* Willd and *Withania somnifera* dunal in rats. Ann NY Acad Sci 1056: 261–278

Bhattacharya A, Muruganandam AV, Kumar V, Bhattacharya SK (2002) Effect of polyherbal formulation, EuMil, on neurochemical pertubations induced by chronic stress. Ind J Exp Biol 40: 1161–1163

Bhutani KK, Paul AT, Fayad W, Linder S (2010) Apoptosis inducing activity of steroidal constituents from Solanum xanthocarpum and Asparagus racemosus. Phytomedicine 17(10): 789-93

Chauhan S, Singh R, Gokhale Y, Lhouvum G, Basu AR (2011) Medicinal Plant Wealth of India, A comprehensive review of selected species, published by 'The Energy and Resources Institute (TERI), prepared for. Government of India: Ministry of Health & Family Welfare

Choudhary BK, Kar A (1992) Mineral contents of *Asparagus racemosus*. Indian Drugs 29(13): 623

Dahanukar SA, Date SG, Karandikar SM (1983) Cytoprotective effect of *Terminalia chebula* and *Asparagus racemosus* on gastric mucosa. Indian Drugs 21: 442-5

Dalvi SS, Nadkarni PM, Gupta KC (1990) Effect of *Asparagus racemosus*on gastric emptying time in normal healthy volunteers. J Postgrad Med 36: 91–94

Datta GK, Sairam K, Priyambada S, debnath PK, Goel RK (2002) Antiulcerogenic activity of Satavari mandur – an Ayurvedic herbo-mineral preparation. Ind J Exp Biol 40: 1173–1177

Devi PAV, Divya PS (2013) Antipyretic activity of ethanol and aqueous extract of root of *A. racemosus* in Yeast induced pyrexia. Asian J Pharm Clin Res. 6: 190–193

Dhuley JN (1997) Effect of some Indian herbs on macrophage functions in ochratoxin A treated mice. J Ethnopharmacol 58: 15–20

Diwanay S, Chitre D, Patwardhan B (2004) Immuno-protection by botanical drugs in cancer chemotherapy. J Ethnopharmacol 90: 49–55

Gautam M, Diwanay S, Gairola S, Shinde Y, Patki P, Patwardhan B (2004) Immunoadjuvant potential of *Asparagus racemosus* aqueous extract in experimental system. J Ethnopharmacol 91: 251–255

Gautam M, Saha S, Bani S, Kaul A, Mishra S, Patil D, Satti NK, Suri KA, Gairola S, Suresh K, Jadhav S (2009) Immunomo-dulatory activity of *Asparagus racemosus*on systemic Th1/Th2 immunity: implications for immuno-adjuvant potential. J Ethnopharmacol 121(2): 241-247

Goel RK, Prabha T, Kumar MM, Prakash dM, Singh G (2006) Teratogenicity of *A. racemosus* willd. Root, a herbal medicine. Indian J exp Biol 44: 570–573

Goel RK, Sairam K (2002) Anti-ulcer drugs from indigenous sources with emphasis on Musa Sapientum, Tamrabhasma, *A. racemosus* and *Zingiber officinale*. Ind J Pharmacol 34: 100–110

Gopumadhavan S, Venkataranganna MV, Rafiq M, Madhumathi BG, Mitra SK (2005) Evaluation of the estrogenic effect of Menosan using the rat models of uterotrophic assay. Med Update 13: 37–41

Goyal RK, Singh J, Lal H (2003) *Asparagus racemosus*—an update. Indian J Med Sci 57: 408–414

Handa SS, Suri OP, Gupta VN, Suri KA, Satti NK, Bhardwaj V, Bedi KL, Khajuria A, Kaul A, Parikh GG, Kulhar P (2003) inventors. Oligospirostanoside, pharmaceutical composition containing novel oligospirostanoside and method for immunomodulation using said oligospirostanoside. United States patent US 6: 649-745

Hayes PY, jahidin Ah, lehmann R, Penman K, Kitching W, de Voss JJ (2006) Asparinins, asparosides, curillins, curillosides and shavatarins: structural clarification with the isolation of shatavarin V, a new steroidal saponin from the root of *Asparagus racemosus*. Tetrahedron lett 47: 8683–8687

Hayes PY, jahidin Ah, lehmann R, Penman K, Kitching W, de Voss JJ (2008) Steroidal saponins from the roots of *Asparagus racemosus*. Phytochemistry 69: 796–804

Hegde GV, Nimbalkar SD, Hegde GS, Naik K (2002) Use of herbal plants for repeat breeding problem in dairy animals. Indian Vet J 79: 861-862

Hussein AA, Badr AM (2008) Influence of antepartum administration of immuno-potentiators on reproductive efficacy of buffalo and viability of their newborn. Vet Ital 44(2): 373 382

Jetmalani Mh, Sabins PB, Gaitonde BB (1967) A study on the pharmacology of various extracts of Shatavari – *A. racemosus* (Willd). J Res Indian Med 2: 1–10

Joglekar GV, Ahuja Rh, Balwani JH (1967) Galactogogue effect of *A. racemosus*. Indian Med J 61: 165

Joshi JDS (1988) Chemistry of Ayurvedic crude drugs: Part VIII: Shatavari 2. Structure elucidation of bio-active shatavarin I and other glycosides. Indian J Chem Section B Organ Chem 27(1): 12-16

Kamat JP, Boloor KK, devasagayam TPA, Venkatachalam SR (2000) Antioxidant properties of *Asparagus racemosus*against damage induced by γ-radiation in rat liver mitochondria. J Ethnopharmacol 71: 425–435

Kamat JP, Venkatachalam, SR (2004) *Asparagus racemosus* and radioprotection. Biotechnology of medicinal plants: Vitalizer and Therapeutic. 77-87

Kant S, Ali N, Chandra G, Siddique RA, Imran M (2014) Effect of shatavari and vitamin E on haemato-biochemical profile of broilers during winter season. Veterinary World. 7(11): 948-951

Kumar MC, Udupa Al, Sammodavardhana K, Rathnakar UP, Shvetha U, Kodancha GP (2010) Acute toxicity and diuretic studies of the roots of *A. racemosus* Willd in rats. West Ind Med J 59: 3–6

Kumari R, Tiwary BK, Prasad A, Ganguly S (2012a) Study on the immuno-modulatory effect of herbal extract of *Asparagus racemosus* willd. in broiler chicks. Global J Res Med Plants & Indigen Med 1(1): 1–6

Kumari R, Tiwary BK, Prasad A, Ganguly S (2012b) *Asparagus racemosus* willd. root extract as herbal nutritional supplement for poultry. Global J Res Med Plants & Indigen Med 1(5): 160–163

Lohar DR, Chaturvedi D and Verma PN (1991) Mineral elements of a few medicinally important plants. Indian Drugs 29: 271-273

Mandal D, Banerjee S, Mondal NB, Chakravarty AK, Sahu NP (2006) Steroidal saponins from the fruits of *Asparagus racemosus*. Phytochemistry 67(13): 1316-21

Mandal SC, Kumar ACK, Lakshmi SM, Sinha S, Murugesan T, Saha BP, Pal M (2000) Antitussive effect of *Asparagus racemosus* root against sulphur dioxide-induced cough in mice. Fitoterapia 71: 686–689

Mandal SC, Nandy A, Pal M, Saha BP (2000b) Evaluation of antibacterial activity of *Asparagus racemosus* Willd. root. Phytother Res 14: 118–119

Mane AG, Kulkarni AN, Korake RL, Bhutkar SS (2012) Effect of supplementation of Ashwagandha (Withania somnifera) and Shatavari (Asparagus racemosus) on growth performance of broilers. Res J Animal Hus & Dairy Sci 3(2): 94-96

Mayo Jl (1998) Black cohosh and chasteberry: herbs valued by women for centuries. Clin Nutr Insights 6: 1–4

Mazumdar BC, Mukhopadhyay PM (2006) Principles and practices of herbal garden. 1st ed. Delhi: Daya Publishing House; p. 225

Mirzaei F (2012) Effect of Herbal Feed Additives on Performance Parameters of Ruminants and especially On Dairy Goat: A Review Int J Agro Vet Med Sci 6(5): 307-331

Mirzaei F, Prasad S (2011) Influence of Dietary Phytoadditive as Polyherbal Combination on Performance of Does and Respective Litters in Crossbred Dairy Goats. Asian-Aust J Anim Sci 24(10): 1386-1392

Mishra A, Niranjan A, Tiwari SK, Prakash D, Pushpangadan S (2005) Nutraceutical composition of *Asparagus racemosus* (Shatavari) grown on partially reclaimed sodic soil. J Med Aroma Plant Sci 27(3): 240-248

Mohanta B, Chakraborty A, Sudarshan M, Dutta RK, Baruah M (2003) Elemental profile in some common medicinal plants of India. Its correlation with traditional therapeutic usage. J Rad Anal Nucl Chem 258(1): 175-179

Moran LA, Serimgeour KG, Horton HR, Ochs RS, Rawn JD (1994) *Biochemistry*, 2nd Edition, I. USA: Neil Patterson

Muruganandam AV, Kumar V, Bhattacharya SK (2002) Effect of poly herbal formulation, EuMIl, on chronic stress-induced homeostatic pertubations in rats. Indian J Exp Biol 40: 1151–1160

Narendranath KA, Mahalingam S, Anuradha V, Rao IS. (1986) Effect of herbal galactogogue (lactare) a pharmacological and clinical observation. Med Surg. 26: 19–22

Onlom C, Khanthawong S, Waranuch N, Ingkaninan K (2014) *In vitro* anti- Malassezia activity and potential use in anti-dandruff formulation of *Asparagus racemosus*. Int J Cosmet Sci 36: 74–78

Padmalatha K, Venkataraman BV, Roopa R (2002) Antianaphylactic effect of dlh-3041 (polyherbal formulation) on rat mesenteric mast cell degranulation. Indian J Pharmcol 34: 119–122

Pandey SK, Sahay A, Pandey RS, Tripathi YB. (2005) Effect of *Asparagus racemosus* rhizome (Shatavari) on mammary gland and genital organs of pregnant rat. Phytother Res 19: 721–724

Parihar MS, hemnani T (2004) Experimental excitotoxicity provokes oxidative damage in mice brain and attenuation by extract of *Asparagus racemosus*. J Neural Transm 111: 1–12

Patel AB, Kanitkar UK (1969) *Asparagus racemosus* willd. – Form bordi, as a galactagogue in buffaloes. Indian Vet J 46: 718–721

Patel IS, Patel RS (2013) Antimicrobial activity of *A. racemosus* wild from leaf extracts – a medicinal plant. Int J Sci Res Publ 3: 1–3

Pattanaik AK, Dutta N, Sharma K, Puneet K, Singh M, Singh A (2009) Influence of *Tinospora cordifolia* as a functional Feed additive on Nutrient Metabolism, Metabolic profile, Antioxidant status and Immune Response of Rams. Proc Anim Nutr Assoc World Conf, 14-17 Feb., New Delhi, India. p. 189

Rao AR (1981) Inhibitory action of *Asparagus racemosus*on dMBA-induced mammary carcinogenesis in rats. Int J Cancer 28: 607–610

Rege NN, Nazareth HM, Isaac A, Karandikar SM, Dahanukar SA (1989) Immuno-therapeutic modulation of intraperitoneal adhesions by *Asparagus racemosus*. J Postgrad Med 35: 199–203

Rege NN, Thatte UM, dahanukar SA (1999) Adaptogenic properties of six rasayana herbs used in Ayurvedic medicine. Phytother Res 13: 275–291

Sabins PB, Gaitonde BB, Jetmalani M (1968) Effect of alcoholic extract of *Asparagus racemosus* on mammary glands of rats. Indian J Exp Biol 6:55-57

Sachdeva H, Sehgal R, Kaur S (2014) *Asparagus racemosus* ameliorates cisplatin induced toxicities and augments its anti-leishmanial activity by immuno-modulation *in vivo*. Parasitol *Int* 63(1): 21-30

Saxena VK, Chourasia S (2001) A new isoflavone from the roots of Asparagus racemosus. Fitoterapia 72(3): 307-9.

Sairam K, Priyambada S, Aryya NC, Goel RK (2003) Gastroduodenal ulcer protective activity of *Asparagus racemosus*: an experimental, bio-chemical and histological study. J Ethnopharmacol. 86: 1–10

Seena K, Kuttan G, Kuttan R (1993) Antitumor activity of selected plant extracts. Amala Research Bulletin 13: 41–45

Sekine T, Ikegami F, Fukasawa N, Kashiwagi Y, Aizawa T, Fujii Y, Ruangrungsi N, Murakoshi I (1995) Structure and relative stereochemistry of a new polycyclic alkaloid, Asparagamine A, showing anti-oxytocin activity, isolated from *Asparagus racemosus*. J Chem Soc Perkin Trans I 4: 391–393

Sekine T, Fukasawa N, Murakoshi I, Ruangrungsi N (1997) A 9, 10-dihydrophenanthrene from Asparagus racemosus. Phytochemistry 44(4): 763-4

Sharma U, Saini R, Kumar N, Singh B (2009) Steroidal saponins from Asparagus racemosus. Chemical and Pharmaceutical Bulletin. 57(8): 890-3

Sharma P, Chauhan PS, Dutt P, Amina M, Suri KA, Dhar KL (2010) A unique immunostimulant steroidal sapogenin acid from the roots of *Asparagus racemosus*. Steroids 76: 358–64

Sharma S, dahanukar SA, Karandikar SM (1985) Effects of long term administration of roots of Ashwagandha and shatavari in rats. Indian drugs 22: 133–139

Sharma S, Ramji S, Kumari S, Bapna JS (1996) Randomized controlled trial os Asparagus racemosus (Shatavari) as a lactogogue in lactational inadequacy. Indian paediatrics 33: 675-7

Singh KP, Singh RH (1986) Clinical trial on Satavari (*Asparagus racemosus* Willd.) in duodenal ulcer disease. J Res Ay Sid 7: 91-100

Somkuwar AP, Khadtare CM, Pawar SD, Gatne MM (2005) Influence of shatavari feeding on milk production in buffaloes. *Pashudhan*. 31(2):3

Subramanian SS, Nair AGR (1968) Chemical components of *Asparagus racemosus*. Curr Sci 37(10): 287-288

Tanwar PS, Rathore SS, Kumar Y (2008) Effect of Shatavari (*Asparagus recemosus*) on milk production in dairy animals. Indian J Anim Res 42: 232-233

Thakur M, Connellan P, Deseo MA, Morris C, Praznik W, Loeppert R, Dixit VK (2012) Characterization and in vitro immuno-modulatory screening of fructo-oligosaccharides of *Asparagus racemosus* Willd. Int J Biol Macromol 50(1): 77-81

Thatte UM, Dahanukar SA (1988) Comparative study of immuno-modulating activity of Indian Medicinal plants. Lithium carbonate and Glucan. Methods Find Exp Clin Pharmacol 10: 639–644

Thatte UM, Dahanukar SA (1989) Immuno-therapeutic modification of experimental infections by Indian medicinal plants. Phytother Res 3: 43–49

Uma B, Prabhakar K, Rajendran S (2009) Anticandidal activity of Asparagus racemosus. Indian J Pharm Sci 71: 342–3

Velavan S, Nagulendran K, Mahesh R, Begum VMH (2007) *In vitro* antioxidant activity of *Asparagus racemosus* root. Pharmacognosy Magazine 3: 26–33

Venkatesan N, Thiyagarajan V, Narayanan S, Arul A, Raja S, Kumar SGV, Rajarajan T, Perianayagam JB (2005). Antidiarrhoeal potential of *A. racemosus* wild root extracts in laboratory animals. J Pharm Pharmaceut Sci 8: 39–46

Visavadiya NP, Narasimhacharya AVRL (2007) Asparagus root regulates cholesterol metabolism and improves antioxidant status in hypercholesteremic rats. Evid. Based Complement. Altern Med 1–8

Whitten PL, Patisaul HB (2001) Cross-species and interassay comparisons of phytoestrogen action. Environ health Perspect 109: 5–20

Wiboonpun N, Phuwapraisirisan P, Tip-pyang S (2004) Identification of antioxidant compound from *Asparagus racemosus*. Phytother Res 18: 771–773.

□□□

Chapter 30

Fenugreek (*Trigonella foenum graecum*)

Sheikh Adil Hamid

Division of Livestock Production and Management, Faculty of Veterinary Sciences and Animal Husbandry, Sher-e-Kashmir University of Agricultural Sciences and Technology, Srinagar-190006, India E-mail: aadilsheikh5@ gmail.com

ABSTRACT

Following the prohibition on usage of antibiotics as growth promoters, the researchers used other alternatives. Now-a-days, phytogenic feed additives like herbs are in vogue and are incorporated in the diet in order to enhance productivity by improvement of digestibility, nutrient absorption and elimination of pathogens residents in the gut. Among the various phytogenics available, this chapter will focus on one such herb known as Fenugreek (*Trigonella foenum graecum*), locally known as Methi. It is mainly cultivated in India, Pakistan and China. It is rich in protein, fat, total carbohydrates and minerals such as calcium, phosphorus, iron, zinc, magnesium, fatty acids predominantly linoleic, linolenic, oleic and palmitic. Fenugreek seeds are the most important and useful part of fenugreek plant having many therapeutic effects like hypoglycaemic, antibacterial, ant-inflammatory, antipyretic, anti-microbial and antioxidant properties. They have a role in improving the performance of poultry birds by their antibacterial activity and positive effect on gut morphology. Besides, they help in decreasing the blood cholesterol levels in poultry, hence have a potential role in prevention of arteriosclerosis.

Keywords: Antioxidant, Fenugreek, growth promoter, immuno-modulator, phytogenic.

30.1 Introduction

Fenugreek (*Trigonella foenum graecum)* locally known as "Methi" is grown mainly in India, Pakistan and China. It is one of the well known spices in human food. Its seeds and green leaves are used in food as well as in medicinal application which is an old practice of human history. Fenugreek has strong spicy and seasoning type sweet flavour (Blank, 1996). Aromatic and flavourful fenugreek is a popular spice and is widely used for well recognized culinary and medicinal properties (Sowmya, 1999). "Kasuri Methi" is very famous for its appetizing fragrance and it is used for culinary preparations (Senthil, 2010). In recent trend, fenugreek is also used as spice adjunct (Srinivasan, 2006). India is a major producer of fenugreek and also a major consumer of it for its culinary uses and medicinal application. Fenugreek grows to a height of about three feet, has three part leaves, the long slender stems bear tripartite, toothed, grey-green obovate leaves, 20-25 mm (3/4-1 in) long. It has long stalked leaves upto 5 cm long stipules triangular, lanceolate, leaflets about 2.5 cms long, obovate to obanceolate. The root is a mass of fingery structures. The sissile axillary flowers are white or pale yellow. The thin, sword-shaped pods are 10-15 cm (4-6 in), with a curved beak-like tip, each carrying 10-20 seeds. The plant radiates a spicy odour which persists on the hands after touching. Flowers are 1-2, axillary, sessile, racemed, whitish or lemon yellow that bloom from June to July. Pod 5.7 cm long with a persistent beak, hairy with 10-20 seeds (Snehlata and Payal, 2012).

Fenugreek seeds are the most important and useful part of fenugreek plant. These seeds are golden-yellow in colour, small in size, hard and have four-faced stone like structure (Altuntas *et al.*, 2005). Fenugreek seed is 3-6 mm long, 2-5 mm wide and 2 mm thick in geometry. Raw fenugreek seeds have maple flavour and bitter taste but by the process of roasting, their bitterness can be reduced and flavour can be enhanced. Fenugreek seeds are used as spices. The whole seed or its ground powder is used in pickles, vegetable dishes and spice powder. Dried seeds are used as condiments. Fenugreek seeds are gummy, fibrous, sticky and gummy in nature. Biologically, its seeds are endospermic in nature (Jani *et al.*, 2009). The fenugreek seeds, as a thumb rule, are harvested 150 to 170 days after_sowing or 30 to 35 days after flowering (Kakani *et al.*, 2009).

30.2 Taxonomy

The taxonomical position of Fenugreek (Flammang *et al.*, 2004) is as follows:

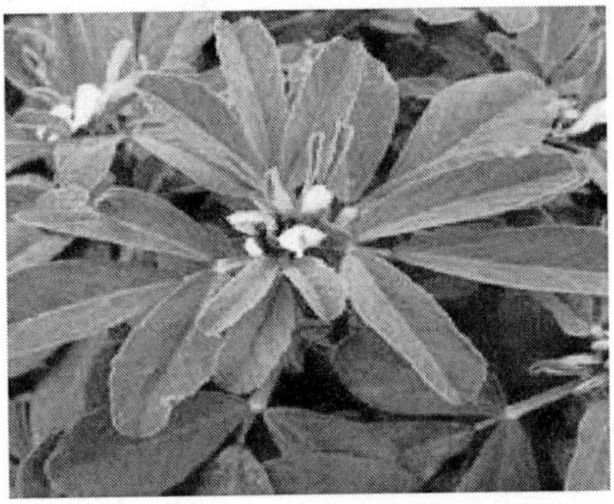

Kingdom	:	Plantae
Division	:	Magnoliophyta
Class	:	Magnoliopsida
Order	:	Fabales
Family	:	Fabaceae
Genus	:	*Trigon*ella
Species	:	*foenum-graecum*

The exact number of species of Fenugreek has been debated. Taxonomists such as Linnaeus suggested that as many as 260 species of Fenugreek may exist, of which a total of only 18 species of *Trigonella* are currently recognized. Most species, including *Trigonella joenum-graecum* L., are diploids with $2n$ = 16 chromosomes. However, some species of Trigonella may contain 18, 28, 30, 32 or 44 chromosomes (Acharya *et al.*, 2007).

30.3 Phytochemistry

The endosperm of the seed is rich in galactomannan, young seeds mainly contain carbohydrates and sugar. Mature seeds content amino acid, fatty acid, vitamins, and saponins. The seeds of fenugreek contain a large quantity of folic acid (84mg/100g). It also contents disogenin, gitogenin, neogitogenin, homorientin saponaretin, neogigogenin, and trigogenin (Rastogi and Mehrotra, 1990). The main chemical constituents of *T. foenum-graecum* are fibers, flavonoids, polysaccharides, saponins, flavonoids and polysaccharides fixed oils and some identified alkaloids viz., trigonelline and choline (Jayaweera, 1981; Yoshikawa *et al.*, 1997).

30.4 Biological Effects of Fenugreek

Fenugreek seed is used in functional food, traditional food, nutraceuticals as well as in physiological utilization such as antibacterial, anticancer, antiulcer, antihelminthic, hypocholesterolemic, hypoglycemic, antioxidant, and antidiabetic agent. It has beneficial influence on digestion and also has the ability to modify food texture (Murlidhar and Goswami, 2012). Fenugreek seeds have many therapeutical effects such as hypoglycaemic, anthelminthic, anti-inflamatory, anti-microbial properties (Basch *et al.*, 2003) and are rich in protein, fat, total carbohydrates and minerals such as calcium, phosphorus, iron, zinc and magnesium (Gupta *et al.*, 1996). Fenugreek also contains lecithin and choline that help to dissolve cholesterol and fatty substances. It also has neurin, biotin, trimethylamine which tends to stimulate the appetite by their action on the nervous system (Michael and Kumawat, 2003).

30.4.1 *Growth Promoter*

Since long Fenugreek is being used as a growth promoter particularly in broiler chicken. Inclusion of Fenugreek seeds in the diet significantly improves the body weight of broiler chicken (Abaza, 2001; Guo *et al.*, 2004; Yatoo *et al.*, 2012). Further, it improves the feed efficiency with reduction in feed cost when used as natural feed additive in broiler chicken diets (Azoua, 2001). Abdel-azeem (2006) reported best results by fenugreek seeds at 0.5% level in the diet of the broiler chicken. Similarly (Weerasingha and Atapattu, 2013 and Mamoun *et al.*, 2014) reported 1% level and Magda (2012) observed 1.5 % inclusion level useful for improving live body weight, body weight gain, feed conversion ratio, protein efficiency ratio, feed consumption and efficiency of energy utilization. Rabia (2010) however reported 3g/kg of feed as best inclusion level for enhancing the performance and body weight of broiler chickens. Raziq (2012) used fenugreek seeds in the water at 10 ml per liter and reported significant increase in the body weight gains of broiler chicken. Aksa *et al.*, 2012 reported that feeding Fenugreek seeds at 3g/kg of feed in broiler chicken significantly increases feed intake due to the presence of galactomannans and neurin which stimulates the appetite and improvement in FCR (feed conversion ratio) due to the beneficial effect on gut microflora. However, the improvement in body weights have been attributed to the presence of essential fatty acids and high quality proteins in the Fenugreek seeds (Murray *et al.*, 1991) and stimulating effect on the digestive system of broiler chicken (Hernandez *et al.*, 2004; Hind *et al.*, 2013). Nevertheless Petit *et al.*, 1993 reported that isolated steroidal saponin fraction of fenugreek seeds increase feed intake and motivation to eat in normal rats. Further, Abo El-Nor (1999) suggested that fenugreek seeds may have an effect on hypothalamus gland to stimulate hungriness center in the brain and increase the desire for eating.

Fenugreek seeds have also been used in the diet of ruminants and encouraging results have been reported. Hassan *et al.*, 2012 used fenugreek seeds in the diets of Sheep and reported a significant increase in the body weights compared to control group and attributed it to high levels of protein in fenugreek seeds which affected the physiological status of animal and resulted in increased body weight gains.

30.4.2 *Reproductive Performance*

Abdul Rahman (2012) investigated the role of fenugreek seeds in the reproductive performance of male broiler chickens. It was found that there was significant ($p<0.05$) activation and improvement in semen quality in aged broiler male chicken. However, when Fenugreek seeds were supplemented in the diets of laying aged breeders, there was seen significant ($p<0.05$) improvement in reproductive performances (Alobaidy, 2012).

30.4.3 *Galactogogue*

Fenugreek seeds have been found to increase the milk yield, when used in the diet of livestock. Ewes fed fenugreek seeds in the diet showed an increase in milk yield which was attributed to stimulatory action of fenugreek seeds in enhancing the appetite and feed intake resulting in an increase in milk production or by stimulation of endogenous hormone sectretion. Increase in milk production was confirmed by increased level of prolactin which is known to have a strong galactopoietic effect on lactation performance (Hassan *et al.*, 2012). Similarly, increase in the milk yield of goats was observed by Balgees Atta Elmnan *et al.* (2013). He reported that the total milk yield during the experimental period responded positively to fenugreek seed supplementation and among the treated groups, goats fed diets having highest per cent of fenugreek seeds (10% and 15%) had a greatest milk yield than those fed the lowest percent of fenugreek seeds (5%) which in turn had highest yield than the control group.

30.4.4 *Medicinal Uses*

The seeds are hot, with a sharp bitter taste; tonic, antipyretic, antihelmenthic, increase the apetite, astringent to the bowels, cure vomiting, bronchitis, remove bad taste from the mouth, useful in heart disease. The plant and seeds are hot and dry, suppurative, aperient, diuretic, useful in dropsy, chronic cough, enlargement of the liver and the spleen. The leaves are useful in external and internal swellings and burns (Prajapati *et al.*, 2003). Further, the polyphenolic extract of fenugreek seed acts as a protective agent against ethanol induced abnormalities in the liver having similar affects as that of silymarin, a known hepatoprotective agent (Kaviarasan and Anuradha, 2007). An anti-inflammatory effect was observed in an animal study which showed that in rats treated with a single dose of fenugreek extract (100 or 200 mg/kg), inhibition of inflammatory swelling was 45% and 62% in the lower and higher dose groups respectively, compared with 100% in untreated animals (Snehlata and Payal, 2012). Fenugreek is also believed to be antihelminthic (ability to cause the evacuation of parasitic intestinal worms) in nature (Murlidhar and Goswami, 2012).

Fenugreek has hypocholesterolemic activity as its consumption in diet reduced triglyceride accumulation in the liver of rats (Basch *et al.*, 2003). Snehlata and Payal (2012) clearly demonstrated the cholesterol-lowering activity of fenugreek in animal studies. In a typical study, fractions of fenugreek seeds were added to the diets of diabetic hypercholesterolemic and normal dogs. The defatted fraction, which contains about 54% fiber and about 5% steroidal saponins, lowered plasma cholesterol, blood glucose, and plasma glucagon levels from pre-treatment values in both groups of dogs. The hypocholesterolemic effect has also been reproduced in rats. Administration of the fiber-rich fraction of fenugreek to diabetic rats lowered total cholesterol, triglycerides, and low density lipoprotein (LDL). They also observed the hypoglycemic effects of fenugreek seeds in dogs. The defatted fraction of the seeds lowered blood glucose levels, plasma glucagons and somatostatin levels; carbohydrate-induced hyperglycemia also was reduced. Singh and Garg (2006) also reported that fenugreek seeds have hypocholesterolemic and even hypoglycemic effect as during the experiment on animals it improved peripheral glucose utilization, contributing to improvement in glucose tolerance and exerts its hypoglycemic effect by acting at the insulin receptor level as well as at the gastrointestinal level. The hypocholesterolemic effect may be due to sapogenins, which increase biliary cholesterol excretion, in turn leading to lowered serum cholesterol levels (Sidhu and Oakenfull, 1986; Sauvaire *et al.*, 1991; Stark and Madar, 1993). The hypoglycemic effect of fenugreek has been attributed to the facts that *in vitro* the amino acid 4-hydroxyisoleucine in fenugreek seeds increased glucose-induced insulin release in rat pancreatic islet cells

(Sauvaire *et al.*, 1998) and this amino acid appeared to act only on pancreatic beta cells, since the levels of somatostatin and glucagon were not altered (Raghuram *et al.*, 1994).

30.4.5 *Immuno-modulatory Effect*

A stimulatory immuno-modulatory effect (as evidenced from body weight, relative thymus weight, cellularity of lymphoid organs, delayed type of hypersensitivity response, plaque forming cell assay, haemagglutination titre, quantitative haemolysis assay, phagocytosis, lymph proliferation and a significant increase in phagocytic index and phagocytic capacity of macrophages) of aqueous extract of fenugreek at three doses 50, 100 and 200 mg per kg of body weight for 10 days on the immune system of Swiss albino mice was observed (Murlidhar and Goswami, 2012).

30.4.6 *Antioxidant Effect*

Fenugreek has powerful antioxidant property that has beneficial effect on liver and pancreas; since antioxidant properties have been linked to health benefits of natural products; such properties are studied with germinated fenugreek seeds which are observed to be more beneficial than dried seeds because of the fact that germinated seed increases the bioavailability of different constituents of fenugreek. An aqueous fraction of fenugreek exhibits the highest antioxidant activity compared to other fractions and the quantity of phenolic and flavonoid compounds are related to antioxidant activity. These studies reveal significant antioxidant activity in germinated fenugreek seeds which may be due to the presence of flavonoids and polyphenols (Balch, 2003). Dixit *et al.* (2005) also reported that fenugreek contains phenolic and flavonoid compounds which help to enhance its antioxidant capacity.

30.4.7 *Gastroprotective Effect*

The aqueous extract and a gel fraction, isolated from the seeds showed significant ulcer protective effects. It has soothing effect on gastric and gastritis ulcer (Srinivasan, 2006). Further, the effect of fenugreek seeds compared to omeprazole was studied on ethanol-induced gastric ulcer. The aqueous extract and a gel fraction isolated from the seeds showed significant ulcer protective effects. The cytoprotective effect of the seeds seemed to be not only due to the anti-secretory action but also to the effects on mucosal glycoproteins. The fenugreek seeds also prevented the rise in lipid peroxidation induced by ethanol presumably by enhancing antioxidant potential of the gastric mucosa thereby lowering mucosal injury. Studies revealed that the soluble gel fraction derived from the seeds was more effective than omeprazole in preventing lesion formation. These observations show that fenugreek seeds possess antiulcer potential (Pandian Suja *et al.*, 2002).

30.5 Adverse Effects

A review of literature on fenugreek reveals no reports of clinically significant harmful adverse effects and it has traditionally been considered safe and well-tolerated as has been reported by Udayasekhara Rao *et al.* (1996) that Short-term (90 days) feeding of fenugreek seeds to rats at levels equivalent to two and four times the therapeutic dose recommended for humans (25 g/day) produced no toxic effects as evidenced by normal liver function tests, lack of any histopathological changes in the liver and no changes in haematological parameter. Muralidhara *et al.* (1999) also investigated toxic effects of debitterized fenugreek powder on acute and subchronic regimes in mice and rats, and could not find any sign of toxicity, mortality, change in body weight, organ weight; upto a maximum dosage of 2-5 g per kg body weight of mice and rat.

30.6 Summary and Conclusions

Fenugreek has many beneficial effects besides improving the growth performance of livestock and poultry without causing any harmful effect on their health. Based on the usefulness of fenugreek as discussed in the chapter, this natural herb (Methi) must be recommended for inclusion in the diets of livestock and poultry for improving their production performance and well being.

References

Abaza IM (2001) The use of some medicinal plants as feed additive in broiler diets. Ph. D thesis submitted to Faculty of Agriculture, Alexandria University, Egypt, pp 3-17.

Abdel-azeem (2006) Effect of using Fenugreek and Fennel seeds as natural feed additives on performance of broiler chicks. Egypt J Nutr Feed 9: 277-297.

Abdul-Rahman SY (2012). Effect of Fenugreek seeds on some physiological characters in broiler breeders male. Mesoptamian J Agric 40: 7-16

Abo El-nor SAH (1999) Influence of fenugreek seeds as a galactogogue on milk yield, milk composition and different blood biochemical of lactating buffaloes during midlactation. Egypt J Dairy Sci 27: 231-238

Acharya SN, Thomas JE, Basu SK (2007) Fenugreek: an "old world" crop for the "new world". Biodiversity 7:1-4

Aksa SB, Alloui N Alloui MN (2012) Utilization of *Fenugreek* (*Trigonella foenum- graecum*) as growth promoter for broiler chickens. J World's Poult Res 2: 25-27

Alobaidy RN (2012) Effect of *Fenugreek Seeds* and *Olive* leaves ration supplementation on productive and physiological performance of laying breeder hen. M.sc. thesis submitted to College of Agriculture and forestry, University of Mosul, Iraq, pp 1-40

Altuntas E, Ozgoz E, Taser OF (2005) Some physical properties of fenugreek *(Trigonella foenum-graceum L.)* seeds. J Food Eng 71:37-43

Azoua HM (2001) Effect of Hot pepper and Fenugreek seeds supplementation on broiler diets. Ph. D. thesis submitted to Faculty of Agriculture, Alexandria University, Egypt, pp 6-55

Balch PA (2003) Prescription for dietary wellness (2nd edn). Penguin group, New York

Balgees Atta Elmnan A, Albekhaita Rewais F, Fadel Elseed AMA, Mahala AG, Amasiab EO (2013). Effect of supplementation of fenugreek (Trigonella foenum -graecum L.) seeds on feed intake, digestibility, N-balance and rumen environment of Nubian Goats. Inter. J. Develop. Sustain. 2(2): 1214-1223

Basch E, Ulbricht C, Kuo G, Szapary P, Smith M (2003) Therapeutic applications of fenugreek. Altern. Med. Rev. 8: 20-27

Blank I (1996) The flavor principle of fenugreek. Nestlé research center. 211th ACS Symposium. New Orleans, pp 24-28

Dixit P, Ghaskadbi S, Mohan H, Devasagayam TP (2005) Antioxidant properties of germinated fenugreek seeds. Phytother Res 19: 977-983

Flammang AM, Cifone MA, Erexson GL, Stankowski LF (2004) Genotoxicity testing of a fenugreek extract. Food Chem Toxic 42: 1769–1775

Guo FC, Kwakel CRP, Soede J, Williams BA (2004) Effect of a Chinese herb medicine formulation, as an alternative for antibiotics, on performance of broilers. Br Poult. Sci. 45: 793-797

Gupta K, Thakral KK, Arora SK, Chowdhary MI (1996) Structural carbohydrate and mineral seeds. Ind. Coca Arecenut species J 20: 120

Hassan SAA, Shaddad SAI, Salih K, Muddither A, Kheder S I, Barsham MA (2012) Effect of oral administration of *Trigonella foenum L.* (Fenugreek seeds) on galactogogue, body weight and hormonal levels in Sudanese desert sheep. J Pharma Biomed Sci 22: 1-4

Hernandez AI, Madrid J, Garcia V (2004) Influence of two plant extracts on broiler performances, digestibility and digestive organs size. Int J Poult Sci 83: 169-174

Hind AA, Saadia AA and Khalid ME (2013) Effect of Different Natural Feed additives Compared to Antibiotic on Performance of Broiler Chicks under High Temperature Environment. Bulletin Envir Pharma Life Sci 2: 139-144

Jani R, Udipi SA, Ghugre PS (2009) Mineral content of complementary foods. Indian J Pediatr 76: 37-44

Jayaweera DMA (1981) Medicinal plant: Part III. Peradeniya, Sri Lanka: Royal Botanic Garden, pp. 225

Kakani RK, Anwer MM, Meena SS, Saxena SN (2009) Advance production technology of fenugreek. NRCSS Tech. Release, pp 1-24

Kaviarasan S, Anuradha CV (2007) Fenugreek *(Trigonella foenum graecum)* seed polyphenols protect liver from alcohol toxicity: a role on hepatic detoxification system and apoptosis. Pharmazie 62: 299-304

Magda EE (2012) Effect of Dietary Fenugreek Seeds (*Trigonella foenum*) as Natural Feed Addition on Broiler Chicks Performance. J. Sci. Tech. 13: 27-31

Mamoun T, Mukhtar A, Mohamed HT (2014) Effect of Fenugreek seed powder on the Performance, Carcass Characteristics and Some Blood Serum Attributes. Adv Res Agri Vety Sci 1: 6-11

Michael D, Kumawat D (2003) Legend and archeology of Fenugreek, constitutions and modern applications of Fenugreek seeds. International Sympozium, USA, pp. 41-42

Muralidhara, Narasimhamurthy K, Viswanatha S, Ramesh BS (1999) Acute and subchronic toxicity assessment of debitterized fenugreek powder in the mouse and rat. Food Chem Toxicol 37: 831-838

Murlidhar M, Goswami TK (2012) A review on the functional properties, nutritional content, medicinal utilization and potential application of fenugreek. J Food Proc Tech 3: 1-10

Murray RK, Granner DK, Mayes PA, Rodwell VW (1991) *The Text Book of Harpers Biochemistry*. 22nd Edition. Applecton and large. Norwalk, Connecticut/Loss Altos, California

Pandian Suja R, Anuradha CV, Viswanathan P (2001) Gastroprotective effect of fenugreek seeds (*Trigonella foenum- graecum*) on experimental gastric ulcer in rats. J Ethnopharmacology 81: 393-397

Petit P, Sauvair Y, Hillaire D (1995) Steroid saponins from Fenugreek seeds : Extraction , purification , and pharmacological investigation on feeding behaviour and plasma. Chol Steroids 60: 674-680

Prajapati P, Sharma and Kumar. 2003. A Handbook of Medicinal Plants- A Complete Source Book", Published by Agrobios (India), pp. 523

Rabia JA (2010) Effect of Using Fenugreek, Parsley and Sweet Basil Seeds as Feed Additives on the Performance of Broiler Chickens. Inter. J. Poult. Sci. 9: 278-282

Raghuram TC, Sharma RD, Sivakumar B (1994) Effect of fenugreek seeds on intravenous glucose disposition in non-insulin dependent diabetic patients. Phytother Res 8: 83-86

Rastogi and Mehrotra BN 1990. Compendium of Indian Medicinal Plants", PID, New Delhi, 1990, volume II, pp 422

Raziq F, Khan S, Naila C, Asad S (2012) Effect of Water Based Infusion of *Lycium, Aloe barbedensis, Pimpinella anisum, Berberis Trigonella foenum-graecum and Allium sativum* on The Performance of Broiler Chicks. Pak Vety J, 32: 593-596

Sauvaire Y, Ribes G, Baccou JC (1991) Implication of steroid saponins and sapogenins in the hypocholesterolemic effect of fenugreek. Lipids 26: 191-197

Sauvaire Y, Petit P, Broca C (1998) 4- Hydroxyisoleucine: a novel amino acid potentiator of insulin secretion. Diabetes 47: 206-210

Senthil A, Mamatha BS, Vishwanath P, Bhat KK, Ravishankar GA (2010) Studies on development and storage stability of instant spice adjunct mix from seaweed. J Food Sci. Tech. 48: 712-717

Sidhu GS, Oakenfull DG (1986) A mechanism for the hypocholesterolaemic activity of saponins. Bri J Nutr 55: 643-649

Singh V, Garg AN (2006) Availability of essential trace elements in Indian cereals, vegetables and spices using INAA and the contribution of spices to daily dietary intake. Food chem. 94: 81-89

Snehlata HS, Payal DR (2011) Fenugreek (*Trigonella foenum-graecum* L.): An Overview. Inter J Current Pharma Rev Res 2: 169-187

Srinivasan K (2006) Fenugreek (*Trigonella foenum-graecum*): A review of health beneficial physiological effects. Food Rev Inter 22: 203-224

Stark A, Madar Z. The effect of an ethanol extract derived from fenugreek (*Trigonella foenum-graecum*) on bile acid absorption and cholesterol levels in rats. Bri J Nutr 69: 277-287

Udayasekhara Rao P, Sesikeran B, Srinivasan Rao P (1996) Short-term nutritional and safety evaluation of fenugreek. Nutr Res 16: 1495–505

Weerasingha AS, Atapattu NSBM (2013) Effects of Fenugreek (*Trigonella foenum-graecum L.*) Seed Powder on growth performance, visceral organ weight, serum cholesterol levels and the nitrogen retention of broiler chicken. Trop Agric Res 24: 289-295

Yatoo MA, Sharma RK, Khan N (2012) Effect of Fenugreek and Black Cumin seeds as Feed Additives on Blood Bio-chemical Profile and Performance of Broilers. Indian J Anim Nut 29: 174-178

Yoshikawa M, Murakami, T, Komatsu H, Murakami N, Yamahara J, Matsuda H (1997) Medicinal Foodstuffs: IV. Fenugreek seeds (1): structures of trigoneosides Ia, Ib, IIb, IIIa and IIIb new furostanol saponins from the seeds of Indian *Trigonella foenum- graecum* L. Chem Pharma Bull 45: 81-87.

❑❑❑